Clinical Pain Management

Cancer Pain

Clinical Pain Management

Cancer Pain

2nd edition

Edited by

Nigel Sykes MA BM BCh FRCGP FRSA
Medical Director and Consultant in Palliative Medicine
St Christopher's Hospice
London, UK

Michael I Bennett MD FRCP
Professor of Palliative Medicine, International Observatory on End of Life Care
Institute for Health Research
Lancaster University
Lancaster, UK

Chun-Su Yuan MD PhD
Cyrus Tang Professor of Anesthesia and Critical Care
Department of Anesthesia and Critical Care
Pritzker School of Medicine
The University of Chicago
Chicago, IL, USA

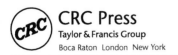

CRC Press
Taylor & Francis Group
Boca Raton London New York

CRC Press is an imprint of the
Taylor & Francis Group, an **informa** business

CRC Press
Taylor & Francis Group
6000 Broken Sound Parkway NW, Suite 300
Boca Raton, FL 33487-2742

First issued in paperback 2019

© 2000 by Taylor & Francis Group, LLC
CRC Press is an imprint of Taylor & Francis Group, an Informa business

No claim to original U.S. Government works

ISBN-13: 978-0-340-94007-5 (hbk)
ISBN-13: 978-1-138-37243-6 (pbk)

Visit the Taylor & Francis Web site at
http://www.taylorandfrancis.com

and the CRC Press Web site at
http://www.crcpress.com

Contents

Contributors   vii

Series preface   xi

Introduction to Clinical Pain Management: Cancer Pain   xiii

How to use this book   xv

Abbreviations   xvii

PART I GENERAL CONSIDERATIONS   **1**

1   Pathophysiology of somatic, visceral, and neuropathic cancer pain   3
     Catherine E Urch and Rie Suzuki

2   Epidemiology of cancer pain   13
     Irene J Higginson, Julie Hearn, and Fliss Murtagh

3   Cancer pain syndromes   27
     Robert Twycross and Michael Bennett

4   History and clinical examination of the cancer pain patient: assessment and measurement   38
     Badi El Osta and Eduardo Bruera

5   Psychological evaluation of patient and family   48
     Barbara Monroe

6   The role of the nonprofessional caregiver in cancer pain management   63
     Christine Miaskowski

7   Teamworking in cancer pain management   71
     Vicky Robinson and Rob George

8   Barriers to cancer pain relief: an international perspective on drug availability and service delivery   81
     Fiona Graham and David Clark

9   Ethical issues in cancer pain management   93
     Fiona Randall

PART II DRUG THERAPIES FOR CANCER PAIN   **101**

10   Clinical pharmacology: principles of analgesic drug management   103
     Stephan A Schug and Kirsten Auret

11   Clinical pharmacology and therapeutics: nonopioids   123
     Victor Pace

12   Clinical pharmacology of opioids: basic pharmacology   151
     Sangeeta R Mehendale and Chun-Su Yuan

13   Clinical pharmacology of opioids: opioid switching and genetic basis for variability in opioid sensitivity   168
     Columba Quigley, Joy Ross, and Julia Riley

14   Clinical pharmacology of opioids: adverse effects of opioids   179
     Juan Manuel Núñez Olarte

15   Clinical pharmacology and therapeutics: drugs for neuropathic pain in cancer   200
     Carina Saxby and Michael Bennett

16   Control of procedure-related pain   213
     Iain Lawrie and Colin Campbell

PART III NON-DRUG THERAPIES FOR CANCER PAIN   223

17   Nerve blocks: chemical and physical neurolytic agents   225
     John E Williams

18   Stimulation-induced analgesia   235
     Mark I Johnson, Stephen G Oxberry, and Karen Robb

19   Radiotherapy   251
     Peter J Hoskin

20   Management of bone pain   256
     Peter J Hoskin

21   Complementary therapies   270
     Jacqueline Filshie and Adrian White

22   Management of breakthrough pain   286
     Giovambattista Zeppetella and Russell K Portenoy

23   Psychological interventions in cancer pain management   296
     T Manoj Kumar, C Venkateswaran, and P Thekkumpurath

24   Control of symptoms other than pain   310
     Emma Hall, Nigel Sykes, and Victor Pace

PART IV CLINICAL MANAGEMENT OF PAIN IN SPECIAL SITUATIONS   343

25   Pediatric cancer pain   345
     John J Collins, Michael M Stevens, and Charles B Berde

26   Cancer pain in older people   359
     Margot Gosney

27   Cancer pain management in the context of substance abuse   379
     Sharon M Weinstein

28   Pain in the dying person   389
     Kate Skinner and Steven Z Pantilat

29   Pain in cancer survivors   399
     W Paul Farquhar-Smith

30   Cancer pain management in the community setting   411
     Margaret Gibbs, Vicky Robinson, Nigel Sykes, and Christine Miaskowski

Index   423

Please note: The table of contents and a combined index for all four volumes in the series can be found on the Clinical Pain Management website at: www.clinicalpainmanagement.co.uk.

Contributors

Kirsten Auret MBBS FRACP FAChPM
Associate Professor in Palliative Medicine, Faculty of Medicine
Dentistry and Health Sciences, University of Western Australia
Perth, Australia

Michael Bennett MD FRCP
Professor of Palliative Medicine
International Observatory on End of Life Care, Institute for
Health Research, Lancaster University, Lancaster, UK

Charles B Berde MD PhD
Chief
Division of Pain Medicine, Children's Hospital, Boston, MA, USA

Eduardo Bruera MD
Chair
Department of Palliative Care and Rehabilitation, MD Anderson
Cancer Center, University of Texas, Houston, TX, USA

Colin Campbell MBChB DRCOG FRCGP FRCP
Consultant in Palliative Medicine
St Catherine's Hospice, Scarborough, UK

David Clark PhD
Director
Institute for Health Research, International Observatory on End
of Life Care, Institute for Health Research, Lancaster University
Lancaster, UK

John J Collins MB BS PhD FRACP
Head
Pain and Palliative Care Service, The Children's Hospital at
Westmead, Sydney, Australia

W Paul Farquhar-Smith MA MB BChir FRCA PhD
Consultant in Pain, Anaesthesia and Intensive Care
Royal Marsden Hospital, London, UK

Jacqueline Filshie MB BS FRCA
Consultant in Anaesthesia and Pain Management
Royal Marsden Hospital, London and Sutton, UK

Rob George MA MD FRCP
Consultant Physician
Meadow House Hospice, Ealing Primary Care Trust
London, UK; and Senior Lecturer, Biomedical Ethics, UCL Medical
School, London, UK

Margaret Gibbs MSc MRPharmS
Specialist Senior Pharmacist
St Christopher's Hospice, Sydenham, UK

Margot Gosney MD FRCP
Professor of Elderly Care Medicine
Institute of Health Sciences, University of Reading
Reading, UK

Fiona Graham MBChB MRCGP MMedSci
Senior Lecturer in General Practice
School of Health and Postgraduate Medicine, University of
Central Lancashire, Preston, UK

Emma Hall MBBS FRCP
Consultant in Palliative Medicine
St Christopher's Hospice, London, UK

Julie Hearn BSc MSc
Head of Clinical Trials
Cancer Research UK
London, UK

Irene J Higginson BMedSci BMBS PhD FFPHM FRCP
Professor of Palliative Care and Policy, Head of Department
King's College London School of Medicine
Department of Palliative Care, Policy and Rehabilitation, Cicely
Saunders Institute, London, UK

Peter J Hoskin MD FRCP FRCR
Consultant Clinical Oncologist, Professor in Clinical Oncology
University College London and Mount Vernon Centre for Cancer
Treatment, Mount Vernon Hospital
Northwood, Middlesex, UK

Mark I Johnson BSc(Hons) PhD
Professor of Pain and Analgesia
Faculty of Health, Leeds Metropolitan University; and
Leeds Pallium Research Group, Leeds, UK

T Manoj Kumar MBBS DPM MD MRCPsych
Consultant in Liaison Psychiatry
Becklin Centre
Leeds, UK

Iain Lawrie MB ChB BSc DipMedEd MRCGP
Consultant in Palliative Medicine
North Manchester General Hospital/St Ann's Hospice
Manchester, UK

Sangeeta R Mehendale PhD
Research Associate
Department of Anesthesia and Critical Care
The University of Chicago
Chicago, IL, USA

Christine Miaskowski RN PhD FAAN
Professor and Associate Dean for Academic Affairs
Department of Physiological Nursing, University of California
San Francisco, CA, USA

Barbara Monroe BA BPhil CQSW
Chief Executive
St Christopher's Hospice, London, UK

Fliss Murtagh MBBS MRCGP MSc
Research Training Fellow
King's College London School of Medicine
Department of Palliative Care, Policy and Rehabilitation
Cicely Saunders Institute
London, UK

Juan Manuel Núñez Olarte
Associate Professor of Medicine
University Complutense of Madrid; and
Head Palliative Care Unit, Hospital General Universitario
Gregorio Marañón
Madrid, Spain

Badi El Osta MD
Chief Fellow
Section of Symptom Control and Palliative Care
Department of Palliative Care and Rehabilitation Medicine
MD Anderson Cancer Center, University of Texas
Houston, TX, USA

Stephen G Oxberry MBChB BSc MRCP
Specialist Registrar in Palliative Medicine
Yorkshire Deanery, University of Leeds; and
Leeds Pallium Research Group
Leeds, UK

Victor Pace LRCP(Ed) LRCP&S(Glasg) FRCS(Ed) FRCP
Consultant in Palliative Medicine
St Christopher's Hospice, London, UK

Steven Z Pantilat MD
Professor of Clinical Medicine
Alan M Kates and John M Burnard Endowed
Chair in Palliative Care; and
Director, Palliative Care Program
Department of Medicine, University of California
San Francisco, CA, USA

Russell K Portenoy MD
Chairman and Gerald J and Dorothy R Friedman Chair in Pain
Medicine and Palliative Care
Department of Pain Medicine and Palliative Care, Beth Israel
Medical Center, New York, USA; and Professor of Neurology and
Anesthesiology, Albert Einstein College of Medicine, Bronx
New York, USA

Columba Quigley MD FRCP
Consultant and Senior Lecturer in Palliative Medicine
Charing Cross Hospital, London, UK

Fiona Randall FRCP PhD
Consultant in Palliative Medicine
The Royal Bournemouth and Christchurch Hospitals NHS
Foundation Trust, Dorset, UK

Julia Riley MBBCh MRCGP FRCP MD
Head of Department Palliative Medicine
Royal Marsden Hospital NHS Trust, London, UK

Karen Robb PhD BSc MCSP
Clinical Specialist Physiotherapist (Oncology)
Physiotherapy Department, Barts Hospital, London, UK

Vicky Robinson RN DN MSc
Consultant Nurse
Palliative Care, Guy's and St Thomas' Hospital NHS Foundation
Trust, Guy's Hospital, London, UK

Joy Ross PhD MRCP
Consultant Palliative Medicine
St Joseph's Hospice; and Honorary Senior Lecturer
Imperial College, London, UK

Carina Saxby MBBcHBAO MRCGP
Specialist Registrar in Palliative Medicine
Yorkshire Deanery, West Yorkshire, UK

Stephan A Schug MD (Cgn) FANZCA FFPMANZCA
Professor and Chair of Anaesthesiology
School of Medicine and Pharmacology
University of Western Australia
Perth, Australia

Kate Skinner MD PhD
Staff Geriatrician
The Jewish Home for the Elderly, San Francisco
CA, USA

Michael M Stevens AM FRACP
Senior Staff Specialist
Oncology Unit, The Children's Hospital at Westmead
Sydney, Australia

Rie Suzuki BSc PhD
Postdoctoral Research Fellow
Department of Pharmacology, University College London
London, UK

Nigel Sykes MA BM BCh FRCP FRCGP
Medical Director and Consultant in Palliative Medicine
St Christopher's Hospice, London, UK

P Thekkumpurath MBBS MRCPsych
Clinical Research Fellow
St Gemma's Hospice, Moortown, Leeds, UK

Robert Twycross DM FRCP
Emeritus Clinical Reader in Palliative Medicine
Oxford University, Oxford, UK

Catherine E Urch BSc BM PhD FRCP
Consultant in Palliative Medicine
Imperial College Healthcare NHS Trust; and Honorary Senior
Lecturer, University College, London, UK

C Venkateswaran MBBS MD
Clinical Research Fellow
St Gemma's Hospice, Moortown, Leeds, UK

Sharon M Weinstein MD
Professor of Anesthesiology, Adjunct Associate Professor of
Neurology and Medicine (Oncology), Director, Pain Medicine and
Palliative Care, University of Utah and VASLCHCS Huntsman
Cancer Institute, Salt Lake City, UT, USA

Adrian White MD BM BCh
Clinical Research Fellow
Peninsula Medical School, Universities of Exeter and Plymouth
Plymouth, UK

John E Williams
Consultant in Anaesthesia and Pain Medicine
Royal Marsden Hospital, London, UK

Chun-Su Yuan MD PhD
Cyrus Tang Professor
Department of Anesthesia and Critical Care, The University of
Chicago, Chicago, IL, USA

Giovambattista Zeppetella BSc MB BS MRCGP FRCP
Medical Director
St Clare Hospice, Hastingwood, Essex; and Honorary Consultant
Princess Alexandra NHS Trust, Harlow, UK

Series preface

Since the successful first edition of *Clinical Pain Management* was published in 2002, the evidence base in many areas of pain medicine has changed substantially, thus creating the need for this second edition. We have retained the central ethos of the first volume in that we have continued to provide comprehensive coverage of pain medicine, with the text geared predominantly to the requirements of those training and practicing in pain medicine and related specialties. The emphasis continues to be on delivering this coverage in a format that is easily accessed and digested by the busy clinician in practice.

As before, *Clinical Pain Management* comprises four volumes. The first three cover the main disciplines of acute, chronic, and cancer pain management, and the fourth volume covers the practical aspects of clinical practice and research. The four volumes can be used independently, while together they give readers all they need to know to deliver a successful pain management service.

Of the 161 chapters in the four volumes, almost a third are brand new to this edition while the chapters that have been retained have been completely revised, in many cases under new authorship. This degree of change reflects ongoing progress in this broad field, where research and development provide a rapidly evolving evidence base. The international flavor of *Clinical Pain Management* remains an important feature, and perusal of the contributor pages will reveal that authors and editors are drawn from a total of 16 countries.

A particularly popular aspect of the first edition was the practice of including a system of simple evidence scoring in most of the chapters. This enables the reader to understand quickly the strength of evidence which supports a particular therapeutic statement or recommendation. This has been retained for the first three volumes, where appropriate. We have, however, improved the system used for scoring evidence from a three point scale used in the first edition and adopted the five point Bandolier system which is in widespread use and will be instantly familiar to many readers (www.jr2.ox.ac.uk/bandolier/band6/b6-5.html).

We have also retained the practice of asking authors to highlight the key references in each chapter. Following feedback from our readers we have added two new features for this edition: first, there are key learning points at the head of each chapter summarizing the most salient points within the chapter; and second, the series is accompanied by a companion website with downloadable figures.

This project would not have been possible without the hard work and commitment of the chapter authors and we are deeply indebted to all of them for their contributions. The volume editors have done a sterling job in diligently editing a large number of chapters, and to them we are also most grateful. Any project of this magnitude would be impossible without substantial support from the publishers – in particular we would like to acknowledge our debt to Jo Koster and Zelah Pengilley at Hodder. They have delivered the project on a tight deadline and ensured that a large number of authors and editors were kept gently, but firmly, "on track."

Andrew SC Rice, Douglas Justins, Toby Newton-John,
Richard F Howard, Christine A Miaskowski
London, Newcastle, and San Francisco

I would also like to add my personal thanks to the Series Editors who have given their time generously and made invaluable contributions through the whole editorial process from the very outset of discussions regarding a second edition in deciding upon the content of each volume and in selecting Volume Editors. More recently, they have provided an important second view in the consideration of all submitted chapters, not to mention stepping in and assisting with first edits where needed. The timely completion of the second edition would not have been possible without this invaluable input.

Andrew SC Rice
Lead Editor

Introduction to Clinical Pain Management: Cancer Pain

In the public mind, and often the professional mind too, cancer is perceived to be an especially painful disease. Worldwide, cancer is becoming more common as western populations age and those of developing countries live long enough to enter the peak years of cancer risk. For these reasons, it was decided to devote a volume of this textbook of pain to the management of cancer-related pain, now extensively revised and updated for this second edition.

It is over 20 years since the analgesic ladder of the World Health Organization placed opioids at the heart of cancer pain management, but too many clinicians still lack confidence in the use of this family of drugs and too many countries lack adequate access to them. This edition examines both issues, but starts with the fundamentals of the pathophysiology of cancer pain and the clinical realities of its epidemiology and diagnostic patterns. Since the first edition, the contribution of genetic variation to the individuality of analgesic and adverse responses to opioids has been increasingly recognized and new material in this area has been included. Other topics in which understanding has advanced are the control of neuropathic pain, often so challenging, and the pharmacology of nonsteroidal anti-inflammatory drugs and, again, these are the subjects of new chapters.

This volume has always recognized that cancer pain is more than a reflection of physical damage from malignancy and the second edition strengthens its coverage of the recognition and management of the psychological dimensions of pain. It has also updated its attention to the broad sweep of issues that arise in the management of malignancy-related pain, from ethics to the use of complementary therapies.

Certain groups of cancer patients have special needs, and here we consider not only children, the elderly, and those with a history of substance abuse, but also include the growing numbers of people who have survived cancer yet are living with the painful sequelae of the disease and its treatment. The reality of cancer pain control is that most of it is conducted in the home because that is where most patients wish to be, and the unique challenges that this presents are addressed from both UK and US perspectives. However, it must be remembered that pain is only one of many symptoms that can arise from cancer, and very many people who contract the disease will still die of it. Accordingly, this volume includes consideration of pain therapy in those who are dying and briefly describes the management of key symptoms other than pain.

The last 40 years have seen major strides in the control of cancer pain and advances continue to be made. As in the first edition, the editors hope that this book may be a help to clinicians in relieving their cancer patients' pain, but we hope also that a third edition will require equally far-reaching revision in order to do justice to the further progress that will by then have been made in bringing relief to the lives of the many thousands of our fellow citizens with cancer.

Nigel Sykes, Michael I Bennett, and Chun-Su Yuan
London, Lancaster, and Chicago

How to use this book

SPECIAL FEATURES

The four volumes of *Clinical Pain Management* incorporate the following special features to aid the readers' understanding and navigation of the text.

Key learning points

Each chapter opens with a set of key learning points which provide readers with an overview of the most salient points within the chapter.

Cross-references

Throughout the chapters in this volume you will find cross-references to chapters in other volumes in the *Clinical Pain Management* series. Each cross-reference will indicate the volume in which the chapter referred to is to be found.

Evidence scoring

In chapters where recommendations for surgical, medical, psychological, and complementary treatment and diagnostic tests are presented, the quality of evidence supporting authors' statements relating to clinical interventions, or the papers themselves, are graded following the Oxford Bandolier system by insertion of the following symbols into the text:

[I]   Strong evidence from at least one published systematic review of multiple well-designed randomized controlled trials
[II]   Strong evidence from at least one published properly designed randomized controlled trial of appropriate size and in an appropriate clinical setting
[III]   Evidence from published well-designed trials without randomization, single group pre-post, cohort, time series, or matched case-controlled studies
[IV]   Evidence from well-designed non-experimental studies from more than one center or research group
[V]   Opinions of respected authorities, based on clinical evidence, descriptive studies or reports of expert consensus committees.

Oxford Bandolier system used by kind permission of Bandolier: www.jr2.ox.ac.uk/Bandolier

Where no grade is inserted, the quality of supporting evidence, if any exists, is of low grade only (e.g. case reports, clinical experience, etc).

Other textbooks devoted to the subject of pain include a tremendous amount of anecdotal and personal recommendations, and it is often difficult to distinguish these from those with an established evidence base. This text is thus unique in allowing the reader the opportunity to do this with confidence.

Reference annotation

The reference lists are annotated with asterisks, where appropriate, to guide readers to key primary papers, major review articles (which contain extensive reference lists), and clinical guidelines. We hope that this feature will render extensive lists of references more useful to the reader and will help to encourage self-directed learning among both trainees and practicing physicians.

A NOTE ON DRUG NAMES

The authors have used the international nonproprietary name (INN) for drugs where possible. If the INN name differs from the US or UK name, authors have used the INN name followed by the US and/or UK name in brackets on first use within a chapter.

Abbreviations

1-Oct	octamer transcription factor-1
6-MNA	6-methoxy, 2-naphtylactic acid
[131I]MIBG	[131]iodine-metaiodobenylguanidine
ACGME	Accreditation Council for Graduate Medical Education
ACS	anorexia cachexia syndrome
ACTH	adrenocorticotropic hormone
ADH	antidiuretic hormone
AIDS	acquired immunodeficiency syndrome
AMPA	alpha-amino-3-hydroxy-5-methylisoxazole-4-proprionic acid
AO	accountable officer
APA	American Psychiatric Association
APC	adenomatous polyposis coli
APS	American Pain Society
ARF	acute renal failure
Asp	aspartic acid
ATC	around-the-clock
BCAA	branched chain amino acids
BPI	Brief Pain Inventory
BPN	brachial plexus neuropathy
CAM	Confusion Assessment Method; or complementary and alternative medicine
CAS	colored analog scale
CBT	cognitive-behavioral therapy
CCK	cholecystokinin
CD	controlled drug
CGRP	calcitonin gene-related peptide
CI	continuous infusion
CIBP	cancer-induced bone pain
CIPN	chemotherapy-induced peripheral neuropathy
Cl	clearance
CM	complementary medicine
CNS	central nervous system; or clinical nurse specialist
COMT	catechol-O-methyltransferase
COPD	chronic obstructive pulmonary disease
COX	cyclooxygenase
COX-2	cyclooxygenase-2
CR	controlled release
CRP	C-reactive protein
CRPS	complex regional pain syndrome
CRS	categorical-rated scale
CSDD	Cornell scale for depression in dementia
CSF	cerebrospinal fluid
CT	computed tomography
DBS	deep brain stimulation
DCOH	dimerization cofactor of HNF1α
DH	Department of Health
DIEP	deep inferior epigastic perforator
DNA	deoxyribonucleic acid
DREZ	dorsal root entry zone
DRG	dorsal root ganglion
DRS	Delirium Rating Scale; or Disability Rating Scale
DSM	Diagnostic and Statistical Manual of Mental Disorders
DSM-IV	*Diagnostic and statistical manual for mental disorders*, vol. IV
DU	duodenal ulcer
DUI	driving under influence
EAPC	European Association for Palliative Care
ECG	electrocardiogram
ECOG	Eastern Cooperative Oncology Group
ECS-CP	Edmonton Classification System for Cancer Pain
EDTMP	ethylene diamine tetraline tetramethyline phosphonic acid
EEG	electroencephalogram
ELNEC	End-of-Life Nursing Education Consortium
EMLA	eutectic mixture of local anesthetics
EORTC	European Organization for Research and Treatment of Cancer
EPA	eicosapentaenoic acid
ERCP	endoscopic retrograde cholangiopancreatography
ESAS	Edmonton Symptom Assessment System
ET	endothelin
FAS	facial affective scale
FBSS	failed back surgery syndrome
FBT	fentanyl buccal tablet

FNSS	failed neck surgery syndrome	NHS	National Health Service
FPS	faces pain scale	NICE	National Institute for Health and Clinical Excellence
FSH	follicle-stimulating hormone	NIH	National Institutes of Health
GABA	gamma-aminobutyric acid	NK1	neurokinin 1
GI	gastrointestinal	NMDA	N-methyl-D-aspartic acid
GP	general practitioner	NNH	number needed to harm
GU	gastric ulcer	NNPC	Neighbourhood Network in Palliative Care
		NNT	number needed to treat
HADS	Hospital Anxiety and Depression Scale	NPY	neuropeptide Y
HCT	home care team	NRPS	nurse-reported pain score
HIV	human immunodeficiency virus	NRS	numerical rating scale
HNF1α	hepatic nuclear factor-1α	NSAID	nonsteroidal anti-inflammatory drug
		NSCLC	nonsmall cell lung cancer
IAHPC	International Association for Hospice and Palliative Care	OAF	osteoclast-activating factor
IAPC	Indian Association of Palliative Care	OD	organizational development
IASP	International Association for the Study of Pain	ONC	oncologist
		ONT	opioid neurotoxicity
ICBN	intercostobrachial nerve	OPG	osteoprotogerin
INCB	International Narcotics Control Board	OTFC	oral transmucosal fentanyl citrate
IOELC	International Observatory on End of Life Care	PAG	periaqueductal gray
IRM	immediate release morphine	PAINAD	pain assessment in advanced dementia
ISCD	International Statistical Classification of Diseases	PBCSP	postbreast cancer surgery pain
		PC	palliative care
i.v.	intravenous	PCA	patient-controlled analgesia
		PCP	primary care physicians
LAS	linear analog scale	PCT	palliative care team; or primary care trust
LC	locus ceruleus		
LH	luteinizing hormone	PD	pharmacodynamic
LMF	lipid-mobilizing factors	PET	positron emission tomography
LOX	lipoxygenase	PGG_2	prostaglandin G_2
LTC	long-term care	PHN	postherpetic neuralgia
		PK	pharmacokinetic
M3G	morphine-3-glucuronide	PLA_2	phospholipase-A_2
M6G	morphine-6-glucuronide	PMF	protein-mobilizing factors
MBS	motor cortex stimulation	PMI	pain management inventory
MDACC	MD Anderson Cancer Center	PMPS	postmastectomy pain syndrome
MDAS	Memorial Delirium Assessment Scale	PNS	peripheral nervous system
MECC	Middle East Cancer Consortium	POX	peroxidase
MEDAL	Multinational Etoricoxib and Diclofenac Arthritis Long-term	PPI	protein-pump inhibitor
		pps	pulses per second
MMAS	Marañón's Myoclonus Assessment Scale	PPSG	Pain and Policy Study Group
MMSE	Mini-Mental State Examination	PSA	prostate specific antigen
MPQ	McGill Pain Questionnaire	PTHrP	parathyroid hormone-related peptide
MR	magnetic resonance	PVG/PAG	periventricular and periaqueductal gray matter
MRI	magnetic resonance imaging		
MSAS 10–18	Memorial Symptom Assessment Scale 10–18	QST	quantitative sensory testing
MST	morphine sulfate tablets		
		RAGE	Radiotherapy Action Group Exposure
NCCN	National Comprehensive Cancer Network	RCT	randomized controlled trial
NCIC-CTC	National Cancer Institute common toxicity criteria	REM	rapid eye movement
		rESS	revised Edmonton Staging System
NCPB	neurolytic celiac plexus block	RF	radiofrequency lesioning
NGO	Non-Government Organization	RR	relative risk

RTOG	Radiotherapy Therapy Oncology Group	THC	Δ9-tetrahydrocannabinol
RVM	rostral ventromedial medulla	TI	therapeutic index
		TMS	transcranial magnetic stimulation
SA	substance abuse	TNF	tumor necrosis factor
SCLC	small cell lung cancer	TRAM	transverse rectus abdominis muscle
SCS	spinal cord stimulation	TSE	transcutaneous spinal electroanalgesia
SIGN	Scottish Intercollegiate Guidelines Network		
SNP	single nucleotide polymorphism	UGT	uridine-diphosphoglucuronosyltransferase
SNRI	serotonin and noradrenergic reuptake inhibitors	UN	United Nations
SP	substance P	VAS	visual analog scale
SPF	Special Prescription Form	VIP	vasoactive intestinal peptide
SRM	slow release morphine	VPG	vomiting pattern generator
SRPS	self-reported pain score	VPL	ventroposterior lateral
SSRI	selective serotonin reuptake inhibitors	VPM	ventroposterior medial
STAS	Support Team Assessment Schedule	VRS	verbal rating scale
SVCO	superior vena caval obstruction		
TCA	tricyclic antidepressants	WDR	wide-dynamic neuron
TENS	transcutaneous electrical nerve stimulation	WHO	World Health Organization

PART I

GENERAL CONSIDERATIONS

1 Pathophysiology of somatic, visceral, and neuropathic cancer pain 3
Catherine E Urch and Rie Suzuki

2 Epidemiology of cancer pain 13
Irene J Higginson, Julie Hearn, and Fliss Murtagh

3 Cancer pain syndromes 27
Robert Twycross and Michael Bennett

4 History and clinical examination of the cancer pain patient: assessment and measurement 38
Badi El Osta and Eduardo Bruera

5 Psychological evaluation of patient and family 48
Barbara Monroe

6 The role of the nonprofessional caregiver in cancer pain management 63
Christine Miaskowski

7 Teamworking in cancer pain management 71
Vicky Robinson and Rob George

8 Barriers to cancer pain relief: an international perspective on drug availability and service delivery 81
Fiona Graham and David Clark

9 Ethical issues in cancer pain management 93
Fiona Randall

Pathophysiology of somatic, visceral, and neuropathic cancer pain

CATHERINE E URCH AND RIE SUZUKI

Introduction   3
Pathophysiology of cancer-induced somatic pain   4
Pathophysiology of cancer-induced neuropathic pain   5
Models of cancer-related neuropathic pain   7
Pathophysiology of cancer-induced visceral pain   9
Conclusions   9
References   9

KEY LEARNING POINTS

- Cancer pain is a mixed mechanism pain.
- It is unique from other pain states in terms of timing, evolution, and complexity.
- Animal models suggest that cancer pain has unique features.
- There are few cancer-induced visceral pain models.

- There is a different sequence of neurotransmitters/receptors/intracellular mechanisms in cancer pain.
- Clinical therapies suggest common end pathways/receptor activation.
- Current translation of therapies from noncancer to cancer pain, in future may target specific cancer-pain targets.

INTRODUCTION

Cancer pain is often labelled as a "mixed mechanism" pain, not easily classified into distinct and discrete etiology or mechanisms. The essential mixed mechanism present in cancer pain may account for some of its unique characteristics. It can only rarely be classified and treated as a pure or exclusive neuropathic or nociceptive pain.[1] In addition, unlike the majority of other pain syndromes, cancer pain is subjected to an ever-changing palate with influences from treatments, the cancer, and time. Thus the changing nature of cancer pain requires the clinician to constantly reassess and reevaluate the new and compound features of the pain. In addition to the nociceptive element of the pain experience, the patient will have complex psychological, spiritual, emotional, and behavioral interpretations of the pain and the meaning of the total pain experience.[2]

Cancer pain is no different from other pain states in many respects. Nociceptive inputs are transmitted by the same Aδ and C fibers, via the same receptors and transduction mechanisms as in other pain states whether acute or chronic, heat, chemical, ischemia, or pressure.[3, 4] All inputs are modulated in the dorsal horn, by which stage it is the interaction and modulation of the afferent inputs, intraneuronal and descending pathways that influence that final output, rather than the clinical diagnosis at the primary afferent,[5, 6, 7] Higher-center interactions, modulation, relay, and output are again the same in cancer as in other chronic or acute pain syndromes.[8, 9] Given the identical pathways, neurotransmitters, and receptors one could ask, is cancer pain a unique pain state requiring different treatments or a merely an extension of more discrete pain syndromes?

Clinical surveys and classifications would suggest there are uniting features of cancer pain and other pain syndromes. Thus, in noncancer pains neuropathic features could be described as being more or less predominant in the overall pain state.[1, 10] In a large series of cancer patients, a similar finding of varying predominance of neuropathic features was found.[11] There is evidence clinically that drugs effective in noncancer pain states, such as opioids, are effective in cancer pain states.[12, 13, 14, 15] The efficacy may be determined rather by the underlying balance of neuronal excitation (inflammatory versus somatic versus neuropathic) rather than the clinical diagnosis. Thus, opioids are reported to be less effective in neuropathic pain than in inflammatory pain, regardless of whether the neuropathic element is caused by a viral deafferentation, surgical transaction, chemotherapy induced, or by direct neuronal destruction by cancer.[16, 17] This would suggest cancer pain is not a "unique pain state," rather an extension of other pain syndromes and therefore models of noncancer neuropathy, inflammation, and visceral pain would have relevance in dissecting the mechanisms in cancer pain. Furthermore, it would suggest that drugs effective in noncancer pain states might be applicable and relevant to cancer pain states. Indeed clinically this is what occurs, with extrapolation from noncancer to cancer.

However, more recent work on chemotherapy-induced neuropathy (which may be considered to be a cancer pain, as it arises out of the treatment of cancer, and it is unclear what role residual or prior presence of cancer pain has) or cancer-induced bone pain may suggest that cancer pain should be considered as the unique pain syndrome.[18, 19, 20] It could be argued that as cancer and the attendant treatments result in mixed pain mechanisms, the resulting neuronal and higher-center stimulation induces a complexity and "chaos" and so produces a unique state. Although fundamentally built from more pure pain states, it evolves to become a pain state in its own right. In the same way as a bract is in essence a simple flower, it is far removed from a complex rose. Although in essence both are flowers, and the resulting evolution, expression, interdependence have made them unique and the outcome will be determined by a multitude of factors. Thus, while in concept they are similar and from the same beginnings, the outcome and features are unique. In a similar way, viral deafferentation pain, such as in herpes zoster, may appear to be the same as paclitaxel (taxol)-chemotherapy induced pain, both reporting similar clinical features and intensity, the mechanisms, treatment, consequences, and impact are different.[21, 22]

This chapter will explore in more depth the pathophysiology of cancer-induced neuropathic, somatic, and visceral pain. Other chapters will deal in more depth with some aspects, such as the physiology of neuropathic pain, and in the consequent treatment of cancer and noncancer pain (see Chapter 1, Applied physiology: neuropathic pain; Chapter 2, Applied physiology: persistent musculoskeletal pain; and Chapter 3, Applied physiology: persistent visceral pain in the *Chronic Pain* volume of this series). Over the past 40 years, there has been an explosion in the level of knowledge and understanding of the neuronal mechanisms and pathways involved in nociception. From the early hypothesis of the "gate theory," through to the growing understanding of the complex modulatory role of the higher central nervous system (CNS) centers in the expression of pain and suffering, the majority of work is in noncancer, either clinically or in animal models. The use of specific models to explore the nature and complexity of cancer pain is relatively new, and in comparison to noncancer pain is poorly understood. Where possible, cancer models will be discussed, although often extrapolations from noncancer have been needed.

PATHOPHYSIOLOGY OF CANCER–INDUCED SOMATIC PAIN

There are few animal models of cancer-induced somatic or nociceptive pain. Until recently, many cancer models of pain required the systemic injection of cancer cells, which resulted in ill and weakened animals, with a variety of nociceptive behaviors. It was difficult to dissect out the mechanism and natural progression of pain, and harder to evaluation drug efficacy. Recently, models of cancer-induced bone pain were developed that allowed growth of a cancer in a predetermined place (in or around a bone), in a fundamentally well animal. The models are all reproducible, consistent, and appear to parallel aspects of the clinical situation. From these models, investigations into the mechanisms (peripheral and central) of the pathophysiology have revealed startling results. These models will be discussed as an example of somatic pain, illustrating the complexity and uniqueness of cancer pain.

Bone pain arising from metastatic carcinoma or primary sarcoma is a common sequela of disease progression. Pain has been reported to occur in up to 80 percent of cases of metastatic bone disease and correlates with reduced quality of life, increased depression, and reduced performance status.[23, 24] Cancer-induced bone pain (CIBP) is a clinical problem with reports of 50–90 percent of patients attending either outpatient pain clinics or requiring hospice admission reporting pain on movement.[25, 26, 27] Schwei *et al.*[28] reported a method of local infusion of cancer (osteosarcoma cells) into a single bone of a mouse. They demonstrated that this method resulted in localized bone pain in a systemically well animal and for the first time provided a model to investigate the pathophysiology of CIBP. The osteosarcoma cells were prepared and infused directly into the medulla of a mouse femur (media injection for the sham groups). Over the subsequent 21 days, the animals were well, but from day 14 onwards demonstrated increasing severe pain behaviors. These were quantified according to limp on walking, flinching or vocalization on palpation, withdrawal threshold to punctate mechanical pressure (von Frey filaments), and spontaneous licking and flinching.

These pain behaviors are taken as correlates of human movement-induced pain, point tenderness, tonic (background) pain, and spontaneous pain, respectively. The animals receiving the intramedullary injection of the sarcoma cells displayed progressively severe nocifensive behavior which correlated with the degree of bone destruction. The sham-operated animals showed no signs of pain behavior. In this early model, the bone was not plugged and a local escape (but not distant metastases) were noted. The bone progressed from normal to pathological fracture and the destruction could be graded on x-ray.[28]

Since 1999, several models using the same principle of local infusion have been described, although now uniformly the bone is plugged after infusion. Models include rat breast carcinoma (MRMT-1 cell line) injection into the tibia, fibrosarcoma, melanoma, adenocarcinoma, prostate cancer within the humerus or femur of mice.[29, 30, 31] In all models, the development parallels the clinical situation with progessive bone destruction (**Figure 1.1**), leading to pathological fracture, accompanying progressive limping, guarding, spontaneous flinching, reduced thresholds to mechanical or cooling stimulus (secondary allodynia).[19, 28] One main difference is the lack of nonpainful metastases, which is a common clinical finding and a situation that may reveal much about the inhibitory controls governing CIBP.

CIBP has been investigated by numerous groups and reveals an interaction between peripheral activation and dorsal horn alterations. In the periphery, tumors invading the medullary space of the bone actively alter the milieu, the normal osteoclast/osteoblast balance, and activate the nociceptive primary afferents via the release of a host of growth factors (such as nerve growth factor, granulocyte colony-stimulating factor), cytokines (such as tumor necrosis factor (TNF)), interleukins (IL)-1, IL-6, chemokines, prostanoids, endothelins and others,[32, 33] and protons (H^+), which reduces the surrounding pH to 5 or below.[34] Invading tumors also elicit a vigorous immune response, albeit ineffective at obliterating the cancer. The invasion of active T cells, macrophages, and natural killer cells adds an inflammatory dimension to the primary afferent activation and interaction.[35] Endothelins (ET) are involved in tumor cell signal transduction, mitogenesis, endothelial growth, and angiogenesis and inflammation and promote pain behaviors when applied to the sciatic nerve via activation of the ET receptors on primary afferents.[36, 37, 38] A mouse model, in which osteolytic connective tissue carcinoma was injected into and on to the calcaneous bone, demonstrated peak pain behaviors found on day ten which correlated with an increase in ET-1 secretion. Furthermore, a blockade of the ET_A receptor reduced nociceptive behavior.[39] In humans, prostate carcinoma has been shown to express high levels of endothelins, the plasma level of which correlates with the severity of pain.[40, 41]

However, as the tumor continues to grow and osteoclasts continue to destroy bone, primary afferents will be destroyed. The tumor may entrap, compress, invade, cause neuronal ischemia, or destroy by direct proteolysis. This will cause direct activation of the primary afferent and "neuropathic" pain. This process has been observed in the murine model of osteosarcoma CIBP.[42] The alterations within damaged peripheral nerves and the subsequent dorsal horn and higher center changes have been discussed in more detail elsewhere. In CIBP primary and secondary peripheral hyperalgesia, characterized by reduced thresholds (to mechanical, thermal, and dynamic stimuli), increased receptive field size and increased area of sensitivity have been demonstrated.[43]

The features of the dorsal horn alteration continue to display a mixture of inflammatory and neuropathic stimuli, resulting in a unique feature. Dynorphin receptors, a prohyperalgesic peptide, were observed to be upregulated in CIBP, neuropathy, and inflammation;[44] however, expected proinflammatory changes such as upregulation of calcitonin gene-related peptide (CGRP), or proneuropathic changes, such as increased neuropeptide Y (NPY), were not.[45, 46] The increased expression of *c-fos* and internalization of substance P (SP)–neurokinin 1 (NK1) receptor complex after noxious stimuli in advanced CIBP demonstrate central sensitization.[47] Furthermore, response to drugs also demonstrate a mixed or unique picture. The dorsal horn neuronal response to CIBP is also unique, with the expected excitation of wide-dynamic neurones (WDR) in the deep lamina, but in addition there appears to be an increase in lamina I WDR neurones.[19, 48] This alteration in WDR from 25 to 50 percent of lamina I neuronal composition may be recruitment of silent neurones or an excitation and alteration in nociceptive specific neurones.[49] The unique nature of CIBP continues in the response to drugs, such as morphine and gabapentin. Morphine is effective in attenuating dorsal horn neuronal response and behavior, to a similar degree as in inflammation;[50] however, other models suggest less responsiveness.[51] Gabapentin is used clinically in neuropathy and in CIBP it attenuates behavioral responses and normalizes the dorsal horn responses.[52]

CIBP has been clinically classified as a somatic nociceptive pain, however work from animal models suggests a more complex picture. While there is undoubtedly inflammatory stimuli within the bone, and corresponding responses within primary afferents and dorsal horn, there is a significant primary afferent destruction/compression resulting in neuropathic elements. The resultant dorsal horn response is unique.

PATHOPHYSIOLOGY OF CANCER–INDUCED NEUROPATHIC PAIN

Neuropathic pain, defined as pain initiated or caused by a primary lesion or dysfunction in the nervous system, is often difficult to manage and poses significant clinical challenges. Although the exact prevalence of neuropathic

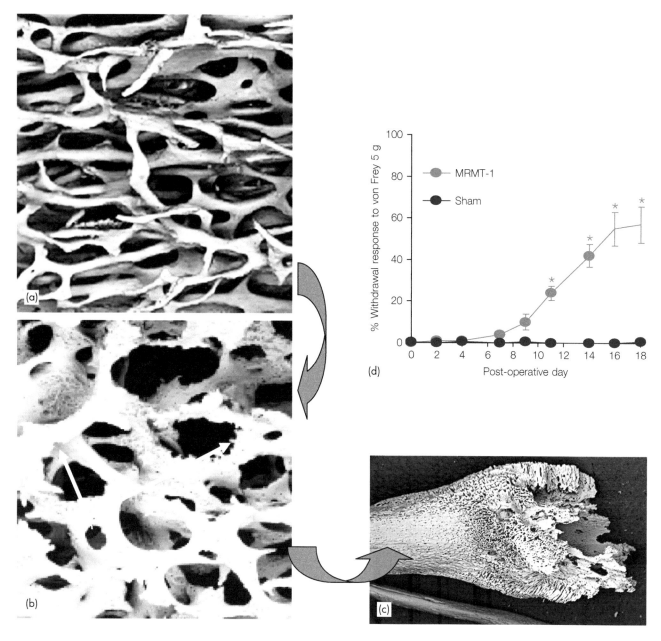

Figure 1.1 The pathological changes that occur within a bone with osteoclast activation secondary to cancer cells. (a) Scanning electron microscope picture of normal trabeculae bone; (b) the arrows indicate the activation of osteoclasts, the loss of smooth trabeculation (R) and bone mass. (b) The femur had been injected with MRMT-1 breast cancer cells 12 days previously. (c) The femur at day 21 after MRMT-1 injection has fractured. The bone can be seen to be extensively destroyed, but also new bone remodelling has occurred. (d) The development of mechanical hyperalgesia over time after intratibial injection of MRMT-1. The graph illustrates the withdrawal of the ipsilateral hindpaw to a nonnoxious stimuli (von Frey hair 5 g). In normal (sham-injected animals) the baseline does not vary as the stimuli continue to be nonnoxious; however, in the MRMT-1-injected animals, the percentage of withdrawals increases from day nine. This correlates with bone destruction as seen in (b) and (c), and from other work (not shown) with alterations in the dorsal horn.

pain in cancer patients remains unknown, it is predicted that at least 15–20 percent of patients are likely to suffer from neuropathic pain during the course of the disease, and an even higher population at advanced stages of the disease. Intractable pain can have a detrimental impact on the overall quality of life; it impairs the patient's ability to perform daily functions, as well as their ability to cope with the disease, further adding to the anxiety, worry, and stress of the afflicted patient and family. This highlights the need for a thorough understanding of the complex cancer syndrome, characteristic of pain symptoms, mechanisms, and treatment options by the health practitioner, and attempts should be made to offer support wherever needed.

Whether due to malignant or nonmalignant origin, neuropathic pain presents with complex multiple symptoms which include a combination of positive and negative signs, such as sensory loss (numbness), spontaneous pain, allodynia, hyperalgesia, and paresthesia.[10, 53, 54] Some of these potential mechanisms have been best studied in animal models involving partial nerve injuries (e.g. sciatic nerve ligation, infraorbital nerve injury), viral infection (varicella zoster virus-induced postherpetic neuralgia (PHN)), systemic chemical injection (streptozocin-induced diabetic neuropathy). However, the availability of cancer-induced models of neuropathy remain limited (see below under Models of cancer-related neuropathic pain).

Neuropathic pain in cancer patients may arise as a result of physical compression of the nerve by the growing tumor or through direct infiltration into the nerve. The spread of colon cancer into the pelvis, for example, may compress the nerve innervating the legs or pelvic structures. Neuropathy may also result secondary to a change in tissue pH (acidosis) or the release of chemical algogens by the tumor, either in areas surrounding the nerve or directly in the nerve itself following tumor infiltration. Paradoxically, neuropathy can also arise as a consequence of cancer-directed therapy, from use of agents with neurotoxic side-effect profiles causing chemical nerve damage. Drugs such as paclitaxel, vincristine, and cisplatin have been widely reported to produce sensory neuropathies, evoking tingling sensations, paresthesias, or numbness in the distal extremities consistent with a glove-and-stocking distribution. In a phase I trial, patients receiving paclitaxel – a plant alkaloid known to produce cytotoxicity through effects on microtubule aggregation – developed symptoms of neuropathy as early as one to three days following treatment.[55] Neurophysiological examination and nerve biopsies often reveal evidence for axonal degeneration, nerve fiber loss, and demyelination.[56] Additionally, surgical interventions involving removal of malignant tumors (e.g. mastectomy, thoracotomy) will commonly result in nerve trauma and deafferentation pain. Patients undergoing mastectomy report a constellation of symptoms, including pain or discomfort in the chest wall, surgical scar, upper arm, and shoulder, which may be suggestive of intercostobrachial nerve damage. Phantom breast tactile sensations may also occur. Finally, radiation-induced fibrosis can injure peripheral nerves (e.g. fibrosis of brachial plexus) causing chronic neuropathic pain that begins months to years following treatment. In debilitated patients, PHN is also a common finding.

MODELS OF CANCER-RELATED NEUROPATHIC PAIN

Despite the existence of a wide range of rodent neuropathy models, there only exist a limited number of animal models involving cancer-related nerve damage. Of these, the most widely studied models involve the use of chemotherapy agents (e.g. paclitaxel) and the inoculation of tumor cells adjacent to peripheral nerves. The different models vary in the use of animal species, tumor types (e.g. sarcoma, mammary carcinoma), choice of chemotherapy agent (e.g. paclitaxel, cisplatin), and tumor inoculation sites (e.g. hindpaw, thigh muscle). One limitation in developing a cancer-induced neuropathy model relates to the technical difficulty in achieving reproducible tumor confinement, preventing its spread to multiple organs, which may otherwise result in a severely ill animal precluding the quantitative assessment of pain. Although the originating source of pain may differ between malignant (e.g. tumor compression) and nonmalignant neuropathic pains (diabetic neuropathy), the mechanisms and neural pathways involved in the generation of the pain state are essentially similar and as such, much of the underlying pathology can be inferred from mechanisms operating in nonmalignant neuropathic pain.

Various mouse models of cancer have been developed that involve the inoculation of murine tumor cells into the hindpaw or the thigh of mice (e.g. squamous cell carcinoma; hepatocarcinoma cells).[57, 58] Spontaneous pain behavior, heat hyperalgesia, and/or mechanical allodynia are readily induced in these models following foot inoculation over varying time courses. In the case of mice injected with the squamous cell carcinoma, pain behaviors displayed an early onset (one to three days after inoculation); however, over 60 percent of mice died within 16 days of surgery and metastasis to the lung was apparent.[57] Despite the tumor progression, there was no sign of tumor infiltration into the nerve, although plantar nerves were clearly encapsulated by tumor cells.[57] The relative contribution of neuropathic damage to the pain behaviors of these mice remains to be studied; however, it would appear that substantial compression of nerves following tumor progression is likely to result in a degree of nerve damage. Other models include inoculation of Meth-A sarcoma cells to the vicinity of the mouse sciatic nerve, which results in the growth of a tumor mass embedding the nerve.[18] Pain behaviors reach a maximum by three weeks post-inoculation, at a time when clear histological signs of nerve damage can be identified. Further immunohistochemical analysis revealed enhanced spinal expression of c-fos (a marker of neuronal activation) and neuropeptides (e.g. substance P, CGRP, dynorphin A), indicating enhanced pain transmission within nociceptive circuits, consistent with behavioral findings.[59] The implantation of mammary adenocarcinoma cells adjacent to the sciatic nerve similarly produces pain behaviors in mice for seven days.[60] In both these animal models, there is a gradual decline of pain behaviors and subsequent appearance of hyposensitivity, which may, in part, correspond to progressive motor paralysis in the animals. Evidence for nerve damage and neural infiltration of immune and malignant cells (with mild edema) would suggest the involvement of neuropathic, as well as inflammatory processes in cancer-induced pain, highlighting the complex pathology of this condition.

The last decade has seen the introduction of a growing number of animal models of sensory neuropathies induced by antineoplastic agents, such as paclitaxel. Paclitaxel is widely used for the treatment of solid tumors and its use is accompanied by side effects including myelosuppression and peripheral neuropathy.[61] While patients may be given treatments to counteract the myelosuppression, no effective agents are available to date for the prevention of nerve damage, making this a major dose-limiting factor. Patients with other predispositions to neuropathy (e.g. previous chemotherapy) or coexisting diabetes or alcohol abuse may, in particular, have high susceptibility to such neurotoxicity. The majority of patients receiving paclitaxel (>50 percent) developed signs of neuropathy by three weeks, which appeared to preferentially affect the sensory, but not motor or autonomic nervous system.[62] Neurological examination classically reveals slower sensory conduction velocities, reduced nerve action potential amplitudes and altered H reflexes.[56] To date, there does not yet exist an effective treatment for chemotherapy-induced neuropathy; however, the availability of new animal models will help shed light on the underlying pathological mechanisms and aid the development of potential therapeutic approaches. With the emergence of paclitaxel- and vincristine-induced models of neuropathy, there has been a growing interest in the molecular, histological, and pharmacological analysis of these models.[62, 63, 64, 65, 66, 67] In a rat model of paclitaxel-induced neuropathy following repeated systemic paclitaxel administration, morphological analysis of the rat sciatic nerves revealed evidence for marked microtubular aggregation within axons which appear to be the primary site of target of this drug.[68, 69] By binding to tubulin of the mitotic spindle, paclitaxel interferes with microtubule dynamics, arresting cellular division and engaging apoptosis.[70] Quantification of paclitaxel tissue concentrations in the rat (peripheral and central nervous system) reveals that systemic paclitaxel readily accesses the peripheral nervous system (PNS) and accumulates in the dorsal root ganglia (DRG).[71] There is evidence to suggest that paclitaxel initiates neuroimmune reactions to evoke proinflammatory cytokine release (e.g. TNF-α, IL-6). In a study in breast cancer patients, the initiation of paclitaxel treatment was accompanied by transient increases in cytokines including IL-8, IL-10, and IL-6.[72] These neuroimmune responses are likely to underlie the flu-like symptoms experienced by patients following therapy with paclitaxel and could additionally contribute to the development of sensory neuropathy.

One confounding factor in the animal models is the detrimental effect of paclitaxel and other chemotherapy drugs (e.g. vincristine) on the animals' general health (e.g. pronounced weight loss, increased mortality) which may be related to the dose, frequency, and route of drug

administration. In a study of vincristine-induced neuropathy, increasing doses of vincristine (1–100 µg/kg/day) was shown to produce increased weight loss in rats, together with a progressive increase in mortality rate.[64] Furthermore, respiratory complications (dyspnea, wheezing) was reported with higher vincristine concentrations.[64] Subsequently, studies have developed protocols for paclitaxel dosing that allowed the progressive assessment of reproducible sensory neuropathy in rats with no significant deterioration of health.[63, 65] While heat sensitivity, as measured by tail flick and hindpaw withdrawal reflex, was reported to be unaltered in one study,[63] Polomano et al.[65] provided detailed characterization of the time-related changes in pain behaviors of these rats. All rats exhibited normal weight gain throughout the duration of the one-month behavioral assay. Paclitaxel-treated rats displayed pronounced heat hyperalgesia, cold and mechanical allodynia symmetrically on both hindpaws, which was maintained for 28 days. However, histological examination of the peripheral nerves or DRG revealed no major abnormalities or signs of degeneration in nerve axons, with the exception of the presence of endoneurial edema in the sciatic nerve.[65]

This raises the question as to what extent axonal degeneration contributes to the development of neuropathic pain behaviors, since the studies by Polomano et al.[65] show demonstrable pain behaviors in the absence of clear nerve pathology, while Cliffer et al.[63] report no changes in (heat) pain sensitivity in rats with severe histopathological damage. Thus, the relationship between pain, sensorimotor function (e.g. electrophysiological diagnosis), and anatomical abnormality is still unclear. The various pathologies observed in animal models (altered pain sensory thresholds, anatomical changes in nerve structure, disruption in nerve conduction, loss of sensory, or motor function) may represent different stages of paclitaxel-induced neuropathy and as such it can be considered to be a graded phenomenon.

There is still limited evidence from animal models regarding the pharmacology of chemotherapy-induced cancer pain models. However, given the evidence for the presence of abnormal heightened excitability in C-nociceptors,[73] as well as central sensitization in the spinal cord following vincristine-induced neuropathy,[74] it could be envisaged that agents acting to attenuate this hyperexcitability may demonstrate some efficacy against behavioral pain end points in preclinical models. The antidepressant venlafaxine was shown to reverse hyperalgesia in a model of vincristine-induced neuropathy,[75] while in another study, ethosuximide, but not morphine or MK-801 (N-methyl-D-aspartic acid (NMDA) receptor antagonist) proved to be effective.[76] In a model of paclitaxel-induced allodynia, gabapentin was shown to reverse mechanical allodynia and this was paralleled by immunohistochemical observations of an upregulation of the gabapentin-binding site (alpha-2 delta subunit of calcium channels),[77] similar to that reported in models of traumatic nerve injury (e.g. spinal nerve ligation, chronic constriction injury).[78] Using animals with vincristine-induced allodynia, Nozaki-Taguchi and colleagues[64] reported the efficacies of several different classes of clinically used drugs, some with proven efficacies in the treatment of peripheral neuropathy. Using a dose of vincristine that causes pronounced allodynia while preserving general health, it was demonstrated that a single dose administration of morphine, lidocaine, mexiletine, and pregabalin produced a reversal of the mechanical hypersensitivity of these animals. More recently, the findings of the above study were further extended to establish a dose–response function to 11 clinically employed drugs to assess their clinical utility in vincristine-induced neuropathy.[79] With the exception of three classes of drugs, including nonsteroidal anti-inflammatory drugs (NSAID) (ibuprofen, acetylsalicylic acid), a COX-2 inhibitor (celecoxib), and an antidepressant (desipramine), the remaining seven agents (lamotrigine, dextromethorphan, gabapentin, acetaminophen, carbamazepine, clonidine, morphine) exerted dose-dependent reversal of mechanical allodynia with varying efficacies and therapeutic indices (TI). Clonidine and morphine were shown to be most potent and safe, with TI values of approximately 1000.[79]

These data could suggest that despite a differing etiology, agents currently used for the treatment of peripheral neuropathic pain may have the potential to show demonstrable efficacies in chemotherapy-induced neuropathy. This remains to be confirmed in future studies. Given the availability of preclinical models, it is expected that further pharmacological characterization and exploration of the underlying mechanisms will follow, which will aid the development of analgesic strategies for the treatment of chemotherapy-induced painful neuropathy.

PATHOPHYSIOLOGY OF CANCER–INDUCED VISCERAL PAIN

The exact prevalence of visceral pain in cancer patients is unclear; however, visceral pain is common and is encountered in patients with primary or metastatic tumor infiltration into the viscera, such as the pancreas, liver, gastrointestinal tract, and lung. Visceral pain is diffuse and poorly localized, and the pain is often referred to distant, and often superficial, somatic structures (e.g. skin), making it difficult to determine the exact source of the pain. Autonomic reflexes, such as nausea and vomiting, may accompany visceral pain, and patients may report the pain as sickening, deep, squeezing, and dull in quality. Visceral structures are unique in that they show exquisite sensitivity to luminal distension, ischemia, or inflammation; however, they are relatively insensitive to other stimuli that would normally evoke intense pain in cutaneous tissues (e.g. burning, cutting). In the colon, for example, the occurrence of visceral pain is largely

dependent on the distending pressure, thus pain will result when the intraluminal pressure exceeds the threshold (40–50 mmHg). In many cases, if the intraluminal pressure does not exceed the pain threshold, the tumor will continue its growth and remain undetected with the result that by the time pain is reported by the patient, there may be significant obstruction of the lumen. In this respect, solid organs are the least sensitive, whereas the serosal membranes of hollow organs are most sensitive. The release of algesic chemical mediators by the tumor may, in some cases, result in the sensitization and activation of nociceptors and this may allow activation of pain pathways at lower thresholds.

To date, our understanding of the characteristics and symptoms of visceral pain have largely come from the clinic, and further dissection of the mechanisms and pathology of this pain state awaits the arrival of an appropriate preclinical model. One model of visceral cancer described to date involves the use of the $Apc^{\Delta716}$ mouse line.[80] Heterozygote mice with mutations in the gene encoding APC (adenomatous polyposis coli) spontaneously developed multiple polyps in the intestinal tract three weeks postnatally, offering the opportunity to allow pharmacological evaluation of compounds such as COX-2 inhibitors[81] and to validate the model as a potential mouse model of colon cancer. The development of pain behaviors in this animal model has not been reported, hence further studies are required to assess whether such a model can be used to study cancer-induced visceral pain.

CONCLUSIONS

It is clear from the above discussion that cancer pain, whilst employing the same basic mechanisms of pain transmission, transduction, neurotransmitters, and receptors, is a complex pain syndrome. The nature of the multiplicity of inducers means that rarely is pain a pure neuropathic, inflammatory, or visceral pain. Rather, cancer pains are perhaps unique in being the essence of interactions, modulations, and interplay from each. In addition, the ever-changing stimuli lead to a complex reemergence of pain, alteration in the balance of pain (for example, from visceral to neuropathic), and consequently complex polypharmacy and nondrug interventions to treat pain. It is clear that extrapolation from noncancer pain physiology is possible; however, further work is needed to elucidate further which aspects of cancer-induced pain are indeed unique.

REFERENCES

* 1. Bennett MI, Smith BH, Torrance N, Lee AJ. Can pain be more or less neuropathic? Comparison of symptom assessment tools with ratings of certainty by clinicains. *Pain.* 2006; **122**: 289–94.

2. Millspaugh CD. Assessment and response to spiritual pain: part I. *Journal of Palliative Medicine.* 2005; **8**: 919–23.

3. Besson JM. The neurobiology of pain. *Lancet.* 1999; **353**: 1610–15.

4. Bridges D, Thompson SW, Rice AS. Mechanisms of neuropathic pain. *British Journal of Anaesthesia.* 2001; **87**: 12–26.

∗ 5. Carpenter KJ, Dickenson AH. Molecular aspects of pain research. *Pharmacogenomics Journal.* 2002; **2**: 87–95.

6. Marples IL, Murray P. Neuropathic pain. *Lancet.* 1999; **354**: 953–4.

∗ 7. Suzuki R, Rygh LJ, Dickenson AH. Bad news from the brain: descending 5-HT pathways that control spinal pain processing. *Trends in Pharmacological Sciences.* 2004; **25**: 613–17.

8. Ploghaus A, Tracey I, Gati JS *et al.* Dissociating pain from its anticipation in the human brain. *Science.* 1999; **284**: 1979–81.

∗ 9. Tracey I. Functional connectivity and pain: how effectively connected is your brain? *Pain.* 2005; **116**: 173–4.

10. Rasmussen PV, Sindrup SH, Jensen TS, Bach FW. Symptoms and signs in patients with suspected neuropathic pain. *Pain.* 2004; **110**: 461–9.

11. Grond S, Radbruch L, Meuser T *et al.* Assessment and treatment of neuropathic cancer pain following WHO guidelines. *Pain.* 1999; **79**: 15–20.

12. Lubbe AS. Opioids in cancer pain. *European Journal of Cancer Care.* 2006; **15**: 208.

13. Foley KM. Advances in cancer pain. *Archives of Neurology.* 1999; **56**: 413–17.

14. Breivik H. Opioids in cancer and chronic non-cancer pain therapy – indications and controversies. *Acta Anaesthesiologica Scandinavica.* 2001; **45**: 1059–66.

15. Bell RF, Wisloff T, Eccleston C, Kalso E. Controlled clinical trials in cancer pain. How controlled should they be? A qualitative systematic review. *British Journal of Cancer.* 2006; **94**: 1559–67.

∗ 16. Mercadante S, Portenoy RK. Opioid poorly-responsive cancer pain. Part 2: Basic mechanisms that could shift dose response for analgesia. *Journal of Pain and Symptom Management.* 2001; **21**: 255–64.

17. Mercadante S, Portenoy RK. Opioid poorly-responsive cancer pain. Part 1: Clinical considerations. *Journal of Pain and Symptom Management.* 2001; **21**: 144–50.

18. Shimoyama M, Tanaka K, Hasue F, Shimoyama N. A mouse model of neuropathic cancer pain. *Pain.* 2002; **99**: 167–74.

∗ 19. Urch CE, Donovan-Rodriguez T, Dickenson AH. Alterations in dorsal horn neurones in a rat model of cancer-induced bone pain. *Pain.* 2003; **106**: 347–56.

∗ 20. Flatters SJ, Bennett GJ. Studies of peripheral sensory nerves in paclitaxel-induced painful peripheral neuropathy: evidence for mitochondrial dysfunction. *Pain.* 2006; **122**: 245–57.

21. Cata JP, Weng HR, Lee BN *et al.* Clinical and experimental findings in humans and animals with chemotherapy-induced peripheral neuropathy. *Minerva Anesthesiologica.* 2006; **72**: 151–69.

22. Boer A, Herder N, Blodorn-Schlicht N *et al.* Refining criteria for diagnosis of cutaneous infections caused by herpes viruses through correlation of morphology with molecular pathology. *Indian Journal of Dermatology, Venereology and Leprology.* 2006; **72**: 270–5.

∗ 23. Coleman RE. Skeletal complications of malignancy. *Cancer,* **80** (Suppl.): 1997: 1588–94.

24. Mercadante S. Malignant bone pain: pathophysiology and treatment. *Pain.* 1997; **69**: 1–18.

∗ 25. Portenoy RK, Hagen NA. Breakthrough pain: definition, prevalence and characteristics. *Pain.* 1990; **41**: 273–81.

∗ 26. Banning A, Sjogren P, Henriksen H. Pain causes in 200 patients referred to a multidisciplinary cancer pain clinic. *Pain.* 1991; **45**: 45–8.

27. Swanwick M, Haworth M, Lennard RF. The prevalence of episodic pain in cancer: a survey of hospice patients on admission. *Palliative Medicine.* 2001; **15**: 9–18.

∗ 28. Schwei MJ, Honore P, Rogers SD *et al.* Neurochemical and cellular reorganization of the spinal cord in a murine model of bone cancer pain. *Journal of Neuroscience.* 1999; **19**: 10886–97.

29. Medhurst SJ, Walker K, Bowes M *et al.* A rat model of bone cancer pain. *Pain.* 2002; **96**: 129–40.

∗ 30. Sabino MA, Luger NM, Mach DB *et al.* Different tumors in bone each give rise to a distinct pattern of skeletal destruction, bone cancer-related pain behaviors and neurochemical changes in the central nervous system. *International Journal of Cancer.* 2003; **104**: 550–8.

∗ 31. Sevcik MA, Ghilardi JR, Peters CM *et al.* Anti-NGF therapy profoundly reduces bone cancer pain and the accompanying increase in markers of peripheral and central sensitization. *Pain.* 2005; **115**: 128–41.

32. Suzuki K, Yamada S. Ascites sarcoma 180, a tumor associated with hypercalcemia, secretes potent bone resorbing factors including transforming growth factor alpha, interleukin 1 alpha and interleukin 6. *Bone and Mineral.* 1994; **27**: 219–33.

∗ 33. Mantyh PW, Clohisy DR, Koltzenburg M, Hunt SP. Molecular mechanisms of cancer pain. *Nature Reviews. Cancer.* 2002; **2**: 201–09.

34. Griffiths JR. Are cancer cells acidic? *British Journal of Cancer.* 1991; **64**: 425–7.

35. Ogmundsdottir HM. Immune reaction to breast cancer: for better or for worse? *Archivum Immunologiae et Therapiae Experimentalis.* 2001; **49** (Suppl 2): S75–81.

36. Asham EH, Loizidou M, Taylor I. Endothelin-1 and tumour development. *European Journal of Surgical Oncology.* 1998; **24**: 57–60.

37. Davar G, Hans G, Fareed MU *et al.* Behavioral signs of acute pain produced by application of endothelin-1 to rat sciatic nerve. *Neuroreport.* 1998; **9**: 2279–83.

∗ 38. De-Melo JD, Tonussi CR, D'Orleans-Juste P, Rae GA. Articular nociception induced by endothelin-1, carrageenan and LPS in naive and previously inflamed knee-joints in the rat: inhibition by endothelin receptor antagonists. *Pain.* 1998; **77**: 261–9.

39. Cain DM, Wacnik PW, Turner M et al. Functional interactions between tumor and peripheral nerve: changes in excitability and morphology of primary afferent fibers in a murine model of cancer pain. *Journal of Neuroscience.* 2001; **21**: 9367–76.

40. Nelson JB, Hedican SP, George DJ et al. Identification of endothelin-1 in the pathophysiology of metastatic adenocarcinoma of the prostate. *Nature Medicine.* 1995; **1**: 944–9.

∗ 41. Lassiter LK, Carducci MA. Endothelin receptor antagonists in the treatment of prostate cancer. *Seminars in Oncology.* 2003; **30**: 678–88.

42. Mantyh PW. A mechanism based understanding of cancer pain. *Pain.* 2002; **96**: 1–2.

43. Herrero JF, Laird JM, Lopez-Garcia JA. Wind-up of spinal cord neurones and pain sensation: much ado about something? *Progress in Neurobiology.* 2000; **61**: 169–203.

44. Honore P, Menning PM, Rogers SD et al. Neurochemical plasticity in persistent inflammatory pain. *Progress in Brain Research.* 2000; **129**: 357–63.

∗ 45. Luger NM, Honore P, Sabino MA et al. Osteoprotegerin diminishes advanced bone cancer pain. *Cancer Research.* 2001; **61**: 4038–47.

46. Honore P, Schwei J, Rogers SD et al. Cellular and neurochemical remodeling of the spinal cord in bone cancer pain. *Progress in Brain Research.* 2000; **129**: 389–97.

47. Honore P, Mantyh PW. Bone cancer pain: from mechanism to model to therapy. *Pain Medicine.* 2000; **1**: 303–09.

∗ 48. Donovan-Rodriguez T, Dickenson AH, Urch CE. Superficial dorsal horn neuronal responses and the emergence of behavioural hyperalgesia in a rat model of cancer-induced bone pain. *Neuroscience Letters.* 2004; **360**: 29–32.

49. Urch CE, Dickenson AH. *In vivo* single unit extracellular recordings from spinal cord neurones of rats. Brain Research. *Brain Research Protocols.* 2003; **12**: 26–34.

∗ 50. Urch CE, Donovan-Rodriguez T, Gordon-Williams R et al. Efficacy of chronic morphine in a rat model of cancer-induced bone pain: behavior and in dorsal horn pathophysiology. *Journal of Pain.* 2005; **6**: 837–45.

∗ 51. Luger NM, Sabino MA, Schwei MJ et al. Efficacy of systemic morphine suggests a fundamental difference in the mechanisms that generate bone cancer vs. inflammatory pain. *Pain.* 2002; **99**: 397–406.

∗ 52. Donovan-Rodriguez T, Dickenson AH, Urch CE. Gabapentin normalizes spinal neuronal responses that correlate with behavior in a rat model of cancer-induced bone pain. *Anesthesiology.* 2005; **102**: 132–40.

∗ 53. Jensen TS, Gottrup H, Sindrup SH, Bach FW. The clinical picture of neuropathic pain. *European Journal of Pharmacology.* 2001; **429**: 1–11.

54. Suzuki R, Dickenson A. Spinal and supraspinal contributions to central sensitization in peripheral neuropathy. *Neurosignals.* 2005; **14**: 175–81.

55. Lipton RB, Apfel SC, Dutcher JP et al. Taxol produces a predominantly sensory neuropathy. *Neurology.* 1989; **39**: 368–73.

56. Sahenk Z, Barohn R, New P, Mendell JR. Taxol neuropathy. Electrodiagnostic and sural nerve biopsy findings. *Archives of Neurology.* 1994; **51**: 726–9.

57. Asai H, Ozaki N, Shinoda M et al. Heat and mechanical hyperalgesia in mice model of cancer pain. *Pain.* 2005; **117**: 19–29.

58. Lee BH, Seong J, Kim UJ et al. Behavioral characteristics of a mouse model of cancer pain. *Yonsei Medical Journal.* 2005; **46**: 252–9.

59. Shimoyama M, Tatsuoka H, Ohtori S et al. Change of dorsal horn neurochemistry in a mouse model of neuropathic cancer pain. *Pain.* 2005; **114**: 221–30.

∗ 60. Eliav E, Tal M, Benoliel R. Experimental malignancy in the rat induces early hypersensitivity indicative of neuritis. *Pain.* 2004; **110**: 727–37.

61. Rowinsky EK. The development and clinical utility of the taxane class of antimicrotubule chemotherapy agents. *Annual Review of Medicine.* 1997; **48**: 353–74.

62. Cavaletti G, Bogliun G, Marzorati L et al. Peripheral neurotoxicity of taxol in patients previously treated with cisplatin. *Cancer.* 1995; **75**: 1141–50.

63. Cliffer KD, Siuciak JA, Carson SR et al. Physiological characterization of Taxol-induced large-fiber sensory neuropathy in the rat. *Annals of Neurology.* 1998; **43**: 46–55.

64. Nozaki-Taguchi N, Chaplan SR, Higuera ES et al. Vincristine-induced allodynia in the rat. *Pain.* 2001; **93**: 69–76.

∗ 65. Polomano RC, Bennett GJ. Chemotherapy-evoked painful peripheral neuropathy. *Pain Medicine.* 2001; **2**: 8–14.

66. Authier N, Gillet JP, Fialip J et al. A new animal model of vincristine-induced nociceptive peripheral neuropathy. *Neurotoxicology.* 2003; **24**: 797–805.

67. Higuera ES, Luo ZD. A rat pain model of vincristine-induced neuropathy. *Methods in Molecular Medicine.* 2004; **99**: 91–8.

68. Cavaletti G, Tredici G, Braga M, Tazzari S. Experimental peripheral neuropathy induced in adult rats by repeated intraperitoneal administration of taxol. *Experimental Neurology.* 1995; **133**: 64–72.

69. Cavaletti G, Cavalletti E, Montaguti P et al. Effect on the peripheral nervous system of the short-term intravenous administration of paclitaxel in the rat. *Neurotoxicology.* 1997; **18**: 137–45.

70. Rowinsky EK, Donehower RC, Jones RJ, Tucker RW. Microtubule changes and cytotoxicity in leukemic cell lines treated with taxol. *Cancer Research.* 1988; **48**: 4093–100.

71. Cavaletti G, Cavalletti E, Oggioni N et al. Distribution of paclitaxel within the nervous system of the rat after repeated intravenous administration. *Neurotoxicology.* 2000; **21**: 389–93.

72. Pusztai L, Mendoza TR, Reuben JM et al. Changes in plasma levels of inflammatory cytokines in response to paclitaxel chemotherapy. *Cytokine.* 2004; **25**: 94–102.

73. Tanner KD, Reichling DB, Levine JD. Nociceptor hyper-responsiveness during vincristine-induced painful

peripheral neuropathy in the rat. *Journal of Neuroscience.* 1998; **18**: 6480–91.

* 74. Weng HR, Cordella JV, Dougherty PM. Changes in sensory processing in the spinal dorsal horn accompany vincristine-induced hyperalgesia and allodynia. *Pain.* 2003; **103**: 131–8.

75. Marchand F, Alloui A, Pelissier T *et al.* Evidence for an antihyperalgesic effect of venlafaxine in vincristine-induced neuropathy in rat. *Brain Research.* 2003; **980**: 117–20.

76. Flatters SJ, Bennett GJ. Ethosuximide reverses paclitaxel- and vincristine-induced painful peripheral neuropathy. *Pain.* 2004; **109**: 150–61.

77. Matsumoto M, Inoue M, Hald A *et al.* Inhibition of paclitaxel-induced A-fiber hypersensitization by gabapentin. *Journal of Pharmacology and Experimental Therapeutics.* 2006; **318**: 735–40.

78. Luo ZD, Calcutt NA, Higuera ES *et al.* Injury type-specific calcium channel alpha 2 delta-1 subunit up-regulation in rat neuropathic pain models correlates with antiallodynic effects of gabapentin. *Journal of Pharmacology and Experimental Therapeutics.* 2002; **303**: 1199–205.

* 79. Lynch 3rd JJ, Wade CL, Zhong CM *et al.* Attenuation of mechanical allodynia by clinically utilized drugs in a rat chemotherapy-induced neuropathic pain model. *Pain.* 2004; **110**: 56–63.

80. Oshima M, Oshima H, Kitagawa K *et al.* Loss of Apc heterozygosity and abnormal tissue building in nascent intestinal polyps in mice carrying a truncated Apc gene. *Proceedings of the National Academy of Sciences of the United States of America.* 1995; **92**: 4482–6.

81. Oshima M, Dinchuk JE, Kargman SL *et al.* Suppression of intestinal polyposis in Apc delta716 knockout mice by inhibition of cyclooxygenase 2 (COX-2). *Cell.* 1996; **87**: 803–09.

2

Epidemiology of cancer pain

IRENE J HIGGINSON, JULIE HEARN, AND FLISS MURTAGH

Introduction	13	Relationships between pain and other factors	18
Assessing the prevalence of pain	13	Future challenges	23
Measurement of pain in epidemiology	14	References	23
The prevalence of cancer pain	14		

KEY LEARNING POINTS

- Pain is generally more prevalent in metastatic disease, and in head and neck, genitourinary, esophageal, and prostate cancers.
- Pain is associated with significantly increased levels of depression, anxiety, hostility, and somatization.

- Most studies of pain prevalence are service-based, not population-based, and reflect variations in service provision.
- Future research needs to focus on population-based studies and interventions which improve accurate assessment and effective treatment.

INTRODUCTION

Pain is defined as "an unpleasant sensory and emotional experience associated with actual or potential tissue damage, or described in terms of such damage."[1] Not only is pain a sensation in a part or parts of the body, but it is also "always unpleasant and therefore an emotional experience."[1] The perception of pain is subjective and is modulated by the patient's mood, the patient's morale, and the meaning of pain for the patient.[2] Moreover, pain is influenced by culture and ethnicity.[3]

Because of the multidimensional nature of pain, it is often useful to think in terms of "total pain," encompassing the physical, psychological, social, and spiritual aspects that influence a person's perception of pain.[4] The concept of "total pain" is pertinent to the understanding of cancer pain in epidemiology, as well as in individual patients.

ASSESSING THE PREVALENCE OF PAIN

An estimated 6.6 million people worldwide die from cancer each year.[5, 6] Despite major improvements in pain control over the last 15 years, cancer-related pain continues to be a significant global public health concern. Exactly how many patients experience pain is difficult to ascertain. Studies to date show a wide variation in the reported prevalence (e.g. Foley,[7] Bonica,[8] Portenoy[9]). This is because prevalence studies are reported in varied settings and patient groups.[10, 11] Usually, prevalence estimates relate to a group of patients referred to a specific service, e.g. a pain clinic. This may mean that many studies concentrate on groups of patients with the most complex problems. Some studies include only those patients who have pain.

In addition, pain is assessed and defined in different ways, and the type of pain is often not well identified. There are no established easily recognized signs of pain, and much reliance is placed on effective communication with the person experiencing pain. In addition, in some instances the prevalence of pain is determined from records of analgesic use. These estimates are likely to be lower than would have been obtained if pain had been systematically assessed. Pain associated with cancer has features of both chronic and acute pain, and can be either the direct or indirect result of the cancer.[12, 13] A patient may have several pains, which can have different causes. Although the site of the tumor influences the characteristics of the pain and the type of intervention,[14] the situation is complicated because the definition of cancer pain also incorporates the pathology of pain (i.e. nociceptive or neuropathic[12]), pain related to the cancer, pain related to the cancer treatment, or pain caused by a concurrent disorder.[15]

MEASUREMENT OF PAIN IN EPIDEMIOLOGY

Any measure of pain must be sufficiently graded to identify changes, clear to both subjects and investigators, easy to score, and have been demonstrated as valid and reliable. Visual analog scales, verbal descriptor scales, and numeric rating scales have been used in a clinical setting to assess pain severity and appear to be broadly equivalent.[16] A more recent example of a numeric rating scale is the Brief Pain Inventory.[17, 18] Numerical rating scales have been endorsed for use in cancer clinical trial instruments because they are easier to understand and easier to score[19] than visual analog scales.

Some general assessment tools include pain alongside other symptoms and problems and thus can be valuable in monitoring pain. As more and more standardized assessment tools become available,[20] comparisons between settings may become feasible. Such measures include the Edmonton Symptom Assessment System (ESAS),[21] the Palliative Care Outcome Scale,[22] the Support Team Assessment Schedule (STAS),[23] and the Memorial Symptom Assessment Scale.[24]

Whether an assessment is carried out by the patient, the physician, the nurse, or the family will obviously affect the data collected. In a study validating an outcome measure for use in palliative care, staff were found to underrate the level of pain and family or carers overrated the level of pain compared with the patient's self-report of pain.[23] However, feedback of patients' assessments may improve professional assessments and thereby improve treatment.

THE PREVALENCE OF CANCER PAIN

The prevalence rates reported here are based on a systematic literature review of prevalence reported elsewhere.[25] Although pain is common in all stages of cancer, it is most common in later rather than early disease, so early and advanced illness are considered separately.

The prevalence of pain in early disease

Table 2.1 shows studies that reported pain in the general adult cancer population. These studies derive from a wide range of countries, including the USA, Europe, Asia, and Africa; the considerable variations between services influence patient selection for each study, and hence the pain prevalence found, especially as almost all studies are service-, rather than population-based. The table also includes three low estimates which determined prevalence from analgesic use (Foley, 29 and 38 percent; Hiraga et al., 33 percent). As a result of the variation in methods of measuring and reporting the data, the values were simply combined to provide a crude overall mean prevalence based on the number of patients in each study and the number reported to be experiencing pain, i.e. a weighted estimate. Excluding these three studies with low estimates provides a weighted (by sample size) mean prevalence of pain of 41 percent (range, 29–85 percent); including them gives a weighted mean prevalence of 35 percent (range, 29–85 percent).

Little evidence exists on the prevalence of pain at or around the time of diagnosis. Vuorinen[32] reported that 35 percent of newly diagnosed patients had experienced pain in the past 2 weeks; Daut and Cleeland[27] reported 18–49 percent of patients had had pain as an early symptom of the disease. Ger et al.[43] found that 38 percent of newly diagnosed cancer patients had pain.

Prevalence of pain in advanced cancer

Table 2.2 shows studies that reported pain prevalence among patients with advanced or terminal cancer. In the majority of cases the data are point prevalence estimates, obtained at referral to a particular service. A study by Mercadante and colleagues (not included in the table) reports prevalence according to performance score, rather than at point of referral.[88] This alternative approach may overcome some of the bias arising from differences in patient selection between services. Period prevalence estimates related mainly to pain over the past week, and occasionally the past two weeks or one month. The combined weighted mean prevalence of pain was 75 percent (range, 53–100 percent). No relationship was found between prevalence and study sample size. The various stages of disease considered and the methods of measurement make it difficult to summarize the data in the tables to provide valid estimates of the prevalence of severe pain, or the proportion of pain affecting or dominating the daily life of patients.

Five studies had used retrospective data collected from bereaved carers of patients with cancer, or from other

Table 2.1 The prevalence of cancer pain in general cancer populations (studies are listed in date order of publication).

Study type	Disease definition and tumor type	Sample size	Prevalence	Reference
Prospective survey	General cancer population	1. 540 2. 397	29% (specified by site) 38% (60% of the terminal patients)	Foley[7]
Prospective survey	General cancer population	237	72%	Trotter et al.[26]
Prospective survey	Breast, prostate, colon, or rectum and three gynecological tumors	667	18–49% had had pain as an early symptom (specified by site); 48% had had pain in the past month Pain was due to the cancer in 56% and 17% of patients with metastatic and nonmetastatic disease respectively Mean scores for worst pain: 4.0 (S.D. 3.6) to 6.7 (S.D. 7.1)[a] Mean scores for average pain: 2.5 (S.D. 3.5) to 5.7 (S.D. 2.1)[a]	Daut and Cleeland[27]
Prospective survey	Lung, pancreas, prostate, and uterine cervix	536	64% with typical pain (specified by site) 30% slight pain, 30% moderate pain, 4% very bad pain 19% had worst pain possible	Greenwald et al.[28]
Prospective survey	General cancer population	240	45% Mean score for present intensity: 2.9 (S.D. 2.5)[a] Mean score for most severe pain in past week: 7.2 (S.D. 2.4) 28% maximal interference, 55% extensive interference	Dorrepaal et al.[29]
Quasi-meta-analysis	General cancer population	14,417	51% patients at all stages 74% patients with advanced/terminal disease	Bonica[30]
Retrospective patient record survey	General cancer population	35,683	32.6% overall In 11.4% before treatment, 24.9% in curative stage, 48.7% in conservative stage, 71.3% in terminal stage	Hiraga et al.[31]
Prospective survey	Newly diagnosed general cancer population	240	35%; a total of 28% still had pain 46% pain related to the cancer, 67% had pain secondary to cancer or its treatment, 18% had unrelated pain	Vuorinen[32]
Prospective survey	General cancer population with intractable pain[b]	1635	99% with continuous pain, 1% with incident or breakthrough pain 3% mild, 11% moderate, 33% severe, 49% very severe/maximal	Grond et al.[10]
Prospective study	Prostate, colon, breast, or ovarian cancer patients	243	64% (specified by site)	Portenoy et al.[33]
Prospective survey	Ovarian cancer patients	151	42% 62% had had pain preceding diagnosis or recurrence Mean severity of pain in general was moderate; mean severity for worst pain was severe 40% experienced any pain almost constantly, 21% experienced worst pain almost constantly Median duration of worst or only pain 2 weeks (range <1–756)	Portenoy et al.[34]

(Continued over)

Table 2.1 The prevalence of cancer pain in general cancer populations (studies are listed in date order of publication) (continued).

Study type	Disease definition and tumor type	Sample size	Prevalence	Reference
Prospective survey	Advanced general cancer population	369	54% with cancer-related pain Mean score for average daily pain: 3.6 (S.D. 2.2) (between mild and moderate) Mean number of hours per day in pain: 9.2 (S.D. 9.1) Mean number of days per week in pain: 4.2 (S.D. 2.8)	Glover et al.[35]
Prospective cross-sectional multicenter survey	General cancer population	605	57% (specified by site), 65% of whom had metastatic disease 69% rated pain as significant (score of 5 or more)[b] 54% rated average pain significant	Larue et al.[36]
Descriptive survey (unclear if it was cross-sectional or prospective)	Ambulatory patients with breast cancer	97	64%, of which 73% was cancer-related Mean score for average daily pain: 3.4 (S.D. 2.3) (mild to moderate) Mean number of hours per day in pain: 8.9 (S.D. 10.1) Mean number of days per week in significant pain: 3.8 (S.D. 3.0)	Miaskowski and Dibble[37]
Prospective survey	Pain clinic cancer population	2266	85% caused by cancer, 17% treatment-related, 9% associated with cancer disease, 9% unrelated 77% had an average pain intensity of severe or worse on previous day 30% had one pain, 39% had two pains, 31% had three or more	Grond et al.[38]
Prospective study	General cancer population all with pain[b]	383	Patients had a mean of 1.8 pain locations and a mean pain duration of 14.2 months (S.D. 33.4) Mean present pain intensity on a numeric rating scale (maximum score 10) was 3.3 (S.D. 2.3); mean average pain intensity over previous week was 4.9 (S.D. 2.1)	De Wit et al.[39]
Randomized controlled trial	General cancer population	438	Pain score – mean 9.9 in treatment group and 11.1 in control group (range 0–40) Prevalence – 42% in treatment group and 36% in control group at pretest and 39% in both groups at post test	Elliott et al.[40]
Retrospective cross-sectional study	General cancer population	13,625	29% reported daily pain	Bernabei et al.[41]
Prospective survey	Patients with recurrent breast or gynecologic cancers	114	70% of patients with breast cancer and 63% of patients with gynecologic cancer had had at least a little pain over the past 4 weeks 51% had mild to moderate pain 62% stated that their pain interfered with their ability to function	Rummans et al.[42]

(Continued over)

Table 2.1 The prevalence of cancer pain in general cancer populations (studies are listed in date order of publication) (continued).

Study type	Disease definition and tumor type	Sample size	Prevalence	Reference
Prospective study	Newly diagnosed general cancer population	296	38% had cancer-related pain; of these, 65% had significant worst pain (i.e. worst pain level scores 5 on a 10-point scale) and 31% had significant average pain (i.e. average pain level scores 5 on a 10-point scale)	Ger et al.[43]
Cross-sectional study	General cancer population	217	64% had pain at some time in the previous 2 weeks	Wells et al.[44]
Prospective cross-sectional international survey	General cancer population all with pain requiring opioid medication	1095	Mean duration of pain: 5.9 months (S.D. 105) 67% reported worst pain intensity over past day was 7 on a 10-point numeric scale 25% experienced two or more pains 80% had pain due to the cancer, 18% had treatment-related pain	Caraceni and Portenoy[45]
Prospective longitudinal study	Patients with cancers of the head and neck	93	48% had pain at admission, 8% severe, 14% in the shoulder 25% had pain at 12 months, 3% severe, 37% in the shoulder 26% had pain at 24 months, 3% severe, 26% in the shoulder	Chaplin and Morton[46]
Prospective study	General cancer population all with pain[b]	593	64% had nociceptive pain, 5% neuropathic pain, 31% mixed Mean intensity on a numeric rating scale (maximum score 100) at admission was 66 (nociceptive), 70 (neuropathic), and 65 (mixed), reducing to 26, 28, and 30 after 3 days, and 18, 21, and 17 at the end of the survey	Grond et al.[47]
Secondary analysis of prospective data from four studies including a clinical trial	Patients with primary lung cancer or cancer metastatic to bone	125	72% had pain McGill Pain Questionnaire total score – mean 19.7 (S.D. 12.5); range 0–53	Berry et al.[48]
Prospective survey	General cancer population (in and out patients)	240	59% had pain (67% of inpatients, 47% of outpatients) Of inpatients, 64% of those with pain had a malignant pain syndrome, 23% a non malignant pain syndrome, and 11% mixed	Chang et al.[49]
Prospective study	Patients with pancreas cancer all with pain[b]	50	The 36 patients in group 1 scored 5.4 (S.D. 0.54) on a pain visual analog scale (maximum score possible 10) The 14 patients in group 2 scored 7.6 (S.D. 0.88)	Rykowski and Hilger[50]
Prospective survey	General cancer population hospitalized for at least 24 hours	258	51.5% had pain, as assessed by physician interview using a structured questionnaire; 29.3% of these had pain thought to be related to the tumour	Ripamonti et al.[51]

(Continued over)

Table 2.1 The prevalence of cancer pain in general cancer populations (studies are listed in date order of publication) (continued).

Study type	Disease definition and tumor type	Sample size	Prevalence	Reference
Prospective survey	General cancer population	263	35.7% had cancer-related pain, as identified by screening questions at interview	Beck and Falkson[52]
Population-based survey	Randomly selected patients from the cancer population	1555	61.6% had cancer-related pain as identified by self-completed questionnaire	Liu et al.[53]
Prospective survey	General cancer population attending oncology outpatients	480	53% had pain 22% had pain which they reported as "quite a bit" or "very much"	Lidstone et al.[54]
Prospective survey	Hospitalized cancer patients	1392	61% had pain, identified using the EORTC-QLQ C30, with almost 30% reporting moderate or severe pain	Rustoen et al.[55]
Prospective survey	General cancer population attending oncology outpatients	480	54% had pain Severe pain was reported by 35% and moderate pain by 35.4% of patients.	Hsieh[56]
Cross-sectional survey	General cancer population, including oncology in and outpatients	178	50% had pain during the previous 24 hours, identified using the Brief Pain Inventory. Moderate to severe pain occurred in 50% of patients surveyed, with 23% reporting severe pain and 33% reporting severe impairment in their ability to work due to pain	Reyes-Gibby et al.[57]

Percentages for severity breakdowns may not equal overall percentages quoted because of missing values.

[a]0 = no pain, 10 = worst pain as assessed by a pain rating scale.

[b]Not included in the calculation of weighted mean prevalence because study population selected to include only those with pain.

Study types: Survey – the main purpose of the study was to survey pain or symptom prevalence; Study – there may have been other reasons for the study, e.g. service evaluation or evaluation of management/control.

informants who could provide information on particular patients.[50, 74, 79, 89, 90] Obviously there are limitations to these data in that the interviews with the bereaved carers or informants took place at least six months after the death of the patient. The data are therefore subject to some recall bias, as well as being subjective assessments. Overall, the estimates were slightly higher than for patient reports (see **Table 2.2**).

The prevalence of pain by primary tumor site and the effect of metastatic disease

Table 2.3 combines studies that provided prevalence data on pain in more than one cancer type in the general adult cancer population. These show a wide range in reported prevalence by tumor site. However, pain appears to be most consistently prevalent among patients with head and neck cancers, genitourinary cancers, cancer of the esophagus, and prostate cancer. In contrast, Foley[7] reported that only 5 percent of patients with leukemia experienced pain. In some instances, the estimates were very varied, e.g. the pain prevalence values for lymphoma ranged from 20 to 87 percent.

Daut and Cleeland[27] found that more pain is usually associated with metastatic than nonmetastatic disease. For example, 64 percent of patients with metastatic breast cancer had pain compared with 40 percent of patients with nonmetastatic disease, a pattern that is consistent throughout cancer types.

RELATIONSHIPS BETWEEN PAIN AND OTHER FACTORS

For many patients, pain is the most feared consequence of cancer.[10, 91, 92] Unrelieved pain causes unnecessary suffering and can be psychologically devastating for the cancer patient.[91] Physical and mental exhaustion may result, along with the loss of hope and undermining of the value of life.[90, 93]

In reviewing the effects of cancer pain on the patient, Bonica[94] summarizes "the physiologic, psychologic, emotional, and sociologic impacts of cancer pain on the patient and family are greater than that of nonmalignant chronic pain." Bonica goes on to state that, if acute pain is the initial symptom of cancer, it is considered the harbinger of a serious illness, and is consequently associated

Table 2.2 The prevalence of cancer pain in patients with advanced or terminal disease, or at the end of life (studies are listed in date order of publication).

Study type	Disease definition and tumour type	Sample size	Prevalence	Reference
Retrospective record review and interviews with general practitioners and carers	Patients who had died from cancer of the pharynx, breast, bronchus, stomach, colon, rectum	279	62%	Ward[58]
Retrospective interview study	Bereaved carers of advanced general cancer population[b]	165	36% had none to mild pain, 31% moderate, 33% had severe to very severe pain	Parkes[59]
Prospective survey	Far-advanced general cancer population, all in pain[d]	100	In only 41% was all pain caused directly by the cancer 90% had had pain for >4 weeks, 57% of these for >16 weeks Of those who had pain for >8 weeks, 77% severe to excruciating 80% had more than one pain, 34% of these had four or more	Twycross[60]
Prospective study	Terminal general cancer population or their primary care persons	1754	69% 19% mild, 21% discomfort, 16% distressing, 7% horrible, 5% excruciating	Morris et al.[61]
Prospective evaluation study	Advanced general cancer population	256	53%	McIllmurray and Warren[62]
Prospective study	Terminal general cancer population[b]	60	Mean scores 53.5 (S.D. 37.5) and 41.9 (S.D. 29.1) for home care and hospital care patients respectively[c]	Ventafridda et al.[63]
Retrospective record review but with prospective data collection	Advanced clinically challenging cancer patients[d]	90	100%, of which 27% mild, 19% mild to moderate, 34% moderate, 20% moderate to severe Major limitation for 94% of those rating pain as moderate to severe	Coyle[64]
Prospective study	Advanced general cancer population	65	68% pain rated as a problem	Higginson et al.[65]
Prospective study	Terminal general cancer population	120	100%	Ventafridda et al.[66]
Prospective survey	Advanced general cancer population	78	71% (specified by site) 24% mild, 40% moderate, 36% severe 60% had one main site of pain, 35% two, 5% three or more	Simpson[67]
Retrospective record review	Advanced cancer population	110	69% 34% related to the primary cancer, 43% related to metastatic disease	Chan and Woodruff[68]
Retrospective record review	Advanced general cancer population who died on the unit	100	99%	Fainsinger et al.[69]
Retrospective interview study	Bereaved carers or informants of people who had died from cancer	383	87% in 1969 84% in 1987	Cartwright[70]
Retrospective record review	Advanced general cancer population over 65 year of age	239	58% with discomfort/pain 12% mild, 18% discomfort, 17% distress, 7% horrible, 6% excruciating	Stein and Miech[71]

(Continued over)

Table 2.2 The prevalence of cancer pain in patients with advanced or terminal disease, or at the end of life (studies are listed in date order of publication) (continued).

Study type	Disease definition and tumour type	Sample size	Prevalence	Reference
Prospective study	Lung cancer patients	52	88%	Mercadante et al.[72]
Prospective study	General advanced cancer population	1000	83% with pain Ranked as most severe symptom out of 30 common symptoms	Donnelly et al.[73]
Prospective survey	Advanced general cancer population	125	74% Over 25%	Ellershaw[74]
Retrospective interview study	Bereaved carers of general cancer population	2018	88%	Addington-Hall and McCarthy[75]
Prospective study	Far-advanced general cancer population	98	64%	Shannon et al.[76]
Prospective survey	Advanced general cancer population, all in pain[d]	111	46% had all pain caused by the cancer, 29% had associated pains, 5% had pain related to the treatment Median score 4 for average pain, median score 6 for worst pain[a] 85% had >1 pain, >40% of these had four or more	Twycross et al.[77]
Prospective study	Advanced cancer population	1640	72% (specified by site) 24% mild, 30% moderate, 21% severe	Vainio and Auvinen[78]
Prospective study	Advanced general cancer population	695	70% (specified by site) 54% mild or moderate, 16% severe or overwhelming	Higginson and Hearn[79]
Retrospective study	Caregivers of general cancer population	170	86% stated pain was a problem; 61% reported a great deal or quite a bit of pain; 25% some or a little 82% reported data on pain relief intervention, 46% of which made pain stop/get better and 56% of which made pain a little better or had no effect or made it worse	Bucher et al.[80]
Retrospective cross-sectional survey	Advanced general cancer population	100	77% had current pain Majority had mild pain 76% had regular analgesics for their pain	Chung et al.[81]
Prospective study	Advanced general cancer population	3577	70.3% had pain at referral Mean intensity on a visual analog scale (maximum score 10) was 4.4 at referral, 2.5 at 1 week, 2.3 in the last week of life	Mercadente[82]
Retrospective cohort study	Advanced cancer patients who subsequently died	223	Pain reported in 66% of all abstracted patient visits 13.2% of patients never had a documented pain complaint 19% had pain complaints documented at each visit Presence of metastases not significantly associated with presence of pain Hospice programs differed in the proportion of visits for which pain was reported (75, 64, and 48%)	Nowels and Lee[83]

(Continued over)

Table 2.2 The prevalence of cancer pain in patients with advanced or terminal disease, or at the end of life (studies are listed in date order of publication) (continued).

Study type	Disease definition and tumour type	Sample size	Prevalence	Reference
Prospective study	Advanced cancer patients admitted to hospice	232	81% had pain at the time of admission Pain severity worsened in the 48 hours before death (prevalence not reported)	Chiu et al.[84]
Retrospective case note review	Patients referred to palliative care services-hospice, community, hospital and outpatients (95% with cancer, and of these 71% had advanced disease)	400	64% had pain at first assessment In the hospice 62% of patients had pain In the community setting 56% had pain In the hospital service 63% had pain In the outpatient service 75% had pain	Potter et al.[85]
Cross-sectional survey	Patients with metastatic cancer or Stage IV lymphoma in hospital for >72 hours for complications not treatment	66	78% of patients had pain (assessed using the Memorial Symptom Assessment Scale)	Tranmer et al.[86]
Prospective survey	In and outpatients with metastatic or recurrent cancer	655	70.8% had some pain in the previous 24 hours 63.6% rated their pain at 5 or higher on a visual analog scale of 0–10	Yun et al.[87]

Percentages for severity breakdowns may not equal overall percentages quoted because of missing values.
[a] 0 = no pain, 10 = worst pain as assessed by a pain rating scale.
[b] Not included in the calculation of weighted mean prevalence because overall prevalence not given.
[c] Scores relate to hours of pain multiplied by a severity coefficient; values can range from 0 to 240.
[d] Not included in the calculation of weighted mean prevalence because study population selected to include only those with pain.
Study types: Survey – the main purpose of the study was to survey pain or symptom prevalence; Study – there may have been other reasons for the study, e.g. service evaluation or evaluation of management/control.

with severe anxiety. However, if the pain is the result of antineoplastic therapy, the physical and emotional reactions are significantly less because of the promise of a successful outcome.

The relationship between pain and psychological well-being is complex. Mood disturbance and beliefs about the meaning of pain in relation to illness can exacerbate perceived pain intensity,[95, 96] and the presence of pain is a major determinant of function and mood.[27] The relationship between pain and psychological distress among patients with cancer has been demonstrated in a range of tumor types.[97, 98, 99, 100] Cancer patients have been reported to develop greater emotional reactions to pain – anxiety, depression, hypochondriasis, somatic focusing, and neuroticism – than patients with nonmalignant chronic pain, presumably because the effects of chronic pain are superimposed on the effects of the cancer itself.[30]

Evidence exists that the cancer patient with pain has significantly increased levels of depression and anxiety (and associated somatization) than the cancer patient without pain.[101, 102, 103, 104] Mood disorders and emotional distress in cancer patients (regardless of the presence of pain) are themselves associated with shorter

survival and increased morbidity,[105] and the precise role of pain in this complex interaction is not clear. Studies of patients with chronic pain (including, but not specifically, cancer pain) show higher levels of depression than in similar populations without pain,[106] but few studies have explored prevalence of depression specifically in cancer patients – where they have, pain is often a less important predictor of depression than other factors, such as anxiety and functional status.[107]

Evidence that pain may cause psychological distress rather than the reverse comes from a study by Spiegel *et al.*,[108] who examined both current and lifetime psychiatric disturbances among 96 patients with cancer from two studies who had high and low pain symptoms. The results suggested that pain in patients with cancer causes substantial depression and anxiety, thereby reducing the patient's capacity to cope with pain and other aspects of the illness. The capacity of pain to precipitate depression and anxiety appears unrelated to prior depression.

One of the most extreme consequences of unrelieved pain in cancer is that uncontrolled pain is a major risk factor in cancer-related suicide.[109, 110, 111, 112] Every attempt should also be made to diagnose and treat

Table 2.3 Prevalence of pain by primary tumor site.[a]

Tumor site	Foley[7] (%)	Daut and Cleeland[27,b] (%)	Greenwald et al.[28] (%)	Simpson[67] (%)	Portenoy et al.[34] (%)	Donnelly et al.[73] (%)	Larue et al.[36] (%)	Vainio and Auvinen[78] (%)	Higginson and Hearn[79] (%)	Chiu et al.[84] (%)	Lidstone et al.[54] (%)	No. studies	Percentage range
Breast	52	64; 40		50	60	89	56	78	76	70	62	10	40–89
Lung	45		71	17			58	74	71	78	68	8	17–78
Prostate		75; 30	56		68	94		83				5	56–94
Genitourinary	70–75			88			58	90	74		40	6	40–90
Lymphoma	20			50			35	87	74		38	6	20–87
Colo-(rectal)		47; 40			62	79	56	79		79		5	40–79
Gastrointestinal	40			50–71					68		58	5	40–68
Cervix[c]		0; 35	56			87				60		4	33–87
Head and neck						91	67	83		87	52	5	52–91
Ovary		59; 39			67	71						3	46–71
Esophagus						77		71				2	71–77
Pancreas			72			85				100		3	72–100
Uterine corpus		40; 14				90						2	30–90
Bladder						85						1	–
Bone	85											1	–
Carcinomatosis				83								1	–
CNS				50							53[d]	2	50–53
Kidney						83						1	–
Leukemia	5											1	–
Melanoma				20								1	–
Multiple myeloma						100						1	–
Oral cavity	80											1	–
Sarcoma				100								1	–
Stomach								74		91		1	–

A special further analysis of the data was undertaken from this study for this chapter.

[a]See **Tables 2.1** and **2.2** for further details on each study (Donnelly et al.,[73] Simpson,[67] Vainio and Auvinen,[78] and Higginson and Hearn[79] report on advanced cancer populations).

[b]Metastatic disease; nonmetastatic disease. Note: An overall percentage was determined for each cancer type from the original article, not given here.

[c]Cervix/cervix-vagina/uterine cervix.

[d]Brain tumors.

CNS, central nervous system.

depression if it exists.[108] Psychiatric symptoms in patients with cancer frequently disappear with adequate pain relief.[113]

FUTURE CHALLENGES

The need to improve cancer pain control, coupled with the increasing number of people living to older ages and living longer with cancer, makes reducing the prevalence of pain at any stage of the disease process of paramount importance. Much more work is needed to study the epidemiology and natural history of cancer pain in general and community populations, rather than in specialist centers, and there is a need for further population-based studies such as that by Liu and colleagues.[53] Standardized assessment tools should be used. Work is also needed to better understand and treat pain in different cultural populations and among older people. As cancer treatments change, so the nature and prevalence of pain in cancer may change, and this will require careful assessment.

Clinicians often do not recognize how frequently pain remains untreated or inadequately managed.[8] It should not be assumed, just because a person has been receiving cancer care or treatment in a healthcare setting, that their pain is being adequately controlled.[79] Continual assessment of the response of the patient's pain complaint is essential to ensure continual pain control and to prevent breakthrough pain. There is also a need for training and education for doctors and nurses at all stages of their careers. The monitoring of pain and knowledge of how to treat cancer pain effectively needs to be extended to all healthcare settings.

REFERENCES

1. International Association for the Study of Pain. Subcommittee on taxonomy of pain terms: a list with definitions and notes on usage. *Pain.* 1979; **6**: 249–52.
∗ 2. Twycross R. Cancer pain classification. *Acta Anaesthesiologica Scandinavica.* 1997; **41**: 141–5.
3. Cleeland CS, Nakamura Y, Mendoza TR *et al.* Dimensions of the impact of cancer pain in a four country sample: new information from multidimensional scaling. *Pain.* 1996; **67**: 267–73.
4. Saunders CM. *The management of terminal illness.* London: Arnold, 1985.
∗ 5. World Health Organization. *The world health report 1996. Fighting disease, fostering development, executive summary.* Geneva: The World Health Organization, 1996.
6. World Health Organization. *Cancer pain relief and palliative care*, 2nd edn. Geneva: World Health Organization, 1996.
7. Foley KM. Pain syndromes in patients with cancer. In: Bonica JJ, Ventafridda V (eds). *Advances in pain research and therapy.* New York, NY: Raven Press, 1979: 59–75.
8. Bonica JJ. Treatment of cancer pain: current status and future needs. In: Fields HL (ed.). *Advances in pain research and therapy.* New York, NY: Raven Press, 1985: 589–616.
9. Portenoy R. Epidemiology syndromes and cancer pain. *Cancer.* 1989; **63**: 2298–307.
10. Grond S, Zech D, Diefenbach C, Bischoff A. Prevalence and pattern of symptoms in patients with cancer pain: a prospective evaluation of 1635 cancer patients referred to a pain clinic. *Journal of Pain and Symptom Management.* 1994; **9**: 372–82.
11. Field GB, Chamberlain C, Urch C *et al.* Evaluation of the support team assessment schedule for the in-patient setting – and its further development. In: de Conno F (ed.). *Proceedings of the IV Congress of the European Association for Palliative Care.* Milan: European Association of Palliative Care, 1997: 99–108.
12. Portenoy R. Cancer pain: pathophysiology and syndromes. *Lancet.* 1992; **39**: 1026–31.
13. Welsh Office NHS Directorate. *Pain, discomfort and palliative care.* Cardiff: Welsh Health Planning Forum, Welsh Office, 1992.
14. Spross JA, McGuire DB, Schmitt RM. Oncology nursing forum position paper on cancer pain: Part 1. *Oncology Nursing Forum.* 1991; **17**: 595–614.
15. World Health Organization. *Cancer pain relief and palliative care.* Geneva: World Health Organization, 1990.
16. Jensen MP, Karoly P, Braver S. The measurement of clinical pain intensity: a comparison of six methods. *Pain.* 1986; **27**: 117–27.
17. Cleeland CS. Pain assessment in cancer. In: Osoba D (ed.). *Effect of cancer of quality of life.* Boca Raton: CRC Press, 1991: 293–306.
18. Cleeland CS, Ladinsky JL, Serlin RC, Nugyen CT. Multidimensional measurement of cancer pain: comparisons of US and Vietnamese patients. *Journal of Pain and Symptom Management.* 1988; **3**: 23–37.
19. Moinpour CM, Feigl P, Metch B *et al.* Quality of life end points in cancer clinical trials: review and recommendations. *Journal of the National Cancer Institute.* 1989; **81**: 485–95.
∗ 20. Hearn J, Higginson IJ. Outcome measures in palliative care for advanced cancer patients: a review. *Journal of Public Health Medicine.* 1997; **19**: 193–9.
21. Bruera E, Kuehn N, Miller MJ *et al.* The Edmonton Symptom Assessment System (ESAS): a simple method for the assessment of palliative care patients. *Journal of Palliative Care.* 1991; **7**: 6–9.
22. Hearn J, Higginson IJ, on behalf of the Palliative Care Audit Project Advisory Group. Development and validation of a core outcome measure for palliative care – The Palliative Care Outcome Scale. *Quality in Healthcare.* 1999; **8**: 219–27.
23. Higginson IJ, McCarthy M. Validity of the Support Team Assessment Schedule: do staffs' ratings reflect those made

by patients or their families. *Palliative Medicine.* 1993; 7: 219–28.

24. Portenoy RK, Thaler HT, Kornblith AB *et al.* The Memorial Symptom Assessment Scale: an instrument for the evaluation of symptom prevalence, characteristics and distress. *European Journal of Cancer.* 1994; **30A**: 1226–36.

25. Hearn J, Higginson IJ. Cancer pain epidemiology: a systematic literature review. In: Portenoy RK, Bruera E (eds). *Cancer pain.* New York, NY: Cambridge University Press, 2003.

26. Trotter JM, Scott R, Macbeth FR *et al.* Problems of oncology outpatients: role of the liaison health visitor. *British Medical Journal (Clinical Research Ed.).* 1981; **282**: 122–4.

27. Daut RL, Cleeland CS. The prevalence and severity of pain in cancer. *Cancer.* 1982; **50**: 1913–18.

28. Greenwald HP, Bonica JJ, Bergner M. The prevalence of pain in four cancers. *Cancer.* 1987; **60**: 2563–9.

29. Dorrepaal KL, Aaronson NK, van Dam FS. Pain experience and pain management among hospitalised cancer patients. *Cancer.* 1989; **63**: 593–8.

30. Bonica JJ. Cancer pain. In: Bonica JJ (ed.). *The management of cancer pain.* Philadelphia, PA: Lea & Febiger, 1990: 400–60.

31. Hiraga K, Mizuguchi T, Takeda F. The incidence of cancer pain and improvement of pain management in Japan. *Postgraduate Medical Journal.* 1991; **67**: S14–25.

32. Vuorinen E. Pain as an early symptom in cancer. *Clinical Journal of Pain.* 1993; **9**: 272–8.

33. Portenoy R, Thaler HT, Kornblith AB *et al.* Symptom prevalence, characteristics and distress in a cancer population. *Quality of Life Research.* 1994; **3**: 183–9.

34. Portenoy RK, Kornblith AB, Wong G *et al.* Pain in ovarian cancer patients – prevalence, characteristics and associated symptoms. *Cancer.* 1994; **74**: 907–15.

35. Glover J, Dibble SL, Dodd MJ, Miaskowski C. Mood states of oncology outpatients: does pain make a difference? *Journal of Pain and Symptom Management.* 1995; **10**: 120–8.

36. Larue F, Colleau SM, Brasseur L, Cleeland CS. Multicentre study of cancer pain and its treatment in France. *British Medical Journal.* 1995; **310**: 1034–7.

37. Miaskowski C, Dibble SL. The problem of pain in outpatients with breast cancer. *Oncology Nursing Forum.* 1995; **22**: 791–7.

38. Grond S, Zech D, Diefenbach C *et al.* Assessment of cancer pain: a prospective evaluation in 2266 cancer patients referred to a pain service. *Pain.* 1996; **64**: 107–14.

39. de Wit R, van Dam F, Zandbelt L *et al.* A Pain Education Program for chronic cancer pain patients: follow-up results from a randomized controlled trial. *Pain.* 1997; **73**: 55–69.

40. Elliott TE, Murray DM, Oken MM *et al.* Improving cancer pain management in communities: main results from a randomized controlled trial. *Journal of Pain and Symptom Management.* 1997; **13**: 191–203.

41. Bernabei R, Gambassi G, Lapane K *et al.* for the SAGE study group. Management of pain in elderly patients with cancer. *Journal of the American Medical Association.* 1998; **279**: 1877–82.

42. Rummans TA, Frost M, Suman VJ *et al.* Quality of life and pain in patients with recurrent breast and gynecologic cancer. *Psychosomatics.* 1998; **39**: 437–45.

43. Ger LP, Ho ST, Wang JJ, Cherng CH. The prevalence and severity of cancer pain: a study of newly-diagnosed cancer patients in Taiwan. *Journal of Pain and Symptom Management.* 1998; **15**: 285–93.

44. Wells N, Johnson RL, Wujick D. Development of a short version of the Barriers Questionnaire. *Journal of Pain and Symptom Management.* 1998; **15**: 285–93.

45. Caraceni A, Portenoy RK, a working group of the IASP Task Force on Cancer Pain. An international survey of cancer pain characteristics and syndromes. *Pain.* 1999; **82**: 263–74.

46. Chaplin JM, Morton RP. A prospective, longitudinal study of pain in head and neck cancer patients. *Head and Neck.* 1999; **21**: 531–7.

47. Grond S, Radbruch L, Meuser T *et al.* Assessment and treatment of neuropathic cancer pain following WHO guidelines. *Pain.* 1999; **79**: 15–20.

48. Berry DL, Wilkie DJ, Huang HY, Blumenstein BA. Cancer pain and common pain: a comparison of patient-reported intensities. *Oncology Nursing Forum.* 1999; **26**: 721–6.

49. Chang VT, Hwang SS, Feuerman M, Kasimis BS. Symptom and quality of life survey of medical oncology patients at a veterans affairs medical center – A role for symptom assessment. *Cancer.* 2000; **88**: 1175–83.

50. Rykowski JJ, Hilger M. Efficacy of neurolytic celiac plexus block in varying locations of pancreatic cancer. *Anesthesiology.* 2000; **92**: 347–54.

51. Ripamonti C, Zecca E, Brunelli C *et al.* Pain experienced by patients hospitalized at the National Cancer Institute of Milan: Research project "Towards a Pain-Free Hospital". *Tumori.* 2000; **86**: 412–18.

52. Beck SL, Falkson G. Prevalence and management of cancer pain in South Africa. *Pain.* 2001; **94**: 75–84.

* 53. Liu Z, Lian Z, Zhou W *et al.* National survey on prevalence of cancer pain. *Chinese Medical Sciences Journal.* 2001; **16**: 175–8.

54. Lidstone V, Butters E, Seed PT *et al.* Symptoms and concerns amongst cancer outpatients: identifying the need for specialist palliative care. *Palliative Medicine.* 2003; **17**: 588–95.

55. Rustoen T, Fossa SD, Skarstein J, Moum T. The impact of demographic and disease-specific variables on pain in cancer patients. *Journal of Pain and Symptom Management.* 2003; **26**: 696–704.

56. Hsieh RK. Pain control in Taiwanese patients with cancer: a multicenter, patient-oriented survey. *Journal of the Formosan Medical Association.* 2005; **104**: 913–19.

57. Reyes-Gibby CC, Duc NB, Yen NP et al. Status of cancer pain in Hanoi, Vietnam: A hospital-wide survey in a tertiary cancer treatment center. *Journal of Pain and Symptom Management.* 2006; **31**: 431–9.

58. Ward AW. Terminal care in malignant disease. *Social Science and Medicine.* 1974; **8**: 413–20.

59. Parkes CM. Home or hospital? Terminal care as seen by surviving spouses. *Journal of the Royal College of General Practitioners.* 1978; **28**: 19–30.

60. Twycross R. Pain in far-advanced cancer. *Pain.* 1982; **14**: 303–10.

61. Morris JN, Mor V, Goldberg RJ et al. The effect of treatment setting and patient characteristics on pain in terminal cancer patients: A report from the National Hospice Study. *Journal of Chronic Disease.* 1986; **39**: 27–35.

62. McIllmurray MB, Warren MR. Evaluation of a new hospice: the relief of symptoms in cancer patients in the first year. *Palliative Medicine.* 1989; **3**: 135–40.

63. Ventafridda V, De Conno F, Vigano A et al. Comparison of home and hospital care of advanced cancer patients. *Tumori.* 1989; **75**: 619–25.

64. Coyle N. The last four weeks of life. *American Journal of Nursing.* 1990; **90**: 75–8.

65. Higginson I, Wade A, McCarthy M. Palliative care: views of patients and their families. *British Medical Journal.* 1990; **301**: 277–81.

66. Ventafridda V, Ripamonti C, De Conno F et al. Symptom prevalence and control during cancer patients' last days of life. *Journal of Palliative Care.* 1990; **6**: 7–11.

67. Simpson M. The use of research to facilitate the creation of a hospital palliative care team. *Palliative Medicine.* 1991; **5**: 122–9.

68. Chan A, Woodruff RK. Palliative care in a general teaching hospital. 1. Assessment of needs. *Medical Journal of Australia.* 1991; **155**: 597–9.

69. Fainsinger RL, Miller MJ, Bruera E et al. Symptom control during the last week of life on a palliative care unit. *Journal of Palliative Care.* 1991; **7**: 5–11.

70. Cartwright A. Changes in life and care in the year before death 1969-1987. *Journal of Public Health Medicine.* 1991; **13**: 81–7.

71. Stein WM, Miech RP. Cancer pain in the elderly hospice patient. *Journal of Pain and Symptom Management.* 1993; **8**: 474–82.

72. Mercadante S, Armata M, Salvaggio L. Pain characteristics of advanced lung cancer patients referred to a palliative care service. *Pain.* 1994; **59**: 141–5.

73. Donnelly S, Walsh D, Rybicki L. The symptoms of advanced cancer: identification of clinical and research priorities by assessment of prevalence and severity. *Journal of Palliative Care.* 1995; **11**: 27–32.

74. Ellershaw JE, Peat SJ, Boys LC. Assessing the effectiveness of a hospital palliative care team. *Palliative Medicine.* 1995; **9**: 145–52.

75. Addington-Hall J, McCarthy M. Dying from cancer: results of a national population-based investigation. *Palliative Medicine.* 1995; **9**: 295–305.

76. Shannon MM, Ryan MA, D'Agostino N, Brescia FJ. Assessment of pain in advanced cancer patients. *Journal of Pain and Symptom Management.* 1995; **10**: 274–8.

77. Twycross R, Harcourt J, Bergl S. A survey of pain in patients with advanced cancer. *Journal of Pain and Symptom Management.* 1996; **12**: 273–82.

78. Vainio A, Auvinen A. Prevalence of symptoms among patients with advanced cancer: an international collaborative study. Symptom Prevalence Group. *Journal of Pain and Symptom Management.* 1996; **12**: 3–10.

79. Higginson IJ, Hearn J. A multi-centre evaluation of cancer pain control by palliative care teams. *Journal of Pain and Symptom Management.* 1997; **14**: 29–35.

80. Bucher JA, Trostle GB, Moore M. Family reports of cancer pain, pain relief, and prescription access. *Cancer Practice.* 1999; **7**: 71–7.

81. Chung JW, Yang JC, Wong TK. The significance of pain among Chinese patients with cancer in Hong Kong. *Acta Anaesthesiologica Sinica.* 1999; **37**: 9–14.

82. Mercadante S. Pain treatment and outcomes for patients with advanced cancer who receive follow-up care at home. *Cancer.* 1999; **85**: 1849–58.

83. Nowels D, Lee JT. Cancer pain management in home hospice settings: a comparison of primary care and oncologic physicians. *Journal of Palliative Care.* 1999; **15**: 5–9.

84. Chiu TY, Hu WY, Chen CY. Prevalence and severity of symptoms in terminal cancer patients: a study in Taiwan. *Supportive Care in Cancer.* 2000; **8**: 311–13.

85. Potter J, Hami F, Bryan T, Quigley C. Symptoms in 400 patients referred to palliative care services: prevalence and patterns. *Palliative Medicine.* 2003; **17**: 310–14.

86. Tranmer JE, Heyland D, Dudgeon D et al. Measuring the symptom experience of seriously ill cancer and noncancer hospitalized patients near the end of life with the memorial symptom assessment scale. *Journal of Pain and Symptom Management.* 2003; **25**: 420–9.

87. Yun YH, Heo DS, Lee IG et al. Multicenter study of pain and its management in patients with advanced cancer in Korea. *Journal of Pain and Symptom Management.* 2003; **25**: 430–7.

∗ 88. Mercadante S, Casuccio A, Fulfaro F. The course of symptom frequency and intensity in advanced cancer patients followed at home. *Journal of Pain and Symptom Management.* 2000; **20**: 104–12.

89. Parkes CM. Terminal care as seen by surviving spouses. *Journal of the Royal College of General Practitioners.* 1978; **28**: 19–30.

90. Cherny NI, Coyle N, Foley KM. The treatment of suffering when patients request elective death. *Journal of Palliative Care.* 1994; **10**: 71–9.

∗ 91. Breitbart W. Cancer pain management guidelines: implications for psycho-oncology. *Psycho-oncology.* 1994; **3**: 103–08.

92. Foley KM. The treatment of cancer pain. *New England Journal of Medicine.* 1985; **313**: 84–95.

93. Twycross RG, Lack SA. *Symptom control in far advanced cancer.* London: Pitman, 1983.

94. Bonica JJ. Evolution and current status of pain programs. *Journal of Pain and Symptom Management.* 1990; **5**: 368–74.

95. Bond MR, Pearson IB. Psychosocial aspects of pain in women with advanced cancer of the cervix. *Journal of Psychosomatic Research.* 1969; **13**: 13–21.

96. Barkwell DP. Ascribed meaning: a critical factor in coping and pain attenuation in patients with cancer-related pain. *Journal of Palliative Care.* 1991; **7**: 5–14.

97. Heim HM, Oei TP. Comparison of prostate cancer patients with and without pain. *Pain.* 1993; **53**: 159–62.

98. Kaasa S, Malt U, Hagen S *et al.* Psychological distress in cancer patients with advanced cancer. *Radiotherapy and Oncology.* 1993; **27**: 93–197.

99. Lancee WJ, Vachon ML, Ghadirian P *et al.* The impact of pain and impaired role performance on distress in persons with cancer. *Canadian Journal of Psychiatry.* 1994; **39**: 617–22.

100. Kelsen DP, Portenoy RK, Thaler HT *et al.* Pain and depression in patients with newly diagnosed pancreas cancer. *Journal of Clinical Oncology.* 1995; **13**: 748–55.

101. Ahles TA, Blanchard EB, Ruckdeschel JC. The multidimensional nature of cancer-related pain. *Pain.* 1983; **17**: 277–88.

102. Ciaramella A, Poli P. Assessment of depression among cancer patients: the role of pain, cancer type and treatment. *Psycho-oncology.* 2001; **10**: 156–65.

103. Thielking PD. Cancer pain and anxiety. *Current Pain and Headache Reports.* 2003; **7**: 249–61.

104. Chaturvedi SK, Maguire GP. Persistent somatization in cancer: a controlled follow up study. *Journal of Psychosomatic Research.* 1998; **45**: 249–56.

105. Evans DL, Charney DS, Lewis L *et al.* Mood disorders in the medically ill: scientific review and recommendations. *Biological Psychiatry.* 2005; **58**: 175–89.

106. Bair MJ, Robinson RL, Katon W, Kroenke K. Depression and pain co-morbidity: a literature review. *Archives of Internal Medicine.* 2003; **163**: 2433–45.

107. Ell K, Sanchez K, Vourlekis B *et al.* Depression, correlates of depression and receipt of depression care among women with breast or gynecologic cancer. *Journal of Clinical Oncology.* 2005; **23**: 3052–60.

108. Spiegel D, Sands S, Koopman C. Pain and depression in patients with cancer. *Cancer.* 1994; **74**: 2570–8.

109. Bolund C. Medical and care factors in suicides by cancer patients in Sweden. *Journal of Psychosocial Oncology.* 1985; **3**: 31–52.

110. Breitbart W. Suicide in the cancer patient. *Oncology.* 1987; **1**: 49–54.

∗111. Cleeland CS. The impact of pain on the patient with cancer. *Cancer.* 1984; **54**: 2635–41.

112. Baile WF, Di Maggio JR, Schapira DV, Janofsky JS. The requests for assistance in dying: the need for psychiatric consultation. *Cancer.* 1993; **72**: 2786–91.

113. Breitbart W. Cancer pain and suicide. In: Foley KM, Bonica JJ, Ventafridda V (eds). *Second International Congress on Cancer Pain: Advances in Pain Research and Therapy.* New York: Raven Press, 1990: 399–412.

3

Cancer pain syndromes

ROBERT TWYCROSS AND MICHAEL BENNETT

Introduction	27	Suprascapular nerve entrapment	32
Cancer bone pain	28	Lumbosacral plexopathy	33
Base of skull metastases	29	Hepatic pain	35
Spinal cord compression	30	Pancreatic pain	35
Meningeal carcinomatosis	31	Intrapelvic pain	35
Unilateral facial pain in cancer of the bronchus	32	Infection	36
Brachial plexopathy	32	References	36

KEY LEARNING POINTS

- Pain is commonly associated with cancer, rising in incidence with advancing disease.
- Patients with cancer often have more than one pain, and pain may be caused by treatment, debility, or concomitant disease rather than cancer itself.
- Cancer bone pain is the most frequent and painful of cancer pain syndromes.

- Pattern recognition of common syndromes, particularly those associated with base of skull metastases and brachial and lumbar nerve plexopathies, can lead to prompt diagnosis and treatment, including improved pain control.
- Recent onset of back pain in a patient with cancer should alert the clinician to the possibility of vertebral metastases, and the need to check for spinal cord compression.

INTRODUCTION

Pain is experienced by 20–50 percent of cancer patients at diagnosis (depending on the primary site) and by up to 75 percent of patients with advanced cancer:[1, 2] Data for the common primary sites or conditions are listed in **Table 3.1**. Pain is:

- moderate or severe in 40–50 percent of patients;
- very severe or excruciating in 25–30 percent of patients.[2]

In a series of over 2000 patients with advanced cancer and pain, it was observed that about:

- one-third had one site of pain;
- one-third had two sites of pain;
- one-third had three or more sites of pain.[3]

Furthermore, not all pain was due to the cancer itself:

- 85 percent of pain was directly attributable to the cancer itself;
- 17 percent of pain was caused by treatment;
- 9 percent of pain was related to the cancer and/or debility;
- 9 percent was caused by a concurrent disorder.[3]

In 15 percent of patients, none of the pain was caused directly by the cancer itself. Common individual causes are shown in **Table 3.2**.

Underlying pain mechanisms are commonly categorized as nociceptive, neuropathic, or a mixture of both. Observational studies have shown that most cancer pain is caused by nociceptive mechanisms. However, in about a

Table 3.1 Prevalence of pain in advanced or terminal cancer.[2]

Primary site of cancer	Patients with pain	
	Mean[a]	Range
Esophagus	87	80–93
Sarcoma	85	75–89
Bone (metastasis)	83	55–96
Pancreas	81	72–100
Bone (primary)	80	70–85
Liver/biliary	79	65–100
Stomach	78	67–93
Cervix uteri	75	40–100
Breast	74	56–100
Bronchus	73	57–88
Ovary	72	49–100
Prostate	72	55–100
Central nervous system	70	55–83
Colon–rectum	70	47–95
Urinary organs	69	62–100
Oral–pharynx	66	54–80
Soft tissue	60	50–82
Lymphomas	58	20–69
Leukemia	54	5–76

[a]Derived from between three and six reports.

Table 3.2 Top ten pains among 211 patients with advanced cancer.

	Type	Cause
1	Bone	
2	Visceral	
3	Neuropathic	Caused by cancer itself
4	Soft tissue	
5	Immobility	
6	Constipation	
7	Myofascial	Related to cancer and/or debility
8	Cramp	
9	Esophagitis	
10	Degeneration of the spine	Concurrent disorder

Data from Sobell House, Oxford, UK.

third of patients, neuropathic mechanisms are involved, generally together with nociceptive ones.[4, 5]

Careful evaluation is necessary to prevent inappropriate treatment and to facilitate optimal management. For example, abdominal pain caused by constipation may be relieved by morphine, but morphine is clearly inappropriate, as is its use for persistent cramp and myofascial pain.

Evaluation of pain in advanced cancer is based primarily on probability and pattern recognition. Awareness of common pain syndromes associated with advanced

cancer is therefore important. It generally allows clinical diagnosis to be made much more rapidly and appropriate treatment started weeks, occasionally months, sooner than might otherwise have been the case.

CANCER BONE PAIN

Bone metastases occur in about 40 percent of patients with lung, renal, and thyroid cancers, and in about 70 percent of patients with breast and prostate cancer.[6] Consequently, bone pain is the most common cause of cancer-related pain.[7] It generally presents as a persistent background pain with exacerbations on movement or activity, often called incident or breakthrough pain.[8] Of 108 patients seen in an oncology clinic with bone pain, 23 percent rated their average pain as severe (7–10 on a scale of 0–10) and 78 percent rated their worst pain as severe.[9] A survey of over 1000 cancer pain patients confirmed that bone pain is one of the most painful cancer pain syndromes, and significantly reduces quality of life.[10]

Vertebral metastases

Metastases to vertebral bodies often cause midline pain (**Table 3.3**).[2, 11, 12] Pain from a vertebral pedicle (a common site of metastasis) may be associated with unilateral nerve root pain. Epidural extension of a paravertebral tumor can also cause unilateral root pain. Disease progression may lead to vertebral body collapse, unilateral or bilateral root pain, and paraplegia or tetraplegia. Common differential diagnoses to consider in cancer patients complaining of neck or back pain are:

- degenerative disk disease; and
- osteoporosis.

Degenerative disk disease is rare at C7, T1, or L1. Radiographic differentiation of osteoporosis from bone metastases may be difficult, particularly in the presence of vertebral body collapse. Ordinary and computed tomography (CT) usually allow a distinction to be made. In osteoporotic vertebral body collapse, tomography usually shows intact vertebral end plates and symmetrical collapse. In metastatic disease, there is erosion of the vertebral end plates, destruction of one or more pedicles, and asymmetrical collapse of the vertebral body. Because the image is based on a signal that reflects tissue chemistry, a magnetic resonance (MR) scan is the radiological investigation of choice to detect a metastasis that is not causing structural deformity (**Figure 3.1**).

With C7–T1 metastases, an associated Horner's syndrome suggests paravertebral disease with involvement of the sympathetic chain. With lumbar metastases, there may be little local pain. Instead, pain is referred to the sacroiliac joint and/or superior posterior iliac crest. Thus,

Table 3.3 Pain syndromes caused by vertebral metastases, spinal cord compression, and meningeal involvement.[2, 11, 12]

Syndrome	Pathophysiology	Characteristics of pain	Concomitants
Vertebrae			
Fracture of odontoid process of C1	Metastasis of odontoid process of C1, pathological fracture and subluxation, compression of spinal cord	Severe neck pain radiating to occiput and vertex of skull, exacerbated by movements of neck, particularly flexion	Progressive sensory, motor, and autonomic dysfunction beginning in upper limb
C7–T1 metastasis	Hematogenous spread of cancer of breast and bronchus; or tumor in paravertebral space, spread to adjacent vertebra and epidural space	Constant aching pain in paraspinal area radiating to both shoulders; unilateral radicular pain (C7–T1) radiating to shoulder and medial aspect of arm	Often tenderness on percussion of spinous process; paresthesia and numbness in fingers 4 and 5; progressive weakness of triceps and hand
Lumbar metastasis	Common site of metastasis from breast, prostate, and other tumors	Aching pain in midback with reference to one or both sacroiliac joints; radicular pain in groins/thighs	Pain may be exacerbated by sitting or lying down and relieved by standing or vice versa
Sacral metastasis	Common site of metastasis from breast, prostate, and other tumors	Aching pain in the sacral and/ or coccygeal region exacerbated by sitting and relieved by walking	Perianal sensory loss; bowel and bladder dysfunction; impotence; may be exacerbated by sitting or lying down and relieved by walking
Epidural spinal cord compression and meninges			
Epidural spinal cord compression	Tumor compression of spinal cord; generally related to vertebral metastasis and collapse	Aching pain and tenderness in the region of involved vertebrae, radicular pain, and garter or cuff distribution of pain in legs	Motor weakness progressing to paraplegia; sensory loss; loss of bowel and bladder function
Meningeal carcinomatosis	Tumor infiltration of the cerebrospinal meninges	Headache, with or without neck stiffness; and pain in the low back and buttocks	Malignant cells in cerebrospinal fluid

when investigating sacroiliac pain, it is important to take radiographs of the whole of the lumbar spine.

Rib metastases

Pathological fractures of the ribs are relatively common in cancers of the breast and prostate, and in multiple myeloma. A rib fracture may well be painless at rest, particularly if a patient is already taking analgesics. The rectus abdominis muscles, however, are attached to the inner aspect of the lower ribs. Thus, when the body is moved from a sitting to a lying position, or vice versa, these muscles tug on a fractured bone and cause transient severe pain. Deep breaths, coughing, laughing, and twisting the trunk also cause severe pain. However, the diagnosis may not be made because the patient simply complains of new severe chest pain. A clinician who is alert to the possibility

of rib metastases will ask the appropriate questions and elicit the classical features of the syndrome.

BASE OF SKULL METASTASES

The base of the skull is roughly the area behind the nose and above the pharynx. There are several syndromes associated with metastases to this area. They share certain features:

- facial paresthesia, dysesthesia, or pain;
- dysfunction of one or more cranial nerves;
- limited diagnostic help from plain radiographs.

The cranial nerves are affected as they pass through or emerge from various foramina in the middle and posterior cranial fossae. The most common cause is a cancer spreading directly from the nasopharynx and metastases

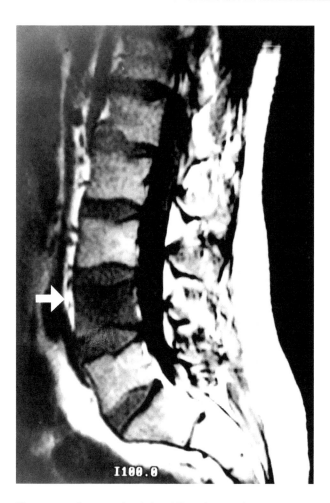

Figure 3.1 An example of the ability of magnetic resonance (MR) scan to detect metastatic disease in bone marrow. This 28-year-old man presented with unremitting low back pain. Clinical examination and conventional radiographs were normal, as was computed tomography. MR scan shows an abnormal signal throughout the L4 vertebral body (arrow). Biopsy showed non-Hodgkin's lymphoma.

from cancers of the breast, bronchus, and prostate. Although headache features prominently in the classical descriptions of these syndromes (**Table 3.4**), some patients complain only of paresthesia or dysesthesia and numbness in the distribution of one or more cranial nerves. When pain is present, this may precede any other symptoms and signs by weeks or months. Sometimes the syndromes occur bilaterally.

Involvement of the hypoglossal nerve (XII) indicates involvement of the neighboring hypoglossal canal. An associated Horner's syndrome indicates extracranial involvement of the sympathetic nerves in proximity to the jugular foramen:

- ipsilateral ptosis;
- constricted pupil;
- enophthalmos;
- reduced facial sweating.

Radiographic investigation is often unrewarding. A plain x-ray is normally no help, but an isotope bone scan or CT may identify the skull metastases (**Figure 3.2**). In about 25 percent of cases, neither of these help and the diagnosis has to be made on clinical evidence alone.[13]

SPINAL CORD COMPRESSION

Spinal cord or cauda equina compression manifests in about 3 percent of all cancer patients.[14] It generally results from the distortion of a vertebral body or pedicle by metastasis. Collapse of the vertebral body is not always a feature. In some cases, the compression is caused by nonvertebral epidural metastasis. In about 70 percent of cases, compression occurs in the thoracic region, in 20 percent of cases in the lumbar spine, and in 10 percent of cases in the cervical spine.[14] Multiple sites of compression occur in about 20 percent of patients. Cancers of the breast, bronchus, and prostate account for over 60 percent of cases. Most others are associated with lymphoma, melanoma, renal cell cancer, myeloma, sarcoma, and head and neck and thyroid cancers.

Pain is the first symptom in > 90 percent of cases and may be present for as little as one day to as long as two years. The nature of the pain varies according to the site of compression. Local pain is not always present and may be masked by previously prescribed analgesics. Local tenderness is common. Root pain is often unilateral in cervical or lumbar compression, but is generally bilateral in patients with a thoracic lesion, particularly if associated with epidural spread.

Some patients experience more pain when lying flat (which is therefore worse at night), whereas in patients with peripheral nerve compression rest usually reduces pain intensity (nights not disturbed by pain). Almost all patients with thoracic cord compression have an upgoing plantar response. Pain may be caused by[15] vertebral metastasis, root compression (radicular pain), and compression of the long tracts of the spinal cord (funicular pain). Radicular and funicular pains are often exacerbated by neck flexion or straight-leg raising, and by coughing, sneezing, or straining. Funicular pain is generally less sharp than radicular pain, has a more diffuse distribution (like a cuff or garter around the thighs, knees, or calves), and is sometimes described as a cold, unpleasant sensation.

Many paraplegics complain of burning, tingling pain (dysesthesia) in areas of the body below the level of the lesion. Descriptions in noncancer paraplegics include severe crushing pressure, vice-like pinching sensations, streams of fire running down the leg to the feet and out of the toes, and a pain like that of a knife being pressed deep into the tissue, twisted around rapidly, and withdrawn all at the same time.[16] These pains may occur after total or partial spinal cord lesions at any level, and are possibly more common with lesions of the cauda equina.[15] The

Table 3.4 Pain syndromes and associated clinical features caused by skull metastases.

Syndrome	Pathophysiology	Characteristics of pain	Concomitants
Cavernous sinus	Metastasis to cavernous sinus	Frontal headache	Dysfunction of cranial nerves III–VI (diplopia, ophthalmoplegia, papilledema)
Sphenoid sinus	Metastasis to sphenoid sinus	Frontal headache radiating to temple with intermittent retro-orbital pain	Dysfunction of cranial nerve VI (diplopia) and nasal stuffiness
Clivus syndrome	Metastasis to clivus of sphenoid bone and basilar part of occipital bone	Vertex headache exacerbated by neck flexion	Dysfunction of cranial nerves VII and IX–XII (facial weakness, hoarseness, dysarthria, dysphagia, trapezius muscle weakness). Begins unilaterally but extends bilaterally
Jugular foramen	Metastasis to jugular foramen	Occipital pain exacerbated by head movement, radiating to the vertex and to shoulder and arm	Dysfunction of cranial nerves IX–XII (hoarseness, dysarthria, dysphagia, trapezius muscle weakness)
Occipital condyle	Metastasis to occipital condyle	Localized occipital pain exacerbated by neck flexion	Dysfunction of cranial nerve XII (paralysis of tongue, dysarthria and buccal dysphagia), weakness of sternomastoid muscle, stiff neck

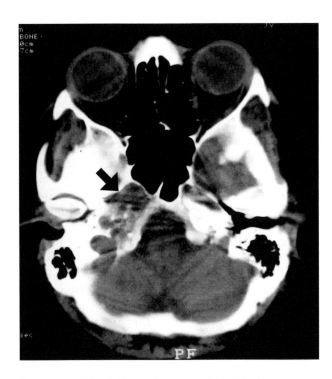

Figure 3.2 This middle-aged woman who had had breast cancer four years earlier presented with paralysis of the right VI and XII nerves. Computed tomography shows metastatic erosion of the apex of the right petrous bone (arrow).

onset of such pains may be immediate, but most occur only after months or years. Because of the long latent period, few patients with malignant paraplegia experience them.

A plain x-ray of the whole spine is essential. In 80 percent of cases it will reveal bone destruction at one or more levels, e.g. loss of a pedicle or vertebral body collapse (usually sparing the intervertebral disk). It may also reveal a soft-tissue mass adjacent to the vertebrae. However, an obvious collapsed vertebra may not be the site of the cord compression. A bone scan does not usually yield additional information. MR imaging is the investigation of choice (**Figure 3.3**), but must not delay treatment. CT with myelography may be helpful if MR imaging is not available.

MENINGEAL CARCINOMATOSIS

Meningeal carcinomatosis occurs as a result of metastatic spread into the cerebrospinal fluid. Numerous metastatic seedlings develop on the meninges of both the brain and the spinal cord. There may also be concomitant invasion of the central nervous system (CNS). In one survey, meningeal infiltration by cancer occurred in about 10 percent of patients with disseminated cancer.[17] In another survey, 90 percent of cases related to:

- breast cancer (>50 percent);
- lung cancer (>25 percent);
- melanoma (12 percent).[18]

Lymphoma is another relatively common cause of meningeal carcinomatosis. Symptoms and signs can be grouped into those involving brain, cranial nerves, and spinal nerves (**Table 3.5**).

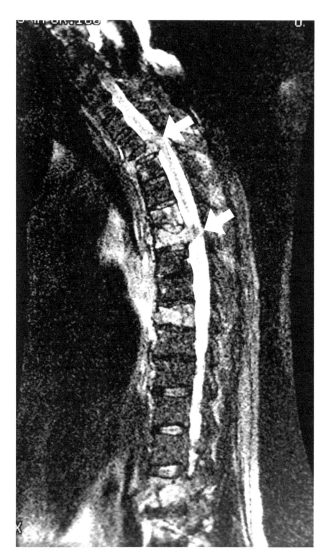

Figure 3.3 An example of the value of magnetic resonance (MR) scan as a noninvasive alternative to myelography in patients with suspected spinal cord compression. This patient with cancer of the prostate had symptoms which appeared clinically to refer to the lower thoracic region. Sagittal MR scan shows altered signal intensity in the bodies of T4, 7, 8, and 11. These indicate active metastases. At two levels (T4 and T8), there has been partial vertebral collapse and tumor extension into the canal, producing significant cord compression (arrows). The patient therefore required radiotherapy covering both levels.

Most patients have symptoms and signs in more than one area at the time of diagnosis. Initial cytological examination of the cerebrospinal fluid was diagnostic in just over half the cases, and eventually became positive in >90 percent.[18]

Headache and back pain are the most common initial features. The headache is often severe and may well be associated with symptoms and signs of meningeal irritation, i.e. nausea, vomiting, photophobia, and neck rigidity. In one series, radicular pain in the buttocks and legs occurred in one-third of cases.[19] Helpful radiological

Table 3.5 Spinal symptoms and signs caused by meningeal metastases from solid tumors (74/90 patients).[18]

Symptoms		Signs	
Lower motor neuron weakness	34	Reflex asymmetry	64
		Weakness	54
Paresthesia	31	Sensory loss	24
Back/neck pain	23	Straight-leg raising	11
Radicular pain	19	Decreased rectal tone	10
Bowel/bladder dysfunction	12	Neck rigidity	7

investigations are myelography, CT myelography, and MR scan with gadolinium enhancement (**Figure 3.4**).

UNILATERAL FACIAL PAIN IN CANCER OF THE BRONCHUS

Unilateral ear and facial pain associated with cancer of the bronchus has been reported.[20] The characteristic features of the pain are initially localized in or around the ear, later more diffuse, and usually no detectable local cause.

The pain is a form of referred pain, relating to a sensory branch of the vagus (nerve of Arnold), which conveys impulses from part of the external auditory canal and a small area of skin behind the ear. In patients not previously known to have lung cancer, finger clubbing may provide a clue to diagnosis.[21]

BRACHIAL PLEXOPATHY

Painful brachial plexopathy in cancer patients may be caused by stretch injury during surgery, transient inflammatory plexopathy (idiopathic or radiation induced), metastasis, and progressive radiation fibrosis.[22]

The pain of brachial plexopathy is usually felt as a burning dysesthetic pain in the ulnar side of the hand (indicating C7–T1 root involvement) and is often accompanied by cramp-like or "crushing" pains in the forearm. Brachial plexopathy is a common complication of Pancoast's tumor (superior pulmonary sulcus syndrome), breast cancer, and lymphoma. Compared with radiation plexopathy, recurrent tumor is more often associated with earlier onset, severe pain, and Horner's syndrome.

SUPRASCAPULAR NERVE ENTRAPMENT

The suprascapular nerve (C5–6) is part of the brachial plexus. *Inter alia*, it carries sensory branches from both the glenohumeral and acromioclavicular joints. It traverses the suprascapular notch which is narrow in some patients. Weakness of the rotatory cuff muscles can result in winging of the scapula and leads to repeated traction

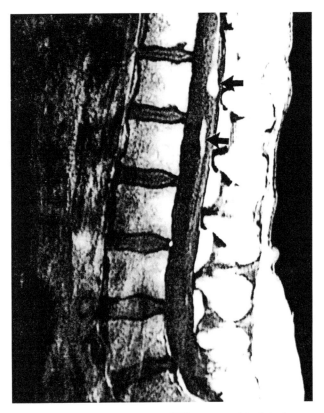

Figure 3.4 Magnetic resonance (MR) scan used to detect cauda equina infiltration. This patient with a previous history of carcinoma of the breast presented with severe sciatica. MR scan was the investigation of choice, because of its ability to distinguish between degenerative disk disease and root compression by vertebral metastases. If neither possibility is demonstrated, gadolinium-enhanced MR scan is required in case the symptoms are caused by metastases in the spinal canal. In this patient, enhanced images showed two plaques of tumor (arrows) infiltrating the roots of the cauda equina.

on the suprascapular nerve. This can lead to inflammation and entrapment with consequential shoulder pain, generally unilateral but occasionally bilateral. Typically, the pain is exacerbated by overhead movement of the arm and when stretching the ipsilateral hand across the thorax and on to the contralateral scapula (Thompson and Kopell test). Tenderness over the suprascapular fossa supports this diagnosis. Risk factors for suprascapular nerve entrapment include:

- weakness and cachexia with winging of the scapula;
- when dyspneic patients lean forward and rest on their arms for long periods, e.g. cancer patients with concurrent chronic obstructive pulmonary disease (COPD);
- excessive use of arms, e.g. in someone with paraplegia or who uses crutches;
- the use of self-propelled wheelchairs;
- upper limb lymphedema, with a heavy arm dragging on the shoulder girdle.[23]

LUMBOSACRAL PLEXOPATHY

Lumbosacral plexopathy presents with sacral and leg pain and associated weakness. Additional inconstant features include leg edema, a palpable mass on rectal examination, and hydronephrosis.[24] Three syndromes have been described:[24]

1. upper (L1–L4), about 30 percent;
2. lower (L4–S3), about 50 percent;
3. upper and lower (L1–S3), about 20 percent.

Most patients report an insidious development of pelvic pain and nerve pain radiating into the leg, followed weeks or months later by sensory symptoms and weakness. Bladder dysfunction and impotence are uncommon.

Lumbar plexopathy ("upper lumbosacral plexopathy") may be caused by a tumor at one of several sites:

- intrathecal (meningeal carcinomatosis);
- epidural (epidural extension of paravertebral tumor, e.g. lymphoma, or associated with spinal cord compression);
- nerve root compression (vertebral collapse);
- paravertebral, i.e. at exit foramina from spinal canal (paravertebral tumor, e.g. lymphoma);
- psoas muscle (malignant psoas syndrome, e.g. melanoma, gynecological cancers, psoas muscle sarcoma);
- renal bed (recurrence of renal cancer);
- retroperitoneum (lymphadenopathy overlying psoas muscle associated with spread of cancer of colon, stomach, adrenal gland, and pancreas);
- retroperitoneum (sarcoma);
- pelvic floor (prostate).[25]

A similar range of possibilities exists for sacral plexopathy. CT is generally helpful. However, the density of muscle and of tumor is similar, and the diagnosis may be made on the basis of an enlarged "muscle" mass. MR scan will clarify if the diagnosis is in doubt.

Renal bed recurrence

Local recurrence of renal cancer after nephrectomy may cause ipsilateral lumbar back pain and L1 and/or L2 nerve compression pain in the ipsilateral groin and/or upper thigh. There is often associated numbness and weakness of iliopsoas muscle manifesting as impaired flexion of the thigh. Activity typically exacerbates the pain. Radiographic investigation may be difficult. Bowel prolapses into the renal bed after nephrectomy and interferes with ultrasound. CT is the best imaging technique in this situation.

Malignant psoas syndrome

Malignant psoas syndrome is a good example of a mixed mechanism pain, both nociceptive (local inflammation and muscle spasm) and neuropathic (lumbosacral plexopathy).[26] The features of this syndrome are:

- clinical evidence of lumbar plexopathy;
- painful fixed flexion of the ipsilateral thigh with exacerbation of pain when extension of the hip is attempted (= a positive psoas test);
- CT evidence of ipsilateral psoas major muscle enlargement (**Figure 3.5**).[27]

Ultrasound is better than CT because muscle and cancer have different echogenicity. MR scan will also distinguish. A painful fixed flexion deformity is also seen with more distal muscle infiltration, i.e. of the iliacus within the pelvis.

Proximally, the psoas major muscle is attached to vertebrae T12–L5. The ventral rami of nerves L1–3 and most of nerve L4 traverse the paravertebral belly of the psoas muscle. Branches give rise to iliohypogastric (L1), ilioinguinal (L1), and genitofemoral (L1–2) nerves, which descend superficially on the surface of the muscle posterior to the iliac fascia and the para-aortic and iliac lymph nodes. Hence, malignant involvement of the psoas muscle results in distribution of pain in these areas.

PERIPHERAL NEUROPATHY

The incidence of peripheral neuropathy as a nonmetastatic (paraneoplastic) manifestation of malignant disease

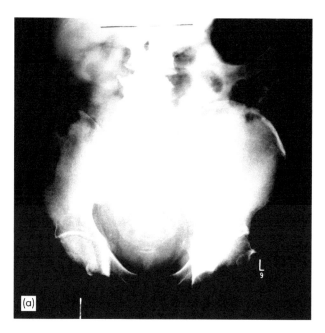

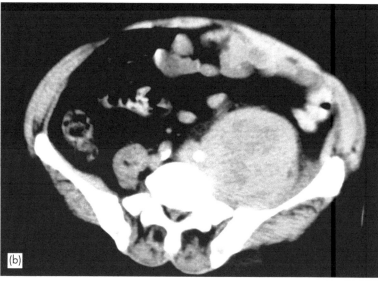

Figure 3.5 (a) Plain x-ray and (b) computed tomography (CT) scan in a patient with severe pain in the anterior left thigh and associated fixed thigh flexion. CT shows massive expansion of the left psoas muscle in the left iliac fossa caused by infiltration by tumor. No abnormality was detectable on the plain x-ray.

is between 1 and 5 percent.[22] It is highest in lung cancer, followed by cancer of the stomach, colon, and breast.[28] A pure sensory neuropathy may be caused by an autoimmune dorsal root ganglionitis. This is most commonly associated with small-cell lung cancer, but is seen occasionally with cancer of the breasts, ovary, and colon.[22]

Cancer may also directly invade a peripheral nerve, for example chest wall or rib lesions may infiltrate intercostal nerves, and paraspinal masses may entrap one or more nerves as they emerge from intervertebral foramina. CT or MR scan usually identifies the tumor. As already noted, paraspinal tumors may extend into the epidural space and also lead to progressive spinal cord compression.

HEPATIC PAIN

Pain is not a constant feature of hepatomegaly. Among 90 patients with advanced cancer and hepatomegaly, less than 40 percent had right hypochondrial pain.[29] When pancreatic cancer patients are excluded (in whom the pain could be pancreatic rather than hepatic), the figure falls to about one-third. The most common pain associated with hepatomegaly is an aching pain in the right hypochondrium. In some patients this is exacerbated by standing or prolonged walking. This is probably caused by traction on the hepatic ligaments. The origins of pain associated with hepatomegaly are stretching of the hepatic capsule; traction on hepatic ligaments (when standing or walking); intrahepatic hemorrhage; outward pressure on rib cage; pinching of abdominal wall; and lumbar spinal strain (as in pregnancy).

Patients occasionally develop rapidly increasing right upper quadrant pain, and present with an "acute abdomen." In patients with advanced cancer, the most likely cause of such pain is hemorrhage into a hepatic secondary with acute distension of the pain-sensitive liver capsule. The pain will diminish as the hematoma resolves and/or the capsule adapts, and analgesic requirements generally return to prehemorrhage levels within a week.

Patients with gross hepatomegaly sometimes complain of discomfort in the lower rib cage, often bilaterally. This may relate to outward pressure on the rib cage. A non-opioid, e.g. paracetamol (acetaminophen), often provides significant relief. A few patients complain of intermittent sharp pains in the right hypochondrium. These are probably caused by the enlarged liver pinching the parietal peritoneum against the lower border of the rib cage. Explanation of the latter, a change of position, and local massage usually provide relief. Some patients with hepatomegaly also complain of backache. This is caused by postural factors and is similar to backache in pregnancy.

PANCREATIC PAIN

As with other primary sites, pain is not a constant feature in pancreatic cancer. Pain relates to obstruction of the pancreatic ducts and to infiltration of pancreatic connective tissue, capillaries, and/or afferent nerves. It occurs in about 90 percent of patients with cancer of the head of the pancreas, particularly if the growth is near the ampulla of Vater.[30] Jaundice is a common accompanying feature. On the other hand, pain occurs in only 10 percent of patients with cancer of the pancreatic body and tail and is generally a late feature.

Pancreatic pain usually occurs in the upper abdomen. It is often said that the pain will be on the right side with cancer of the head of the pancreas and on the left with cancer of the tail. This is not always the case.[31] The patient usually experiences constant pain, which becomes increasingly severe over a period of time. As with other causes of epigastric pain, in some patients the pain is eased by bending forward and exacerbated by lying supine.

Pain may also be experienced in the back. It is typically midline in the upper lumbar and lower thoracic region. It may spread laterally to right and left, particularly if severe. Unless there is coexistent degenerative spinal disease, there is no bone tenderness or restriction of spinal movement. The presence of back pain may indicate spread into the retroperitoneum and para-aortic nodes; penetration into paravertebral muscles; and referred pain from the pancreas itself.

INTRAPELVIC PAIN

Intrapelvic pain was present in 11 percent of a series of 350 patients with advanced cancer.[29] In over half, the pain was associated with recurrent cancer of the colon or rectum. A quarter had malignancies of the female reproductive tract, and 1 percent had extra-abdominal primaries.

The pattern of pain associated with intrapelvic malignant disease varies. Central hypogastric pain is relatively common in patients with cancers of the bladder and uterus. It is also seen in patients with colorectal cancer, particularly if adherent to or invading the bladder or uterus. More common is pain in the iliac fossae. This is typically unilateral and associated with local recurrence adherent to the lateral pelvic wall. Sometimes the patient becomes bedbound because walking exacerbates the pain. This suggests attachment to, or infiltration of, the ipsilateral iliopsoas muscle by the cancer.

Presacral recurrence often leads to lumbosacral plexopathy. Pain may be felt in the perineum or external genitalia rather than the legs. Severe intrapelvic pain often radiates to the upper thighs in a diffuse manner. Pain may also be referred to the lumbar region, as in some non-malignant gynecologic disorders.

Rectal pain is another type of intrapelvic malignant pain. It may be experienced even if the rectum has been excised surgically. If a local recurrence is present, the patient may complain of discomfort on sitting. This may be mild and described as a feeling of "pressure," or it may be severe enough to prevent the patient from sitting down. The reverse is also seen: no pain when sitting but an increasingly severe dragging pain when standing for more than a few minutes or after walking some 50–100 m. This type of pain may relate to a deeper recurrence with adherence to myofascial structures.

A painful sensation of rectal fullness is occasionally a problem. It is similar to the discomfort felt by normal subjects when experiencing an intense urgent desire to defecate. Such pain is generally related to a local tumor in the unresected rectum or to involvement of the presacral plexus by recurrent tumor. Rarely, it is a phantom phenomenon after rectal excision. Severe stabbing pains ("like a red-hot poker") are occasionally reported. These may relate to spasm of the rectum or the pelvic floor. This type of pain can make the patient distraught.

After perineal resection for rectal cancer, most early-onset pains (within a few weeks of surgery) are postoperative neuropathic pains, and late-onset pain (after more than three months) almost invariably indicates recurrence.[32] In many patients, the pain may develop months before the recurrence becomes apparent (median six months).[33]

In one study, nearly two-thirds of patients described early-onset pain as shooting, bursting, or a tight ache. In most, the pain was mild to moderate, intermittent, and spontaneous.[32] Fewer than 5 percent obtained good relief from nonopioids and opioids. The late-onset pain was mainly sharp, aching, and often severe and continuous, located deeper within the pelvis and was typically exacerbated by pressure and sitting.[32] In contrast to the early-onset group, over half of the patients responded well to nonopioids and opioids.

Phantom bladder pain is rare. It probably occurs only after cystectomy when the patient has had considerable preoperative bladder pain either from the tumor itself or from intractable cystitis. Phantom bladder symptoms (bladder distension and a desire to void) are described more frequently. They occur after cystectomy and cord transection and in patients on hemodialysis.[34]

Bladder spasm

Spasm of the detrusor muscle manifests as a deep painful sensation lasting several minutes or up to half an hour in the suprapubic region and/or referred to the tip of the penis. Frequency depends on the cause. Irritation of the trigone by infection or cancer may act as a trigger. Investigation may include bacterial cultures (to identify infection); cystoscopy (to detect intravesical cancer); and MR scan (to detect intramural and extravesical cancer).

INFECTION

Infection was the cause of pain in 4 percent of nearly 300 patients referred to a pain relief service in a cancer hospital.[35] Infection in or around a tumor can lead to a rapid increase in pain, but is not always thought of as a possible cause. However, one report describes seven patients with head and neck cancer in whom infection was responsible for some or all of their pain.[36] All the patients had large tumor masses with ulceration and necrosis, together with swelling, induration, and erythema of the surrounding tissue. In each case, pain had previously been well controlled with an oral opioid, and then increased considerably over a few days. In three of the patients, a change was noted in the appearance of the tumor, two had a leukocytosis and one was febrile. Empirical treatment with antibiotics resulted in pain relief within three days in all seven patients.[36]

REFERENCES

1. Kane RL, Wales J, Bernstein L et al. A randomised controlled trial of hospice care. Lancet. 1984; 1: 890–4.

* 2. Bonica JJ. Cancer pain: current status and future needs. In: Bonica JJ (ed.). The management of pain, 2nd edn. Philadelphia, PA: Lea & Febiger, 1990: 400–55.

* 3. Grond S, Zech D, Diefenbach C et al. Assessment of cancer pain: a prospective evaluation in 2266 cancer patients referred to a pain service. Pain. 1996; 64: 107–14.

4. Grond S, Radbruch L, Meuser T et al. Assessment and treatment of neuropathic cancer pain following WHO guidelines. Pain. 1999; 79: 15–20.

5. Caraceni A, Portenoy RK. An international survey of cancer pain characteristics and syndromes. IASP Task Force on Cancer Pain. Pain. 1999; 82: 263–74.

6. Chow E, Hoskin P, van der Linden Y et al. Quality of life and symptom end points in palliative bone metastases trials. Clinical Oncology. 2006; 18: 67–69.

7. Mercadante S. Malignant bone pain: pathophysiology and treatment. Pain. 1997; 69: 1–18.

8. McQuay HJ, Jadad AR. Incident pain. Palliative Medicine. 1994; 21: 17–24.

9. Janjan NA, Payne R, Gillis T et al. Presenting symptoms in patients referred to a multidisciplinary clinic for bone metastases. Journal of Pain and Symptom Management. 1998; 16: 171–8.

10. Portenoy RK, Payne D, Jacobsen P. Breakthrough pain: characteristics and impact in patients with cancer pain. Pain. 1999; 81: 129–34.

* 11. Foley KM. Pain syndromes in patients with cancer. In: Bonica JJ, Ventafridda VV (eds). Advances in pain research and therapy, vol. 2. New York: Raven Press, 1979: 59–75.

* 12. Portenoy RK. Cancer pain: epidemiology and syndromes. Cancer. 1989; 63: 2298–307.

13. Greenberg HS, Deck MDF, Vikram B *et al*. Metastasis to the base of the skull: clinical findings in 43 patients. *Neurology.* 1981; **31**: 530–7.

∗ 14. Kramer JA. Spinal cord compression in malignancy. *Palliative Medicine.* 1992; **6**: 202–11.

15. Guttman L. *Spinal injuries: comprehensive management and research*. Oxford: Blackwell Scientific Publications, 1973.

16. Davis L, Martin J. Studies upon spinal cord injuries. II. The nature and treatment of pain. *Journal of Neurosurgery.* 1947; **4**: 483–91.

17. Posner JB, Chernik NL. Intracranial metastases from systemic cancer. *Advances in Neurology.* 1978; **19**: 579–92.

∗ 18. Wasserstrom WR, Glass JP, Posner JB. Diagnosis and treatment of leptomeningeal metastases from solid tumours: experience with 90 patients. *Cancer.* 1982; **49**: 759–72.

19. Olson ME, Chernik NL, Posner JB. Infiltration of the leptomeninges by systemic cancer: a clinical and pathologic study. *Archives of Neurology.* 1974; **30**: 122–37.

20. Bindoff L, Heseltine D. Unilateral facial pain in patients with lung cancer: a referred pain via the vagus. *Lancet.* 1988; **1**: 812–15.

21. Schoenen J, Broux R, Moonen G. Unilateral facial pain as the first symptom of lung cancer: are there diagnostic clues? *Cephalagia.* 1992; **12**: 178–9.

22. Kelly JB, Payne R. Pain syndromes in the cancer patient. *Neurologic Clinics.* 1991; **9**: 937–53.

23. Penn J, Zbigniew Z. Shoulder pain? Is it suprascapular nerve entrapment? *European Journal of Palliative Care.* 2006; **13**: 98–100.

24. Jaeckle KA, Young DF, Foley KM. The natural history of lumbosacral plexopathy in cancer. *Neurology.* 1985; **35**: 8–15.

25. Ladha SS, Spinner RJ, Suarez GA *et al*. Neoplastic lumbosacral radiculopathy in prostate cancer by direct perineural spread: an unusual entity. *Muscle Nerve.* 2006; **34**: 659–65.

26. Agar M, Broadbent A, Chye R. The management of malignant psoas syndrome: case reports and literature review. *Journal of Pain and Symptom Management.* 2004; **28**: 282–93.

27. Stevens J, Gonet YM. Malignant psoas syndrome: recognition of an oncologic entity. *Australasian Radiology.* 1990; **34**: 150–4.

∗ 28. McLeod JG. Carcinomatous neuropathy. In: Dyck PJ, Thomas PK, Lambert EH, Bunge R (eds). *Peripheral neuropathy.* Philadelphia, PA: WB Saunders, 1984: 2180.

29. Bains M, Kirkham SR. Carcinoma involving bone and soft tissue. In: Wall PD, Melzack R (eds). *Textbook of pain.* Edinburgh: Churchill Livingstone, 1989: 590–7.

30. MacFarlane DA, Thomas LP. *Textbook of surgery.* Edinburgh: Churchill Livingstone, 1964.

31. Krech RL, Walsh D. Symptoms of pancreatic cancer. *Journal of Pain and Symptom Management.* 1991; **6**: 360–7.

32. Boas RA, Schug SA, Acland RH. Perineal pain after rectal amputation: a 5 year follow up. *Pain.* 1993; **52**: 67–70.

33. Radbruch L, Zech D, Grond S *et al*. Perineal pain and rectal carcinoma – prevalence in local tumour recurrence. *Medizinische Klinik.* 1991; **86**: 180–5.

34. Dorpat TL. Phantom sensations of internal organs. *Comprehensive Psychiatry.* 1971; **12**: 27–35.

35. Gonzalez GR, Foley KM, Portenoy RK. Evaluative skills necessary for a cancer pain consultant. American Pain Society Meeting, Phoenix, AZ, 1989.

36. Bruera E, MacDonald RN. Intractable pain in patients with advanced head and neck tumours: a possible role of local infection. *Cancer Treatment Reports.* 1986; **70**: 691–2.

4

History and clinical examination of the cancer pain patient: assessment and measurement

BADI EL OSTA AND EDUARDO BRUERA

Introduction	38	Integration of pain and other symptoms	44
Evaluation of patients with cancer pain	39	Summary and conclusions	44
Characterization of the cancer pain syndrome	41	References	45
Pain evaluation	41		

KEY LEARNING POINTS

- A thorough history and physical examination is necessary for the diagnosis of the cause of pain.
- Classifying pain enables physicians to better delineate pathophysiology and facilitates treatment efficacy.
- The multidimensional treatment of pain is of great importance.

- Neuropathic and incident pain, psychological distress, addictive behavior, and cognitive function can make pain treatment challenging.
- Many tools have been validated for pain clinical assessment and research purposes.

INTRODUCTION

Pain occurs in 60–80 percent of patients with advanced cancer before death.[1, 2] During the 1970s and early 1980s, a number of authors demonstrated that patients with cancer pain were inadequately managed.[3, 4] As a result, organizations such as the International Association for the Study of Pain, the World Health Organization, and other intergovernmental and nongovernmental organizations launched major initiatives promoting the education of healthcare professionals and the lay public on cancer pain management.[4, 5, 6] Initial guidelines and scholarly reviews focused on dispelling existing myths and on proposing simple yet effective treatments. The assessment of pain was generally discussed in a very simple way, with emphasis on the need for an appropriate assessment of the "mechanics" of pain: location, radiation, character, intensity, syndromal presentation, and nerve pathways involved in the conduction of nociceptive stimuli.

During recent years, it has become more evident that the optimal evaluation of the patient with cancer pain requires a multidimensional assessment of the pain syndrome, the patient's clinical, psychological, and psychiatric characteristics, and a number of social and family variables. A number of prognostic factors have been identified that have a major impact on the nature of the pain complaint and on the response to treatment.

In the following, we will initially discuss the evaluation of patients with cancer pain along with the different aspects of the assessment of the pain syndrome and the need to integrate the pain with other common symptoms in patients with advanced cancer. Finally, areas for future research will be discussed.

EVALUATION OF PATIENTS WITH CANCER PAIN

History

Table 4.1 summarizes the main components of the medical history in patients with cancer pain. It is crucial to have a good understanding of the underlying cancer (primary site, histology, and anatomical extent), as well as the current disease status. In patients with advanced cancer, the likelihood is higher that the pain is due to locally advanced or metastatic cancer. However, in up to one-fifth of these patients the pain is due to other causes, such as cancer treatments or unrelated, often premorbid, problems.[1] In addition, some specific primary sites and histologies are more likely to metastasize to specific areas of the body than others (e.g. prostate cancer to bones, small-cell lung cancer to the brain).

Previous cancer treatments should be reviewed in depth. Some antineoplastic treatments, such as aggressive surgery, chemotherapy, or radiation therapy, are capable of causing chronic pain syndromes. Alternatively, some patients may potentially benefit from specific antineoplastic interventions, such as hormonal therapy or radiation therapy.

Most patients with cancer pain have advanced disease and a variety of other devastating physical symptoms and psychosocial sequelae,[7] some of which, such as anxiety or depression, may impact on the expression of pain intensity. Other symptoms, such as nausea and confusion, will influence the choice of therapeutic interventions for pain treatment. Therefore, it is of great importance to consider pain within the context of the other physical and psychosocial symptoms and to monitor the effects of pain and its treatment on these other symptoms.

The presence of other pain syndromes, due either to cancer or to chronic nonmalignant pain, may provide important information about patients' coping strategies and their prior responses to analgesic therapies.

A history of alcohol or drug abuse is an independent poor prognostic factor for pain control.[8] Patients should

Table 4.1 Medical history in patients with cancer pain.

Medical history	
Cancer stage:	Primary site
	Histology
	Anatomical extent
Previous cancer treatment	
Cancer pain syndrome	
Other physical symptoms	
Previous pain syndromes and treatment	
Psychosocial assessment	
History of alcoholism/drug abuse	
Assessment of cognitive function/delirium	
Other medical conditions	

routinely undergo screening assessments for alcohol, such as the CAGE questionnaire,[9] and an assessment of a history of drug use.

One of the most important aspects of the psychosocial assessment is the presence or significant history of mood disorders.[10] Depression occurs in approximately 25 percent of patients with advanced cancer.[11] Mood disorders are likely to be intensified by cancer pain. On the other hand, the expression of pain and other somatic symptoms can be higher in patients with mood disorders.[8] A number of tools can be used for the assessment of the presence and intensity of depression.[12] Recent research suggests that simple assessments such as a visual analog scale (VAS) or the question "Are you depressed?" can be as reliable as more complex and time-consuming instruments in cancer patients.[13] Vignaroli et al.[14] have evaluated the screening performance of the Edmonton Symptom Assessment System (ESAS)[15, 16] for depression and anxiety compared to that measured by the Hospital Anxiety and Depression Scale (HADS).[17] The diagnosis of anxiety or depression is made when a patient scores 8 or more on HADS. Of the 216 cancer patients analyzed, this retrospective study showed that the ideal cutoff point of ESAS for the screening for depression and anxiety in palliative care is 2 out of 10 with sensitivity of 77 percent and specificity of 55 percent for depression, and with sensitivity of 86 percent and specificity of 56 percent for anxiety. Patients with a depression or anxiety score of ≥2/10 on the ESAS should undergo further evaluation of depression and anxiety.

Cognitive failure is a frequent finding in patients with advanced cancer,[18] occurring in more than 80 percent of patients before death.[19, 20] The presence of cognitive failure makes the assessment of intensity and other dimensions of pain very difficult. In addition, cognitive failure may be aggravated by pharmacological interventions for the management of pain, and, therefore, a regular screening of cognitive function and delirium should be performed.[20]

Three of the more commonly applied tools are the Folstein Mini-Mental State Examination (MMSE), the Memorial Delirium Assessment Scale (MDAS), and the Delirium Rating Scale (DRS). No single tool is relied on exclusively to establish a definitive diagnosis of delirium in all cases. An individual patient's score, whether normal or abnormal, must be correlated with the clinical situation.

The MMSE, devised by Folstein et al.,[21] comprises 11 questions that assess five general areas of cognition: orientation, registration, attention and calculation, recall, and language. A score of <24 out of 30 is generally indicative of cognitive dysfunction, although this score is generally corrected to reflect age and educational level.[22] The MMSE has several advantages in that it is among the most frequently used tests in the clinical evaluation of delirium and has been validated for use in patients with advanced cancer. It is familiar to many clinicians, and can be administered with very little training by most health-care professionals. It is quick to complete, taking an average of five to ten minutes, and its numerical score quantifies cognitive impairment, which can then be compared over time in a given patient, allowing evaluation of the efficacy of various management strategies. The MMSE is limited by the fact that it is simply a screening tool for cognitive dysfunction and therefore cannot differentiate between delirium and other cognitive disorders, such as dementia. In addition, the MMSE cannot detect the other dimension of delirium, such as awareness and perceptual disturbance, delusions, and psychomotor agitation.[23] Therefore, two patients with equal scores may look quite different clinically, one being in severe distress with multiple hallucinations and severe agitation and the other being hypoactive in appearance.

The MDAS, developed by Breitbart et al.,[24] is a ten-item, four-point observer-rated scale designed to quantify the severity of delirium in medically ill patients and assess disturbances in awareness, orientation, short-term memory, digit span, attention capacity, organized thinking, perception, delusions, psychomotor activity, and arousal in a way reflecting all the main diagnostic criteria according to the *Diagnostic and statistical manual for mental disorders*, vol. IV (DSM-IV) of the American Psychiatric Association. Each of the ten items is rated from 0 (none) to 3 (severe). Originally tested in a heterogeneous population of cancer and noncancer patients,[24] the MDAS has been used and validated for screening and diagnosis of delirium in cancer patients.[25] Although its reported administration time is approximately ten minutes, additional time is required for review and discussion with family members and nursing staff. Studies have shown that the MDAS is able to distinguish patients with delirium from those with other cognitive or noncognitive psychiatric disorders.[24] Fadul et al.[26] presented a retrospective study on 31 palliative care professionals after they have received a training session on the MDAS. The correct diagnosis was achieved in 96.8 percent ($n = 30$) despite an overall percentage error of 31 percent for orientation, short-term memory, digit span and 45 percent for all other items ($p < 0.001$). The percentage of error did not differ between physicians, nurses, and other palliative care professionals ($p > 0.99$). The MDAS can be applied routinely in a palliative care setting. However, future research with larger samples is needed to assess whether the training of healthcare professionals will have a stable effect over time and to further confirm their study result. In our clinical setting, this tool has replaced the MMSE for the assessment and monitoring of delirium.

The Disability Rating Scale (DRS) is a ten-item rating scale assessing a broad range of delirium symptomatology. It is suitably easy to administer and, although suggested as a suitable scale for the assessment of delirium severity, it has been validated more for use as a diagnostic tool. A limitation is its failure to assess some features considered essential to the diagnosis of delirium, including inattention, disorganized thinking, and clouding of consciousness.

An ideal clinical tool will be used regularly and repetitively on all patients. A "perfect tool," if used only rarely, is of no practical benefit. Regular assessment, even of patients who appear cognitively intact, is essential for timely identification and management, especially as mild delirium of recent onset has the greatest potential for reversibility.

Finally, a number of other medical conditions influence optimal pain management. The presence of renal failure may have implications for the accumulation of active opioid metabolites or the safe administration of nonsteroidal anti-inflammatory drugs. Patients with borderline cognitive function or dementia may have difficulties tolerating opioids or adjuvant drugs, such as tricyclic antidepressants or anticonvulsants. Patients with acute or chronic infection or diabetes may be poor candidates for corticosteroids. In summary, clinicians need to have a complete understanding of the patient's medical and psychiatric condition in order to establish a safe and effective therapeutic plan.

Physical examination

Patients with cancer pain should undergo a complete physical examination, the results of which, when combined with those of a thorough history, are sufficient to reach an appropriate diagnosis of the cause of pain in the majority of patients.[27] In addition, the physical examination reveals important information about the anatomic extent of tumor spread and the overall physical condition of the patient. For example, patients who are confused, profoundly cachectic, and who are non-ambulatory are unlikely to benefit from aggressive orthopedic reconstruction of the spine or long bones and are probably more appropriately treated with less aggressive, essentially pharmacologic, interventions.

Investigations

Even in seriously ill patients, ancillary laboratory and imaging investigations are sometimes extremely useful in clarifying the causes of pain and aiding the selection of analgesic interventions. Plain x-rays and bone scans contribute to decision-making regarding the appropriateness of radiation therapy and orthopedic procedures in patients with bone pain. Computed tomography and magnetic resonance imaging can help determine the cause of intrathoracic and intra-abdominal pain syndromes, and magnetic resonance imaging is essential to confirm the early diagnosis of epidural spinal cord compression.

CHARACTERIZATION OF THE CANCER PAIN SYNDROME

Table 4.2 summarizes the main factors that should be considered in characterizing the cancer pain syndrome. The location, radiation, descriptors, duration, and onset of the pain syndrome will provide important clues as to the pathophysiology and underlying cause of pain. Nociceptive pain is defined as pain that arises from activation of peripheral nociceptors. The nervous system is fundamentally intact, and complaints of pain usually correlate well with the extent of tissue damage (i.e. tumor invasion of bone or soft tissue[28]). Two subgroups of nociceptive pain are recognized.

1. **Somatic**: patients usually describe a discrete pain location and commonly use descriptors such as aching, sharp, stabbing, or throbbing. Typical examples of somatic nociceptive pains are those related to bone metastases or infiltration of the skin and soft tissues by cancer.
2. **Visceral**: because of the distribution and convergence of nociceptors, these pain syndromes are usually described more vaguely with regards to both location and quality. Patients usually use descriptors such as tugging, cramping, or pressure. Pain is usually associated with tumor invasion of intra-abdominal or intrathoracic organs, distension, or compression, and pain signals are conducted by the afferent autonomic nervous system.

Neuropathic pain is defined as pain caused by aberrant somatosensory processing,[28] and in cancer patients this is most frequently due to tumor involvement of peripheral nerves, roots, or spinal cord. Patients most commonly describe this pain as burning, numb, shock-like, or electrical. Pain is usually located in the trajectory of the involved nerves and is frequently accompanied by corresponding motor and/or sensory abnormalities. For example, a patient with lung cancer and burning pain in the right hemithorax radiating along the intercostal space arising after a thoracotomy is likely to be experiencing neuropathic pain due to a postthoracotomy syndrome.

Table 4.2 Cancer pain syndrome assessment.

Assessment
Cause (tumor, treatment, unrelated)
Location(s) – radiation
Descriptors
Intensity – aggravating factors, relieving factors
Duration and onset
Previous analgesic treatments
Functional and psychological impairment

Alternatively, continuous stabbing pain that is well localized and with no radiation which preceded the thoracotomy is more likely to reflect nociceptive pain due to involvement of the pleural space or bone by the primary tumor.

Careful assessment of previous therapies decreases the likelihood of using drugs or interventions that were previously found to be ineffective or poorly tolerated. Specifically, common opioid side effects, such as sedation, constipation, and nausea should be assessed.

In patients with multiple sites of pain, it is particularly important to assess each site separately and to carefully record the different characteristics. Often, the pathophysiology and cause of each pain is quite different, and this will require different approaches in a given patient.

PAIN EVALUATION

In recent years, it has become evident that the appropriate evaluation of pain requires the regular assessment of intensity, insight into its multidimensional features, an appreciation of the patient's clinical and psychosocial characteristics, and consideration of prognostic factors that may have a major impact on treatment outcome, thus helping to focus care. It has also become apparent that the features should be considered in the context of the other major symptom complexes that are also very common in patients with advanced cancer. Unfortunately, there is evidence that pain is usually poorly assessed by clinicians.[29, 30, 31]

Intensity

It is crucial to assess and monitor the intensity of pain. This can be accomplished using VAS, verbal scales, and numerical scales or more complex pain questionnaires. Some of the most commonly used instruments for the measurement of pain intensity are as follows:

- Edmonton Symptom Assessment System;[15, 16]
- Brief Pain Inventory (BPI);[32]
- Memorial Pain Assessment Card;[33]
- McGill Pain Questionnaire (MPQ);[34]
- verbal descriptors;
- numerical scales;
- VASs;
- facial scales (pediatrics).[35]

Most of these instruments and techniques are considered reliable for the assessment of the intensity of pain. The choice of instrument depends largely on the patient population and the setting in which care is delivered. In some regions of the world where the rate of illiteracy is high, facial scales, colored circles, or pictures of fruits of different size can be used to describe the intensity of pain at a given time.

The commonly used instruments described above measure the intensity of pain at a given time only. Of the more comprehensive instruments, we will describe the BPI,[32] the MPQ,[33] and the Memorial Pain Assessment Card.[34]

The BPI can be administered by a healthcare professional or may be self-administered. The longer version takes approximately 15 minutes to complete while a shorter version requires just a few minutes. The BPI includes a graphic representation of the location of pain and a group of qualitative pain descriptors. The severity of pain is assessed using VAS for pain at its best and worst, and on average. The perceived level of interference with normal activities (life enjoyment, work, mood, sleep, walking, relationships with others) is also reported. There is ample evidence that the BPI is cross-culturally valid.[32, 36]

The MPQ is one of the oldest and best-established pain assessment instruments.[33] Patients are required to select terms used to describe pain from a list. The descriptors are then organized into sensory, affective, or evaluative dimensions. The MPQ also provides a graphic display of pain location. This instrument has been used in patients with cancer pain,[37] and in recent years a short form of the MPQ has been found to be a valuable tool in patients with chronic cancer pain.[38]

The Memorial Pain Assessment Card can be completed in less than one minute and is easily understood by patients.[34] It consists of a small card that is folded so that four separate measures can be performed. It contains scales intended for the measurement of pain intensity, pain relief, and mood, as well as a set of descriptors. It is valid and effective for clinical use and is recommended both for the clinical assessment of individual patients and as an outcome measure for clinical trials.[34]

The Edmonton Symptom Assessment System is a group of ten VAS for ten different symptoms, including pain intensity. This tool allows for a very rapid (approximately one minute) assessment of pain, mood, and other physical symptoms. The results are reported in a graph that is kept in the patient's chart. This tool has been found to be reliable for individual patient treatment,[15, 16, 39] as well as for clinical research and program evaluation.[16, 40]

One major limitation of the more complex instruments is that, because of their length, they cannot easily be administered repeatedly. The appropriate frequency of measurement of pain has not been determined in prospective research. In acute care settings, assessment takes place usually once or twice a day. In chronic care settings, in which patients are assumed to be more stable, assessment is usually performed three times a week. Finally, in patients managed by home care or ambulatory care, assessment usually takes place at the time of the patient's clinic or hospital visit. Some simple instruments, such as numerical scales, can also be utilized reliably by telephone.

An important aspect of effective pain assessment and monitoring is a graphic display of pain intensity in the patient's chart.[15] In the past, it became apparent that a regular graphic display of the patient's vital signs greatly assisted in recognizing abnormalities that required correction. Regular reporting of laboratory results and x-rays in the medical records also make visible the number of factors not readily accessible to physical examination. An appropriate format for recording pain and other symptoms renders the patient's distress more visible and assists the team in the overall planning and monitoring of quality of care.[40, 41]

Multidimensional pain assessment

At the present time, nociception occurring at the level of the primary or metastatic cancer site cannot be measured. Cortical perception of pain is also not measurable. Thus, all pain measurement is based on the patient's expression of pain intensity and distress. This expression is influenced by factors that modulate the level of nociception, perception, and expression. Therapeutic interventions can be conceived of as targeting pain production at each level of nociception perception and expression.

In the past, cancer pain and hospice groups used a more unidimensional methodology. This approach considered that "pain is what the patient calls pain and has the intensity the patient reports." This was frequently considered to mean that 100 percent of a given patient's expression of pain was due to nociception and, therefore, treatable with analgesic drugs. This rather simplistic approach could result in massive doses of opioids, opioid-related toxicity, and excessive reliance on pharmacological approaches compared with that which may result when nonpharmacological approaches to pain control are integrated.

Table 4.3 summarizes the components of pain expression in two different patients reporting bony metastatic pain with an intensity of 8/10. In the case of patient 1, in whom the overwhelming majority of the pain expression relates to nociception, opioid analgesics are likely to be highly effective. In the case of patient 2, a major part of the pain expression is due to somatization related to depression and to severe aggravation of pain with minimal movements. This second patient is much less likely to respond to simple increases in opioid doses. A combination of counseling, with or without antidepressant therapy, and the consideration of radiation therapy or orthopedic procedures to the painful bony area will likely be required in order to achieve a significant decrease in the expression of pain. These cases are examples of how multidimensional assessment can help in the recognition of the relative contribution of different dimensions to the patient's expression, thereby assisting in the planning of care.

A positive history of alcoholism or drug abuse indicates a higher risk for coping chemically. Alcoholism occurs in 5–15 percent of the general population and in approximately 20 percent of hospitalized patients.[42] Unfortunately, in more than two-thirds of patients the

Table 4.3 Components of pain expression in two different patients.

Component (%)	Patient 1 (intensity 8/10)	Patient 2 (intensity 8/10)
Nociception	80	30
Somatization	5	30
Chemical coping	5	10
Incidental component	10	30
	100	100

diagnosis is not made in a timely manner.[9, 42] Four-item questionnaires, such as the CAGE, are extremely simple and result in an accurate diagnosis of alcoholism.[9, 42] A history of alcoholism is a major prognostic factor for the development of rapid opioid dose escalation and the occurrence of opioid-related neurotoxicity.[8] However, when patients undergo regular screening for alcoholism and are offered multidimensional and multidisciplinary support, both pain intensity and overall opioid use are not significantly different among alcoholic patients compared with those with no history of alcoholism.[9]

Somatization, either as a primary coping strategy or as a result of affective disorders such as anxiety or depression, is also an independent poor prognostic factor in patients with cancer pain.[8] The appropriate assessment and management of affective disorders with both pharmacological and nonpharmacological techniques, including appropriate counseling of patients with a history of somatization, can result in improved symptom control and satisfaction with care.

In noncommunicative patients with delirium or dementia, behavioral scales and third-party assessments have been proposed for the assessment of pain.[43] Unfortunately, validation of these tools following traditionally accepted criteria is elusive because of the characteristics of the patient population. Communicative patients with dementia are probably less able to recall, interpret, and articulate their experience and, consequently, are less likely to report pain[44] than patients without delirium. One of the main potential confounders for the measurement of pain in people with delirium and dementia is memory impairment, as pain experienced at one moment may soon be forgotten.[45, 46] A comprehensive study in 51 control subjects and 44 patients with dementia concluded that dementia is capable of influencing not only the report, but also the experience of pain.[46]

A number of authors have reported cases of communicative demented patients who appeared to have diminished or absent self-reporting of pain.[45] Behaviors displayed by the patients suggested that decreased pain perception rather than expression was the main reason for decreased self-reporting.[45, 47]

Agitated behavior caused by factors other than pain may be misinterpreted as pain and mistakenly treated with opioid analgesics, a phenomenon that has been observed in patients with agitated delirium related to cancer.[48] Decreased or absent self-reporting of pain may make the diagnosis of acute complications such as fractures, dental problems, urinary retention, or other acute intercurrent events difficult. Finally, the presence of cognitive failure significantly increases the likelihood of neurotoxicity from both opioids and most adjuvant analgesic drugs.

Neuropathic pain has been described as a syndrome in which there is commonly a reduced responsiveness to opioid analgesics.[8, 49] The recognition of neuropathic pain should assist clinicians in deciding on the use of adjuvant analgesic drugs and early referral to specialized pain services.

Incident pain or "breakthrough" pain has been defined as a transitory increase in pain that occurs in one context of ongoing pain of moderate intensity or less. Opioid titration in patients with pain or breakthrough pain is typically difficult because of rapidly changing levels of pain and dose requirements.

Staging of pain (the development of a common language)

After the recognition of the poor quality of pain control in diverse populations,[3] intensive educational efforts have resulted in significant improvement in the management of cancer pain during recent years, although results reported by different groups remain variable. Some original papers describe extremely good results after the use of relatively low doses of opioids.[50, 51, 52] More recent studies have suggested that, even after using doses of opioids five or six times higher, 10–30 percent of patients are still unable to achieve adequate pain control.[53, 54, 55, 56] One likely explanation for such varied results is the absence of a homogeneous method for the assessment of pain intensity and pain relief. Another explanation for some diverse findings is the differing characteristics of patients treated by different groups. The relative prevalence of patients with more severe or otherwise distinct pain syndromes in a given sample could have a major impact on treatment outcome.

The recognition of poor prognostic features has led to the development of staging systems for different primary tumors, which has been a major advance in cancer research and treatment.[57, 58] These systems have required frequent changes as knowledge of the biology of cancer developed, but have allowed researchers to speak a common language and practitioners to apply the results of their research in a logical and predictable fashion.

The precise definition of patient characteristics in clinical research trials results in an accurate interpretation of data, successful application of therapies, and the subsequent formulation of more advanced clinical research studies. In the clinical field, the early recognition of patients with poor prognostic features results in better planning of care by ensuring faster referral to specialized services.

Unfortunately, such systems are not available for cancer pain. Most publications describe patients as having "pain due to cancer," although this statement is probably as simplistic and difficult to assess and interpret as "carcinoma of the breast." In patients with breast cancer, we know that estrogen and progesterone receptors, positive or negative axillary nodes, histological characteristics of the primary tumor, neoplastic status, and pattern of dissemination are all of prognostic importance. In pain, too, the factors described in **Table 4.3** can influence prognosis and management. The presence or absence of these and perhaps other factors will have a major effect on the results of treatment.

The revised Edmonton Staging System (rESS) was developed by Fainsinger et al.[59] to overcome some limitations in relation to definitions and terminology of the elements of the Edmonton Staging System. It is a validated and clinically acceptable tool for pain classification and cancer pain populations' comparison in research studies.[59] It has a good predictive value and a moderate to high interrater reliability (ranging from 0.67 for pain mechanism to 0.95 for presence of addiction).[59, 60] It consists of five features: mechanism of pain, presence or absence of incidental pain, presence or absence of psychological distress and addictive behavior, and level of cognitive function. In a multicenter study involving 746 advanced cancer patients, Fainsinger et al.[59] found that younger patients (<60 years), as well as patients with neuropathic pain, incidental pain, psychological distress, or addiction, required longer time periods to achieve stable pain control ($p < 0.05$) based on a univariate Cox regression analysis. In a subsequent multivariate Cox regression analysis, only younger patients (<60), neuropathic, and incidental pain were significantly associated with time to reach stable pain control ($p \leq 0.05$). Patients with neuropathic pain, incidental pain, psychological distress, or addiction ended up on higher morphine equivalent daily dose ($p < 0.001$). In another validation study, Nekolaichuck et al.[60] have revised the definitions for incidental pain, psychological distress, addictive behavior, and cognitive function of the rESS based on palliative medicine and pain specialists feedback. The name of the rESS was changed then to Edmonton Classification System for Cancer Pain (ECS-CP) (**Table 4.4**).

It is through the development of staging systems such as the ECS-CP that a common language and methodology for both clinical research and treatment planning can be established.

INTEGRATION OF PAIN AND OTHER SYMPTOMS

Pain is only one of many symptoms experienced by cancer patients.[7] It is important to assess pain within the context of other symptoms for a number of reasons. Pain may not necessarily be the symptom that is having the greatest impact on a patient's quality of life at a given point in time. Pain intensity may have an impact on other physical symptoms, such as fatigue or mobility, or on psychosocial symptoms, such as depression or anxiety. Alternatively, psychosocial symptoms may have an impact on the patient's expression of pain.[8]

The treatment of pain may lead directly to a worsening of other symptoms, such as nausea, constipation, and delirium. The ESAS,[15, 16] STAS,[61] and a number of other tools allow for simultaneous assessment and monitoring of multiple symptoms. These tools involve the completion of a panel of VAS or numerical scales at regular intervals by the patient or, if the patient is cognitively impaired, a nurse.

One of the pivotal clinical challenges in cancer pain management is to maximize the impact on the patient's pain expression, while minimizing the worsening of coexisting symptoms and production of new symptoms.

SUMMARY AND CONCLUSIONS

In recent years, there has been increased emphasis on the importance of appropriate clinical assessment of patients with cancer pain. All patients complaining of cancer pain should undergo a complete medical history and physical examination. It is important to determine the cancer stage and previous treatments, to characterize each pain syndrome, and to assess contextual psychosocial issues and other medical conditions. Even in very ill patients, imaging studies may contribute important information for clinical decision-making. There are excellent and simple instruments for assessing and monitoring pain intensity. The most useful instruments for cancer patients are those that assess multiple symptoms and allow for a graphic display of data. The multiple dimensions that modulate the nociceptive production, cortical perception, and expression of pain should be considered in each patient. Clinicians should remember that the expression of pain intensity is a multidimensional construct that results from the relative contribution of many factors. Appropriate multimodal pain management will consider the relative contribution of these factors in a given patient at a given time. Finally, in cancer patients, pain occurs within the context of a number of devastating physical and psychosocial symptoms. Some of those symptoms are more common and may be more intense than pain itself. Because of the relative impact of pain and its treatment on other symptoms, they should be regularly measured.

Unfortunately, the available body of knowledge on the appropriate assessment of pain is not applied in the routine treatment of cancer patients. The main future challenge in this area is to ensure that patients have access to these evaluations on a regular basis.

Table 4.4 Edmonton Classification System for cancer pain (ECS-CP) definitions of terms.

Classification	Description
1. Mechanism of pain	
No	No pain syndrome
Nc	Any nociceptive combination of visceral and/or bone or soft tissue pain
Ne	Neuropathic pain syndrome with or without any combination of nociceptive pain
Nx	Insufficient information to classify
2. Incident pain	
Pain can be defined as incident pain when a patient has background pain of no more than moderate intensity with intermittent episodes of moderate to severe pain, usually having a rapid onset and often a known trigger	
Io	No incident pain
Ii	Incident pain present
Ix	Insufficient information to classify
3. Psychological distress	
Psychological distress, within the context of the pain experience, is defined as a patient's inner state of suffering resulting from physical, psychological, social, spiritual, and/or practical factors that may compromise the patient's coping ability and complicate the expression of pain and/or other symptoms	
Po	No psychological distress
Pp	Psychological distress present
Px	Insufficient information to classify
4. Addictive behavior	
Addiction is a primary, chronic, neurobiologic disease, with genetic, psychosocial and environmental factors influencing its development and manifestations. It is characterized by behaviors that include one or more of the following: impaired control over drug use, compulsive use, continued use despite harm, and craving	
Ao	No addictive behavior
Aa	Addictive behavior present
Ax	Insufficient information to classify
5. Cognitive function	
Co	No impairment
Ci	Partial impairment
Cu	Total impairment
Cx	Insufficient information to classify
ECS-CP profile:	_____ (combination of the five circled responses, one for each category)

Reproduced by kind permission of Dr Robin Fainsinger from www.palliative.org/PC/ClinicalInfo/AssessmentTools/AssessmentToolsIDX.

REFERENCES

1. Levy MH. Pharmacologic treatment of cancer pain. *New England Journal of Medicine.* 1996; **335**: 1124–32.

2. Bruera E, Watanabe S. New developments in the assessment of pain in cancer patients. *Supportive Care in Cancer.* 1994; **2**: 312–18.

3. Marks RM, Sachar EJ. Undertreatment of medical inpatients with narcotic analgesics. *Annals of Internal Medicine.* 1973; **78**: 173–81.

* 4. World Health Organization Expert Committee Report. *Cancer pain relief and palliative care.* Technical Series 804. Geneva: World Health Organization, 1990.

5. US Department of Health and Human Services. *Management of cancer pain. Clinical practice guidelines.* AHCPR Publications, No. 94-0592, March 1994.

6. World Health Organization. *Cancer pain relief,* 2nd edn. Geneva: World Health Organization, 1996: 43.

* 7. Bruera E, Neumann CM. Respective limits of palliative care and oncology in the supportive care of cancer patients. *Supportive Care in Cancer.* 1999; **7**: 321–7.

* 8. Bruera E, Schoeller T, Wenk R *et al.* A prospective multi-centre assessment of the Edmonton Staging System for cancer pain. *Journal of Pain and Symptom Management.* 1995; **10**: 348–55.

9. Bruera E, Moyano J, Seifert L *et al.* The frequency of alcoholism among patients with pain due to terminal cancer. *Journal of Pain and Symptom Management.* 1995; **10**: 599–603.

* 10. Breitbart W, Bruera E, Chochinov H, Lynch M. Neuropsychiatric syndromes and psychological symptoms in patients with advanced cancer. *Journal of Pain and Symptom Management.* 1995; **10**: 131–41.

* 11. Breitbart W, Chochinov HM, Passik S. Psychiatric aspects of palliative care. In: Doyle D, Hanks GWC, MacDonald N (eds). *Oxford Textbook of Palliative Medicine,* 2nd edn. Oxford: Oxford University Press, 1998: 933–54.

12. Lynch ME. The assessment and prevalence of affective disorders in advanced cancer. *Journal of Palliative Care.* 1995; **11**: 10–18.

* 13. Chochinov HM, Wilson KG, Enns M, Lander S. "Are you depressed?" Screening for depression in the terminally ill. *American Journal of Psychiatry.* 1997; **154**: 674–6.

* 14. Vignaroli E, Pace EA, Willey J *et al.* The Edmonton Symptom Assessment System as a screening tool for depression and anxiety. *Journal of Palliative Medicine.* 2006; **9**: 296–303.

15. Bruera E, Kuehn N, Miller MJ *et al.* The Edmonton Symptom Assessment System (ESAS): a simple method for the assessment of palliative care patients. *Journal of Palliative Care.* 1991; **7**: 6–9.

* 16. Chang VT, Hwang SS, Feuerman M. Validation of the Edmonton Symptom Assessment Scale. *Cancer.* 2000; **88**: 2164–71.

17. Bjelland I, Dahl AA, Haug TT, Neckelmann D. The validity of the Hospital Anxiety and Depression Scale. An updated literature review. *Journal of Psychosomatic Research.* 2002; **52**: 69–77.

18. Pereira J, Hanson J, Bruera E. The frequency and clinical course of cognitive impairment in patients with terminal cancer. *Cancer.* 1997; **79**: 835–42.

19. Massie MJ, Holland J, Glass E. Delirium in terminally ill cancer patients. *American Journal of Psychiatry.* 1983; **140**: 1048–50.

20. Pereira J, Hanson J, Bruera E. The frequency and clinical course of cognitive impairment in patients with terminal cancer. *Cancer.* 1997; **79**: 835–42.

* 21. Folstein MF, Folstein S, McHugh PR. "Mini-mental state": a practical method for grading the cognitive state of patients for the clinician. *Journal of Psychiatric Research.* 1975; **12**: 189–98.

22. Crum RM, Anthony JC, Bassett SS, Folstein MF. Population-based norms for the mini-mental state examination by age and educational level. *Journal of the American Medical Association.* 1993; **269**: 2386–91.

23. Anthony JC, LeResche L, Niaz U *et al.* Limits of the 'Mini-Mental State' as a screening test for dementia and delirium among hospital patients. *Psychological Medicine.* 1982; **12**: 397–408.

* 24. Breitbart W, Rosenfeld B, Roth A *et al.* The Memorial Delirium Assessment scale. *Journal of Pain and Symptom Management.* 1997; **13**: 128–37.

* 25. Lawlor PG, Nekolaichuk C, Gagnon B *et al.* Clinical utility, factor analysis, and further validation of the memorial delirium assessment scale in patients with advanced cancer: Assessing delirium in advanced cancer. *Cancer.* 2000; **88**: 2859–67.

26. Fadul N, Kaur G, Zhang T *et al.* 16th International Congress on Care of the Terminally Ill. Montreal, Canada, 2006.

* 27. Cherny N. Cancer pain: principles of assessment and syndromes. In: Berger A, Portenoy RK, Weissman DE (eds). *Principles and practice of supportive oncology.* Philadelphia, PA: Lippincott-Raven, 1998: 3–42.

28. Portenoy RK. The physical examination in cancer pain assessment. *Seminars in Oncology Nursing.* 1997; **13**: 25–9.

29. Sloan PA, Donnelly MB, Schwartz RW. Cancer pain assessment and management by housestaff. *Pain.* 1996; **67**: 475–81.

30. Grossman SA. Assessment of cancer pain: a continuous challenge. *Supportive Care in Cancer.* 1994; **2**: 105–10.

31. Grossman SA, Sheidler VR, Swedeen K *et al.* Correlation of patient and caregiver ratings of cancer pain. *Journal of Pain and Symptom Management.* 1991; **6**: 53–7.

* 32. Cleeland CS, Ryan KM. Pain assessment: global use of the Brief Pain Inventory. *Annals of the Academy of Medicine, Singapore.* 1994; **23**: 129–38.

* 33. Melzack R. The short-form McGill pain questionnaire. *Pain.* 1987; **30**: 191–7.

34. Fishman B, Pasternak S, Wallenstein SL *et al.* The memorial pain assessment card: a valid instrument for the evaluation of cancer pain. *Cancer.* 1987; **60**: 1151–8.

* 35. McGrath PA. Pain control. In: Doyle D, Hanks GWC, MacDonald N (eds). *Oxford textbook of palliative medicine,* 2nd edn. Oxford: Oxford University Press, 1998: 1013–31.

36. Caraceni A, Mendoza TR, Mencaglia E *et al.* A validation study of an Italian version of the Brief Pain Inventory (Breve Questionario per al Valutazione del Dolore). *Pain.* 1996; **65**: 87–92.

37. Graham C, Bond SS, Gerkovich MM, Cook MR. Use of the McGill Pain Questionnaire in the assessment of cancer pain: replicability and consistency. *Pain.* 1980; **8**: 377–87.

38. Dudgeon D, Raubertas RF, Rosenthal SN. The short-form McGill Pain Questionnaire in chronic cancer pain. *Journal of Pain and Symptom Management.* 1993; **8**: 191–5.

39. Glare P, Virik K. Independent prospective validation of the PaP score in terminally patients referred to a hospital-based palliative medicine consultation service. *Journal of Pain and Symptom Management.* 2001; **22**: 891–8.

* 40. Bruera E, MacDonald S. Audi Methods: the Edmonton symptom assessment system. In: Higginson I (ed.). *Clinical audit in palliative care.* Oxford: Radcliffe Medical Press, 1993: 61–77.

* 41. Foley KM. Supportive care and quality of life. In: De Vita VT, Hellman S, Rosenberg SA (eds). *Cancer principles and practice of oncology,* 5th edn. Philadelphia, PA: Lippincott-Raven, 1997: 2807–41.

42. Moore RD, Bone LR, Geller G *et al.* Prevalence, detection, and treatment of alcoholism in hospitalized patients. *Journal of the American Medical Association.* 1989; **261**: 403–7.

43. Baker A, Bowring L, Brignell A, Kafford D. Chronic pain management in cognitively impaired patients: a preliminary research project. *Perspectives.* 1996; **20**: 4–8.

44. Farrell MJ, Katz B, Helme RD. The impact of dementia on the pain experience. *Pain.* 1996; **67**: 7–15.

* 45. Fisher-Morris M, Gelletly A. The experience and expression of pain in Alzheimer patients. *Age and Ageing.* 1997; **26**: 497–500.

46. Porter FL, Malhotra KM, Wolf CM *et al.* Dementia and response to pain in the elderly. *Pain.* 1996; **68**: 413–21.

47. Robinson D, Bucci J, Fenn H. Pain assessment in the Alzheimer's patient. *Journal of the American Geriatrics Society.* 1995; **43**: 318–19.

48. Bruera E, Fainsinger R, Miller MJ, Kuehn N. The assessment of pain intensity in patients with cognitive failure: a preliminary report. *Journal of Pain and Symptom Management.* 1992; **7**: 267–70.

49. Portenoy RK, Foley KM, Inturrisi CE. The nature of opioid responsiveness and its implications for neuropathic pain: new hypothesis derived from studies of opioid infusion. *Pain.* 1990; **43**: 273–86.

50. Lamerton R. *Care of the dying.* New York, NY: Penguin, 1980.

51. Mount B. Medical applications of heroin. *Canadian Medical Association Journal.* 1979; **120**: 405–7.

52. Twycross R. Opioids. In: Wall P, Melzack R (eds). *Textbook of pain.* Edinburgh: Churchill Livingstone, 1984: 686–701.

53. Banning A, Stugren P, Henriksen H. Treatment outcome in a multidisciplinary cancer pain clinic. *Pain.* 1991; **47**: 129–34.

54. Bruera E, Brenneis C, Michaud M, MacDonald RN. Influence of the pain and symptom control team (PSCT) on the patterns of treatment of pain and other symptoms in a cancer center. *Journal of Pain and Symptom Management.* 1989; **4**: 112–16.

* 55. Coyle N, Adelhart J, Foley KM, Portenoy RK. Character of terminal illness in the advanced cancer patient: pain and other symptoms during the last four weeks of life. *Journal of Pain and Symptom Management.* 1990; **5**: 83–93.

* 56. Grond S, Zech D, Schug SA *et al.* Validation of World Health Organization guidelines for cancer pain relief during the last days and hours of life. *Journal of Pain and Symptom Management.* 1991; **6**: 411–22.

57. American Joint Committee for Cancer Staging and End Result Reporting. *Manual of staging of cancer.* Chicago, IL: American Joint Committee for Cancer Staging and End Result Reporting.

58. Paterson AHG. Clinical staging and its prognostic significance. In: Stall B (ed.). *Pointers to cancer prognosis.* Dordrecht: Nijhoff, 1988: 37–48.

* 59. Fainsinger RL, Nekolaichuk CL, Lawlor PG *et al.* A multicenter study of the revised Edmonton Staging System for classifying cancer pain in advanced cancer patients. *Journal of Pain and Symptom Management.* 2005; **29**: 224–37.

* 60. Nekolaichuk CL, Fainsinger RL, Lawlor PG. A validation study of a pain classification system for advanced cancer patients using content experts: the Edmonton Classification System for Cancer Pain. *Palliative Medicine.* 2005; **19**: 466–76.

* 61. Higginson I. Audit methods: validation and in-patient use. In: Higginson I (ed.). *Clinical audit in palliative care.* Oxford: Radcliffe Medical Press, 1993: 48–54.

5

Psychological evaluation of patient and family

BARBARA MONROE

Introduction	48	Children	54
What is special about cancer pain?	49	Sexuality and intimacy	55
Coping and adaptation	49	Assessment and coping mechanisms	55
Assessment	50	Risk assessment for depression, suicide, and anxiety	56
The importance of effective communication skills	52	Conclusions	58
The importance of the family	52	References	58
Family assessment – practical steps	53		

KEY LEARNING POINTS

- The individual's experience of pain is a complex and multidimensional phenomenon.
- Psychological distress is key in the patient's experience of cancer.
- Social support is a key factor in maintaining coping and promoting adaptation; it also strongly influences care options.
- Pain assessments must include screening for psychological distress and social support.

- Family and informal carers should be involved in assessments and treatment plans and may also need support in their own right.
- Attention to effective and appropriate communication is vital.
- Psychological interventions add usefully to physical treatments for pain.
- Depression and anxiety are common in patients with cancer. Effective screening and appropriate treatment can help to prevent adverse consequences for patients.

INTRODUCTION

The individual's experience of pain is a multidimensional phenomenon with physiological, sensory, behavioral, cognitive, and affective components and therefore demands a multidimensional assessment. To acknowledge the role of psychological factors in pain[1] in no way denies the physical component and the need to treat. It is, however, increasingly recognized that physical modalities alone may not be sufficient to help those who fear the meaning of pain and feel a sense of decreased control over their lives. Gamsa's[2] thorough review of the psychological

factors in chronic pain concludes that, "systematic studies show that anxiety and depression contribute to pain, that certain personality disorders and cognitive styles are associated with chronic pain and that in some cases pain is maintained by psychological rewards." There is evidence that psychological approaches have added useful interventions to physical treatments in multidisciplinary pain clinics[3] and in oncology and palliative care settings.[4, 5, 6, 7] Psychological distress is key in the patient's experience of cancer.[8, 9, 10] It interacts with physical distress and perhaps survival.[11, 12] It is influenced by perceptions of family and social support, attributions of meaning and hope, and the perceived degree of personal control. Zaza and Baine's review[13] of cancer pain and psychosocial factors found strong evidence of an association between increased pain and increased distress and moderate evidence for an association with decreased levels of social activity and support. They conclude that good pain assessment should include screening for psychological distress.

An acknowledgement of the links between psychological state and pain should not be used to manage the frustrations of healthcare providers at the failure of pharmacological efforts by shifting the "blame" to the patient with an alternative diagnosis that attributes pain to psychological causes. It is clear, however, that attention to the emotional and psychological distress that forms part of the cancer experience for patients and those close to them can diminish suffering, improve quality of life, and prevent problems in bereavement. It is also important that healthcare professionals can distinguish between normal reactions of adjustment to a life-threatening illness and symptoms of clinical psychiatric disorders that are amenable to treatment.

WHAT IS SPECIAL ABOUT CANCER PAIN?

Public attitudes to cancer pain are important.[14] There is a widespread understanding that cancer is potentially fatal and inevitably painful alongside an expectation that any pain may be untreatable. There is evidence that the belief that pain signifies disease progression is associated with elevated pain intensity.[15, 16] The process by which pain is appraised and interpreted is likely to be a function of psychological, as well as physical factors. Turk et al.[17] conclude that the variability in the occurrence of pain in patients with metastases, as well as across cancer diagnoses, seems to suggest that disease progression is only one of the factors accounting for the pain experienced by cancer patients. Beliefs, meaning, expectations, and mood will play an important role in modulating the pain experience of cancer patients.[18] In Barkwell's study,[19] patients with cancer were divided into three groups according to the meaning they attributed to their disease: challenge, punishment, enemy. Those who saw their illness as a punishment experienced more pain and depression. Another study demonstrated a link between high levels of hope and high levels of coping.[20] Evidence suggests that patients who believe they can control their pain, avoid catastrophizing about their condition, and believe they are not severely disabled, appear to function better than those who do not.[21, 22] Cognitive behavioral therapy is emerging as a useful treatment option.[23, 24]

In general, it is clear that social support is a key factor in maintaining coping and promoting adaptation in the cancer patient.[25, 26] Higher mortality rates have been recorded for cancer patients in the first year after the loss of a spouse, and it was noted that those who were married survived longer than single patients.[27, 28] There is substantial evidence for links between patient and family functioning. Patients with high pain scores tend to express more anxiety about the future of their families,[29] and in turn there is concordance between levels of anxiety in family and patient.[30] There are also links between family depression and patient disability and symptoms.[31] A two-year follow up of over 600 newly diagnosed cancer patients found a strong relationship between the number and severity of unresolved concerns in the patients and the later development of anxiety disorder and depressive illness.[32] Another study found that the majority of cancer patients express most concern about their family's future and their own loss of independence, the number of concerns being clearly related to the degree of their psychological distress.[33] This is in contrast to an earlier study of hospice patients in which pain and symptom control were found to be the most important concern,[34] a difference that might be partly explained by deficits in communication skills. Evidence showed that hospice patients had a strong bias to selectively disclose physical symptoms and that nurses did not elicit or register patients' concerns accurately.[35] Unsatisfactory pain relief has also been correlated with relatives who had limited information about the death and found it hard to discuss the issues with clinical staff.[36] There are suggestions that longer illness duration is related to lessened mood disturbance and that a rapid course of terminal illness may lead to diminished well-being.[37] When pain in dying patients is lessened, their ability to adapt psychologically is increased. This cluster of results clearly highlights the necessity to assess patients' social and familial networks and any concerns they may have about them. It also emphasizes that, as the quality of life of patients and families is intertwined, the patient and family should be treated as the unit of care.

All of the studies confirm that pain is a complex phenomenon and that helping people with cancer pain needs much more than skilled drug prescribing.[38] Good pain control will take into account the society and culture of the patient,[39] will seek to understand the psychological processes of the individual in coping with stress, and will provide excellent communication and support where appropriate to patient and family. It is important to remember that with appropriate pain and symptom interventions and good social support, some dying patients score levels of self-esteem and well-being similar to those of healthy populations.[40]

COPING AND ADAPTATION

A diagnosis of cancer brings huge losses, both actual and potential, not only for the individual with cancer, but also for those close to him or her: loss of physical health, body image, independence, career and status, normal family life, predictability, self-esteem, motivation, meaning, and sometimes interpersonal relationships. Most profoundly, patients will experience a draining diminution in their self-confidence and their ability to control their own lives.[41] Saunders[42] created the concept of total pain (social, emotional, physical, and spiritual) to describe the experience of suffering. It is usefully extended in the World Health Organization (WHO) components of pain diagram (**Figure 5.1**).

The individual exists in a context in which body, mind, and spirit combine with family and broader relationship networks, community, and society. This framework is helpfully encapsulated in **Figure 5.2**.

Lazarus and Folkman[45] defined coping as individuals' efforts to manage demands that are perceived as likely to exceed their resources. Behaviors are usually aimed at problem-solving by altering the relationship between the person and his or her environment, changing the perception of events, or changing the environment itself. Denial, anger, avoidance, regression, rationalization, intellectualization, and attachment are all common coping mechanisms. Whether a coping strategy is determined to be helpful or unhelpful is often a question of viewpoint.[46] No one way of coping is inherently more desirable; the important issue is whether it is effective for patients and not damaging to those close to them. Weisman[47] suggests that adaptive coping involves

confronting problems, revising plans, keeping communication open, a willingness to use the assistance of others, and the ability to maintain an appropriate sense of optimism and hope. The ability to cope successfully with any crisis depends on having various kinds of resources, for example personal, social, medical, and financial. The extent and availability of such resources will influence adaptation. Variables such as social class, socioeconomic status, culture and ethnicity, age, gender, phase and nature of illness, and the behavior of healthcare providers will also influence the availability and choice of coping mechanisms and styles.[48]

ASSESSMENT

The National Council for Palliative Care[49] provides a helpful definition of psychosocial care, stating that it is "concerned with the psychological and emotional well-being of the patient and their family/carers, including issues of self esteem, insight into, and adaptation to the illness and its consequences, communication, social functioning and relationships." The objective of the psychological assessment is to maximize effective intervention, which will be aimed at reducing the impact of

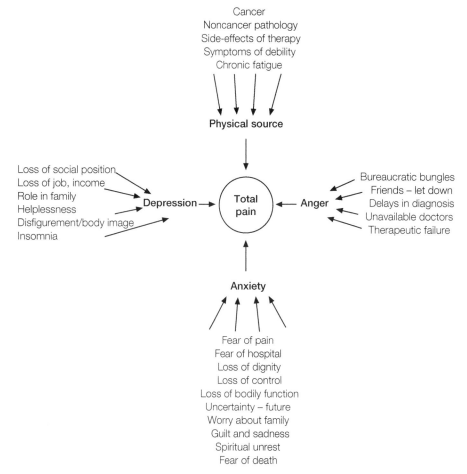

Figure 5.1 Components of pain (after World Health Organization).[43]

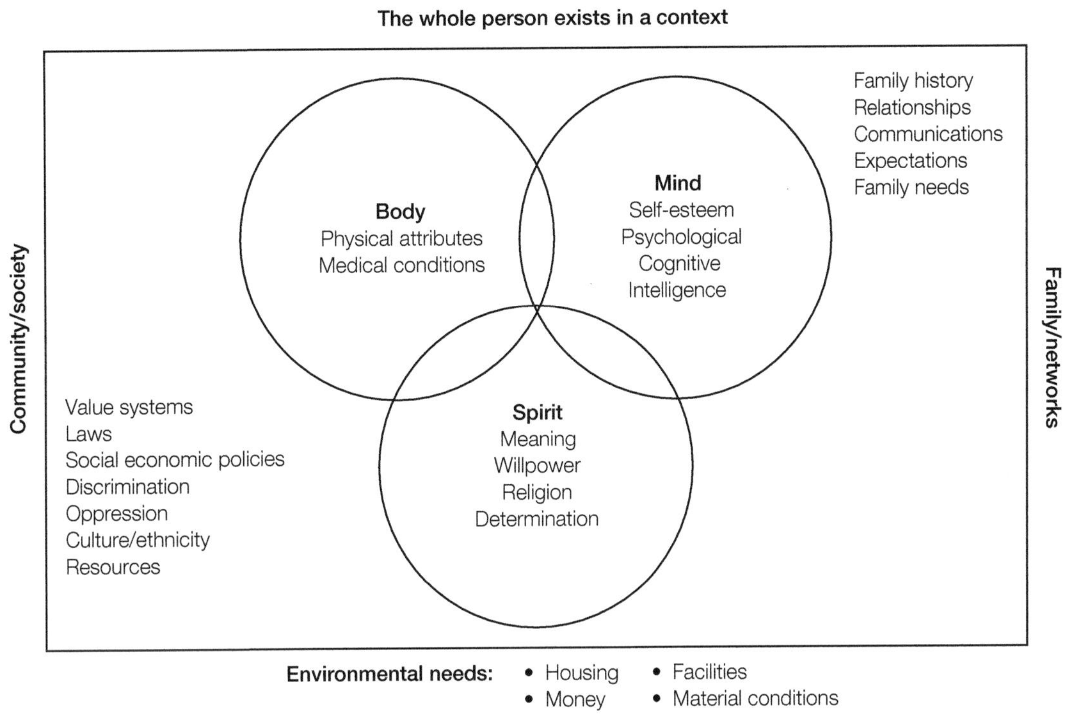

The whole person exists in a context

Figure 5.2 Framework for holistic assessment (redrawn from Oliviere *et al.*[44] with permission).

existing losses, preventing further losses, promoting coping, and providing a sense of control and engagement in the decision-making process. Options will be maximized if individuals are given an adequate flow of information at the pace of their choosing and an opportunity to express and, where possible, share their feelings and help to preserve relationships.[44] Assessment is not a one-off process.[45] Assessments should be made early and often. People change their minds and circumstances alter. It is often part of an indistinguishable cycle with intervention; indeed, the assessment process itself will often be therapeutic. The aim is to create a partnership between the patient and those close to him or her and the healthcare team.

Randall and Downie[50] have emphasized the moral and ethical issues evident in questioning individuals and those close to them about personal and sensitive information. It is important to agree with the ill person and the family the reason for enquiries, to obtain consent, and to check on it at regular intervals: "Please let me know if there is something I ask that you would rather not discuss." Patients should always be asked if they would like to be seen alone or with someone else and, if so, with whom. It is also important to discuss confidentiality and with whom information may be shared, both within the patient's family and friendship network and within the professional team. Good professional recording and communication are vital if effective care is to be achieved and duplication of enquiry avoided. The use of genograms and ecomaps can assist healthcare professionals to

record information in a clear, easily updated manner that leaves the patient in control of the material disclosed.[44, 51] Such pictorial mapping generates additional information about roles, patterns of communication, and losses and gaps in care.[52, 53]

Assessments may be informal or follow predetermined formats, including the use of questionnaires such as the Hospital Anxiety and Depression Scale. It may be helpful to think of psychological risk assessment divided into: (1) predisposing factors, such as previous unresolved losses; and (2) perpetuating factors, such as long-standing marital difficulties. Whatever the format, assessments will contain four main perspectives: (1) the individual, (2) the family and those close to the individual, (3) physical resources, and (4) social resources.[54]

The individual

A psychosocial assessment aims to discover what changes the patient thinks the illness has brought, who or what currently provides support, any gaps in the support network, and the patient's reaction to the illness and its implications for his or her values, beliefs, and aims.

Helpful questions include: What worries you most about your illness? What is helping most at the moment? What has kept you going at other difficult times? Has being ill made any difference to what you believe in? What is the worst thing at the moment? Is there anyone you are especially worried about?

Family, friends, and carers

An assessment will cover:

- the effect of the illness on family roles and relationships;
- personal histories of family members and any likely impact on caring capacity;
- life cycle issues for the family, e.g. births, children leaving home, retirement;
- previous crises and how they were handled and additional concurrent crises, e.g. job loss;
- the presence of other vulnerable individuals in the family, e.g. someone with a learning disability, a dependent elderly relative.

Physical resources

Assumptions must not be made about the physical resources available to individuals. Housing, money, employment, and unmet physical needs, such as the lack of a commode, can become the most important concerns of the patient or family.[55, 56] They will often not be disclosed unless specifically enquired about by the professional as patients may assume that they are not appropriate subject matter. Patients threatened with eviction for rent arrears because they can no longer work will find it difficult to approach symptom control and treatment compliance in a straightforward way.

Social resources

The patient and family must be set within a context of their community and social network, which may include:

- informal and formal caring resources, e.g. neighbors, churches, social and healthcare agencies;
- culture and ethnicity – there may be specific requirements or difficulties based on religious or cultural expectations;[57, 58, 59]
- potential discrimination – some groups in society are less able than others to voice their needs, e.g. the very poor, the profoundly deaf, those with learning disabilities.[60]

All of the above will be set within the laws and value systems of the particular society.

THE IMPORTANCE OF EFFECTIVE COMMUNICATION SKILLS

Effective assessments and intervention depend on effective communication. Respect and a nonjudgmental attitude are the key to establishing trust. Patients are clear about what they want from healthcare professionals: respect, approachability, to be listened to, an unhurried attitude, prompt appointments, repeated explanations of treatments and their side effects, continuity of care, honesty, referrals to other specialists, and sensitivity to psychological issues.[61] Despite Randall and Downie's[50] rather sanguine view of communication skills in health care professionals – "Genuine professional concern for the patient's welfare will naturally lead to effective communication" – numerous studies have demonstrated deficits in their assessment and communication skills.[62, 63, 64] Effective communication is a repeated process that returns control to the patient and helps the family to regain confidence.[65] Unhelpful communication can imply that the truth is too dangerous to share or confronts people with a truth for which they are unprepared or which they are unwilling to receive. Information should be offered in a variety of forms (verbal, written, taped) and interpreters provided where appropriate.[66] It must always be remembered that patients have the right not to know information.

Attention to the beginning and ending of meetings can increase the efficacy of assessment and intervention. It is important, for example, to consider who should attend – patient, family, friends, relevant professionals – and to make proper introductions. On closure there should be a time warning and a "catch all" – "We've got about five minutes left, is there anything else that's important for you to mention?" Decisions and agreements should be clearly summarized and the time and date of the next meeting confirmed.

THE IMPORTANCE OF THE FAMILY

Family and friends are important as informal carers for patients with cancer. Increasing numbers of patients are receiving the majority of their care at home. A systematic review of the factors influencing home deaths in cancer patients indicated that two strong determinants were living with relatives and having extended family support.[67] Regarded as a resource to the patient and as potential coworkers with the professional team, it is important that friends and family are supported if they are to continue with their task. Furthermore, depression and anxiety in the family are linked to patient difficulties. The burden of caring has been described in many studies, and there are reports of increased risk of physical and psychological morbidity among carers.[68, 69] Caregivers face conflicting demands and conflicting advice; they often have to put their own lives on hold.[70]

A study that examined the concerns of informal carers during the palliative care phase found that 84 percent reported above normal levels of psychological distress and 41 percent experienced high levels of strain related to caregiving.[71] Life restrictions, emotional distress, and limited support were among the reported causes of strain. Unmet practical needs are also cited as a source of stress in many studies, along with the failure of healthcare professionals to meet carers' learning needs adequately.[72, 73] It is also clear that, if their educational needs about patient care remain unmet, family members can become a barrier to effective symptom management rather than a means of supporting patient compliance.[74, 75] It is, however, important to note that many carers see caring as a natural extension of existing relationships and report satisfaction and fulfillment in caring tasks.[76, 77]

The family and those close to the patient may also be viewed as co-clients.[78] Care for the family has an important preventive health component as family members will live on into a future shaped in part by their experience of the patient's illness and perhaps death. As Parkes[79] memorably reminds us, "Cancer can affect a family in much the same way as it invades the body, causing it to deteriorate if left untreated." The family is a complex system that changes over time. It has a past and a future that exert pressures on the present. Patients will also belong to other networks of relationships, some of which may be more significant than those with biological links. Unless a clear assessment is undertaken, help for the family can get lost in anxiety for the patient. Family life deteriorates along with the patient, but patient and family members will have different needs at different times. Family members may require different types of support and sometimes have conflicting agendas. Internal and external cultural expectations about the roles, rights, and responsibilities of individual family members will also have an impact.[80] Changes in family structure, e.g. divorce, separation, stepfamilies, geographic distance, which are increasingly common, may add to the burden of informal carers. The literature[81, 82, 83] is clear about their needs, which are listed below.

- Adequate nursing support and confident, committed family doctors providing coordinated care.
- Access to specialist care where appropriate.
- The assurance that good symptom control is being given to the patient.
- Knowledge of available support and advocacy to obtain it in time, including practical help with household tasks, personal care and equipment and financial support where necessary.
- Access, where appropriate, to respite care, either as an inpatient or as a home-sitting service. Many will be struggling with rapid and frightening changes in the physical needs and capacities of the ill person and the consequent physical caring tasks.
- Knowledge about the illness and training in skills to enhance patient comfort.
- Emotional support directed specifically at the carer.

Ideally, individual time for an assessment and response to carers' needs should be negotiated at the start of the relationship between the professional and patient and family so that it is accepted as a normal part of the contract. If separate meetings are offered only when difficulties arise, they may cause suspicion and guilt.

There are relatively few studies about the psychological state of families of a terminally ill patient, although Kristjanson[84] has produced a useful review. Most studies have examined morbidity after bereavement,[85] although in an important study of families affected by cancer, Kissane et al.[86] demonstrated a relationship between family functioning during the illness and adaptive grief outcome. The study found spouses' perception of overall family coping as being poor to be correlated with greater grief intensity and depression and poorer social adjustment. Family coping that was perceived as adaptive was linked with a good outcome. This research indicates both the need for an assessment of family functioning as part of good clinical care in order to identify families at risk and the importance of collaborative partnership. What counts is individuals' own view of whether or not they are coping as a family. Professionals must therefore find out from the family how they view themselves and their difficulties. Kissane and colleagues[87] have developed a short self-administered family relationships index to identify families at risk. Their research indicates positive outcomes for limited, focused family sessions provided to at risk families.[88]

Significant factors which seem to predispose a family to emotional risk include:[89]

- recent diagnosis of advanced illness;
- anger about delays in diagnosis or treatment;
- close dependent relationship with the ill person;
- other dependants in the family, e.g. children, elderly parents;
- carer isolated with little perceived support;
- carer unable to be realistic about the patient's prognosis;
- previous or current mental health problems or previous losses, especially if recent;
- evidence of dependency on drugs or alcohol;
- practical difficulties such as housing or finance;
- estranged family members or significant conflict within the family;
- history of abuse or trauma.

FAMILY ASSESSMENT – PRACTICAL STEPS

A family assessment should include the following steps.

1. Find out how everyone defines the problem, but be neutral. Every individual will need to feel that the professional understands their point of view.
2. Consider the impact of the illness on roles and tasks and any care gaps.
3. Does the illness challenge the belief structure of the family? Has it brought unfinished business to the fore?

4. Anticipate and acknowledge differences and conflicts of need. "You are both feeling lonely and resentful. You want to help your mother but you are worried about giving up your job. You would like to go home to your daughter but you are anxious about the burden this might place on her."
5. Help people negotiate and compromise, which often means assisting them to find a dignified way to retreat from fixed positions.
6. Facilitate the sharing of emotional pain and anxiety. Generalization may help. "Many families tell us … What is it like for you?"
7. Be realistic and encourage a focus on concrete and achievable goals.
8. Recognize and respect family coping mechanisms.
9. Outline clearly the resources available to the family and find out which they would like to use. Do not coerce them.

CHILDREN

Many research studies have made clear the cost of inadequate support and involvement for children facing serious illness in someone close to them.[90, 91, 92, 93] Children may respond with emotional and behavioral disturbance at the time, throughout childhood, and on into adulthood. When the likely outcome of the illness is death, studies confirm the importance of children's predeath experiences in mediating and influencing the course and outcome of bereavement.[94] Significant factors include the openness of communication in the family, the relationship of the child with the ill person, the availability of community support, and the extent to which the child's parenting needs have continued to be met. When someone in the family is very ill, everyone is affected, including children. However, adults' desires to protect children often leave children confused and alone with their fears and fantasies, which may be much worse than the reality. Children are always aware when something significant is happening in the family; they overhear conversations, are aware of body language and practical changes, and often pick up adult gossip from school friends. They also sense adult anxiety. However, they do not always ask unprompted questions, sometimes keeping their worries to themselves out of a desire to protect the adults and family life.

Children need:

- respect and acknowledgement;
- information that is clear, simple, truthful, and repeated about what is happening and why and what might happen next;
- reassurance about practical issues and about their own care;
- reassurance that nothing they did or said made the illness happen;

- a chance to talk about feelings with adults who are prepared to share theirs;
- appropriate involvement in helping the patient.

Parents have good reasons for feeling anxious about talking to their children, and these are often shared by professionals. They are often struggling to maintain their own control in the midst of uncertainty and strong emotion. They may underestimate what a child understands or worry that saying the wrong thing may make matters worse. It is often important to support parents with their own emotional needs before they can contemplate addressing those of their children. The aim should always be to help parents to talk to their own children themselves, to give them the confidence and skills to begin to assess and meet their own children's needs. Christ et al.'s research[95] demonstrates the value of giving parents information about their children's developmental needs. Sandler et al.'s studies[96] show promise for a family-based cognitive behavioral intervention.

Helping parents to talk to children

The following guidance should be given to parents.[97, 98]

- Acknowledge that it will feel uncomfortable and distressing.
- Reassure them that information does not need to be given all at one time, but step by step, using age-appropriate vocabulary and not being afraid to say "I don't know." Offer suggestions about possible explanations.
- Warn parents not to be surprised if children change the subject or focus on the practical. "What's for tea?"
- Help them to understand and respond to their children's emotions and sometimes changed behavior. For example, children may be angry at having their routines upset. They may become more clingy or more naughty.
- Help parents to involve other people in their child's network: friends, relatives, teachers.
- Offer parents resources, such as booklets to read themselves and books to read with their children.
- Parents need to think about:
  - What their children know already. It often helps to start with children's own observations so that any misapprehensions can be corrected. For example, "What have you noticed that's different about mummy? Why do you think mummy is ill?"
  - What they want their children to know, e.g. what the doctors have said, what the treatment is, and what the side effects might be.
  - What the children want to know, remembering that they may not ask, e.g. "Is it my fault? Is cancer catching? Will daddy die?"

- Always work with what seems manageable and comfortable to parents themselves. There is no one right way, only the way that is right for them and their family.

SEXUALITY AND INTIMACY

Studies have documented the importance of sexuality as a quality of life issue for patients and their partners.[99] There is a large body of evidence confirming that sexual behaviors, self concepts, and relationships are deeply affected in many adults with disease.[100, 101] Studies also confirm the efficacy of sexual counseling programs[102] alongside a conviction among healthcare professionals that sexuality is an integral part of their responsibility toward patients and those close to them.[103, 104] Yet research also demonstrates that professionals seldom address the issue.[105, 106] There remains a gap between theory and practice. It is clearly inappropriate to expect every healthcare professional to be a specialist in sexual counseling. However, the responsibility for making an assessment of whether or not this is an important area for the individual belongs to all[107] and evidence suggests that many cancer patients prefer to receive information and support from their generic team.[108]

Potential sexual problems relating to illness fall into two linked categories: (1) mechanical problems that are the direct physical consequences of illness or treatment and (2) the emotional consequences of the illness, including changes in the way people feel about themselves and each other and their body image. Professionals need to be able to initiate dialog and discussion, to identify and assess need, and to provide first-line help with the offer of referral on for specialist support if appropriate.[109] It is important to avoid assumptions, for example that sex is less important to older people or to someone not currently in a relationship. Individuals and those close to them need time to come to terms with their illness and its implications. Anticipation and honest discussion can reduce anxiety, so information should be given in advance wherever possible, in both verbal and written form.

Most people will not ask for help spontaneously. Learning to ask is the professional's responsibility. A recent study suggested that when this was done the majority of patients with advanced cancer actively wished to discuss this aspect of their lives.[110]

Taking a sexual history

The following approach may be helpful.

1. See people separately and together.
2. Use questions that move from the general to the specific. "How has your illness/treatment affected your work/home/sex life?"
3. Use questions that give permission. "Do you have any worries about the sexual side of things?"
4. Use phrasing that implies that most people experience these kinds of doubts. "People often have questions they'd like to ask about the sexual side of life."
5. Find an appropriate and understandable vocabulary for the individual.
6. "In what ways has your illness changed the way you feel about yourself as a man/woman/partner?"
7. "How long have you been together? Has the physical side of your relationship been important to you/your partner?"
8. "In what ways has your illness changed the way you can get close to your partner?"
9. "What do you want most from your partner at the moment? What do you think your partner's reaction would be?"

Professionals should always be alert to the possibility of violent or abusive relationships.[111]

ASSESSMENT AND COPING MECHANISMS

Denial

Some patients, or those close to them, may deny the diagnosis or the implications of the disease. Denial is a phase of the coping process that revises or reinterprets a portion of a painful reality. Professionals should tackle denial carefully and consider whose problem it is. People are only at risk when their denial of their symptoms or issues around their illness is so persistent that it jeopardizes aspects of their physical well-being and ultimate prognosis, or the well-being of those close to them.[47]

Questions to ask include:

- is denial affecting help-seeking behavior and compliance?
- is denial reducing emotional distress?
- is denial leaving the patient in immediate, persistent, or extreme anxiety?
- is the denial temporary or persistent? Many people move in and out of denial;
- has the information about the diagnosis or treatment been given in a way that is clearly understandable?
- have any underlying major psychiatric disorders or organic mental disorders been excluded?

"What if?" questions may help those in denial as they allow the maintenance of some distance from the painful truth. "Imagine for a moment that you weren't around to look after your children. In those circumstances who would you want to be involved?" Other approaches might include image work, art, or music therapy, or very gentle probing. "I know you like to look on the bright side of things but are there ever moments when you find yourself thinking less positive thoughts?"

Anger

Extreme anger can make it hard to assess what is important for the patient or what might be potentially helpful interventions. Strategies to manage anger include the following.[112]

- Remember that anger is an energy that can be positively harnessed.
- Invite people to sit down in a quiet place. Speak calmly. "Can you explain to me why you are feeling like this?"
- Avoid becoming defensive or patronizing.
- Acknowledge the anger, legitimizing it where appropriate. Be honest if a mistake has been made.
- Recognize the feelings that may be underneath anger: loneliness, fear, a sense of injustice.
- Encourage expression. "Just how angry have you been?"
- Try to suggest a coping strategy, e.g. registering a complaint, talking to a relative.
- Assess the danger to yourself and stop the interview if there is a risk of physical aggression.

RISK ASSESSMENT FOR DEPRESSION, SUICIDE, AND ANXIETY

Depression

Depression is a common symptom among cancer patients, although reports of its prevalence vary enormously.[40, 113] A systematic review of depression amongst patients with advanced cancer suggests that it is very common in that population.[114] There are strong links between poor functional capacity and depression and between depression and chronic pain.[115, 116] Failure to recognize depression can enormously increase physical and psychological suffering for both patients and those close to them. Severe depression can make symptom management more difficult, reduce compliance, and lead to death wishes or a desire for euthanasia.[117] Some research suggests that patients with depression in the context of serious illness may have a shorter life expectancy.[118] It is important to distinguish between depressed mood, which is often present as part of a natural adjustment reaction, and depressive illness, which is a clinical entity and severely disabling condition that may be potentially life-threatening because of the associated risk of suicide[119] and which benefits from antidepressant therapy and psychological support. It is always important to rule out depression due to a medical condition, e.g. hypercalcemia, hypothyroidism.

A major depressive episode, as widely accepted and encapsulated in the DSM-IV,[120] can be described as the presence of depressed mood or loss of interest or pleasure lasting most of the day, for at least two weeks, in the presence of four or more of the following:

- significant loss or increase of appetite/weight;
- psychomotor retardation or agitation almost every day;
- loss of energy or fatigue nearly every day;
- feelings of worthlessness or excessive or inappropriate guilt nearly every day;
- impaired concentration or memory nearly every day;
- recurrent thoughts of death;
- recurrent suicidal ideation.

In the case of patients with severe depression it is important to start drug treatment and then to provide other supportive interventions, such as cognitive therapy, relaxation therapy, and personal counseling.[121] One of the difficulties with the quoted criteria is that several of them are somatic in nature and can be confused with the symptoms of cancer itself, such as loss of weight and energy. It is therefore important to consider them within the context of the physical illness. Various writers have suggested distinctive features of depression in cancer patients, such as social withdrawal, complete failure to respond to good news or funny situations, persistent tearfulness, a feeling of being a burden when this is obviously not the case, chronic pain resistant to treatment, and perceiving the illness as a punishment.[122, 123]

Healthcare workers assessing depression should not make assumptions. The patient must be asked directly: "Do you feel depressed?" Hotopf[124] offers a helpful list of key questions to elicit a patient's narrative of illness and suggests the variant, "Have you been depressed most of the time in the last two weeks?" Several studies have demonstrated that, although medical personnel are good at picking up pain and physical problems, they are much less effective in detecting psychosocial problems.[35] In one study, 58 percent of patients identified problems not mentioned by professionals, and 52 percent of these were psychosocial.[125] It therefore follows that a careful history from both patient and close family or friends is essential, including whether the symptoms represent a change from previous functioning. Predisposing factors are:

- a past personal or family history of depressive illness;
- a previous suicide attempt;
- lack of social support;
- recent stressful events;
- alcohol or other substance abuse.

Diagnostic instruments, such as the Present State Examination and structured clinical interviews, are designed to aid differential diagnosis, but they are time-consuming to administer and require special training. Screening instruments such as the Goldberg Health Questionnaire are also available, but these, too, take time to administer. Another possibility is the use of a self-rating instrument such as the Hospital Anxiety and Depression Scale (HADS). Moorey et al.[126] tested the HADS in 560 patients with cancer and concluded that it "seemed to be the best instrument for rapid evaluation of psychological interventions in patients with physical illness." Although the instrument was originally designed to measure severity of anxiety and depression, studies to validate its use as a screening instrument for depression in cancer patients have been carried out.[127] These studies have highlighted some of the drawbacks such as the false-positive and -negative results that emerge with self-screening and the ambiguity of several of the items in patients with poor performance status. General screening questions can play an important role: "How is your morale these days considering what has happened? What can you tell me about how discouraged you ordinarily get?"[47]

More recent research[128] has cast doubt on Chochinov's study[129] of the use of the single question on depression as a reliable diagnostic test.

Suicide

Cancer patients are at an increased risk of suicide relative to the general population, particularly in the final stage of illness.[130, 131] Screening for depressive illness is vital as depression is a factor in 50 percent of all suicides.[132] Uncontrolled pain is also a very important risk factor.[133, 134] Hopelessness is the key variable that links suicide and depression in the general population. In the face of cancer, loss of control and a sense of helplessness are significant factors in suicide vulnerability, as is fatigue.

EVALUATION OF SUICIDE RISK

The following guidelines may be helpful.

- Never be afraid to ask. "How low have you been? Have you ever thought of ending your life? How? When did you think of doing it? What has stopped you?"
- Take threats seriously. Offer appropriate follow up and avoid prohibiting statements such as "You shouldn't talk like that."
- Recognize despair. This gives people a sense of relief and lets them know they are being taken seriously.
- Check for consistency over time. Some episodes are brief and do not reflect a sustained and committed desire to die.
- Discussing suicide openly can acknowledge the individual's need to retain a sense of control over aspects of his or her death and also allow a fuller discussion about preventable fears and anxieties, such as "How will I die? "How might my symptoms be managed?"

- Patients may also need to discuss existential anxieties such as fears of punishment. "What will happen to me after death?"
- Clinicians should also be aware of the danger of the first few weeks on antidepressants, which can lift retardation before improving mood, so that people have the energy to act while remaining very low in spirit.

If suicidal risk is present, it is important to refer the patient to a psychiatrist for a professional consultation. However, it is rarely appropriate to refer patients to specialist psychiatric units. According to Breitbart and Krivo,[135] "The goal of the intervention should not be to prevent suicide at all costs, but to prevent suicide that is driven by desperation," reminding professionals that the vast majority of cancer patients who express suicidal ideation do so while suffering unrecognized and untreated psychiatric disturbances and poorly controlled physical symptoms, especially pain.

Anxiety

Anxiety is a common response to a fear-provoking diagnosis and an uncertain future. However, if present at a clinical level, it can be disabling and is potentially responsive to an active drug regimen.[121] At any level anxiety can reduce the threshold to physical suffering, especially pain, and make the disclosure and resolution of significant practical and emotional concerns much more difficult.[136] Anxiety and depression often occur together, and both will need to be attended to in many situations with cancer patients.[47, 137, 138] A clinical anxiety state may include phobic disorders such as claustrophobia, and panic attacks may occur in stressful situations.

Predisposing factors include:

- a past or family history of an anxiety disorder;
- poor social support;
- recent receipt of bad news;
- previous alcohol or substance abuse;
- unstable environment in childhood/early experience of separation;
- overprotection by family or partner;
- previous experience of a distressing death.

A clinical anxiety state is often indicated when the patient reports feeling extremely apprehensive or tense and sometimes tormented and unable to make decisions. It is dominating and intrusive in quality and will often be self-described as significantly different from normal mood. This mood will have persisted for more than two weeks for more than 50 percent of the time. It will be accompanied by the presence of other anxiety-related symptoms, which can be considered to fall into in four categories.

1. Psychological apprehension: feelings of dread, threat, fear, worries over trivia, irritability.
2. Somatic and autonomic: tremor, diarrhea, sweating, nausea.
3. Vigilance and scanning: poor concentration, insomnia, fatigue on waking, distractability.
4. Motor tension and behavioral symptoms: shakiness, trembling, muscle aches, fatigue, restlessness, angry outbursts, demands for attention, clinging.

It is always important to exclude organic causes such as endocrine and metabolic disorders, alcohol withdrawal, chronic dementing illness, acute confusional state, and drug-induced motor restlessness.

Upon diagnosis of a clinical anxiety state, appropriate pharmacology is essential, with psychotherapeutic support such as cognitive–behavioral therapy, aromatherapy, and relaxation techniques, as well as general emotional support for patient and family.

CONCLUSIONS

Psychological distress is key in the patient and family's experience of cancer and interacts with physical distress.[46, 139] Good pain relief is multidimensional and demands a careful, multifaceted, often multiprofessional, approach that does not need to be hugely sophisticated but knows when to call in specialists. The husband of a woman who died of breast cancer declared that in his opinion, "The great deficits in cancer care lie in communication and the psychological care of patient and family."[140] Skills in psychological evaluation are vital if these deficits are to be remedied. Excellent pharmacology, appropriate information, and emotional support are equally important in our efforts to help those with cancer.

REFERENCES

1. Dworkin RH, Breitbart WS (eds). *Psychosocial aspects of pain: a handbook for health care providers.* Seattle: IASP Press, 2004.
* 2. Gamsa A. The role of psychological factors in chronic pain. II. A critical appraisal. *Pain.* 1994; **57**: 17–29.
* 3. Flor H, Fydrich T, Turk DC. Efficacy of multidisciplinary pain treatment centres: a meta-analytic review. *Pain.* 1992; **49**: 221–30.
* 4. Fallowfield L. Psychosocial interventions in cancer. *British Medical Journal.* 1995; **311**: 1316–17.
* 5. Devine EC. Meta-analysis of the effect of psychoeducational interventions on pain in adults with cancer. *Oncology Nursing Forum.* 2003; **30**: 75–89.
6. Keefe FJ, Abernethy AP, Campbell L. Psychological approaches to understanding and treating disease-related pain. *Annual Review of Psychology.* 2005; **56**: 601–30.
* 7. Meyer TJ, Mark MM. Effects of psychosocial interventions with adult cancer patients: a meta-analysis of randomized experiments. *Health Psychology.* 1995; **14**: 101–08.
* 8. Fawzy FI, Fawzy NW, Arndt LA, Pasnau RO. Critical review of psychosocial interventions in cancer care. *Archives of General Psychiatry.* 1995; **52**: 100–13.
9. Fawzy FI, Fawzy NW, Canada AL. Psychosocial treatment of cancer: an update. *Current Opinion in Psychiatry.* 1998; **52**: 601–5.
* 10. Vachon M, Kristjanson L, Higginson I. Psychosocial issues in palliative care: the patient, the family and the process and outcome of care. *Journal of Pain and Symptom Management.* 1995; **10**: 142–50.
11. Spiegel D, Bloom J, Kraemer HC, Gotheil E. Effect of psychosocial treatment on survival of patients with metastatic cancer. *Lancet.* 1989; **2**: 888–91.
12. Fawzy FI, Fawzy NW, Hyun CS *et al.* Effects of an early structured psychiatric intervention. *Archives of General Psychiatry.* 1993; **50**: 681–9.
* 13. Zaza C, Baine N. Cancer pain and psychosocial factors: a critical review of the literature. *Journal of Pain and Symptom Management.* 2002; **24**: 526–42.
14. Levin DN, Cleeland CS, Dar R. Public attitudes toward cancer pain. *Cancer.* 1985; **56**: 2337–9.
15. Daut RL, Cleeland CS. The prevalence and severity of pain in cancer. *Cancer.* 1982; **50**: 1913–18.
16. Spiegel D, Bloom JR. Pain in metastatic breast cancer. *Cancer.* 1983; **52**: 341–5.
17. Turk DC, Sist TC, Okifuji A *et al.* Adaptation to metastatic cancer pain, regional/local cancer pain and non-cancer pain: role of psychological and behavioural factors. *Pain.* 1998; **74**: 247–56.
18. Jensen MP, Turner JA, Romano JM. Changes in beliefs, catastrophizing and coping are associated with improvement in multidisciplinary pain treatment. *Clinical Psychology.* 2001; **69**: 655–62.
19. Barkwell DP. Ascribed meaning: a critical factor in coping and pain attenuation in patients with cancer-related pain. *Journal of Palliative Care.* 1991; **7**: 5–14.
* 20. Herth K. Fostering hope in terminally-ill people. *Journal of Advanced Nursing.* 1990; **15**: 1250–9.
* 21. Jensen MP, Turner JA, Romano JM, Karoly P. Coping with chronic pain: a critical review of the literature. *Pain.* 1991; **47**: 249–83.
22. Sullivan MJ, Thorne B, Haythornthwaite JA *et al.* Theoretical perspectives on the relation between catastrophizing and pain. *Clinical Journal of Pain.* 2001; **17**: 52–64.
* 23. Morley S, Eccleston C, Williams A. Systematic review and meta-analysis of randomized controlled trials of cognitive behaviour therapy and behavior therapy for chronic pain in adults, excluding headache. *Pain.* 1999; **80**: 1–13.
24. Waters SJ, Campbell LC, Keefe FJ, Carson JW. The essence of cognitive-behavioral pain management. In: Dworkin RH,

Breitbart WS (eds). *Psychosocial aspects of pain: a handbook for healthcare providers.* Seattle: IASP Press, 2004: 261–83.

25. Strang P. Emotional and social aspects of cancer pain. *Acta Oncologica.* 1992; **31**: 323–6.

26. Willey C, Silliman RA. The impact of disease on the social support experiences of cancer patients. *Journal of Psychosocial Oncology.* 1990; **8**: 79–95.

27. Goodwin JS, Hunt WC, Key CR, Samet JM. The effect of marital status on stage, treatment and survival of cancer patients. *Journal of the American Medical Association.* 1987; **258**: 3125–30.

∗ 28. Redd WH, Silberfarb PM, Andersen BL. Physiologic and psychobehavioural research in oncology. *Cancer.* 1991; **67** (Suppl.): 813–22.

29. Strang P. Existential consequences of unrelieved cancer pain. *Palliative Medicine.* 1997; **11**: 299–305.

30. Hodgson C, Higginson I, McDonnell M, Butters E. Family anxiety in advanced cancer: a multicentre prospective study in Ireland. *British Journal of Cancer.* 1997; **76**: 1211–14.

31. Kurtz ME, Kurtz JC, Given CW, Given B. Relationship of caregiver reactions and depression to cancer patients' symptoms, functional states and depression – a longitudinal view. *Social Science Medicine.* 1995; **40**: 837–46.

32. Parle M, Jones B, Maguire P. Maladaptive coping and affective disorders among cancer patients. *Psychological Medicine.* 1996; **26**: 735–44.

33. Heaven CM, Maguire P. The relationship between patients' concerns and psychological distress in a hospice setting. *Psycho-oncology.* 1998; **7**: 502–7.

34. Higginson IJ, McCarthy M. Measuring symptoms in terminal cancer: are pain and dyspnoea controlled? *Journal of the Royal Society of Medicine.* 1989; **82**: 264–7.

35. Heaven CM, Maguire P. Disclosure of concerns by hospice patients and their identification by nurses. *Palliative Medicine.* 1997; **11**: 283–90.

36. Miettinen T, Tilvis R, Karppi P, Arve S. Why is the pain relief of dying patients often unsuccessful? The relatives perspectives. *Palliative Medicine.* 1998; **12**: 429–35.

37. Dobratz MC. Analysis of variables that impact psychological adaptation in home hospice patients. *Hospice Journal.* 1995; **10**: 75–88.

38. Davidson P. Facilitating coping with cancer pain. *Palliative Medicine.* 1988; **2**: 107–14.

39. Otis JD, Cardella LA, Kerns RD. The influence of family and culture on pain. In: Dworkin RH, Breitbart WS (eds). *Psychosocial aspects of pain: a handbook for healthcare providers.* Seattle: IASP Press, 2004: 29–46.

40. Bukberg J, Penman D, Holland JC. Depression in hospitalised cancer patients. *Psychosomatic Medicine.* 1984; **46**: 199–211.

41. Northouse PG, Northouse LL. Communication and cancer: issues confronting patients, health professionals and family members. *Journal of Psychosocial Oncology.* 1987; **5**: 17–46.

42. Saunders C. Introduction – history and challenge. In: Saunders C, Sykes N (eds). *The management of terminal malignant disease*, 3rd edn. London: Edward Arnold, 1993: 1–14.

43. World Health Organization. *Cancer pain relief and palliative care.* Report of a WHO Expert Committee. WHO Technical Report Series 804. Geneva: World Health Organization, 1990: 21.

44. Oliviere D, Hargreaves R, Monroe B. Assessment. In: *Good practices in palliative care: a psychosocial perspective.* Aldershot: Ashgate, 1997: 25–48.

45. Lazarus RS, Folkman S. Coping and adaptation. In: Gentry WD (eds). *The handbook of behavioural medicine.* New York: Guilford, 1984: 282–325.

∗ 46. Vachon M. The emotional problems of the patient in palliative medicine. In: Doyle D, Hanks G, Cherny N, Calman K (eds). *Oxford textbook of palliative medicine*, 3rd edn. Oxford: Oxford University Press, 2004: 961–85.

47. Weisman A. *The coping capacity.* New York: Human Sciences Press, 1986.

48. Field D, Hockey J, Small N (eds). *Death, gender and ethnicity.* London: Routledge, 1997.

49. National Council for Hospice and Specialist Palliative Care Services. *Feeling better: psychosocial care in specialist palliative care.* A discussion paper. Occasional paper 13. London: NCHSPCS, 1997.

50. Randall F, Downie RS. *Palliative care ethics. A companion for all specialties*, 2nd edn. Oxford: Oxford University Press, 1999.

51. Sheldon F. Mapping the support networks. In: *Psychosocial palliative care: good practice in the care of the dying and bereaved.* Cheltenham: Stanley Thornes, 1997: 79–80.

52. Kirschling JM (ed). *Family-based palliative care.* New York: Howarth Press, 1990.

53. McGoldrick M, Gerson R. *Genograms in family assessment.* New York: Norton, 1985.

∗ 54. Monroe B. Social work in palliative medicine. In: Doyle D, Hanks G, Cherny N, Calman K (eds). *Oxford textbook of palliative medicine*, 3rd edn. Oxford: Oxford University Press, 2004: 1007–17.

55. Levy J, Payne M. Audit of welfare benefits advocacy in a palliative care setting. *European Journal of Palliative Care.* 2006; **13**: 15–17.

56. Hughes A. Poverty and palliative care in the US: issues facing the urban poor. *International Journal of Palliative Nursing.* 2005; **11**: 6–13.

57. Oliviere D. Culture and ethnicity. *European Journal of Palliative Care.* 1999; **6**: 53–6.

58. Sheldon F. The cultural and spiritual context of death and bereavement. In: *Psychosocial palliative care – good practice in the care of the dying and bereaved.* Cheltenham: Stanley Thornes, 1997: 17–34.

59. Payne S, Chapman A, Holloway M *et al.* Chinese community views: promoting cultural competence in

palliative care. *Journal of Palliative Care.* 2005; **21**: 111–16.

60. McEnhill L. Disability. In: Oliviere D, Monroe B (eds). *Death, dying and social differences.* Oxford: Oxford University Press, 2004: 97–118.

61. National Cancer Alliance. *Patient-centred cancer services? What patients say.* Oxford: National Cancer Alliance, 1996.

62. Stedeford A. Couples facing death. II. Unsatisfactory communication. *British Medical Journal.* 1981; **283**: 1098–101.

63. Maguire P. Barriers to psychological care of the dying. *British Medical Journal.* 1985; **291**: 1711–13.

64. Chan A, Woodruff RK. Communicating with patients with advanced cancer. *Journal of Palliative Care.* 1997; **13**: 29–33.

∗ 65. Fallowfield L. Communication with the patient and family in palliative medicine. In: Doyle D, Hanks G, Cherny N, Calman K (eds). *Oxford textbook of palliative medicine,* 3rd edn. Oxford: Oxford University Press, 2004: 101–07.

66. Hogbin B, Fallowfield L. Getting it taped – the bad news consultation with cancer patients in a general surgical outpatients department. *British Journal of Hospital Medicine.* 1989; **41**: 330–3.

∗ 67. Gomes B, Higginson IJ. Factors influencing death at home in terminally ill patients with cancer: systematic review. *British Medical Journal.* 2006; **332**: 515–21.

∗ 68. Kinsella G, Cooper B, Picton C. A review of the measurement of caregiver and family burden in palliative care. *Journal of Palliative Care.* 1998; **14**: 37–45.

69. Hinton J. Can home care maintain an acceptable quality of life for patients with terminal cancer and their relatives? *Palliative Medicine.* 1994; **8**: 83–96.

70. Hull M. Sources of stress for hospice care-giving families. In: Kirschling J (ed). *Family-based palliative care.* New York: Howarth, 1990.

71. Payne S, Smith P, Dean S. Identifying the concerns of informal carers in palliative care. *Palliative Medicine.* 1999; **13**: 37–44.

72. Hudson P. The educational needs of lay carers. *European Journal of Palliative Care.* 1998; **5**: 183–6.

73. Kristjanson L, Leis A, Koop P *et al.* Family members' care expectations, care perceptions, and satisfaction with advanced cancer care. *Journal of Palliative Care.* 1997; 1: 5–13.

74. Panke JT, Ferrell BR. Emotional problems in the family. In: Doyle D, Hanks G, Cherny N, Calman K (eds). *Oxford textbook of palliative medicine,* 3rd edn. Oxford: Oxford University Press, 2004: 985–92.

∗ 75. Harding R, Higginson IJ. What is the best way to help caregivers in cancer and palliative care? A systematic literature review of interventions and their effectiveness. *Palliative Medicine.* 2003; **17**: 63–74.

76. Thomas C, Morris SM. Informal carers in cancer contexts. *European Journal of Cancer Care.* 2002; **11**: 178–82.

77. Payne S. Carers and caregivers. In: Oliviere D, Monroe B (eds). *Death, dying and social differences.* Oxford: Oxford University Press, 2004: 181–98.

78. Twigg J. Models of carers: how do social care agencies conceptualise their relationship with informal carers? *Journal of Social Policy.* 1989; **18**: 53–66.

79. Parkes CM. The emotional impact of cancer on patients and their families. *Journal of Oncology and Laryngology.* 1975; **89**: 1271–9.

80. Die-Trill M. The patient from a different culture. In: Holland JC (ed). *Psycho-oncology.* Oxford: Oxford University Press, 1998: 857–66.

81. Sykes N, Pearson S, Chell S. Quality of care: the carer's perspective. *Palliative Medicine.* 1992; **6**: 227–36.

82. Thorpe G. Enabling more dying people to remain at home. *British Medical Journal.* 1993; **307**: 915–18.

∗ 83. Neale B. Informal palliative care: a review of research on needs, standards and service evaluation. Occasional Paper No. 3. Sheffield: Trent Palliative Care Centre, 1991.

∗ 84. Kristjanson LJ. The family's cancer journey: a literature review. *Cancer Nursing.* 1994; **17**: 1–17.

∗ 85. Kissane D, Bloch S. Family grief. *British Journal of Psychiatry.* 1994; **164**: 728–40.

∗ 86. Kissane D, Bloch S, McKenzie D. Family coping and bereavement outcome. *Palliative Medicine.* 1997; **11**: 191–201.

∗ 87. Kissane DW, Bloch S. *Family focused grief therapy. A model of family-centred care during palliative care and bereavement.* Buckingham: Open University Press, 2002.

88. Kissane DW, McKenzie M. Psychosocial morbidity associated with patterns of family functioning in palliative care: baseline data from the Family Focused Grief Therapy controlled trial. *Palliative Medicine.* 2003; **17**: 527–37.

89. Oliviere D, Hargreaves R, Monroe B. Working with families. In: *Good practices in palliative care: a psychosocial perspective.* Aldershot: Ashgate, 1998: 54.

90. Black D. Childhood bereavement: distress and long term sequelae can be lessened by early intervention. *British Medical Journal.* 1996; **312**: 1496.

91. Christ GH. *Healing children's grief: surviving a parent's death from cancer.* Oxford: Oxford University Press, 2000.

92. Weller RA, Weller EB, Fristad MA, Bowes BM. Depression in recently bereaved prepubertal children. *American Journal of Psychiatry.* 1991; **148**: 1536–40.

93. Silverman PR. *Never too young to know. Death in children's lives.* Oxford: Oxford University Press, 2000.

94. Worden WJ. *Children and grief. When a parent dies.* New York: Guilford Press, 1996.

95. Christ GH, Raveis VH, Siegel K *et al.* Evaluation of a preventive intervention for bereaved children. *Journal of Social Work in End-of-Life and Palliative Care.* 2005; 1: 57–81.

96. Sandler I, Ayers T, Wolchik S *et al.* The Family Bereavement Program: efficacy evaluation of a therapy-based prevention program for parentally bereaved children and adolescents. *Journal of Consulting and Clinical Psychology.* 2003; **71**: 587–600.

97. Monroe B. It is impossible not to communicate – helping the grieving family. In: Smith S, Pennells M (eds).

Interventions with bereaved children. London: Jessica Kingsley, 1995: 87–106.

98. Monroe B, Kraus J (eds). *Brief interventions with bereaved children.* Oxford: Oxford University Press, 2005.

* 99. Fallowfield L. The quality of life: sexual function and body image following cancer therapy. *Cancer Topics.* 1992; **9**: 20–1.

100. Schover LR. Sexual dysfunction. In: Holland JC (ed). *Psycho-oncology.* Oxford: Oxford University Press, 1998: 494–9.

101. Nishimoto P. Sex and sexuality in the cancer patient. *Nurse Practitioner Forum.* 1995; **6**: 221–7.

102. Capone MA, Good RS, Westie KS, Jacobsen AF. Psychosocial rehabilitation of gynaecologic oncology patients. *Archives of Physical Medicine and Rehabilitation.* 1980; **61**: 12–32.

103. Gamel C, Davis BD, Hengeveld M. Nurses' provision of teaching and counselling on sexuality: a review of the literature. *Journal of Advanced Nursing.* 1993; **18**: 1219–27.

104. Waterhouse J, Metcalfe M. Attitudes towards nurses discussing sexual concerns with patients. *Journal of Advanced Nursing.* 1991; **16**: 1048–54.

105. Vincent CE, Vincent B, Greiss FC, Linton EB. Some marital concomitants of carcinoma of the cervix. *Southern Medical Journal.* 1975; **68**: 552–8.

106. Stausmire JM. Sexuality at the end of life. *American Journal of Hospice and Palliative Care.* 2004; **21**: 33–9.

107. Monroe B. A sexual-sensitive approach to palliative care. In: Oliviere D, Hargreaves R, Monroe B (eds). *Good practices in palliative care: a psychosocial perspective.* Aldershot: Ashgate, 1997: 96–111.

108. Schover LR. Sexual rehabilitation after treatment for prostate cancer. *Cancer.* 1993; **71**: 1024–30.

109. Cort E, Monroe B, Oliviere D. Couples in palliative care. *Sexual and Relationship Therapy.* 2004; **19**: 337–54.

110. Ananth H, Jones L, King M, Tookman A. The impact of cancer on sexual function: a controlled study. *Palliative Medicine.* 2003; **17**: 202–05.

111. Payne M. Adult protection cases in a hospice: an audit. *Journal of Adult Protection.* 2005; **7**: 4–12.

112. Faulkner A, Maguire P, Regnard C. The angry person. In: Regnard C, Hockley J (eds). *Flow diagrams in advanced cancer and other diseases.* London: Edward Arnold, 1995: 81–5.

113. Lansky SB, List MA, Hermann CA *et al.* Absence of major depressive disorder in female cancer patients. *Journal of Clinical Oncology.* 1985; **3**: 1553–60.

114. Hotopf M, Ly KL, Chidgey J, Addington Hall J. Depression in advanced disease – a systematic review 1: Prevalence and case finding. *Palliative Medicine.* 2002; **16**: 81–97.

115. Foley KM. The treatment of cancer pain. *New England Journal of Medicine.* 1985; **313**: 84–95.

116. Glover J, Dibble SL, Dodd MJ, Miaskowski C. Mood states of oncology outpatients: does pain make a difference? *Journal of Pain and Symptom Management.* 1995; **10**: 120–8.

117. Breitbart W, Rosenfeld B, Pessin H *et al.* Depression, hopelessness and desire for hastened death in terminally ill patients with cancer. *Journal of the American Medical Association.* 2000; **284**: 2907–11.

118. Watson M, Haviland JS, Greer S *et al.* Influence of psychological response on survival in breast cancer: a population-based case control study. *Lancet.* 1999; **354**: 1331–6.

119. Brugha TS. Depression in the terminally ill. *British Journal of Hospital Medicine.* 1993; **50**: 175–81.

120. American Psychiatric Association. *DSM-IV casebook: a learning companion to the diagnostic and statistical manual of the American Psychiatric Association.* Washington, DC: American Psychiatric Association, 1994.

*121. Breitbart W, Chochinov M, Passik S. Psychiatric symptoms in palliative medicine. In: Doyle D, Hanks G, Cherny N, Calman K (eds). *Oxford textbook of palliative medicine.* Oxford: Oxford University Press, 2004: 746–74.

122. Endicott J. Measurement of depression in patients with cancer. *Cancer.* 1984; **53** (Suppl.): 2243–9.

123. Casey P. Depression in the dying – disorder or distress? *Progress in Palliative Care.* 1994; **2**: 1–3.

124. Hotopf M. Depression, sadness, hopelessness and suicide. In: Sykes N, Edmonds P, Wiles J (eds). *Management of advanced disease.* London: Arnold, 2004: 106–18.

125. Rathbone GV, Horsley S, Goacher J. A self evaluated assessment suitable for seriously ill hospice patients. *Palliative Medicine.* 1994; **8**: 29–34.

126. Moorey S, Greer S, Watson M *et al.* The factor structure and factor stability of the hospital anxiety and depression scale in patients with cancer. *British Journal of Psychiatry.* 1991; **158**: 255–9.

127. Robaye E. Screening for adjustment disorders and major depressive disorders in cancer in-patients. *British Journal of Psychiatry.* 1990; **156**: 79–83.

128. Williams M, Dennis M, Taylor F. Is asking patients in palliative care, "Are you depressed?" appropriate? Prospective study. *British Medical Journal.* 2003; **327**: 372–3.

129. Chochinov H, Wilson K, Enns M, Lander S. Are you depressed? Screening for depression in the terminally ill. *American Journal of Psychiatry.* 1997; **154**: 674–6.

130. Breitbart W. Cancer pain and suicide. In: Foley K, Bonica JJ, Ventafridda V *et al.* (eds). *Advances in pain research and therapy,* vol. 16. New York: Raven Press, 1990: 399–412.

131. Bolund C. Suicide and cancer. *Journal of Psychosocial Oncology.* 1985; **3**: 31–52.

132. Fox BH, Stanek EJ, Boyd SC, Flannery JT. Suicide rates among cancer patients in Connecticut. *Journal of Chronic Diseases.* 1982; **35**: 85–100.

133. Cutler F, Reynolds D. An eight year survey of hospital suicides. *Suicide, Life Threatening Behaviour.* 1971; **1**: 184–201.

134. Guze S, Robins E. Suicide and primary affective disorders. *British Journal of Psychiatry.* 1970; **117**: 437–8.

135. Breitbart W, Krivo S. Suicide. In: Holland JC (ed). *Psycho-oncology.* Oxford: Oxford University Press, 1998: 541–7.

136. Maguire P, Faulkner A, Regnard C. The anxious person. In: Regnard C, Hockley J (eds). *Flow diagrams in advanced cancer and other diseases.* London: Edward Arnold, 1995: 73–6.

137. McCartney CF, Cahill P, Larson DB *et al.* Effect of psychiatric liaison program on consultation rates and on detection of minor psychiatric disorders in cancer patients. *American Journal of Psychiatry.* 1989; 7: 898–901.

138. Carroll BT, Kathol RG, Noyes R *et al.* Screening for depression and anxiety in cancer patients using the hospital anxiety and depression scale. *General Hospital Psychiatry.* 1993; **15**: 69–74.

139. Foley KM. Acute and chronic cancer pain syndromes. In: Doyle D, Hanks G, Cherny N, Calman K (eds). *Oxford textbook of palliative medicine.* Oxford: Oxford University Press, 2004: 298–316.

140. Sinclair S. Bereavement services: a service user's perspective. Paper presented at the European Association of Palliative Care Congress. London, September 1997.

6

The role of the nonprofessional caregiver in cancer pain management

CHRISTINE MIASKOWSKI

Introduction	63	Difficulties in implementing a pain management regimen in the home	66
Congruence in patients' and family caregivers' perceptions of the cancer pain experience	64	Caregiver skills and cancer pain management	66
Family caregivers' perceptions of the barriers to effective cancer pain management	64	Implications for clinical practice	68
The impact of the cancer pain experience on the family caregiver	65	Implications for research	68
		References	68

KEY LEARNING POINTS

- The shift in cancer care from the inpatient to the outpatient setting has placed a tremendous burden on patients and their family caregivers.
- One of the most frequently cited concerns of family caregivers of oncology patients is pain management.
- Most family caregivers overestimate the intensity of the patient's cancer pain.
- Family caregivers perceive a significant number of barriers to effective cancer pain management, including concerns about addiction and concerns about the side effects of analgesic medications.

- Family caregivers who care for patients in pain experience increased psychological distress and decreased quality of life.
- Family caregivers face numerous difficulties with the implementation of an effective pain management plan at home.
- Family caregivers need ongoing education and coaching to develop optimal approaches to care for patients with cancer pain.

INTRODUCTION

Throughout the world, dramatic increases in the aging population and cost containment policies in health care have shifted the care of patients with cancer from the inpatient to the outpatient setting. This shift in care has placed an enormous burden on patients and their family members to manage cancer pain in the home environment.[1, 2, 3] As noted by Ferrell and colleagues,[2] one of the

most frequently cited concerns of family members of oncology patients is the management of cancer pain.

While the definition of a family caregiver varies, in this chapter, the terms "caregiving" and "family caregiver" are defined broadly. Caregiving includes the informal (i.e. unpaid) care provided by family members that goes beyond the customary and normative social support provided in social relationships.[3] Likewise, while the family caregiver was originally conceptualized as a person related by marriage or blood who lived with the patient, in many studies of cancer pain management, family caregivers were defined as the individual determined by the patient to be most involved in their care.[4, 5, 6, 7, 8, 9, 10]

An examination of the literature on the role of the nonprofessional (i.e. family) caregiver in cancer pain management determined that the research has focused on:

- congruence in patients' and family caregivers' perceptions of the cancer pain experience;
- family caregivers' perceptions of the barriers to effective cancer pain management;
- the impact of the cancer pain experience on the family caregiver; and
- difficulties that patients and family caregivers have in implementing pain management regimens in their homes.

More recently, work by Schumacher and colleagues[1, 11] has focused on the need to understand and identify the skills that family caregivers need to care for someone with a life-threatening or chronic illness. The purpose of this chapter is to summarize the research findings in the four areas listed above. In addition, Schumacher's work on the concept of family caregiving skill will be applied to cancer pain management. The chapter concludes with a discussion of clinical implications and directions for future research.

CONGRUENCE IN PATIENTS' AND FAMILY CAREGIVERS' PERCEPTIONS OF THE CANCER PAIN EXPERIENCE

Several studies have evaluated for congruence between patients' and family caregivers' ratings of cancer pain.[4, 5, 12, 13, 14, 15, 16, 17][IV] In one of the earliest studies, Ferrell and colleagues[12] reported that family caregivers greatly overestimated the patients' pain intensity (i.e. 69.9 (caregiver rating) compared to 45.5 (patient rating) using a 0 to 10 visual analog scale). In addition, family caregivers rated the patients' pain to be extremely distressing to the patient, as well as for themselves. Work by Clipp and George[16] determined that almost without exception family caregivers perceived patients as having more pain than the patients themselves reported. In another study of oncology outpatients and their family caregivers,[5] only 30 percent of the patient–family caregiver dyads were congruent in their perception of the intensity of the pain that the patient was experiencing. In the remaining 70 percent of the dyads who were noncongruent in their perceptions of the patients' pain, 74.5 percent overestimated the patients' pain (i.e. average discrepancy was 35.5 mm (s.d. = 22.9; range, 11–97 mm) and 25.5 percent underestimated that patients' pain (i.e. average discrepancy was 38.2 mm (s.d. = 22.5; range, 12–94 mm). These findings were confirmed in a study of hospitalized oncology patients and their family caregivers in Taiwan,[13] as well as in a study of hospice patients and their family caregivers.[17] While the majority of the evidence suggests that family caregivers tend to overestimate their family members' pain, in a recent study of hospice patients and their family caregivers,[15] the family caregivers underestimated the amount of pain that the patients were experiencing.

Two studies have tried to determine the factors that were associated with being in a noncongruent dyad. In one study,[13] family caregivers in noncongruent dyads were more likely to be older and less educated. In addition, patients in these noncongruent dyads reported higher pain intensity scores, higher pain interference scores, and poorer functional status scores. In another study,[14] family caregivers who perceived their family member to be in a great deal of distress as a result of their pain, who associated greater efforts at pain relief with greater levels of pain, and who were themselves distressed by the patient's pain, had the most inaccurate estimates of the patients' pain.

It is interesting to note that in all of the studies listed above, all of the patients were able to self-report their level of pain intensity. The fact that in most cases family caregivers' perceptions of the pain experience were not in concert with their family members suggests that, in these dyads, effective communication about pain and pain management did not occur. Clinicians need to assess patients' and family caregivers' perceptions of and communications about the patients' pain experience. Clinicians need to encourage patients and family caregivers to communicate about the patients' pain and to work together to improve cancer pain management.

Misinterpretation of the patients' pain experience by family caregivers could result in undertreatment or overtreatment of the patients' pain. In addition, a lack of congruence between the patients and family caregivers about the patients' pain experience (i.e. both the intensity and distress associated with the pain) could lead to unnecessary feelings of distress and burden. These feelings could be relieved through more effective communication about the patients' and family caregivers' perceptions of the pain experience, as well as discussions of their fears and concerns.

FAMILY CAREGIVERS' PERCEPTIONS OF THE BARRIERS TO EFFECTIVE CANCER PAIN MANAGEMENT

Several studies have evaluated barriers to effective cancer pain management in family caregivers in Australia,[18] Taiwan,[19, 20, 21] and the United States.[22] In all of these studies, several different versions of the Barriers questionnaire[23] were used to evaluate family caregivers' perceptions of barriers to effective cancer pain management. The original Barriers questionnaire had 27 items and was scored into eight subscales that evaluated beliefs that affected one's willingness to communicate about pain and beliefs that interfered with the use of opioids to manage pain. The eight subscales measured were:

1. fear of opioid side effects;
2. fear of addiction;
3. the belief that increasing pain signifies disease progression;
4. fear of injections;
5. concern about the development of tolerance to analgesic medications;
6. believing that "good" patients do not complain about pain;
7. the belief that reporting pain may distract the physician from treating or curing the cancer; and
8. fatalism or believing that pain is inevitable with cancer and cannot be relieved.

In the Australian study,[18] the major concerns or barriers that family caregivers reported were concerns about the addictiveness of analgesic medications; concerns that their family members' experience of pain was a sign of progressive disease, and concerns about the side effects of analgesic medications, particularly constipation. In the study in Taiwan with family caregivers of oncology outpatients,[19] the subscales with the highest barrier scores were concerns that pain was a sign of disease progression, concerns about the development of tolerance to analgesic medications, concerns about side effects, and concerns about addiction. In the other study conducted in Taiwan with family caregivers of hospice patients,[21] the subscales with the highest barrier scores were concerns that cancer pain indicated disease progression, concerns about side effects, and the belief that pain medications are better given on an as-needed basis rather than around the clock. This last scale was added specifically to the Taiwanese version of the Barriers questionnaire. Finally, in the study in the United States,[22] the subscales with the highest barrier scores were concerns about side effects, concerns about addiction, and concerns that cancer pain indicated disease progression.

Findings from these five international studies[18, 19, 20, 21, 22][IV] suggest that family caregivers have significant concerns that may interfere with effective cancer pain management. Across these five studies, concerns about addiction and about the side effects of analgesic medications appear to be universal among family caregivers. Additional research is needed to determine how these perceived barriers in family caregivers impact the care of the patient with cancer pain.

THE IMPACT OF THE CANCER PAIN EXPERIENCE ON THE FAMILY CAREGIVER

Pain is a major source of concern for family caregivers. The suffering of the patient leads to family suffering.[24] In one study of nonterminal advanced cancer patients receiving outpatient treatment,[25] 80 percent of the patients experienced pain and 65 percent of their family caregivers were extremely concerned about the pain. Therefore, it is not surprising that assistance with pain management is frequently cited as a healthcare need by cancer patients and their family caregivers.[26, 27]

One of the first studies that evaluated the impact of cancer pain on family caregivers was undertaken by Miaskowski and colleagues.[6] Differences in mood states, health status, and caregiver strain between family caregivers of oncology outpatients were compared with and without cancer pain. In this study, a convenience sample of 86 family caregivers of patients with cancer pain and 42 caregivers of pain-free patients completed a number of self-report questionnaires. Family caregivers of patients with cancer pain reported significantly higher depression and anxiety scores than family caregivers of pain-free patients. Although family caregivers of patients with pain had lower health status scores and higher caregiver strain scores, these differences were not statistically significant. These findings suggest that clinicians need to assess the psychological needs of family caregivers who are caring for patients with cancer pain.

Ferrell and colleagues[2] conducted a study that was designed to describe the experience of cancer pain management from the perspective of the family caregiver and to measure the impact of the patient's pain on the family caregiver's quality of life. The major findings from this study suggested that family caregivers who care for a cancer patient with pain:

- experience sleep disturbances and fatigue;
- experience depression and anxiety;
- experience a sense of uncertainty;
- reported that caregiving imposed a financial burden because of changes in the patient's income, changes in their own income, and additional cancer-related expenses (e.g. medical expenses, out-of-pocket costs for pain medications, out-of-pocket expenses for alternative pain relief treatments);
- estimated that they devoted over 12 hours per day to the care of the patient and that three hours per day were devoted to pain management activities.

More recent work has focused on an evaluation of the impact of caring for palliative care patients on family caregivers.[28, 29, 30, 31] As in previous reports, caring for a palliative care patient resulted in increased psychological distress and decreased quality of life for the family caregiver. Findings from all of these studies suggest that family caregivers who care for patients in pain experience a significant amount of stress that results in mood disturbances and decreases in quality of life. More research is needed to determine the most effective approaches to assist family caregivers to care for patients with cancer pain and to decrease the stress associated with this care.

DIFFICULTIES IN IMPLEMENTING A PAIN MANAGEMENT REGIMEN IN THE HOME

With the shift in cancer care from the inpatient to the outpatient setting, the majority of cancer pain management is undertaken in the patient's home. While several studies have evaluated the effectiveness of interventions to change patients and family caregivers knowledge[32, 33, 34, 35] and behaviors,[36, 37, 38, 39, 40, 41, 42, 43] only one study has identified difficulties that patients and family caregivers have in implementing a pain management regimen at home.[44][IV]

As part of a large randomized clinical trial that evaluated the effectiveness of a self-care intervention to improve cancer pain management,[36, 45] data were obtained from audiotaped and transcribed interactions between the intervention nurses and patients and family caregivers on the difficulties that they faced in putting a cancer pain management regimen into practice at home.[44] The seven difficulties are summarized in **Table 6.1**.

While a large amount of literature has been published on barriers to effective cancer pain management,[21, 23, 46, 47, 48] no studies have evaluated the practical difficulties that patients and their family caregivers face in implementing a cancer pain management regimen in their homes. It is interesting to note that none of the difficulties that were reported by patients and family caregivers focused on fears of addiction, tolerance, or physical dependence. Rather the difficulties identified through this qualitative analysis[44] represent ongoing challenges that patients and their family caregivers face on a day-to-day basis. The analysis indicated that putting a pain management regimen into practice at home is an ongoing problem-solving process in which a variety of difficulties with pain management may be encountered and must be dealt with on an ongoing basis.

In order to improve cancer pain management and make it easier for family caregivers to manage pain at home, clinicians need to engage with patients and family caregivers in the following ways:

- perform ongoing pain assessments and schedule regular times for communication with patients and family caregivers about pain management;
- evaluate on an ongoing basis the specific difficulties that patients and family caregivers have with pain management;
- brainstorm with patients and family caregivers about problem-solving strategies to effectively manage these difficulties;
- evaluate the efficacy of strategies employed and revise these strategies to optimize the pain management plan.

The provision of information about cancer pain management to patients and their family caregivers may not be sufficient to improve pain control in the home care setting. Patients and their family caregivers require ongoing assistance with problem-solving to optimize their pain management regimen. This ongoing assistance requires that clinicians be available to assist with problem-solving and to modify the pain management plan as necessary.

CAREGIVER SKILLS AND CANCER PAIN MANAGEMENT

Work by Schumacher and colleagues[1, 11] suggests that family caregivers of patients with cancer require an unprecedented level of skill to provide safe and effective care. Yet, evidence exists that family caregivers are not prepared to provide this level of care and that this lack of preparation evokes feelings of uncertainty, inadequacy, fear, anxiety, and even terror.[49, 50]

According to Schumacher and colleagues,[11][IV] family caregiving involves a wide array of cognitive, behavioral,

Table 6.1 Difficulties putting pain management regimens into practice at home.

Difficulty	Examples
Obtaining the prescribed medication(s)	Analgesic medications were not stocked in the pharmacy
	Lack of insurance coverage for analgesic medications
Accessing information	Inability to obtain basic and practical information about pain management from clinicians
Tailoring prescribed medication regimens to meet individual needs	Inability to find the optimal dose and/or timing of analgesic medications
Managing side effects	Most troubling side effect was constipation
	Some patients reported a cascade of side effects
Cognitively processing complex information	Patients complained of difficulties thinking analytically and/or difficulties with memory
Managing new or unusual pain	When pain deviated from its normal pattern, patients and family caregivers reported difficulties with pain management
Managing multiple symptoms simultaneously	Patients reported difficulties managing multiple symptoms related to their cancer treatment and their pain management regimens

and interpersonal processes and subprocesses. These processes include:

- monitoring;
- interpreting;
- making decisions;
- taking action;
- making adjustments;
- accessing resources;
- providing hands-on care;
- working together with the ill person;
- navigating the healthcare system.

Based on their interviews with family caregivers of patients with cancer,[11] it appears that considerable interindividual variability exists in caregivers' successful use of these processes and subprocesses. While the research studies that derived these processes were undertaken with family caregivers of patients undergoing cancer treatment, they can be applied to family caregivers of oncology patients with cancer pain. The definitions for the nine processes and some examples of subprocesses that might be specific to family caregivers who are caring for patients with cancer pain are listed in **Table 6.2**.

Based on Schumacher's work in family caregivers of oncology patients,[1, 11, 51, 52, 53][IV] as well as work by others primarily in gerontology,[54, 55, 56, 57, 58][IV] family caregiving is an extremely complex process that requires family caregivers to have a large number of different skills. Schumacher defined family caregiving skill as the ability to engage effectively and smoothly in the nine caregiving processes listed in **Table 6.2**.[1] The development of skillful caregiving is complex and involves much more than simply the willingness or motivation to follow instructions. It requires that family caregivers receive education and training to be able to care for the patient with cancer pain. However, brief periods of instruction may not be sufficient to provide the family caregiver with the requisite knowledge and skills needed to provide the most effective and safe care to the patient with pain.

Little is known about the requisite knowledge and skills that family caregivers need to effectively perform cancer pain management. As noted above, several studies have identified the barriers to effective cancer pain management that family caregivers perceive.[20, 22, 59] However, only one intervention study was found that documented the effects of a pain education program with patients and family caregivers.[20][II] In this study, the pain

Table 6.2 Examples of family caregiving processes and subprocesses related to pain management.

Caregiving processes	Examples of subprocesses specific to pain management
Monitoring is the process of observing how the care receiver is doing	Performing daily pain assessments Keeping a pain diary
Interpreting is the process of making sense out of what is observed	Making a judgment that pain intensity has increased based on changes in the patient's behavior
Making decisions is defined as the process of choosing a course of action based on one's observations and interpretations of the situation	Weighing advantages and disadvantages of increasing the patient's dose of pain medication within the parameters of the analgesic prescription
Taking action is defined as the process of carrying out caregiving decisions and instructions	Taking into account the side effects of the analgesic medications in relationship to the other medications the patient is taking
Making adjustments is defined as the process of progressively refining caregiving actions until a strategy that works well is found	Timing the patient's activity in relationship to analgesic intake Developing routine procedures for the management of breakthrough pain
Accessing resources is defined as a process of obtaining what is needed to provide care, including information, equipment, and supplies for home use, help with housework, and assistance with personal care	Providing the patient with a walker to assist with ambulation Trying different nonpharmacologic pain management interventions to find the most effective one Asking clinicians questions about how to improve the patient's pain management Accessing the internet for information on analgesic medications
Providing hands-on care is defined as the process of carrying out nursing and medical procedures	Filling the patient's pillbox to facilitate adherence with the analgesic regimen Giving the patient a massage or a backrub
Working together with the ill person is defined as the process of sharing illness-related care in a way that was sensitive to the personhood of both the care receiver and the caregiver	Developing a routine around analgesic intake with the patient Discussing the patient's fears and concerns about analgesic medications
Navigating the healthcare system is defined as the process of ensuring that the care receiver's needs are adequately met	Determining which oncology clinician provides the best pain management Advocating for patient's pain management needs

education intervention was conducted with both the patient and the family caregiver over a period of 30 to 40 minutes in the inpatient setting. Two follow-up visits were held at two and four weeks after the intervention in the outpatient clinic. The information that was part of the educational program addressed specific concerns of Taiwanese patients and their family caregivers related to reporting pain and using analgesics. In addition, specific barriers to effective cancer pain management were addressed. Patients and family caregivers who received the educational intervention had significant reductions in their barrier scores. In addition, patients in the experimental group reported significantly lower pain intensity and pain interference scores at the end of the study.

Additional research is warranted to determine the specific knowledge and skills that family caregivers need to provide safe and effective cancer pain management at home. At a minimum, family caregivers should receive education and skills training, as well as a written pain management plan, that addresses the following areas:

- the causes of the patient's pain;
- the types and rationales for the various analgesic medications;
- instructions for having the prescriptions for analgesics filled;
- specific instructions for how to dose and titrate the analgesic medications;
- instructions on how to manage analgesic side effects;
- instructions for storage and safe keeping of medications;
- instructions on who to call if pain is not relieved or increases in intensity or if side effects occur; and
- instructions on when and how to use nonpharmacologic approaches for cancer pain management.[60]

IMPLICATIONS FOR CLINICAL PRACTICE

Based on the limited amount of literature on the role of family caregivers in cancer pain management, it is clear that family caregivers play a significant role in cancer pain management. At a minimum, clinicians need to assess family caregivers knowledge of cancer pain management and their perceived barriers to cancer pain management. Ideally, education about pain management should be provided to the patient and the family caregiver together. In addition, clinicians should assure family caregivers that they will assist them to develop an effective pain management plan for the patient. Family caregivers need to understand that education about pain management will be an ongoing part of the patient's care. Family caregivers should be encouraged to call clinicians if they have questions or concerns about the pain management plan.

IMPLICATIONS FOR RESEARCH

Current trends in the healthcare system are placing increased burdens on patients and family caregivers. Future research needs to identify how perceived barriers on the part of family caregivers impact their management of the patients' pain. In addition, descriptive longitudinal studies are needed to evaluate the impact of caring for a patient with cancer pain on the physical and emotional health of the family caregiver. Finally, studies are needed to determine the most effective interventions to assist family caregivers to develop the skills they need to provide the most effective care to patients with cancer pain.

REFERENCES

* 1. Schumacher KL, Stewart BJ, Archbold PG et al. Family caregiving skill: development of the concept. *Research in Nursing and Health.* 2000; **23**: 191–203.
2. Ferrell BR, Grant M, Borneman T et al. Family caregiving in cancer pain management. *Journal of Palliative Medicine.* 1999; **2**: 185–95.
3. Hauser JM, Kramer BJ. Family caregivers in palliative care. *Clinics in Geriatric Medicine.* 2004; **20**: 671–88.
4. Yeager KA, Miaskowski C, Dibble SL, Wallhagen M. Differences in pain knowledge and perception of the pain experience between outpatients with cancer and their family caregivers. *Oncology Nursing Forum.* 1995; **22**: 1235–41.
5. Miaskowski C, Zimmer EF, Barrett KM et al. Differences in patients' and family caregivers' perceptions of the pain experience influence patient and caregiver outcomes. *Pain.* 1997; **72**: 217–26.
6. Miaskowski C, Kragness L, Dibble S, Wallhagen M. Differences in mood states, health status, and caregiver strain between family caregivers of oncology outpatients with and without cancer-related pain. *Journal of Pain and Symptom Management.* 1997; **13**: 138–47.
7. Riley-Doucet C. Beliefs about the controllability of pain: congruence between older adults with cancer and their family caregivers. *Journal of Family Nursing.* 2005; **11**: 225–41.
8. Oi-Ling K, Man-Wah DT, Kam-Hung DN. Symptom distress as rated by advanced cancer patients, caregivers and physicians in the last week of life. *Palliative Medicine.* 2005; **19**: 228–33.
9. Keefe FJ, Lipkus I, Lefebvre JC et al. The social context of gastrointestinal cancer pain: a preliminary study examining the relation of patient pain catastrophizing to patient perceptions of social support and caregiver stress and negative responses. *Pain.* 2003; **103**: 151–6.
10. Porter LS, Keefe FJ, Hurwitz H, Faber M. Disclosure between patients with gastrointestinal cancer and their spouses. *Psycho-Oncology.* 2005; **14**: 1030–42.

* 11. Schumacher KL, Beidler SM, Beeber AS, Gambino P. A transactional model of cancer family caregiving skill. *Advances in Nursing Science.* 2006; **29**: 271–86.

12. Ferrell BR, Ferrell BA, Rhiner M, Grant M. Family factors influencing cancer pain management. *Postgraduate Medical Journal.* 1991; **67** (Suppl. 2): S64–9.

13. Lin CC. Congruity of cancer pain perceptions between Taiwanese patients and family caregivers: relationship to patients' concerns about reporting pain and using analgesics. *Journal of Pain and Symptom Management.* 2001; **21**: 18–26.

14. Redinbaugh EM, Baum A, DeMoss C et al. Factors associated with the accuracy of family caregiver estimates of patient pain. *Journal of Pain and Symptom Management.* 2002; **23**: 31–8.

15. Tu MS, Chiou CP. Perceptual consistency of pain and quality of life between hospice cancer patients and family caregivers: a pilot study. *International Journal of Clinical Practice.* 2007; **61**: 1686–91.

16. Clipp EC, George LK. Patients with cancer and their spouse caregivers. Perceptions of the illness experience. *Cancer.* 1992; **69**: 1074–9.

17. McMillan SC, Moody LE. Hospice patient and caregiver congruence in reporting patients' symptom intensity. *Cancer Nursing.* 2003; **26**: 113–18.

18. Aranda S, Yates P, Edwards H et al. Barriers to effective cancer pain management: a survey of Australian family caregivers. *European Journal of Cancer Care.* 2004; **13**: 336–43.

19. Lin CC. Barriers to the analgesic management of cancer pain: a comparison of attitudes of Taiwanese patients and their family caregivers. *Pain.* 2000; **88**: 7–14.

20. Lin CC, Chou PL, Wu SL et al. Long-term effectiveness of a patient and family pain education program on overcoming barriers to management of cancer pain. *Pain.* 2006; **122**: 271–81.

21. Lin CC, Wang P, Lai YL et al. Identifying attitudinal barriers to family management of cancer pain in palliative care in Taiwan. *Palliative Medicine.* 2000; **14**: 463–70.

22. Vallerand AH, Collins-Bohler D, Templin T, Hasenau SM. Knowledge of and barriers to pain management in caregivers of cancer patients receiving homecare. *Cancer Nursing.* 2007; **30**: 31–7.

23. Ward SE, Goldberg N, Miller-McCauley V et al. Patient-related barriers to management of cancer pain. *Pain.* 1993; **52**: 319–24.

* 24. Ferrell BR, Rhiner M, Cohen MZ, Grant M. Pain as a metaphor for illness. Part I: Impact of cancer pain on family caregivers. *Oncology Nursing Forum.* 1991; **18**: 1303–09.

25. Perry GR, Roades de Meneses M. Cancer patients at home: needs and coping styles of primary caregivers. *Home Healthcare Nurse.* 1989; **7**: 27–30.

* 26. Ferrell BR, Cohen MZ, Rhiner M, Rozek A. Pain as a metaphor for illness. Part II: Family caregivers' management of pain. *Oncology Nursing Forum.* 1991; **18**: 1315–21.

27. Ferrell BR, Taylor EJ, Grant M et al. Pain management at home. Struggle, comfort, and mission. *Cancer Nursing.* 1993; **16**: 169–78.

28. Grov EK, Dahl AA, Fossa SD et al. Global quality of life in primary caregivers of patients with cancer in palliative phase staying at home. *Supportive Care in Cancer.* 2006; **14**: 943–51.

29. Grov EK, Dahl AA, Moum T, Fossa SD. Anxiety, depression, and quality of life in caregivers of patients with cancer in late palliative phase. *Annals of Oncology.* 2005; **16**: 1185–91.

30. Grov EK, Fossa SD, Sorebo O, Dahl AA. Primary caregivers of cancer patients in the palliative phase: a path analysis of variables influencing their burden. *Social Science and Medicine.* 2006; **63**: 2429–39.

31. Valdimarsdottir U, Helgason AR, Furst CJ et al. The unrecognised cost of cancer patients' unrelieved symptoms:a nationwide follow-up of their surviving partners. *British Journal of Cancer.* 2002; **86**: 1540–5.

32. Clotfelter CE. The effect of an educational intervention on decreasing pain intensity in elderly people with cancer. *Oncology Nursing Forum.* 1999; **26**: 27–33.

33. Ferrell BR, Grant M, Chan J et al. The impact of cancer pain education on family caregivers of elderly patients. *Oncology Nursing Forum.* 1995; **22**: 1211–18.

34. Glajchen M, Moul JW. Teleconferencing as a method of educating men about managing advanced prostate cancer and pain. *Journal of Psychosocial Oncology.* 1996; **14**: 73–87.

35. Walker JR. A study to develop and assess the value of a leaflet on pain control for patients taking MST in the community. *Palliative Medicine.* 1992; **6**: 65–73.

* 36. Miaskowski C, Dodd M, West C et al. Randomized clinical trial of the effectiveness of a self-care intervention to improve cancer pain management. *Journal of Clinical Oncology.* 2004; **22**: 1713–20.

37. Dalton J. Education for pain management: A pilot study. *Patient Education and Counseling.* 1987; **9**: 155–65.

38. de Wit R, van Dam F, Zandbelt L et al. A pain education program for chronic cancer pain patients: follow-up results from a randomized controlled trial. *Pain.* 1997; **73**: 55–69.

39. Ferrell BR, Ferrell BA, Ahn C, Tran K. Pain management for elderly patients with cancer at home. *Cancer.* 1994; **74** (7 Suppl): 2139–46.

40. Oliver JW, Kravitz RL, Kaplan SH, Meyers FJ. Individualized patient education and coaching to improve pain control among cancer outpatients. *Journal of Clinical Oncology.* 2001; **19**: 2206–12.

41. Rimer B, Levy MH, Keintz MK et al. Enhancing cancer pain control regimens through patient education. *Patient Education and Counseling.* 1987; **10**: 267–77.

42. Ward S, Donovan HS, Owen B et al. An individualized intervention to overcome patient-related barriers to pain management in women with gynecologic cancers. *Research in Nursing and Health.* 2000; **23**: 393–405.

43. Wells N, Hepworth JT, Murphy BA *et al.* Improving cancer pain management through patient and family education. *Journal of Pain and Symptom Management.* 2003; **25**: 344–56.

∗ 44. Schumacher KL, Koresawa S, West C *et al.* Putting cancer pain management regimens into practice at home. *Journal of Pain and Symptom Management.* 2002; **23**: 369–82.

45. West CM, Dodd MJ, Paul SM *et al.* The PRO-SELF(c): Pain Control Program – an effective approach for cancer pain management. *Oncology Nursing Forum.* 2003; **30**: 65–73.

46. Gunnarsdottir S, Donovan HS, Serlin RC *et al.* Patient-related barriers to pain management: the Barriers Questionnaire II (BQ-II). *Pain.* 2002; **99**: 385–96.

47. Almog YJ, Anglin MD, Fisher DG. Alcohol and heroin use patterns of narcotics addicts: gender and ethnic differences. *American Journal of Drug and Alcohol Abuse.* 1993; **19**: 219–38.

48. Lai YH, Keefe FJ, Sun WZ *et al.* Relationship between pain-specific beliefs and adherence to analgesic regimens in Taiwanese cancer patients: a preliminary study. *Journal of Pain and Symptom Management.* 2002; **24**: 415–23.

49. Stetz KM, Brown MA. Taking care: caregiving to persons with cancer and AIDS. *Cancer Nursing.* 1997; **20**: 12–22.

50. McLane L, Jones K, Lydiatt W *et al.* Taking away the fear: a grounded theory study of cooperative care in the treatment of head and neck cancer. *Psycho-Oncology.* 2003; **12**: 474–90.

51. Schumacher KL. Reconceptualizing family caregiving: family-based illness care during chemotherapy. *Research in Nursing and Health.* 1996; **19**: 261–71.

52. Schumacher KL. Family caregiver role acquisition: role-making through situated interaction. *Scholarly Inquiry for Nursing Practice.* 1995; **9**: 211–26.

53. Schumacher KL, Stewart BJ, Archbold PG. Conceptualization and measurement of doing family caregiving well. *Image – the Journal of Nursing Scholarship.* 1998; **30**: 63–9.

54. Bowers BJ. Intergenerational caregiving: adult caregivers and their aging parents. *Advances in Nursing Science.* 1987; **9**: 20–31.

55. Given BA, Given CW. Family caregiving for the elderly. *Annual Review of Nursing Research.* 1991; **9**: 77–101.

56. Albert SM. Do family caregivers recognize malnutrition in the frail elderly? *Journal of the American Geriatrics Society.* 1993; **41**: 617–22.

57. Brown MA, Stetz K. The labor of caregiving: a theoretical model of caregiving during potentially fatal illness. *Qualitative Health Research.* 1999; **9**: 182–97.

58. Corcoran MA. Management decisions made by caregiver spouses of persons with Alzheimer's disease. *American Journal of Occupational Therapy.* 1994; **48**: 38–45.

59. Vallerand AH, Saunders MM, Anthony M. Perceptions of control over pain by patients with cancer and their caregivers. *Pain Management Nursing.* 2007; **8**: 55–63.

60. Miaskowski C, Cleary J, Burney R *et al. Guideline for the management of cancer pain in adults and children.* Glenview, IL: American Pain Society, 2005.

7

Teamworking in cancer pain management

VICKY ROBINSON AND ROB GEORGE

Setting the scene	71	Conclusion	80
Some theory	74	References	80
Reviewing our scenarios	77		

KEY LEARNING POINTS

- Teamwork is a key element in the successful management of pain and other symptoms in cancer patients.
- Whilst every clinician brings their own skill set to a situation, many of these are transferable to others in the team.

- Successful teamwork is dependent on good relationships, clear tasks, and defined end points.
- Teams are never static – they are always changing and conflict is inevitable at times.
- Organizational development (OD) methods can help in understanding the dynamic nature of teams.

No man is an Island, entire of it self; every man is a piece of the Continent, a part of the main; if a clod be washed away by the sea, Europe is the less, as well as if a promontory were, as well as if a manor of thy friends or of thine own were; any man's death diminishes me, because I am involved in Mankind; and therefore never send to know for whom the bell tolls; it tolls for thee.

John Donne
Devotions upon Emergent Occasions (1624)
"Meditation XVII"

ignorant of the elements of effective teamwork is perilous in such a complex area as pain management. Read on!

In order to maintain accessibility and relevance for clinicians, our exploration begins with two slightly stereotypical examples of teams in action. We then use them to:

- contextualize and examine some theories of teamwork;
- offer a framework for those with a strategic role in the formation and development of clinical teams; and
- give readers who have responsibility for leading and managing teams the confidence to influence change processes where their team is weak or dysfunctional.

SETTING THE SCENE

Two views of teamwork

Teamworking and interdisciplinary practice are modern mantras. One may therefore be forgiven for viewing this chapter as a sop to political correctness. However, to be

James's team

It is Friday afternoon in the breast clinic of a large teaching hospital. Dr James Moss, the consultant oncologist, is proud of this clinic. It was his idea to draw counseling, nursing, and medicine together in one place.

After all, no one can be all things to all people and he had fought hard for the space and staffing necessary. Still, here they all are: a multidisciplinary team in action. In the department each Friday afternoon, apart from James, are a cancer counselor (Linda), a breast care nurse (Julie), and when requested a specialist palliative nurse.

Soon it will be 4 p.m. He simply *must* leave by then. The boys are so looking forward to one of their few weekends away sailing. If he is late, they will not get to the coast by seven. Work takes enough of his life as it is. He simply can't break his promise this time.

At 3:40 p.m. Janet Cooper walks in with her husband Colin. She looks awful. Janet was diagnosed with breast cancer just after her 40th birthday two years ago and has done very well given the aggressiveness of her disease, although she now has widespread liver and bone metastases. She has just had radiotherapy to her hip and chemotherapy starts on Monday. Colin has taken the day off work to come to the hospital with her. James greets them at the door smiling. "Twenty minutes: plenty of time," he thinks.

Janet sits down and bursts into tears. The pain in her side is not responding to simple analgesia. Could she have something stronger? James glances at Colin, and feels a flood of sorrow as he thinks "I can't take away their hope, but she is unlikely to see Christmas. I'll have to start some morphine too, just whilst we're waiting for the radiotherapy to work." He still couldn't prescribe morphine without feeling he'd lost – irrational, but there it is.

"I'll get Linda to see them. They need to talk. Linda's such a brick, a real expert at this stuff. I just don't know how she copes with all these tales of woe. Still, that's what a team's for – horses for courses."

James Moss writes the prescription and reassures Janet and Colin that the radiotherapy and chemotherapy really will help and that he is going to ask the cancer counselor to see them both. Three fifty p.m. Perfect. James knocks on Linda's door on his way out.

"Linda, can you talk to Janet and Colin Cooper for me. Two year history, nasty disease, bone and liver mets. I've just started her on morphine for pain control. She's taking the whole thing quite badly. I think they both suspect that this could be the beginning of the end, although I've reassured them that this course of radiotherapy and chemo will make her much better."

"I've arranged to see them both again in six weeks time after the chemo' has finished. Can you keep an eye on her and do your stuff for me until then. My secretary's got the notes – all the information you need is there."

Julie makes to say something, but James is already out of the door. He shakes off a strange feeling of melancholy as he hurries down the corridor. However, he quickly reassures himself:

"That's what I like. Someone to pick up the psychological bit. Good teamwork. It really is excellent to have a holistic service."

Linda fumes. "Here we go again: another shot in the dark. Why do I always feel that I have to pick up all the pieces? I'll talk to Julie first to see if she knows the patient." Linda sails into Julie's office and slumps in the chair.

"Can I talk to you? He's done it again: a typical Friday afternoon catastrophe on my doorstep. I don't know them, I haven't been introduced, and I didn't hear what he said. I'm not clairvoyant you know. How many times do I have to tell him? We're going to have to sit him down and pin back his ears back you know." Julie just nods and shrugs at the right moments as there is no point in trying to interrupt Linda when she is in full flood, but it does seem she has a point. What neither knows is that, whilst he would never admit it, James Moss finds Linda very intimidating when she is in the room with him and a patient – she makes him feel so inadequate that he stumbles over simple interactions and he doesn't quite know how to deal with it. Subconsciously he will do almost anything to avoid joint consultations.

James' team is coming up to its first anniversary – it is still very young. Referring on to another professional is not teamwork, it is only the beginning of teamwork – James doesn't know that, but he is also saddled with his inhibitions with Linda – this will come out sooner or later. Equally Linda does not make his task easy or her difficulties clear. James will probably be mortified when he hears of the tension he is causing. Teams only form once there is open communication. We will come back to this.

The experienced team

This second scenario highlights something else: the need for a breadth of experience and the professional affiliations and backgrounds required to help a young man who is dying from disseminated malignancy.

Steve is a 28-year-old artist, engaged to Jenny. He was referred to the local interdisciplinary specialist palliative care team (PCT) by his general practitioner (GP) following a left below knee amputation for an aggressive osteosarcoma. Six weeks following surgery, Steve was diagnosed with liver metastases. His GP is asking for advice on how to manage Steve's phantom limb pain, and for some general support for Jenny and for Steve's parents. The team discusses the case at referral and decides on a joint assessment by one of the more experienced clinical nurse specialists (CNS) and a team doctor.

His phantom limb pain is well controlled with appropriate neuropathic agents and Steve says that this isn't the issue. He wants a second opinion on treatment for his cancer.

"You are not here to discuss my death. I was told that you were coming to advise on treating my pain. It's obvious that you should do this by treating my cancer." It is clear that there is a lot of tension in the family.

Over the next few weeks and several hours of tirades against doctors the CNS learns several things. Jenny is four months pregnant, and Steve's own parents had lost a child, Jason, at the age of nine. This was before Steve was born and was never spoken of. Steve was therefore feeling guilty and very angry at the prospect of "deserting" his family so soon.

"I simply refuse to give in to this." He sobs.

The case is clearly complex and operates at several levels beyond Steve's pain. It is also affecting the clinicians who are involved and threatens to draw them into the family's vortex of fear and anxiety. Here, the strength of teamwork should offer a check and a protection for the CNS and GP as well as a framework for managing the case. Here is what happens.

The referral by the GP for assistance with Steve's phantom limb pain also legitimizes his need for some personal support in managing the case. On feeding back, this is brought up with the GP (who is used to working with specialist palliative care). He is quite open about the distress that the case is causing the practice. He has known the family for 30 years and was involved at the time of Jason's death. "I've been looking for an excuse to get you guys involved – there is too much going on for me to handle on my own and I feel part of it."

The CNS presents Steve and his family at the large interdisciplinary team meeting and the GP attends too. She too confesses to feeling helpless and asks for assistance in deciding the most effective strategy now that the complexity of the family dynamic has emerged. After half an hour's discussion, there is a clear game-plan and contingent approaches should one or more of the family fail to cope or should the disease progress unexpectedly.

It is self-evident that this case is beyond one practitioner and both clinicians, who are familiar with teamwork, know it. The human problems associated with managing pain and uncertainty are "up front" with Steve: denial, fear of addressing the meaning of pain and symptoms, unresolved matters from the past, etc. Complex problems require more than one brain and more than one discipline. In this mature team, however, whilst mechanisms are in place for calm and controlled management of this type of case, it has taken nine years to get there.

The need for teamworking in cancer

ISSUES FOR THE PATIENT

People with malignant disease perceive pain to tell them that the cancer is alive and well, and they are not. It is a powerful message, a reminder of mortality, the prospect of suffering and of a future lost. When patients told Cicely Saunders, "all of me is wrong" or "it all hurts," she defined the concept of "total pain,"[1] referring to the physical, emotional, social, and spiritual disease experienced at times by cancer patients and their families. The experience may well precipitate a crisis or be a watershed.

It raises questions of mortality, existence, priorities, and relationships that need emotional or psychological support, ranging from an effective listening ear through to an expert intervention from a psychologist, psychiatrist, specialist social worker, or spiritual care advisor in more difficult cases.

Pain also raises practical questions: "how am I going to manage if I have to give up work, or how do I get out of bed, up and down stairs, to and from hospital appointments, etc.?" Practical assessment and intervention from an occupational therapist or physiotherapist or social support from family and friends can make a measurable difference in a patient's ability to cope with increasing disability.

In 2004, Gysels and Higginson undertook a systematic review of the literature on teamwork in palliative care as part of the work for the National Institute for Health and Clinical Excellence's (NICE) Guidance for Supportive and Palliative Care for People with Cancer.[2] They found evidence strongly in support of specialist palliative care teams working in homes, hospitals, and hospices as a means to improve outcomes such as pain, symptom control, and satisfaction. They call for more research to examine the various skill mixes.

ISSUES FOR THE CLINICIAN

Donne was right that "No man is an island," especially when we are working with people facing crisis. Pain does something to us. It is not hard to imagine the pain and suffering being experienced by our two cases. The experience of pain signals that something is happening inside. For doctors in particular, whose imperative so often is to cure a patient, acknowledging the feelings of helplessness and sadness that accompany progressive disease can be a very hard thing to do.

To benefit fully from team life, one must come to acknowledge that we need not only each other's professional expertise, but also each other for professional companionship. This enables us to share the burden of often impossibly difficult and sometimes tragic situations – situations that at times challenge us as people as well as professionals.

Our overriding obligation to such patients must be to ensure that we provide a caring environment in which the diverse facets of a patient's pain can be managed. We must ensure appropriate information, choice, and therapeutic diversity for all our patients through involving individuals from different professional backgrounds who each take a different approach to pain management.

Both our cameos demonstrate the need for more than one professional to be involved in caring for a patient and family. We can also say that both scenarios demonstrate a team approach. But what are the key differences between James's team and the experienced team? The following section will take us through some of the theories of teamwork and look at some of the problems and pitfalls, which must be overcome to become a successful team. Having visited the theories, we shall return to our cameos.

SOME THEORY

So what is a team?

We all know what a team is. It is a group of people who work together to achieve a common goal that cannot be achieved alone. Each individual usually has a specific role and brings a unique talent, whilst being able to "turn their hand" to another skill. Sports like football demonstrate this.

The equivalent in clinical practice is interdisciplinary care. A doctor is not a counselor and vice versa. Nor is a nurse a psychologist. Each has skills specific to their professions, but some are transferable. Good team players, whilst knowing their own area and general limitations, should be able to perform the basics of their colleagues' areas. Functioning together their effectiveness far exceeds that of an individual, provided they understand each other's personal and professional skills and help each other to recognize and develop their strengths and abilities within the group. However, it needs more than just a collection of well meaning professionals to deliver interdisciplinary care effectively. What is necessary?

For the diverse needs of patients with pain to be addressed seamlessly and effectively, a team far more easily achieves them. This is one of the foundations on which specialist palliative care and hospice services are built, and now is required in all cancer centers across the UK. However, much of the evidence in support of teamworking in cancer pain and palliative care still remains anecdotal[3, 4] despite some objective evidence that bereaved carers perceived better pain and symptom management, financial help, and information on local services when there was a specialist interdisciplinary team involved.[5]

From research we find two essential groups of ingredients aside from the people: one to do with the job in hand (the task), and the other to do with managing the problems that arise when people work together (the relationships). Both areas must be understood, developed, and fostered. This takes both time and effort. We now come onto this.

What makes a team succeed?

CLARITY

The overarching theme around tasks and operations is the need for clarity and consistency. The majority of research relevant to us has been undertaken in primary care and mental health. Basically, the themes are common and there are no real surprises, perhaps with the exception of evaluation and accountability, which Field and West emphasize.[6] This is perhaps because they refer to mature teams and demonstrate the end points of a time-consuming growth process (**Table 7.1**).

VARIETY

Equally, it is not surprising that teams comprising people with identical characteristics do not work well. In fact, having the brightest people in a team in no way

Table 7.1 What makes a team succeed?

Firth-Cozens[7]	McGrath[8] (Mental Health)	Field and West[6] (Primary Care)
Staff		
Staff with diverse skills and knowledge	Competent and committed staff	Individuals' contributions should be identifiable
	Agreed definitions of members roles,	
	Open communication systems and shared information	
Tasks		
A common goal	Goals and priorities must be agreed	Group goals must be clear
	There should be a task-centered, problem solving approach	The team's task is interesting in itself
		Individual tasks should be intrinsically rewarding
Relationships		
Staff who accept and manage conflict	Staff who are self critical, self-managing, and able to cope with conflict	Individuals who feel that their own work is essential to the success of the team
Staff who work towards unity	Participative management	Individuals who are subject to evaluation
Support for team members	An environment that is supportive,	Inbuilt performance feedback as part of goals setting
Opportunities for individuals to develop	informal, and member-orientated, creative and stimulating	

guarantees that it will be the best team. This is because the most effective teams have members who express characteristics that fulfill a variety of roles and behaviors necessary for balance. Within reason, the presence of these is as important to a good team as the caliber of its members. Meredith Belbin (**Table 7.2**) has carried out the most comprehensive study of this area.[9]

Belbin's work is essential reading for anyone interested in increasing effectiveness and understanding the essential ingredients for a successful team.[9] It is one of the few pieces of organizational development research of this kind that has stood the test of time to prove itself to be both valid and reliable.

In short, there are eight roles necessary to a team performing at its peak. This does not mean that an effective team has to have eight members, as one person can take two and occasionally three roles. Note also that a person may fulfill different roles in different groups or circumstances. The roles according to Belbin are tabulated (+). First, you will be able to see how certain roles are clustered and can be met by one person, and second, whilst people tend to have one or two "natural roles," they are not fixed. For example, in one group, one may function principally as the shaper and in another as the resource investigator if a more effective shaper is present or if there is no resource investigator in the second group.

So far then, we see that teams need different types of people with clearly defined roles, both technically and within the organic world of that team.

Support and peer supervision

PEER SUPERVISION

Everyone acknowledges that cancer and palliative care are stressful[10] areas of work and clinicians need peer-support and supervision. Not surprisingly, they are much-valued

characteristics of a good working environment.[6] We see this between the lines in the experienced team and explicitly in Linda's support from her colleague Julie. Social support at work has also been identified as a crucial stress-reducing factor.[11, 12] However, this is a two-edged sword as those working in hospice environments have identified. Vachon[10] found that over 70 percent of stress in hospice staff was attributed to organizational or role issues rather than relationships with patients and families or working with death and dying!

West[13] has helpfully described four types of social support in the team environment.

1. Emotional support – the "shoulder to cry on."
2. Informational support – someone who can point you in the right direction.
3. Instrumental support – practical help in times of heavy workload or simply "helping each other out."
4. Appraisal support – different perspectives on a given problem, not necessarily solution-generating.

A useful note here is that it is often these types of support that cross the barriers of role suspicion, historical hierarchies, and "ownership" of patients to forge a team where loyalty and affiliation are balanced properly between the team and ones profession. We see this, for example, with the CNS and GP in the experienced team.

TIME

Whilst it is common sense that a group of people who know what they are doing and why, can manage the aggravations and pressures of working together and still develop and keep the principal goal in view will be a good team, the time investment to get to this point is considerable. Five years is generally considered necessary

Table 7.2 Belbin's team roles.

Role	Description
Chairman/Coordinator	Coordinating role, focusing and balancing the group and its judgments. This person is not necessarily the brightest in a group or oddly, the leader. Doctors are often forced into this role, but frequently do it badly
Company person	A practical person, good at administration and implementing decisions
Teamworker	The engine room of the team, people who are loyal, committed, and noncompetitors and good at bridging conflicts and disputes
Completer-finisher	The person who makes sure projects are completed and kept on schedule. A very important role and often seen in administrators
Monitor–evaluator	The team analyst, who always spots the problems, is bright and slightly one-step back
Shaper	The natural leader who drives ahead with an idea and can be quite ruthless and inclined to take umbrage
Plant	Another intellectual who often works alone, but comes up with the ideas
Resource investigator	The charismatic member, entrepreneurial and popular who knows where to get what is needed, but is poor on follow through.

from inception to reach this stage. Furthermore, it does not stop there: teams go through cycles of function and dysfunction as members leave, new ones join, and as the tasks and goals change over time. A team is never static and the building process is never over!

The downsides of teamwork and how may it fail

> If you work on a team, then you will have to be prepared to show your battle scars
>
> Dame Cicely Saunders, Founder of the Modern Hospice Movement

TIME

On the one hand, time is essential to building teams, but on the other it is often at a premium, both overall (above) and as part of daily practice. Interdisciplinary teamwork is slower than working alone, but whilst decision-making can take longer, the quality of a decision made by a team is likely to be higher than that of an average team member.[13] In this regard, teamworking is inefficient. That said, Payne argues that our work will be happier and more successful if we all pay attention to teamwork all the time as part of our practice.[14]

CONFLICT AND COMMUNICATION BREAKDOWN

Furthermore, team members do not always agree. Indeed, performing teams need a degree of conflict/tension – overt and covert to maintain creativity and momentum. Without it there is no force for change. If this tension is not managed well or communication is allowed to deteriorate, people will polarize to their profession, form cliques, or withdraw. Any which way, trouble comes when we stop communicating and healthy tensions turn to civil war. It is here that the social links will work to maintain team integrity and where good management is necessary.

At such times in a team's developmental cycles, it does seem easier to go it alone, but so often our poor communication is the root of team tensions or poor service delivery. In reality, problems such as these are occupational hazards and a function of historical barriers between primary, secondary, and tertiary care, between professions, and between professionals and patients and families. This leads us to an important warning.

PROBLEMS WITH POWER, STATUS, AND COMMUNICATION

Amongst colleagues

It would be naive and irresponsible were we not to say that most times, effective teamwork requires professional or organizational status to be set aside. Much has been written over the years about the power-based relationships between caring professions. For example, the stereotypical doctor/nurse relationship portrays the nurse as subservient handmaiden to the doctor's masculine authority and sacred medical knowledge. If one enters the worlds of cancer, pain management, or palliative care and holds to these stereotypes, not only will one be a bad team member, but also a real obstruction to good patient care and partnership. We see shades of this in James Moss.

With our patients

From first presentation to discharge home it is quite usual for a patient to come into contact with at least 13 different professionals. The deluge of information can be confusing and distressing if different sources conflict or are inconsistent. This is a major risk with uncoordinated teamwork. The best solution on the one hand is to ensure that patients feel that they too are part of the team. Yet, on the other, reasonable differences in professional opinion around optimum treatments may be the last thing a patient needs to experience. It is at times like this that the quality and maturity of teamworking will find the necessary balance between disclosure and paternalism and the team will be comfortable with the need, on occasions, to plan behind closed doors.

Absent planning and maintenance

One of the major obstacles to the formation and functioning of teams within acute settings in particular has been the lack of strategic planning and investment in the new team development. A documented, though little discussed, example of this was the Charing Cross experience.[15]

Briefly, the palliative care support services at the hospital had a short and dysfunctional life and were disbanded. The authors highlighted their areas of difficulty, which led to their team's collapse within the overall problems of a hospital ill-designed architecturally, medically, or socially for a team approach to care. Compare their list of problems with **Table 7.1**:

- an amorphous team;
- understaffing, with only one full-time member (a nurse);
- no designated leader or role clarity;
- no clear referral criteria;
- lack of common office space;
- poor communication; and
- underfunding from senior management with other priorities.

The Charing Cross gives us a very clear message: without planning and development a team will fail and because the structure and constituency of teams differs between organizations, there can be no shortcut or "off the shelf solution." We now come to this.

Planning and developing a team

In these days of outcome measures there is little room for throwing resources at organizations and leaving them to get on with it. Any service development strategy must be justifiable, evidence-based, and take into account the need for in-built team development strategies that promote the development of good characteristics.

PLANNING

Øvretveit[16] suggests a useful model to assist those responsible for designing multidisciplinary services. Although he refers to community care, it transfers easily to any sector of health care. He stresses that teams should not be set up before a survey of local need. He stresses that these will not only focus development on local need, but will also foster genuine long-term commitment from senior managers and consultants.

Table 7.3 emphasizes two elements. The left hand column defines and analyzes each element of need from various perspectives and the right hand column lists the mechanisms that are necessary to make sense of the analysis in a coherent and doable organizational mechanism that demands accurate information, clear communication, and care planning. This next section offers some clues on how to achieve this.

PROCESSES: ORGANIZATIONAL DEVELOPMENT

> We trained very hard, but it seemed that every time we were beginning to form up into teams, we would be reorganised. I was to learn in later life that we tend to meet any new situation by reorganising and a wonderful method it can be for creating the illusion of progress, while producing confusion, inefficiency and demoralisation.
>
> Caius Petronius (AD66)

Petronius is highlighting the need for time and opportunity that must be given to allow teams to pass through their developmental phase and stabilize. This is the value of OD.

OD refers to those efforts intended to improve an organization's culture and processes as a group and between individuals in the group. Essentially, this means that one needs to use techniques and skills that foster relationships that will help people work well together.[17]

Teambuilding is the best known aspect of OD. Some consider it to be the single most important element.[18] Its aim is to improve team effectiveness by enabling teams to diagnose how they work together and improve their skills and effectiveness. However, for those readers who go cold at the prospect of playing silly games with colleagues, take heart! Guzzo and Shea[19] found that teambuilding has a positive effect on team members' attitudes to and perceptions of each other, but does not increase team performance! Despite this, there are some essential elements of organizational development strategy which must exist if the team is to develop in a healthy way (**Table 7.4**). However, what managers will find is that, once again, time is the key, combined with objectives and, in extreme circumstances external help from an expert. **Table 7.4** lists the type of OD technique that may be of value, using Tuckman's natural stages of team development.[20] We refer interested readers to the literature.[13, 18, 21]

Summary

The theory so far has told us that there is more to a team than a group of professionals. It should be clear, not just from this chapter, that patients with cancer need more than one discipline and this is best delivered by a team. Studies in palliative care and bereaved relatives seem to confirm this. Secondly, whilst elements of good teamwork are common sense, clarity about roles and tasks, and the development of stable, flexible, and accountable team life needs time, skilled management, and hard work. Thirdly, the task never ends and regardless of the ingredients, teams will cycle through phases of internal conflict, consolidation, and performance (the apocryphal forming, storming, norming, and performing). With these data, we can now return to our two examples of teams at work.

REVIEWING OUR SCENARIOS

James's team

We have just a small snapshot of James's team but let's assume that it is representative of many groups of

Table 7.3 A model for designing a multidisciplinary service.

Elements to be analyzed separately	The means to bring coherence
Assessment of need and the services to meet the need	Care plans
Level of need of individuals, communities, and populations	Information systems
The different types of need	Organizational structures
The various perspectives as to need, e.g. those of the patient, carers, and various professionals	Representatives operating in relationships of trust and understanding

Reprinted from Ref. 16, with permisssion.

Table 7.4 Tuckman's natural stages of team development and behaviors.

Stage of development	Associated member behavior	Objective	Process and developmental need
Forming	Polite, enquiring, avoiding conflict	Agree on team's mission statement and setting of initial objectives	Strong internal leadership through meetings, brainstorming, and objective setting. An emphasis on unity and desire to be part of the group
Storming	Emotions begin to emerge as underlying conflicts begin to surface, some withdraw	Agree on rules of engagement, e.g. operational policy within the team, decision making process and establish leadership	Emerging differences of opinion amongst members sometimes involving a challenge to leadership when external help may be needed
Norming	Mutual respect, shared responsibilities	Improve internal relationships and test relationships with others outside the team	Personal and group evaluation, recognizes the strength of diversity whilst maintaining core values. The values rather than the wish to be part of the group begin to maintain unity
Performing	Maturity and mutual acceptance (warts and all!)	Productive and seeking to do better.	Understanding that none of us is as good as all of us. Celebrating the achievements of the team rather than the individuals. Striving together to improve.

Reprinted from Ref. 20, with permission.

clinicians working together. From these we can take one of two views.

1. This is a team in its early stages of development; or
2. This is a group of professionals working in the same place at the same time, rather than a team.

From either reading, it falls short of teamwork. The patient and her husband were left with a prescription for a very strong painkiller and were told that they needed to see a counselor. Communication is at best poor between doctor and nurse, there seems to be little understanding of each other's roles, there are no clear rules/protocols for case review or management, and it appears that there is no agreed time or format to discuss difficulties.

James's perception was that he had given plenty of his time to the patient, that he had nothing more to offer as a doctor, and needed to hand over the psychological and emotional care to the counselor. Linda's view was that he yet again was shirking his responsibilities as a team member in communicating with her and his patient the real truth about what was happening. Both are of course right. Where things have failed is in communication and an agreed modus operandi (an operational policy to use management-speak). What is encouraging is that these problems are soluble using basic approaches with open discussion, negotiation, and an agreed framework of accountability within the team. With some candid discussion, both Linda and James will realize that both of them needs to change. What they need is help to do this.

Let's look at an alternative scenario.

Janet walks in to the consulting room, sits down and bursts into tears, saying that the pain in her side is not responding to the painkillers. James glances at Colin, thinking to himself, "I can't take away their hope. Her chances of surviving more than six months are less than 10 percent. I'm going to need some help with this one."

Addressing them together, he might say, "We all know that the success of treatment are uncertain in the long term, but we do need to wait to see how well the radiotherapy controls the pain. In the mean time we can try stronger painkillers."

"This is a very difficult time and I can see how terribly anxious you both are this afternoon. I think there are other strategies we need to look at to help you both to cope with this situation, but I cannot do this on my own. Fortunately I am part of a team and with your permission, I'd like to take some advice from Linda, our counselor. May I ask her in to introduce you? You can then have an initial chat with her and we will all meet for a full discussion next week."

"Can I suggest that over the next few days you sit down together and write down all the questions you have for us and when you come back next Friday, we can sit down together with Linda to answer them all to the best of our ability."

In taking this approach, James has first fulfilled his medical role in addressing the physical pain. Second, he is beginning to introduce other team members and their skills to help this couple cope with advancing disease and the pain of loss, change, and uncertainty. However, he has given some very important signals to Janet and Colin:

- he understands that they are in crisis, he is taking things seriously, and he wants to keep a close eye on things;
- they haven't got to wait another month to the next appointment;
- he doesn't know everything; and
- he works as part of a team.

"On your way out, make sure that you tell reception that you want a long appointment with Linda and I. That will ensure that we have sufficient time together to come up with a game plan."

James then calls Linda in and makes the introductions. This takes a few moments longer, though he is still able to leave at 4 p.m., but this time everyone is clear about what is going on.

A long appointment is a thirty-minute one as opposed to a ten-minute one. As part of their team development strategy, they had agreed on criteria for joint consultations in which they had agreed their mutual roles for such interactions. This has resulted in a highly effective working relationship; it provides a safer environment for patients to ask difficult questions of the doctor. The team counselor is then able to give a further thirty minutes, if necessary, to look at more specific psycho-emotional issues with the patient. Mutual cases are then discussed at the regular interdisciplinary team meetings, which provide an environment for peer support and supervision.

By now we hope that you have concluded on the one hand that James's team demonstrates poor teamwork, but on the other hand, for it to be good, it does not require a completely different approach or group therapy, just common sense and communication. This is a young team about to enter the storming stage. **Figure 7.1** illustrates the conflict management and strategies that the team may need.

The experienced team

Scenario 2 encapsulates the work of a team that has been in existence for more than five years. The apparent ease of

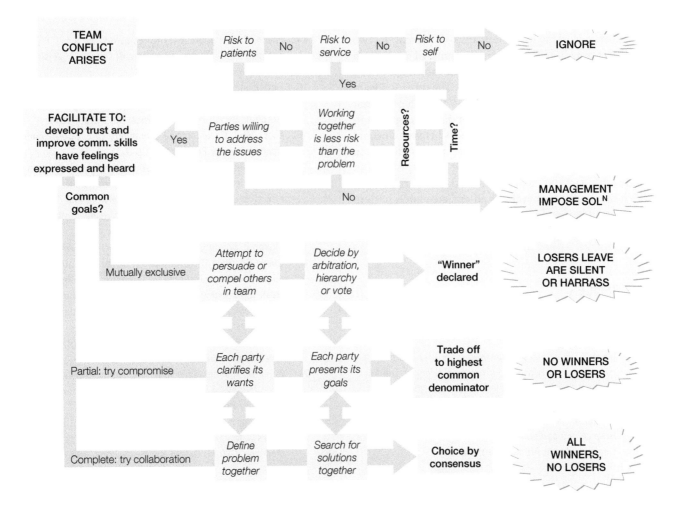

Figure 7.1 Strategies for conflict management. Adapted with permission from Cummings I. Interdisciplinary Teamworking. In: Doyle D, Hanks G, MacDonald N (eds.) *Oxford Textbook of Palliative Medicine.* OUP, 1999, p28.

assessment, the inclusion of the GP (and later the district nurses and hospital consultant) are only possible because of the structures that surround clinical practice: the team has clear referral criteria and goals, a mission statement, minimum standards of communication, clinical practice, notekeeping, a strong sense of corporate identity, and a clearly negotiated relationship between team members and those outside the team.[22]

This does not mean that this kind of team is perfect, but the existence of checks and balances to engage complex problems minimizes the risk of patient or staff morbidity from poor communication. Needless to say this has developed over the years, needed hard work, and more than a little give and take. It is however, as a highly functional team, at risk of complacency, and unthinking routine based in the belief that their way is the right way simply because it is the way that they do things.

Sooner or later, this team will begin to dysfunction and the arrival of a new member will expose it.

CONCLUSION

In this chapter we have attempted to illustrate how teamworking can make a difference to our patient care and our own working lives. Our cameos represent the two poles of teamwork. One extreme claims to be a team because they are in the same place at the same time once a week and make referrals to each other. The other is a team because they are so interdependent that they cannot function without each other. Each has strengths and weaknesses and there are infinite shades between one and the other. It is also worth saying that any one team can operate along the spectrum according to the problem in hand and in fact the most experienced teams are those in which the modus operandi is fluid and adaptable, both to the environment and to the problems in hand. Only you will know at which point to balance your team.

REFERENCES

1. Saunders CM. The last frontier. *Frontier.* 1966. Winter: 183–6.
2. Gysels M, Higginson I. *Improving supportive and palliative care for adults with cancer: research evidence.* London: National Institute for Clinical Excellence, 2004: 215. Available from: www.nice.org.uk
3. Dunlop R, Hockley J. National. In: Saunders C (ed.). *Hospice and palliative care. An interdisciplinary approach.* London: Edward Arnold, 1990: 14.
4. Sheldon F. Teamwork and palliative care. Is it effective? In: Sheldon F (ed.). *Psychosocial palliative care.* Cheltenham: Stanley Thornes, 1997: 112.
5. Jones RVH. Teams and terminal cancer at home: do patients and carers benefit? *Journal of Interprofessional Care.* 1993; **7**: 239–44.
6. Field R, West M. Teamwork in primary health care. 1 Perspectives from practices. *Journal of Interprofessional Care.* 1995; **9**: 122–30.
7. Firth-Cozens J. Building teams for effective audit. *Quality in Health Care.* 1992; **1**: 252–5.
8. McGrath M. *Multidisciplinary teams.* Aldershot: Gower, 1991.
9. Belbin M. *Management teams: why they succeed or fail.* Oxford: Butterworth-Heinemann, 1994.
10. Vachon MLS. Staff stress in hospice/palliative care: a review. *Palliative Medicine.* 1995; **9**: 91–122.
11. Cooper CL, Mitchell S. Nursing the critically ill and dying. *Human Relations.* 1990; **43**: 297–311.
12. Mallett K, Price JH, Jurs SG, Slenker S. Relationships amongst burnout, death anxiety and social support in hospice and critical care nurses. *Psychological Reports.* 1991; **68**: 1347–59.
13. West M. *Effective teamwork.* Leicester: BPS Books, 1994: 66.
14. Payne M. Two approaches to teamwork. In: Speck P (ed.). *Teamwork in palliative care.* Oxford: Oxford University Press, 2006: 118.
15. Herxheimer I, Maclean D *et al.* The short life of a terminal care support team: the experience at Charing Cross Hospital. *British Medical Journal.* 1985; **290**: 1877–9.
16. Øvretveit J. *Co-ordinating community care.* Buckingham: Open University Press, 1993: 26–7.
17. Iles P, Auluck R. From organisational to interorganisational development in nursing practice: improving the effectiveness of interdisciplinary teamwork and collaboration. *Journal of Advanced Nursing.* 1990; **15**: 50–8.
18. Moxon P. *Building a better team.* Aldershot: Gower, 1993.
19. Guzzo RA, Shea GP. Group performance and intergroup relations in organizations. In: Dunnette MD, Hough LM (eds). *Handbook of industrial and organisational psychology.* Palo Alto, CA: Consulting Psychologists Press, 1992: 269.
20. Tuckman BW. Development sequence in small groups. *Psychological Bulletin.* 1965; **63**: 384–99.
21. Payne M. Teambuilding: how, why and where? In: Speck P (ed.). *Teamwork in palliative care.* Oxford: Oxford University Press, 2006: 117–36.
22. Cummings I. Interdisciplinary teamworking. In: Doyle D, Hanks G, MacDonald N (eds). *Oxford textbook of palliative medicine.* Oxford: Oxford University Press, 1999: 28.

8

Barriers to cancer pain relief: an international perspective on drug availability and service delivery

FIONA GRAHAM AND DAVID CLARK

Introduction	81	Patterns of service development	85
Drug availability	82	Conclusions	89
The principle of balance	84	References	90

KEY LEARNING POINTS

- Cancer pain remains unrelieved, particularly in resource-poor settings, worldwide.
- The main barriers to cancer pain relief are lack of opioids, inadequate education, and government indifference to the issue.
- The principle of "balance" is essential in opioid regulation.

- Cancer pain and palliative care services across the world remain weakly developed and have limited coverage.
- Cancer pain and palliative care services must be locally appropriate and sustainable.
- Awareness of, and engagement with, issues is essential for all with an interest in achieving a cancer pain-free world.

INTRODUCTION

Around the world, cancer is increasing and it is having a differential impact in poorer countries. Of the estimated ten million people[1] who are diagnosed every year, over half are living in the developing world and many will have incurable disease at the time of diagnosis. By 2020, it is estimated that the incidence of cancer will double.[2] The global burden of cancer will increase from 10 to 24 million over the next 50 years and 17 million of these will be in developing countries.[3]

Cancer pain is common. Two-thirds of those with advanced disease, and a third of those undergoing active treatment, suffer pain.[4] Until earlier referral and diagnosis occur and standard therapies are able to be deployed for the majority of those with cancer, pain relief and palliative care will remain the most relevant provision for large numbers

affected. Meanwhile, both cancer and palliative care remain relatively low priorities on the global health agenda.[5]

In this chapter, we examine how cancer pain has developed as a field of interest, going on to highlight the particular problem of drug availability. We describe in detail the work of the Pain and Policy Studies Group in Wisconsin, USA and show how its research and development program is having an impact on opioid availability in a number of different countries and resource settings.[6] In order to gain a better understanding of related service developments, we also draw on studies undertaken by the International Observatory on End of Life Care at Lancaster University, UK as part of its global development program.[7] The chapter contains a number of case studies and illustrations that highlight the barriers to cancer pain relief, as well as some of the approaches that have been found to overcome these.

Before the 1970s, cancer pain had received little international attention as either a clinical or a public health problem and was often regarded as an inevitable, not fully controllable, consequence of the disease.[8, 9] The spread of modern hospice and palliative care and the creation of the professional field of pain studies encouraged a small number of pioneering oncologists to organize the first International Symposium on Cancer Pain, held in 1978.[10] Research presented at this and subsequent conferences suggested that physicians had the means to relieve even severe cancer pain and that the principal factors contributing to poor pain management were legal barriers against opioid use and poor dissemination of available knowledge about pain management. In 1982, the World Health Organization (WHO) enlisted the aid of palliative care leaders, cancer pain specialists, and pharmaceutical manufacturers to develop a global Programme for Cancer Pain Relief, based on a three-step analgesic ladder with the use of adjuvant therapies, and incorporating the use of strong opioids as the third step.[11] WHO representatives launched an international initiative to remove legal sanctions against opioid importation and use, relying on national coordinating centers to organize professional education and to disseminate the core principles of the pain management. The WHO programme met with only partial success, however. Opioid consumption between 1984 and 1993 rose dramatically in ten industrialized countries, but showed much smaller increases in the rest of the world[12] and significant differences in the pattern and the extent of opioid use continued to be observed within and between global regions.[13]

Effective management of cancer pain needs to be multifaceted and should be informed by the concept of "total pain," as described by Cicely Saunders, founder of the modern hospice movement, with its recognition of the physical, psychological, social, and spiritual dimensions of pain.[14] Drug treatment, however, remains the mainstay of cancer pain relief. Since 1986, the WHO analgesic ladder[15] has provided a deliberately simple framework for the progressive treatment of malignant pain.[11] Its originators hoped it would lead to a world free of cancer pain, though they acknowledge now that this has not come to pass.[16] There are many reasons for this, including reluctance on the part of physicians to prescribe strong opioids, fear among healthcare professionals and the public about addiction and abuse, lack of state and national government engagement with the issue of cancer pain, and a lack of availability of essential drugs due to stringent regulation and economic factors.

Recognition of these issues led the WHO to develop its concept of "foundation measures" to promote the implementation of cancer pain relief programs. These highlight the importance of three key factors essential if cancer pain is to be overcome: education, government policy, and drug availability.[4]

Education needs to be wide ranging to achieve these aims. Clearly, healthcare professionals must be trained in the appropriate and safe use of analgesic drugs, particularly opioids, but this can be difficult if the dominant culture in their workplace is to view these as dangerous drugs of misuse. Education, therefore, needs to begin by addressing these fears. Paradoxically, a useful starting point for these discussions is the Single Convention on Narcotic Drugs 1961 (amended 1972) which recognized "… that the medical use of narcotic drugs continues to be indispensable for the relief of pain and suffering."[17]

Policymakers, drug regulators, and the general public also need to be more aware that opioid drugs, such as morphine, have an essential place in the management of pain – one that cannot be sacrificed because of any potential for diversion and misuse.

Government policy, whether at state or national level, has to recognize and emphasize the importance of the effective management of cancer pain, which should be seen as a priority. Similarly, the availability of essential drugs is crucial in efforts for the relief of pain in cancer. In some regions of the world, access to appropriate drugs is taken for granted, but in many more these are simply unavailable. The reasons for this are complex, but engagement with them is essential for anyone who concurs with the vision of a world free of cancer pain. As Liliana de Lima, of the International Association for Hospice and Palliative Care (IAHPC) has reflected:

> In so far as improving access to opioids is an international effort, we are all affected to some degree by the decisions and actions taken by others. We need to become aware that opioid availability is not just a local issue, but rather one with no borders. All stakeholders in this process, including patients, professionals, multilateral organizations, the pharmaceutical industry, policymakers, and healthcare professionals, need to be included in the development of strategies to improve this situation.[18]

DRUG AVAILABILITY

Key to the effective implementation of the WHO analgesic ladder is the availability of the medication necessary at each of the three steps. It is both fruitless and frustrating for practitioners to be trained in the effective management of pain and to then lack the tools to implement that knowledge. Economic factors can sometimes limit the availability of analgesics recommended on the first two steps of the ladder but, in reality, it is the lack of the step three analgesics, principally morphine, which results in the most suffering. The major reason for this is regulation and its interpretation.

The Single Convention on Narcotic Drugs[17] is an international treaty that seeks to ensure that all United Nations (UN) member countries take steps to prevent the abuse of narcotic drugs while ensuring adequate availability for medical and scientific use. Derived from the Greek *narke* (numbness)[19] narcotics are, essentially, substances which induce drowsiness. The term "narcotic drug" however, has a legal significance denoting any substance, natural or synthetic, listed in schedules I and II of the 1961 Convention. The International Narcotics Control Board (INCB) was created by the convention for its implementation. The remit of the Single Convention is to promote governmental compliance with the treaties.

Currently, the Single Convention exercises control over 116 narcotic drugs. These are grouped into four schedules depending on their therapeutic effectiveness and propensity for misuse, with Schedule I drugs, such as morphine, fentanyl, and opium, subject to the most stringent controls. The WHO is charged with assessing whether the list should be added to or amended. States that are signatories to the Convention agree to implement its terms locally and to cooperate with other states in achieving its aims, principally to ensure that the production, trade, and distribution of narcotic drugs is properly managed and is for scientific and medical purposes only. They must also recognize the authority of the international control organs: the Commission on Narcotic Drugs of the Economic and Social Council and the INCB.

The commission is concerned with all aspects of the Convention, particularly with respect to amending the schedules, identifying issues relevant to the functions of the INCB, and communicating with parties outside the convention to encourage adoption of similar measures.

The board consists of 13 members including three with a medical, pharmacological, or pharmaceutical background from a list of at least five nominated by the WHO. The remaining ten are elected from a list compiled by both members and nonmembers of the UN. They serve for five years. Each year, states must provide the board with estimates of their drug requirements and statistics related to the production and consumption, import and export, seizure and disposal, and stocks of drugs, as well as details of areas where the opium poppy is cultivated. Using these data, the manufacture and importation of each drug is limited depending on the sum of the quantities that are:

- consumed for medical and scientific purposes;
- used for the manufacture of other drugs not covered by the Convention and those in Schedule III;
- exported;
- added to the stock to bring it to the level of the relevant estimate;
- required for special purposes, within the limit of the relevant estimate.

Countries where the opium poppy is grown also need to establish a national opium agency which designates areas for cultivation and licences the producers. Licences are also needed for the manufacture, trade, and distribution of drugs, except when this is carried out by a state enterprise. Medical prescriptions are required for the supply of drugs, unless legally available over the counter and, if deemed necessary, Schedule I drugs may need to be prescribed on official forms. Export of drugs is forbidden unless in accordance with the laws of the importing country and within the estimates of need for that country. Complicated arrangements exist for import and export to happen. Organizations and professional individuals utilizing the drugs therapeutically are required to keep scrupulous records and governments must ensure illicit traffic is avoided.

Given the level of control exercised over narcotic drugs, it is not difficult to understand why some, from healthcare practitioners through to national governments, make the decision that obtaining and prescribing these drugs is too onerous. Because of the potential for abuse, regulation is necessary, but this can exist in harmony with adequate supplies for medical need. Indeed, the INCB is committed to assisting governments to achieve a more balanced approach[20] as the following examples illustrate.

Regulation in Italy

Towards the end of the 1990s, the INCB became increasingly troubled about the low levels of morphine consumption in Italy, a country with a relatively high per capita income. Indeed, the INCB annual report for 2000 stated:

> The Board remains concerned about the low levels of consumption of morphine for medical purposes in Italy, which may be indicative of insufficient availability of the drug for pain management purposes.[21]

Efforts had been made to address the problem with little success, until 1998 when a study[22] revealed that, although lack of physician education and cultural prejudices were implicated in the problem, there were major difficulties related to the prescribing of drugs. The necessary piece of documentation, the Special Prescription Form (SPF) was complex, with three parts, and the amount that could be supplied was strictly limited. In addition, physicians and pharmacists were liable to severe penalties in the event of any technical error. These factors, it was postulated, dissuaded doctors from prescribing the necessary drugs to combat pain effectively. As a result of the study and through new legislation, a simplified prescription was developed which required that the necessary information be entered only once in a way which bore more resemblance to the standard Italian script, thus decreasing any stigma related to the prescribing of opioid medication. The maximum supply available on one prescription increased from eight days to one month and sanctions against physicians and pharmacists became more lenient. With these measures, and an enlightened program of physician and public education about cancer pain funded by the Drug Department of the Italian Ministry of Health, the basis for a more relevant and appropriate approach to the management of cancer-related pain in Italy has been established.

Regulation in India

In India in the early 1980s, increasing medical use of opioids gave rise to fears about diversion and drug misuse. The 1985 Narcotic Drugs and Psychotropic Substances Act was passed in response. The Act established new licencing requirements, with states developing their own procedures to conform to the law. The procedures became so complex that institutions seeking to purchase morphine from a neighboring state required five different licences from two different departments in each state, which took time and energy to procure, and all of which had to be valid for shipment to proceed. The result was that physicians and hospitals stopped trying to obtain these drugs and India's consumption of morphine fell by 97 percent between 1985 and 1997. The INCB recognized that this decline indicated that opioids were no longer available for legitimate use and charged the Indian Government with the responsibility to tackle the problem. A WHO demonstration project in Kerala, India, was able to show that when prescribing practices, stock security, and record maintenance were scrupulous, making opioids available for cancer pain did not lead to diversion or misuse.[23] Armed with this information, practitioners from the demonstration project, the Pain and Palliative Care Society, and the Indian Association for Palliative Care were able to lobby state and national government officials into a commitment to maintain a minimum stock of morphine for medical use. In the meantime, many patients had suffered unnecessary pain witnessed by Professor Rajagopal, from the demonstration project:

> To communicate the intensity of the dread felt by staff and patients when a morphine shipment was delayed and the joy when the morphine finally arrived is not possible.[23]

THE PRINCIPLE OF BALANCE

The principle of balance is a concept that applies to ensuring that opioid analgesic drugs are available for legitimate medical use, notably pain relief, whilst preventing their diversion for illicit purposes. The idea has been developed by David Joranson and colleagues at the Pain and Policy Study Group (PPSG), Madison, WI, USA. Joranson's work has been important and influential in the field and, although we highlight some of the work here, readers are directed for further detail to the PPSG website, which is an invaluable resource.[6]

The Pain and Policy Studies Group was established by Joranson in 1996. The group is part of the University of Wisconsin Comprehensive Cancer Center within the School of Medicine and Public Health. It investigates national and international opioid policy and has developed guidelines and undertaken workshops essential to the implementation of any meaningful change in government policy. To date, the PPSG has provided technical assistance to governments and nongovernmental organizations in Africa, Asia, Europe, and Latin America. As a WHO Collaborating Center, it began in 1998 to develop guidelines for governments to assess their opioid regulation policies. An international working group of experts was convened to review these guidelines, including representatives from Italy, China, India, Nigeria, Japan, Saudi Arabia, and the Americas. This resulted in the WHO document *Achieving a balance in national opioids control policy: guidelines for assessment,*[24] subsequently endorsed by the INCB,[25] and which consists of a self-assessment checklist of 16 guidelines within three areas:

1. assessing national policy;
2. estimating annual opioid requirements;
3. ensuring an effective system for distributing drugs to patients.

The guidelines, which are available in some 14 languages, also emphasize the importance of regulators, governments, and practitioners working together to achieve a balanced approach to regulation and availability.

Having developed the guidelines, the next step was to put them into action. To simply send them to the relevant national regulators was unlikely to produce rapid results so the team developed a workshop approach, bringing together both regulators and clinicians to consider the guidelines within their own local contexts. The first of these workshops was held in Quinto, Ecuador in 2000, with representatives from Peru, Bolivia, Chile, Venezuela, Ecuador, and Colombia. A follow-up meeting in 2002 found evidence of progress: Venezuela had held a national workshop to highlight the importance of opioid availability and, in Colombia, a National Network of Pain Relief charged with educating doctors in the appropriate medical use of opioids had been established.[26] There was, however, evidence to support the impression that achieving policy change was a long process with much patience and perseverance required.

The case of Romania illustrates that through this approach, along with enthusiasm, determination, and support, tangible changes can be made to government policy on opioid availability. In 2002 the PPSG, in collaboration with the WHO regional office and the Open Society Institute, held one of its workshops in Budapest, Hungary attended by representatives from Bulgaria, Croatia, Hungary, Lithuania, Poland, and Romania. Romania was chosen as a pilot country for follow up. It had very restrictive policies on the use of opioids, which dated from more than 35 years earlier at the time of the Ceausescu regime. Yet, within its pioneering palliative care services, there were healthcare professionals who were highly motivated to lobby for and to initiate change[27] and within the Ministry of Health there was a willingness to engage with the issues. The ministry established a Commission of Specialists in Pain Therapy and Palliative Care, charged with identifying and clarifying the main barriers to effective cancer pain relief in Romania. This group worked closely with the team from the PPSG which undertook a comprehensive review of the country's existing regulations and, in summer 2003 presented its recommendations for change to the Ministry of Health. These recommendations included the removal of government restrictions on the maximum doses of opioids and simplification in the process of drug authorization for longer-term prescribing. They also requested that more than one opioid could be prescribed on one form and that change in drugs and doses could be determined by patient need. The Ministry of Health was also asked to clarify various points about effective record keeping, responsibility for submission of statistics to the INCB, and which opioids were to be licenced for importation and manufacture in Romania. In addition, the ministry was asked to make the effective management of cancer pain a high priority and to work with the Ministry of Education to ensure pain treatment formed an integral part of the training of health professionals. Drafting new legislation based on the recommendations then started and, whilst this proved challenging for all involved, the proposed law passed both houses of the Romanian parliament in November 2005. As Daniela Mosoiu, hospice physician and a key figure in effecting the changes commented:

> We hope that the Romania project will serve as a positive example of how an outdated and restrictive national antinarcotics law can be reformed into one that embodies the essential principle of balance, retaining essential control over the security and distribution of controlled drugs, while allowing physicians to practice modern pain medicine and care for their patients.[27]

PATTERNS OF SERVICE DEVELOPMENT

Just as innovations in cancer pain relief began to get underway from the 1970s onwards, significant strides were also being made in the global development of palliative care, which in many areas had a strong emphasis on the care of patients with cancer and gave attention to the effective management of pain and other symptoms. It was the work of Dr Cicely Saunders, first developed in St Joseph's Hospice in Hackney, east London that was to prove most consequential, for it was she who began to

forge a peculiarly modern philosophy of terminal care. Through systematic attention to patient narratives, listening carefully to stories of illness, disease, and suffering, she evolved the concept of "total pain".[14] This view of pain moved beyond the physical to encompass the social, emotional, even spiritual aspects of suffering – captured so comprehensively by the patient who told her, "All of me is wrong."[28] However, it was also linked to a pragmatic approach to pain management. Her message was simple, "constant pain needs constant control."[29] Analgesics should be employed in a method of regular giving which would ensure that pain was prevented in advance, rather than alleviated once it had become established; and they should be used progressively, from mild, to moderate to strong.

Having established the modern science and art of caring for patients with advanced malignant disease, Cicely Saunders went on to found the world's first modern hospice, combining clinical care, teaching, and research at St Christopher's in south London, which opened in 1967. Immediately it became a source of inspiration to others and was also firmly established in an international network. The correspondence of Dr Saunders shows clearly how it attracted the interests of clinicians from many countries who were eager to develop their practical skills through work on the wards of the hospice.[30] It quickly sought to establish itself as a center of excellence in a new field of care. Its success was phenomenal and it soon became the stimulus for an expansive phase of hospice and palliative care development, not only in Britain, but also around the world.

From the outset, ideas developed at St Christopher's were applied differently in other places and contexts. Within a decade it was accepted that the principles of hospice care for cancer patients could be practiced in many settings: in specialist inpatient units, but also in home care and day care services; likewise, hospital units and support teams were established that brought the new thinking about the care of those with advanced malignant disease into the very heartlands of acute cancer medicine. Modern hospice developments took place first in affluent countries, but in time they also gained a hold in poorer countries, often supported by mentoring and twinning arrangements with more established hospices in the west. By the mid-1990s, a process of maturation was in evidence in some countries, but elsewhere growth was slow and a source of disappointment to palliative care activists.

Yet all around the world there are examples of innovative services seeking to address the problem of cancer pain. The difficulties they face in achieving their goals are complex in character and can be found in rich and poor countries alike. Close working relationships within the field of palliative care have been important to success in many places and the efforts of pain specialists interested in malignancies have also been vital. Drawing on studies undertaken by the International Observatory on End of

Life Care (IOELC),[7] we highlight here the particular example of access to cancer pain relief in selected settings.

In the context of wider palliative care development, an analysis of the global situation of palliative care,[31] led by Michael Wright, reveals striking variations both between and within world regions. The study categorizes hospice-palliative care development, country by country, throughout the world using a four-part typology. The four categories are:

1. no identified hospice-palliative care activity;
2. capacity building activity, but no service;
3. localized palliative care provision;
4. countries where palliative care activities are approaching integration with mainstream service providers.

Palliative care services were found in 115/234 countries. The total numbers of countries in each category were: no identified activity 78 (33 percent), capacity building 41 (18 percent), localized provision 80 (34 percent), and approaching integration 35 (15 percent).

This typology differentiates levels of palliative care development in both hemispheres and in rich and poor settings. In category four, hospice-palliative care services are characterized by: a countrywide critical mass of activists; a range of providers and service types; a broad awareness of palliative care on the part of both health professionals and local communities; a measure of integration of palliative care services with mainstream service providers; the availability of strong pain-relieving drugs; palliative care influence on policy; the development of recognized education centers; academic links with universities; the performance of research; and the existence of a national association. Category three countries are characterized by the development of a critical mass of activists in one or more locations, the establishment of a hospice-palliative care service, the growth of local support, the sourcing of funding, the availability of morphine, and the provision of training by hospice and palliative care organizations. In category two, there is evidence of a range of capacity building activities designed to create the organizational, workforce, and policy capacity for hospice-palliative care services to develop, albeit with no current services identified. Finally, in 78 countries there is no contemporary evidence of palliative care interest.

Although half of the world's countries have a palliative care service, development remains extremely patchy and seems to be driven more by local contingencies and the involvement of specific leaders and innovators, rather than on the basis of population need or public health principles. For example, in North America, both Canada and the USA are in category four (approaching integration), whereas in Greenland, no palliative care activity could be identified. In Latin America, the two southernmost countries, Argentina and Chile, fall into category

four. Costa Rica, however, stands alone in category four among the countries of Central America and the Caribbean. In Western Europe, with the exception of Portugal, Luxembourg, and a few small countries, such as Andorra, all countries are in category four. In Central and Eastern Europe, however, with the exception of Hungary, Poland, Romania, and Slovenia, all countries are in category three, localized provision. In Western Asia and the Middle East, only Israel is in category four, whilst in many countries throughout the region, no service could be identified. In Africa, only Uganda, Kenya, and South Africa have achieved a level of integration with wider health services. In 32 of the 48 African countries, no service could be identified. In the Asia Pacific region, a patchwork of initiatives was identified, but only a small number of countries is approaching integration with wider health services. In Oceania, only Australia and New Zealand have achieved such integration.

We now highlight these issues in more depth in three case studies: India,[32] a study led by Liz McDermott, the six countries in the Middle East,[33] led by Amanda Bingley and Africa,[34] led by Michael Wright.

India

In the Indian example, a country in the localized provision category of development, we see a picture of mixed fortunes.

In India, it is estimated that one million new cases of cancer occur each year, with over 80 percent presenting at stage III and IV.[35] Two-thirds of patients with cancer are "incurable"[36, 37, 38] and approximately one million people are experiencing cancer pain every year.[39] It is difficult to assess the exact requirement for palliative care because of inadequate disease registration, cultural stigma, and communication problems.

The IOELC review conducted in 2005–2006 set out to assess the current state of palliative care in India, mapping the existence of services state by state and exploring the perspectives and experiences of those involved. One hundred and thirty-five hospice and palliative care services were identified in 16 states. These are usually concentrated in large cities, with the exception of the state of Kerala, where they are much more widespread. Nongovernment organizations, public and private hospitals, and hospices are the predominant sources of provision. There are 19 states or union territories in which no palliative care provision could be identified. Development of services is uneven, with greater provision evident in the south than the north.

The history of palliative care in India began in 1975 when the government initiated a National Cancer Control Programme. By 1984, this plan was modified to make pain relief one of the basic services to be delivered at primary healthcare level, although it has not been readily translated into extensive service provision.[40]

In 1986, Professor D'Souza opened the first Indian hospice, Shanti Avedna Ashram, in Mumbai, Maharashtra, central India.[41] Concurrently, pain clinics were established (at the Regional Cancer Centre, Trivandrum, Kerala and at Kidwai Memorial Institute of Oncology, Bangalore, Karnataka) and oral morphine was made available, free of charge, for the first time.[35, 42, 43]

From the 1990s onwards, there was a significant increase in the momentum of development of hospice and palliative care provision in India. This was demonstrated by an expansion in the number of services, as well as other key events and initiatives. The few services established were able to act as examples of the ways in which care could be offered to people at the end of their lives. Of significance was the establishment in 1993 of the Indian Association of Palliative Care (IAPC), during a workshop arranged with the guidance of WHO and the Government of India,[44] and in 1995 the IAPC set up a Palliative Care Drugs Committee and Educational Task Force.[45]

The mid to late 1990s saw a range of developmental activities. CanSupport was founded by Harmala Gupta in Delhi to provide the first free palliative care home care support service in north India. In Pune, Maharasthra, the Cipla Cancer Palliative Care Centre was established which, in consultation with Cancer Relief India, developed a new concept of a "living" palliative care center[46] with 50 beds arranged round a quadrangle with a children's playground in the middle. In addition, the Pain and Palliative Care Clinic was established at Medical College Hospital in Calicut, Kerala.

At the beginning of the 1990s, north Kerala did not have any palliative care facilities and there was only an outpatient pain clinic in Trivandrum, south Kerala. In 1993, a small group of doctors and social activists, all personally involved in the terminal care of cancer patients, organized an outpatient palliative care service at Calicut Medical College providing for both the physical and emotional needs of patients. It aimed to be free and accessible to poor patients in a context that was "adapted to the Indian scenario."[37]

In June 1996, a homecare service was set up with the aim of "delivering palliative care to the patients who are unable to reach the hospital, to empower patients to care for themselves and to empower the family to care for patients."[47] The homecare service was delivered by a doctor and some trained volunteers. In the first year of operation, the homecare team made 340 visits and concluded that home-based, volunteer-delivered palliative care may be the most suitable way to deliver palliative care to people in need in that area of Kerala.

The success of the home care program led to the Neighbourhood Network in Palliative Care (NNPC) initiative in 2001, which attempts to develop a sustainable community-led service capable of offering comprehensive long-term care (LTC) and palliative care (PC) to those in need.[48] In this program, volunteers from the local community are trained to identify problems of the chronically ill in their area and to intervene effectively, with active support from a network of trained professionals. The NNPC programs appear to have been very successful in the areas where they have been launched. In Malapurum, a poor district in Kerala with a population of four million, the coverage of LTC and PC rose to 70 percent in two years. There is an NNPC clinic roughly every 10 km which means patients should not have to travel more than 5 km. The concept took ten years to evolve and is now being subject to careful evaluation.

Finally, there are three government-funded centers which have been successful at providing and developing hospice and palliative care provision in India: Kidwai Memorial Institute of Oncology, Bangalore; Trivandurum Regional Cancer Centre, Kerala; and Tata Memorial Cancer Hospital, Mumbai. These centers run palliative care courses and raise awareness of palliative care in their area, as Dr Cherian Koshy of Trivandurum comments:

> We have been able to train a sizeable number of doctors who have gone through the one month hands-on training, which equips them to stock morphine. And we also have frequent training programs, one day, two day, three day, short training programs. We have quite a large number of nurses who have been trained. And this message of palliative care I think has already become a movement in our state. And we even have medical students coming... and people are aware about this philosophy of palliative care.[49]

The Middle East

In 2005, a study by the IOELC identified a total of 69 palliative care services across the six member countries of the Middle East Cancer Consortium (MECC).[33] The Palestinian Authority and Turkey were described as in the initial capacity building stage of palliative care development. Jordan and Egypt were identified as providing localized provision and Cyprus and Israel were considered to be approaching integration.

Home care services are the most common type of palliative care service provision in the region, although there is no home care in Egypt, Palestinian Authority, or Turkey. In Cyprus, two charities provide all the specialist services in the Greek Cypriot south and one provides some limited support in the Turkish Cypriot north.

In Israel, there is one major Non-Government Organization (NGO) that provides funding towards several services, educational and research activity, and public education programs. In the Palestinian Authority, one NGO offers psychosocial support for women with breast cancer at the end of life, as well as support for breast cancer survivors and other health-related services.

Of the 11 hospice inpatient palliative care units in the region, seven are freestanding (Cyprus, one; Egypt, two; and Israel, four). The remaining four units are dedicated specialist beds based within hospital oncology wards in Israel and Jordan. These kinds of specialist inpatient units are distinct from hospital-based consultation services offered at the end of life. In such situations, professionals who are aware of the principles of palliative medicine or who have completed some specialist training provide pain and symptom management. They are often constrained from developing full palliative care services because of limited resources, a lack of trained staff, and little support from colleagues. In 2005, this type of provision was the only service available in Turkey, although there were some motivated oncologists working to develop more comprehensive services in several major hospitals. In the Palestinian Authority and Egypt, this kind of service continues to be the main type of provision.

Opioids are reported to be available in all MECC countries. Cyprus, Egypt, Israel, Jordan, and Turkey make annual returns of data on opioid preparation and consumption, as sovereign states and members of the INCB. The Palestinian Authority is not an acceded party to the conventions of the INCB and therefore has no published figures for the consumption of narcotic drugs. A limited range of opioids is available for use in oncology units in the West Bank and Gaza Strip, although choice and availability of drugs cannot be guaranteed.[50]

The range of available drugs varies in different countries, but all MECC members report access and usage of common generic opioids used in palliative care, including codeine and generic morphine preparations. Healthcare professionals across the region note a general trend away from the use of morphine and an increase in use of more expensive proprietary opioids, in particular transdermal fentanyl. INCB data confirm anecdotal reports, from physicians and oncologists in the region, who observe widespread prescribing of fentanyl preparations, notably highest in Israel and Turkey, but widely used in Cyprus and Egypt. In Israel, physicians also note an increase in use of other opioid derivatives, such as hydrocodone and oxycodone.

All MECC member countries now have some form of government legislation for opioid availability and prescribing powers for physicians. Quantities permitted per prescription range from sufficient medication (of any appropriate strength) for three days up to ten days supply. In Israel, the maximum (and exception) at any one time is a 30-day supply. As part of opioid awareness and education, Israel, Cyprus, and Jordan routinely include pharmacists in their palliative care training courses. The increase in training opportunities in Israel and Cyprus has resulted in markedly less antagonism and phobia from healthcare professionals and consequently their patients. Opioid phobia, however, remains a considerable barrier to adequate opioid prescribing in Turkey and Jordan.

Education and training in palliative care is available internationally at postgraduate and fellowship level for all healthcare professionals in the MECC region who have the means to travel, or are supported through NGO or other charitable funding. Israel, with the most integrated palliative care services, is the only country in MECC that has some core training units in palliative care for medical students, and has also developed a national specialist postgraduate qualification in the subject. Cyprus, Israel, and Jordan have short units during core nursing training and Egypt has some palliative care training in development for core nursing education. International opportunities in palliative care education are a vital part of raising awareness and providing access to training courses for all MECC members – in the case of physicians in the Palestinian Authority and Egypt, such opportunities represent the only viable training option.

Despite a varied picture in terms of population patterns, healthcare systems, palliative care needs, and stages of palliative care service development, Cyprus, Egypt, Israel, Jordan, the Palestinian Authority, and Turkey share many of the major barriers to service development: lack of training, resources, problems with government legislation, and insecure funding. Cyprus and Israel have the most advanced development and Jordan and Egypt have some localized provision, albeit more developed in Jordan than Egypt. The Palestinian Authority and Turkey are capacity building, although the Palestinian Authority lacks any real resources for service development or pain and symptom management. In contrast, Turkey is experiencing increasing awareness of palliative care with Turkish cancer and pain specialists becoming active in palliative care service development.

Africa

Several initiatives are underway to promote the development of hospice and palliative care in Africa. WHO is involved in a joint palliative care project for cancer and HIV/AIDS patients in the five countries of Botswana, Ethiopia, Tanzania, Uganda, and Zimbabwe.[51] The Diana, Princess of Wales Memorial Fund has supported palliative care initiatives in the nine countries of Ethiopia, Kenya, Malawi, Rwanda, South Africa, Tanzania, Uganda, Zambia, and Zimbabwe.[52] The Foundation for Hospices in sub-Saharan Africa,[53] now a part of the National Hospice and Palliative Care Organization in the USA,[54] has a growing program of twinning schemes. The Open Society Institute has a grant support program for southern Africa.[55] An evidence base for the African palliative care context is also beginning to emerge with analyses of models of service delivery[56] and an appraisal of the literature relating to services in sub-Saharan Africa.[57]

The history of hospice development in Africa stretches back to the late 1970s, when services first appeared in

Zimbabwe and in South Africa. Island Hospice was founded in Harare in May 1979 and had developed 17 regional branches by 1997.[58] In the late 1970s, hospice initiatives were also developing in South Africa – in Johannesburg, Port Elizabeth, Cape Town, and Durban. The visit of Cicely Saunders to South Africa in 1979 added impetus to these developments and within a year or two hospice organizations were operating in a variety of settings throughout the country. After the start made in these two countries, it was another decade before hospice and palliative care developments began to occur elsewhere in Africa: in Kenya and Swaziland (1990); Botswana, Tanzania, and Zambia (1992); Uganda (1993); Sierra Leone (1994); Morocco (1995); Congo-Brazzaville and Nigeria (1996); Malawi (1997); Egypt (2001), and the Gambia (2004).

The IOELC[34] review identified 136 hospice and palliative care organizations in 15 countries, an area with a population of 407 million people. The vast majority of these are nongovernment, charitable, and faith-based organizations. Over half (76) were found in South Africa, which has more such organizations than all of the other African countries combined (**Table 8.1**).

Although in South Africa there are 37 organizations with free-standing hospice inpatient facilities, 8/15 countries with hospice-palliative care in Africa have no such facility and, in general, there is an emphasis on the development of home care services. These are found in 14/15 countries and are provided by 111 of the 136 organizations identified. Forty-nine organizations have hospital-based services, found in 11/15 countries. Day care services and clinics are run by 87 organizations in 14/15 countries.

This limited development of hospice-palliative care organizations is also reflected in the low level of opioid use across the continent (**Figure 8.1**).[59] Yet, whilst a clear match exists between the country with the most reported defined daily doses of morphine and that with the most hospice and palliative care services (South Africa), it is difficult to explain why Namibia, the Central African Republic, and Tunisia report higher morphine use than other countries when the review could identify no hospice or palliative care services in those countries. Across Africa there are many reported problems of morphine availability and these are exacerbated by fears of using the drug, both on the part of practitioners and patients.

Nevertheless, there are some examples of outstanding success in tackling the problem of morphine availability. In Uganda, morphine for cancer and HIV/AIDS patients is provided free of charge by the government and, in a groundbreaking innovation of March 2004, a Statutory Instrument[60] was signed by the Minister of Health authorizing palliative care nurses and clinical officers to prescribe morphine.

CONCLUSIONS

The problems we have described in this chapter are not those of poverty and underdevelopment alone, though such factors play their part. Many countries still have hugely inadequate supplies of appropriate pain medication, even though this can be made available at low cost. Some governments put in place draconian measures to limit the manufacture, sale, transportation, storage, and

Table 8.1 Hospice and palliative care: organizational provision in Africa (15 countries).

Country	No. of organizations	No. of known branches	Organizations making inpatient provision		Organizations making outpatient provision	
			Hospice	Hospital	Home care	Day care/clinic
Botswana	3	0	0	1	3	3
Congo	1	0	0	1	1	0
Egypt	3	0	2	1	1	1
Kenya	8	3	0	6	8	6
Malawi	5	0	0	4	2	3
Morocco	1	0	0	1	0	1
Nigeria	2	0	0	1	1	1
Sierra Leone	1	0	1	0	1	1
South Africa	76	42	37	19	61	49
Swaziland	4	0	1	0	3	2
Tanzania	4	0	0	3	3	3
The Gambia	1	0	0	0	1	1
Uganda	8	124	2	6	7	6
Zambia	6	0	6	0	6	6
Zimbabwe	13	6	2	6	13	4
Total	136	175	51	49	111	87

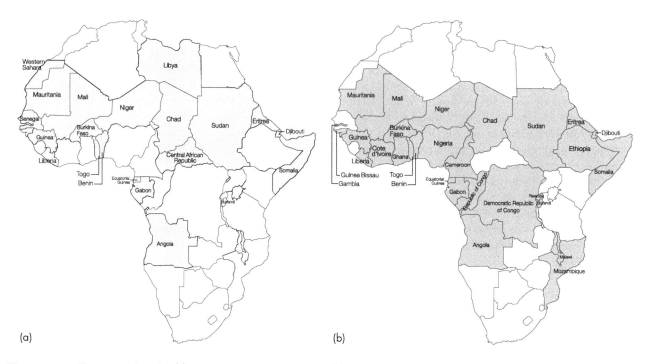

(a)　　　　　　　　　　　　　　　　　　　(b)

Figure 8.1 African countries with (a) no reported morphine use and (b) those with no known palliative care.

prescription of strong opioid drugs. Too often the balance between "regulation" and "availability" is tipped in favor of the regulators, to the extent that simple pain-relieving measures are largely unavailable. The problem is compounded by clinicians made nervous about prescribing strong painkillers for risk of social opprobrium, or even prosecution. The world of cancer pain and palliative care services is divided between the "haves" with access to a range of appropriate medications and the knowledge and will to use them – whilst the "have nots" are denied even simple formulations. The underdevelopment of cancer pain and palliative care services globally does a disservice to those who could benefit from improved provision and is frankly unjust. Good care for cancer patients, including the relief of pain at the end of life and the opportunity for a dignified death, should be regarded as basic human rights to which everyone should have access when the time comes.

REFERENCES

1. Sikora K (ed.). *World Health Organization Programme on Cancer Control: Developing a global strategy for cancer.* Geneva: WHO, 1998.

2. Selva C. International control of opioids for medical use. *European Journal of Palliative Care.* 1997; **4**: 194–8.

3. Parkin DM, Bray FI, Devesa SS. Cancer burden in the year 2000: the global picture. *European Journal of Cancer.* 2001; **37**: 4–66.

∗ 4. World Health Organization. *Cancer pain relief with a guide to opioid availability*, 2nd edn. Geneva: World Health Organization, 1996.

5. Sloan A, Gelband H (eds). *Cancer control opportunities in low and middle income countries.* Washington: The National Academic Press, 2007.

∗ 6. Pain and Policies Studies Group, University of Wisconsin; last updated: December 4, 2007; cited December 2007. Available from: www.painpolicy.wisc.edu.

∗ 7. International Observatory on End of Life Care. Lancaster University, UK; cited December 2007. Available from: www.eolc-observatory.net.

8. Seymour J, Clark D, Winslow M. Pain and palliative care: the emergence of new specialties. *Journal of Pain and Symptom Management.* 2005; **29**: 2–13.

9. Seymour J, Clark D. The modern history of morphine use in cancer pain. *European Journal of Palliative Care.* 2005; **12**: 152–5.

10. Bonica JJ, Ventafridda V. *International Symposium on Pain of Advanced Cancer.* New York: Raven Press, 1979.

11. Meldrum M. The ladder and the clock: cancer pain and public policy at the end of the twentieth century. *Journal of Pain and Symptom Management.* 2005; **29**: 41–54.

12. Stjernsward J, Joranson DE. Opioid availability and cancer pain – An unnecessary tragedy. *Supportive Care in Cancer.* 1995; **3**: 157–8.

13. Seymour J, Clark D. The modern history of morphine use in cancer pain. *European Journal of Palliative Care.* 2005; **12**: 152–5.

14. Clark D. 'Total pain', disciplinary power and the body in the work of Cicely Saunders 1958–67. *Social Science and Medicine.* 1999; **49**: 727–36.

15. World Health Organization. *Cancer pain relief.* Geneva: World Health Organization, 1986.

16. Swerdlow M. Memorandum of meeting with Jan Stjernsward, May 22–25, 1981. In: Mark Swerdlow Papers,

John C Liebeskind History of Pain Collection, Louise M Darling Biomedical Library, UCLA.

* 17. United Nations. Single convention on narcotic drugs, 1961. Geneva: United Nations 1973. Available at www.incb.org/incb/convention_1961.

18. De Lima L. Opioid availability in Latin America as a global problem: a new strategy with regional and national effects. *Innovations in End-of-Life Care.* 2003; **5**: 97–103.

19. *Compact Oxford English Dictionary.* Oxford: Oxford University Press, 2003.

20. Pain and Policy Studies Group. *Improving availability of essential pain medicines for cancer and HIV/Aids: Report for 2005.* Madison, WI: University of Wisconsin Comprehensive Cancer Centre.

21. International Narcotics Control Board. *Report of the International Narcotics Control Board for 1999.* New York: United Nations, Available at www.icnb.org/e/ind_ar.

22. Blengini C, Joranson DE, Ryan KM. Italy reforms national policy for cancer pain relief and opioids. *European Journal of Cancer Care.* 2003; **12**: 28–34.

* 23. Rajagopal MR, Joranson DE, Gilson AM. Medical use, misuse, and diversion of opioids in India. *Lancet.* 2001; **358**: 139–43.

24. World Health Organization. *Achieving a balance in national opioids control policy.* Geneva: World Health Organization, 2000.

25. International Narcotics Control Board. *Report of the International Narcotics Control Board for 2001.* New York: United Nations, 2002.

26. Joranson DE. Improving availability of opioid pain medications: testing the principle of balance in Latin America. *Innovations in End-of-Life Care.* 2003; **5**: 105–14.

* 27. Mosoiu D, Ryan K, Joranson D, Garthwaite J. Reform of drug control policy in Romania. *Lancet.* 2006; **367**: 2110–17.

28. Saunders C. *Care of patients suffering from terminal illness at St Joseph's Hospice.* Hackney, London: Nursing Mirror, Vol. 14, 1964: vii–x.

29. Saunders C. Drug treatment in the terminal stages of cancer. *Current Medicine and Drugs.* 1960; **1**: 16–28.

30. Clark D. *Cicely Saunders founder of the hospice movement. Selected letters 1959–1999.* Oxford: Oxford University Press, 2002.

31. Wright M, Wood J, Lynch T, Clark D. Mapping levels of palliative care development: A global view. *Journal of Pain and Symptom Management* (in press).

32. International Observatory on End of Life Care. Lancaster University, UK; cited December 2007. Available from: www.eolc-observatory.net/global_analysis/india.htm.

33. International Observatory on End of Life Care. Lancaster University, UK; cited December 2007. Available from: www.eolc-observatory.net/global_analysis/mecc.htm.

* 34. Wright M, Clark D. *Hospice and palliative care in Africa: a review of developments and challenges.* Oxford: Oxford University Press, 2006.

35. Seamark D, Ajithakumari K, Burn G et al. Palliative care in India. *Journal of the Royal Society of Medicine.* 2000; **93**: 292–5.

36. Sebastian P, Varghese C, Sankaranarayanan R et al. Evaluation of symptomatology in planning palliative care. *Palliative Medicine.* 1993; **7**: 27–34.

37. Kumar S, Rajagopal MR. Palliative care in Kerala. Problems at presentation in 440 patients with advanced cancer in a south Indian state. *Palliative Medicine.* 1996; **10**: 293–8.

38. Vijayaram S, Ramamani PV, Chandrashekhar NS et al. Continuing care for cancer pain relief with oral morphine solution. One-year experience in a regional cancer center. *Cancer.* 1990; **66**: 1590–5.

39. Stjernsward J, Stanley K, Tsechkovski M. Cancer pain relief: an urgent public health problem in India. *Clinical Journal of Pain.* 1985; **1**: 95–7.

40. Rajagopal MR, Venkateswaran. Palliative care in India: Successes and limitations. *Journal of Pain and Palliative Care Pharmacotherapy.* 2003; **17**: 121–8.

41. Shanti Avedna Sadan. *A light in the darkness.* Mumbai: Shanti Avedna Sadan, 2005.

42. Burn GL. A personal initiative to improve palliative care in India. *Palliative Medicine.* 1990; **4**: 257–9.

43. Vijayaram S, Bhargava K, Ramamani M et al. Experience with oral morphine for cancer pain relief. *Journal of Pain and Symptom Management.* 1989; **4**: 130–4.

44. Bhatia MT. President's message. *Indian Journal of Palliative Care.* 1996; **2**: 3–5.

45. Indian Association of Palliative Care. Resolutions adopted in the IIND International Conference of the Indian Association of Palliative Care held in Ahmedabad 6.2.95 to 8.2.95. *Indian Journal of Palliative Care.* 1995; **2**: 54.

46. Burn G. A personal initiative to improve palliative care in India: 10 years on. *Palliative Medicine.* 2001; **15**: 159–62.

47. Ajithakumari K, Sureshkumar K, Rajagopal MR. Palliative home care – the Calicut experience. *Palliative Medicine.* 1997; **11**: 451–4.

48. Kumar S. Learning from low income countries: what are the lessons? Palliative care can be delivered through neighbourhood networks. *British Medical Journal.* 2004; **329**: 1184.

49. Interview with Dr Cherian Koshy 12/11/04 by Lucy Selman. Summary available www.eolc-observatory.net/global_analysis/india_oral_histories.

50. 2006 data on access and availability of medications in Gaza and the West Bank available in the WHO Health Crisis in Action Report, July 2006 (see updated information on the WHO weblink http://millenniumindicators.un.org/unsd/mi/mi_results.asp?crID=275&fID=r15).

51. World Health Organization. *Community health approach to palliative care for HIV/AIDS and cancer patients in sub-Saharan Africa.* Geneva: World Health Organization, 2004: 8. Available from: http://whqlibdoc.who.int/publications/2004/9241591498.pdf.

52. The Diana, Princess of Wales Memorial Fund. The work continues; cited December 2007. Available from: www.theworkcontinues.org.

53. Foundation for Hospices in sub-Saharan Africa, Alexandria, VA, USA; cited December 2007. Available from: www.fhssa.org.

54. National Hospice and Palliative Care Organisation. Advancing care at the end of life. Alexandria, VA, USA; cited December 2007. Available from: www.nhpco.org.

55. Open Society Institute. New York, NY, USA; cited December 2007. Available from: www.soros.org.

56. Harding R, Stewart K, Marconi K *et al.* Current HIV/AIDS end-of-life care in sub-Saharan Africa: a survey of models, services, challenges and priorities. *BMC Public Health.* 2003; 3: 33.

57. Harding R, Higginson I. *Palliative care in sub-Saharan Africa. An appraisal.* London: King's College and Diana, Princess of Wales Memorial Fund, 2004. See www.theworkcontinues.org/causes/pall_library.

58. McElvaine D. Zimbabwe: the Island Hospice experience. In: Saunders C, Kastenbaum R (eds). *Hospice care on the international scene.* New York: Springer, 1997: 52.

59. International Narcotics Control Board. Narcotic drugs: estimated world requirements for 2004. Statistics for 2002. New York: United Nations, 2004.

60. Ministry of Health, Republic of Uganda. Statutory instruments 2004: 24 The National Drug Authority (Prescription and Supply of Certain Narcotic Analgesic Drugs) Regulations, 2004. Ministry of Health, 2004.

9

Ethical issues in cancer pain management

FIONA RANDALL

Introduction	93	Decision-making for adult patients who lack capacity	96
Education of healthcare professional and patient on issues of pain control	94	The relief of pain and the prolongation of life	97
Consent for pain relief	94	Conclusions	99
"Total pain"	95	References	99
The role of relatives in decision-making for patients who have capacity	95		

KEY LEARNING POINTS

- There is an obligation upon healthcare professionals to be competent in pain relief and to provide adequate analgesia; they are also obliged not to impose treatment without consent.
- Professionals should not offer or provide treatments that will confer overall harm yet there is usually a personal element to assessment of harm and benefit.
- They are obliged to seek consent, but yet must not force unwanted information on patients in the process, nor deny pain control to those who do not wish to be fully informed.
- When gravely ill patients have pain which is unusually difficult to control, it occasionally happens that we

foresee that the adverse effects of adequate medication might shorten life. In this situation, the doctrine of double effect may be used to justify the provision of adequate analgesia if, but only if, all of the following conditions are met:
  - the adverse effects are foreseen, but not intended;
  - the bad effect (shortening of life) must not be the means to the good effect (relief of suffering);
  - the good effect of relief of suffering must outweigh the bad effect of shortening of life (condition of proportionality).

INTRODUCTION

The essential aims of all health care are: the relief of suffering, the prolongation of life, and the restoration of function. There is therefore an ethical requirement that all who are engaged in health care should promote these aims. Since the relief of pain is an important aspect of the relief of suffering, there is an ethical requirement to relieve pain to the extent that that is possible. These aims seem uncontroversial, but in the clinical situation controversy can arise because they can conflict with other

ethical requirements of health care and they can conflict with each other. This chapter discusses six ethical complexities which arise:

1. in the education of healthcare professionals and patients on issues of pain relief;
2. in the process of obtaining consent from the patient for pain relief;
3. in the idea of "total pain" and what the healthcare professionals can reasonably be expected to do;

4. in the role of relatives in decision-making for patients with capacity;
5. over decision-making for patients who lack capacity;
6. in the possible conflict between the relief of pain and the prolongation of life.

EDUCATION OF HEALTHCARE PROFESSIONAL AND PATIENT ON ISSUES OF PAIN CONTROL

As pain control is an intrinsic part of the healthcare professional role, the importance accorded by professionals to pain relief is a moral issue in itself. It is therefore strange and morally questionable that, in general, a low priority is given to education about pain relief in undergraduate and postgraduate medical education, especially when compared with the priority given to life-prolonging measures. The low priority given to pain control in education is reflected in doctors' attitudes to the importance of pain relief. However, since it is an intrinsic aim of health care that doctors have an obligation to be competent at a basic level in pain control and an obligation to provide the treatment that achieves pain control, doctors and nurses with specialist knowledge and experience should take every opportunity to pass that knowledge on to others and should also try to encourage others to strive continuously to achieve the best possible pain control in all patients.

Patients also frequently lack knowledge of the methods of pain control and the adverse consequences of unrelieved pain. They are often reluctant to take appropriate analgesics. There are four common reasons for this. (1) They may not have been told the diagnosis and possible prognosis. This raises the ethical issue of adequately informed consent which is discussed below under Consent for pain relief. (2) They may have been told that they have advanced malignant disease, but may not believe the information they have been given. By refusing the analgesic they may be attempting to sustain the belief that they do not have the disease. (3) They may fear they will become addicted to morphine or tolerant to it, fears which will be especially influential if they also believe that they will get better. (4) Patients may refuse optimal analgesia for fear it will "mask" the pain and so detract from attempts to monitor and treat the disease. All four misunderstandings require sensitive explanation regarding the true state of affairs.

Apart from the formal ethical requirement to obtain consent for a treatment, there is a good therapeutic reason for educating the patient in pain control. It is that pain control is most likely to be successful when patients understand their illness and the ways in which the medication is intended to alleviate pain. They will then be able to cooperate with healthcare professionals, and pain control can become a partnership.

The education of both healthcare professional and patient is therefore an ethical preliminary to pain control.[1]

CONSENT FOR PAIN RELIEF

Seeking consent to treatment with appropriate analgesic regimens usually entails a discussion about the clinical circumstances in general – it is not just a matter of asking the patient to take morphine. Of course, patients may decline analgesia, or may occasionally want to retain a degree of pain as a yardstick of how the illness is going, but doctors and nurses should make sure that a refusal of analgesia is made only after the patient has had the opportunity to comprehend the medical facts of the situation. In other words, by offering information, doctors and nurses should endeavor to ensure that refusal of consent is informed, and that consent given is adequately informed.

Seeking adequately informed consent from patients includes informing them about the harms and risks of treatment, and this includes the side effects of medications.[2] It is possible to become so overwhelmed by a desire to relieve the patient's pain that we lose sight of the parallel obligation to inform patients of the significant side effects of the drugs or procedures. This happens particularly when it seems to the professionals that the benefit of pain relief far outweighs the harm of a particular side effect, such as constipation or sedation. Some drugs (for example nonsteroidal anti-inflammatory agents) are associated with a multitude of side effects, some of which are serious and not uncommon, especially in the context of advanced malignancy. In particular, gastrointestinal hemorrhage and renal failure may be precipitated by their use. Since clinicians strive to achieve pain control, and because they consider that the benefits of drugs outweigh their harms in the circumstance, it is easy for them to fail to mention serious and relatively common side effects that present harms or risks.

There is a professional view of the importance of these harms and risks in the circumstances, and this view is based on value judgment, as well as factual information. However, we know that patients place different values on various harms and benefits, so that what may seem to the professional to be an acceptable harm or risk may not be acceptable to the patient. Therefore, even if the professional considers that the benefits of an analgesic outweigh the side effects, it can be argued that the professional should mention common side effects to the patient, because the latter may consider certain adverse effects as particularly undesirable.[3]

For example, whereas some patients would rather be completely pain free, even if this means being drowsy, others would rather accept some pain, for instance on movement, rather than feel sedated by the analgesics. Patients need to be offered the chance to participate fully in decision-making regarding analgesia, because full participation increases the chance of establishing the best regimen for them. Therefore, professionals have a moral obligation to try to enable patients to have a basic understanding of their illness and painkillers so that they can work together with their doctors to overcome the pain.

Healthcare professionals have a clear obligation not to harm patients in terms of increasing suffering or causing threat to life, and so should not provide treatments whose associated harms and risks in these respects outweigh their benefits in the clinical circumstances. At the same time, we have already acknowledged that the patient's own assessment of the importance of those harms and risks is of crucial relevance in the decision. For example, a nerve block may alleviate pain but at the cost of rendering a limb numb, and there may be other risks of loss of function through misadventure. The patient may or may not consider a numb and possibly weak limb to be better than a painful one, whereas the doctor, from experience, may know that other patients often find a numb and useless limb more distressing than a painful one. Patient and doctor between them need to weigh up the harms, risks, and benefits. If agreement is not reached then, in the final analysis, the doctor can and should decline to provide a treatment requested by the patient if the doctor considers that the harms and risks outweigh possible benefits, and the doctor should not insist on treatment which the patient refuses.[4, 5]

The right to give informed consent and to be fully involved in decision-making regarding pain control should not be transformed into a duty. In other words, giving fully informed consent should not become a condition of receiving adequate pain control. It seems intuitively wrong that patients who do not want much information should have to have it forced upon them and thus be forced to give fully informed consent before pain control is provided. Some patients, especially those who are terminally ill and exhausted, do not wish to be fully informed or involved in decision-making, and it seems reasonable to respect their choice in this regard. They may state that they do not want to discuss all the details of their illness or to receive a list of side effects of medications. Instead, they may want professionals to offer what they consider is the best option and then they choose to accept that option on less information than would be regarded as adequate for fully informed consent. It seems reasonable that such patients should be able to choose the extent of their involvement in decision-making. They are responsible then for that choice.[6]

"TOTAL PAIN"

The multifactorial etiology of pain has come to be appreciated, and the concept of "total pain" has been generally accepted.[7, 8] Indeed, as our understanding of the physiology of pain improves, it is becoming clear that cognitive and emotional factors do influence pain pathways. Total pain is a concept relating to distress that includes emotional, social, and spiritual components, as well as the purely physical pain aspect of the pathology. For terminally ill patients and those suffering chronic pain, professionals are increasingly encouraged to consider that the aim is to alleviate total pain, which, of course, entails addressing emotional, social, and spiritual sources of distress. This goes way beyond the traditional remit of health care, and it raises some moral issues. For example, is it realistic to imply that professionals can alleviate nonphysical sources of distress? How cost-effective in terms of resources (especially professional time) is it to attempt to do this? Has the patient given any form of consent to interventions designed to alleviate emotional, social, or spiritual distress?

In particular, in the context of palliative care, it is generally considered that professionals should try to alleviate emotional and social pain[9] and that doing so entails knowing how the patient and family are adjusting to the whole illness scenario and how it is affecting their relationships with each other. All of this entails questioning the patient and family about intimate relationships. Such questioning is unjustifiably intrusive if the patient has not requested such assistance, or at least given consent freely to discussions about his or her very private affairs. It is all too easy, especially if buoyed up by an almost missionary zeal to alleviate total pain, for professionals to intrude into patients' private affairs under the (probably misguided) impression that we can alleviate emotional, social, and spiritual distress. Our motivation to alleviate these components of total pain should not drive us to intervene without the patient's consent, just as our motivation to alleviate the physical component of pain with analgesics does not justify treating the patient without his or her consent.[10]

THE ROLE OF RELATIVES IN DECISION-MAKING FOR PATIENTS WHO HAVE CAPACITY

In western society, the wishes of the adult patient who has decision-making capacity are currently considered to override those of their relatives as far as treatment decisions are concerned. There is a moral imperative for healthcare professionals to uphold the patient's rights to information and to consent to or refuse treatment, and to protect patients from coercion by (usually well-meaning) relatives.

In contrast, in some other cultures the relatives' views are considered to be as important as, or sometimes more important than, those of the patient. In these cultures, knowledge of the diagnosis may be given to the relatives and withheld from the patient. Of course, in these cultures patients will be aware that this is occurring as they will be familiar with the culture. Where the views of relatives are given priority in this way, the relatives may make decisions on behalf of the patient. When those from such cultures are being treated in a western environment, then they become subject to the ethical and legal requirements of the west.

DECISION-MAKING FOR ADULT PATIENTS WHO LACK CAPACITY

At the end of life, many patients will be unable to make decisions for themselves, by reason of confusion or diminished consciousness. When it is clear that the illness will result in death and that further attempts to prolong life are unlikely to succeed, the moral obligation to relieve pain logically supersedes any obligation to continue to strive to prolong life. Healthcare professionals should then make the patient's comfort their first priority.[11] They will then wish to provide an analgesic regimen that will enable the patient to be comfortable, but without causing more sedation than is necessary to achieve this. However, since the patient lacks capacity to consent to or refuse treatment options, the question arises as to who should have authority to make treatment decisions on the patient's behalf.

In western society, when the patient's wishes are not known and cannot be ascertained, relatives may or may not be given decision-making authority on behalf of the patient, depending on the law of the country concerned. For example, under the Mental Capacity Act 2005 in England, relatives do not normally have decision-making authority and so cannot consent to or refuse treatment on behalf of the patient. However, provision is made for patients, when they have capacity, to appoint a relative as an "attorney" with authority to make specified decisions on the patient's behalf when the patient loses capacity.[12] In contrast, in some other countries, including the USA, relatives can routinely consent to or refuse treatment on behalf of the patient, and may be expected to take this responsibility.

However, it should be noted that relatives cannot force the healthcare team to give treatment that the professionals consider is inappropriate because of an adverse balance of harms and risks to benefits.[13] In other words, relatives cannot insist that the patient be given a treatment (for example excessive sedation) that has very little chance of benefit, in comparison with more major and/or more certain harms and risks.

The differences between the laws of various countries reflect the fact that there are moral arguments both for and against giving relatives decision-making authority for patients who lack capacity. Such decision-making authority enables and perhaps requires relatives to consent to or refuse an analgesic regimen on behalf of the patient. The policy regarding decision-making for patients who lack capacity is generally decided on the basis of two issues: first, who is likely to make decisions that most accord with what is best for the patient; and second, who can be said to have some sort of entitlement to make decisions for the patient.

It can be argued that the healthcare professionals are better placed, on the grounds of professional knowledge and experience, to know what is the best analgesic regimen for the patient. On the other hand, relatives are likely to have a better knowledge of the patient's previously expressed wishes and values. Ideally, healthcare professionals and relatives should work together to formulate the analgesic regimen that best accords with attaining comfort without going against the patient's known values. Disagreement about an analgesic regimen is uncommon, but if relatives refuse the analgesic regimen considered most appropriate by the healthcare team the consequences for the patient may be very serious. Therefore, in some countries, such as the UK, decision-making authority for patients who lack capacity normally lies with the healthcare team and not with the relatives.

However, in other countries decision-making authority lies with the relatives, who can therefore refuse the analgesic regimen on behalf of the patient. They might do this if they believed it would or might shorten life. Decision-making authority may be granted to relatives because of a view that they are entitled in some way to make decisions for the patient. Such an entitlement may be based on the idea of an ownership or property right, but this idea is intuitively unattractive. It is more plausible to base an entitlement for relatives to make decisions on behalf of incompetent patients on the idea that such a policy affirms and fosters intimate relationships between family members. Alternatively, it may be thought that relatives may be most likely to decide in the patient's best interests, but where pain control is concerned it must be admitted that the knowledge and experience of the healthcare professionals make them more likely to know what regimen is most likely to be effective.

Regardless of whether the healthcare team or the relatives are granted legal decision-making authority for patients who lack capacity, there is a moral duty for both parties to work together to try to achieve the analgesic regimen that will enable the patient to be comfortable, while at the same time respecting as far as possible the patient's previously stated values.

Some patients make oral or written statements while they have capacity in order to influence treatment decisions that may arise later when they lack capacity to make those decisions. Such statements are called "advance statements," or may be referred to as "living wills." A doctor presented with an advance statement has to decide (as far as possible) whether the patient had capacity when it was made and whether it was intended to apply to the circumstances that have actually arisen. The legal status of advance statements varies in different countries. Concerns may arise that patients should not be able to refuse adequate pain control in advance; for this reason the Mental Capacity Act in the UK stipulates that a patient cannot refuse measures essential for pain relief, seen as "basic care," via an advance statement.[14] It would be extraordinarily rare for patients to state that they did not want to be pain free at the end of their lives, or for them to want their relatives and carers to see them distressed at this time.

Fortunately, when adequate explanation is given to relatives, agreement about treatment is normally reached without conflict, and patients at the end of life can and should be as free of distress as current medical knowledge allows.

THE RELIEF OF PAIN AND THE PROLONGATION OF LIFE

Healthcare professionals must achieve a delicate moral balance between their obligations.

- There is an obligation to strive to alleviate pain, yet there is an obligation not to impose treatment without consent.
- Treatments should not be offered or provided that will confer overall harm, yet there is usually a personal element to assessment of harm and benefit.
- There is an obligation to seek consent, but professionals must not force unwanted information on patients in the process, nor deny pain control to those who do not wish to be fully informed.

If all these obligations are accepted by healthcare professionals and the delicate moral balances required are achieved, there will still remain those moral problems that occur when there is a conflict between the main aims in health care and their corresponding obligations. The most common conflict in the area of pain control is that which is perceived to occur between the obligation to relieve suffering and the obligation to prolong life.

The scenario, often reported dramatically in the media, in which a patient with a terminal illness has pain and distress which has been difficult to control and it is found that drug regimens that effectively alleviate the pain also inevitably result in sedation with possible shortening of life, is familiar to all. Unfortunately, one would be led to believe by the media, certainly in the UK, that such situations are the norm, if indeed pain can be controlled at all. Those reading this book will be aware that with good pain control such situations are not common,[15] but they do still occur and treatment decisions have to be made.

Everyone is bound by the laws of our communities and countries. The vast majority of communities and countries have laws that prohibit one person from intentionally causing the death of another. Intentionally causing the death of another person, i.e. killing another person, is a major offence and is punishable by law. This law quite rightly applies to doctors and nurses, and indeed it could be argued that it must apply particularly to doctors and nurses, who are entrusted with the care of their patients and who are normally considered to have an obligation to try to prolong life. So, although doctors and nurses have a moral obligation to alleviate pain, they also have moral and legal obligations not intentionally to cause the deaths of their patients. The legal prohibition is to do with both intention and causation and it reflects the consensus that there is a moral prohibition against intentionally causing the death of another. Thus, in most countries, there are legal and moral prohibitions against healthcare professionals intentionally causing the deaths of their patients.

Returning to the problem scenario, occasionally it happens when a patient is terminally ill that the drug regimen required to alleviate distress will have other effects, such as sedation or respiratory depression, which in the context of the patient's grave illness will possibly hasten death. However, doctors are morally and legally prohibited from intentionally causing the patient's death. At the same time, they have an obligation to relieve suffering. What can be done to resolve these conflicting obligations?

Two main approaches are commonly used to justify the use of a drug regimen given to alleviate distress in those terminally ill when it may result in hastening death. The first or "common-sense" approach is to argue that on the basis of a relatively simple balance of benefits to harms and risks, the analgesic regimen is morally justified, and the second is to use a more complex philosophical approach called "double effect." If we begin with the common-sense approach, one might say that the benefit of freedom from pain in the context of a terminal illness outweighs the harms of sedation and the risk of shortening life. Of course, the patient's views are essential in assessing the benefit of pain relief, the harm of sedation, and the risk of earlier death. Some dying patients like and want a degree of sedation; others do not like it and do not want it. Some want to live as long as possible, and want potentially life-prolonging treatments to be attempted; others do not.[3]

It is generally accepted that when a patient who is terminally ill wants to be free of pain, even at the cost of sedation and possible shortening of life, then the necessary drug regimen should be provided, even if it may result in death slightly earlier. When the patient is unable to take part in decision-making, doctors may take this view and implement the drug regimen on the basis of the patient's overall benefit. Patients, doctors, and the law in the UK accept this practice and consider it to be morally, as well as legally justified in the circumstances. It is also reasonable to conclude that the analgesic regimen was not the fundamental cause of the patient's death – the illness is considered the primary or fundamental cause of the patient's death, although it is acknowledged that death may occur slightly earlier as a result of the side effects of sedation.

The second is a philosophical approach called the rule or doctrine of "double effect."[16] It can be invoked in circumstances in which a single act has two anticipated effects, one good (such as pain relief) and one bad (such as earlier death). It can then be argued that the act may be morally justifiable if the bad effect is not intended although it is foreseen. This rule or doctrine is sometimes used to justify the use of drug regimens to prevent distress, which is considered the good effect, even if that may entail a risk of shortening life, which is considered a bad effect. The doctrine of double effect relies upon the distinction between intending the good effect of treatment and foreseeing but not intending the bad or adverse effect.

The doctrine of double effect has four conditions which must be satisfied if the doctrine is to justify the action. They are as follows.

1. The act itself must be good. Pain control is a good act.
2. The agent must intend only the good effect, i.e. pain relief.
3. The bad effect (shortening of life) must not be the means to the good effect (relief of suffering).
4. The good effect must outweigh the bad effect.

This complex argument involves two assumptions which require discussion; the distinction between intending and foreseeing, and a view of what causes death.[17]

First, the moral distinction between intended and foreseen effects of treatment is accepted in medical practice. Virtually all treatments have foreseen harms and risks. Although healthcare professionals intend the benefits from treatments, the fact that they foresee side effects and risks does not mean that they intend those harms and risks in the sense of wanting, seeking, or aiming at those harms and risks. For example, surgeons do not intend the discomfort and anxiety that accompany an operation, although they foresee them. Similarly, oncologists do not intend the adverse effects of chemotherapy, such as nausea, although they foresee them. In both cases, it is generally accepted that the doctors intend only the benefits, and that they foresee but do not intend the harms and risks.

Intention is itself a highly complex psychological concept which has been much discussed in moral philosophy. Intention has to do with planning towards the outcome, or wanting, desiring, or willing that outcome. This is how it is understood in ordinary usage, when its meaning is distinguished from the concept of foreseeing but not aiming at, willing, or planning a consequence or effect. Complex philosophical arguments can be constructed to defend or reject the existence of a distinction between intending and foreseeing a consequence of an action. They are usually based on difficult borderline examples and are not relevant to the ordinary clinical situation in which healthcare professionals and the public accept the distinction at face value. Almost every treatment has side effects, but it is generally accepted that healthcare professionals intend only the beneficial effects of treatment and not the side effects, although the latter may be foreseen.

The public acceptance of the moral distinction between intending and foreseeing effects of treatment is based on trust in the integrity of healthcare professionals. In return, professionals have to be worthy of that trust. This entails being clear in our thinking and being honest with ourselves and others about our intentions. In health care, the aim of a treatment is the effect which is intended. We cannot be clear and honest about our intentions unless we have thought clearly and been honest with ourselves about our aim in providing the treatment.

Turning secondly from the intention to causality, the issue of what actually causes death must also be discussed. In the situation described, the cause of death is the terminal illness, and not the drug regimen given to alleviate distress or even the absence of more life-prolonging technology. This is certainly the case if the same drug regimen given to a fitter person would not cause death. Similarly, the cause of death of a patient who dies of renal failure is in fact renal failure and not the absence of a renal transplant or dialysis. Issues around causality are very complex philosophically, but for the public, the law, and healthcare professionals a more common-sense approach is needed and is accepted.

The essential aims of health care are the relief of suffering and the prolongation of life. I have stressed that there is always a moral obligation for healthcare professionals to minimize suffering. In contrast, the aim of prolonging life must be seen in the light of the inevitability of human death, so that for all people there comes a time when further attempts to prolong or sustain life by means of health care will fail. Thus, there is not always a moral obligation to strive to prolong or sustain life. On the other hand, healthcare professionals must not intentionally shorten the life of their patients or cause their deaths, because the prohibition against killing to which the vast majority of societies subscribe must be upheld, especially where vulnerable people such as patients are concerned.

Euthanasia, defined as an intentional act that brings about the death of the patient in order to alleviate suffering, cannot be justified by the doctrine of double effect. The doctrine will not justify an intentional act of killing, which euthanasia is, because the good effect (relief of suffering) is brought about by means of the bad effect (the death of the patient). Moreover, the bad effect is clearly intended (as opposed to foreseen). Thus, the conditions of the doctrine of double effect are not satisfied by euthanasia. So the doctrine cannot be used to justify euthanasia.

At the end of life, there is a moral obligation to provide good pain relief using adequate doses of clinically appropriate analgesics, sometimes supplemented by judicious use of sedatives, such as benzodiazepines. However, since the death of the patient is foreseen, doctors and nurses sometimes fear that the patient's death may wrongly be attributed to the provision of analgesia and for this reason they lack the courage to prescribe and provide analgesics necessary to achieve relief of pain. This failure to provide adequate and appropriate analgesia at the end of life is a moral failure, and it should be regarded as culpable. It should be seen as just as culpable as failure to provide life-prolonging treatment in circumstances where that treatment would be life sustaining. Patients need to be able to trust that their doctors will do all that is clinically appropriate and necessary to relieve pain at the end of life. Healthcare professionals must have the knowledge, skills, and courage to achieve this aim. So there is a moral obligation to acquire the knowledge and skills to provide effective pain relief, and a further obligation to have the courage, compassion, and equanimity to provide the best possible analgesic regime at the end of life.

It is obvious that very fine moral lines exist in all these matters. Harms and risks of treatment must be carefully weighed against benefits, and distinctions are sometimes finely drawn. Yet this must be so, for moral decision-making in medicine is very complex, and cannot be simplified by any theory into a simple formula that will give the answer when applied to the particular situation. So communities and healthcare professionals agree some basic legal and moral rules (such as the doctrine of double effect). Within the necessary constraints of those rules it is for patients and their doctors to work out the best course of action in each particular clinical situation.

One may be held blameworthy in health care for what one has not done, as well as for what one has done. Thus, doctors and nurses might be considered blameworthy for not relieving the patient's pain. The fact that the doctor and nurses did not do something does not mean that no blame may be attributed to that decision. Similarly, one may be praised for making a correct decision to withhold an inappropriate treatment, just as one may be praised for giving an appropriate treatment. So the issue of rightness or wrongness of a treatment decision, and the corresponding attribution of praise or blame, cannot be simplified into a distinction between doing and not doing something.

CONCLUSIONS

- Relief of suffering is an essential aim of health care but, as in all other areas of medicine, is accompanied by an obligation not to cause harm.
- There is an obligation upon healthcare professionals to attain competence in pain control.
- There is a requirement for honest discussion with patients about the risks and benefits of proposed pain therapies.
- There should be acceptance of the patient's right to consent to or refuse therapies offered and to indicate the level of information they desire for decision-making.

- An understanding of the multifactorial nature of the pain experienced should be balanced by a parallel understanding of the need for consent to intrusive personal enquiry.
- At the end of life, as death is inevitable, the obligation to relieve suffering must ultimately outweigh the obligation to attempt to prolong life when a conflict of obligations arises.
- With competent use of pain therapies, the risk of shortening life in order to relieve suffering arises occasionally, not frequently.
- Where it is foreseen that adequate pain relief might shorten life, it may legitimately be considered that this risk is outweighed by the benefit of comfort; this decision belongs primarily to the patient who has capacity, not the healthcare professional.
- Adverse effects of treatment can be foreseen without being intended.
- The cause of death remains the disease which has given rise to the situation necessitating the treatment, not the treatment itself.
- For the doctrine of double effect to be invoked legitimately, the shortening of life must not be the means to relieve pain. The doctrine cannot justify euthanasia.
- Moral culpability applies equally to the failure to provide a necessary treatment such as adequate analgesia at the end of life and to the giving of an inappropriate treatment.

REFERENCES

1. Breitbart W, Payne D, Passik K. Psychological and psychiatric interventions in pain control. In: Doyle D, Hanks G, Cherny N et al. (eds). *Oxford textbook of palliative medicine*, 3rd edn. Oxford: Oxford University Press, 2005: 428.

* 2. General Medical Council. Seeking patients' consent: the ethical considerations. London: Greater Medical Council Publications, 1998: paras 4–6.

3. Foley K. Acute and chronic cancer pain syndromes. In: Doyle D, Hanks G, Cherny N et al. (eds). *Oxford textbook of palliative medicine*, 3rd edn. Oxford: Oxford University Press, 2005: 303.

4. Randall F, Downie RS. Autonomy, dignity, respect and the patient-centred approach. In: *The philosophy of palliative care: critique and reconstruction*. Oxford: Oxford University Press, 2006: 63.

5. Foley K. Acute and chronic cancer pain syndromes. In: Doyle D, Hanks G, Cherny N et al. (eds). *Oxford textbook of palliative medicine*, 3rd edn. Oxford: Oxford University Press, 2005: 302.

6. Randall F, Downie RS. Autonomy, dignity, respect and the patient-centred approach. In: *The philosophy of palliative*

care: critique and reconstruction. Oxford: Oxford University Press, 2006: 64.

7. Foley K. Acute and chronic cancer pain syndromes. In: Doyle D, Hanks G, Cherny N *et al.* (eds). *Oxford textbook of palliative medicine*, 3rd edn. Oxford: Oxford University Press, 2005: 300.

* 8. Breitbart W, Payne D, Passik K. Psychological and psychiatric interventions in pain control. In: Doyle D, Hanks G, Cherny N *et al.* (eds). *Oxford textbook of palliative medicine*, 3rd edn. Oxford: Oxford University Press, 2005: 425–6.

9. Foley K. Acute and chronic cancer pain syndromes. In: Doyle D, Hanks G, Cherny N (eds). *Oxford textbook of palliative medicine*, 3rd edn. Oxford: Oxford University Press, 2005: 301.

* 10. Randall F, Downie RS. Assessment and treatment of psychosocial and spiritual problems. In: *The philosophy of palliative care: critique and reconstruction.* Oxford: Oxford University Press, 2006: 149–60.

11. Foley K. Acute and chronic cancer pain syndromes. In: Doyle D, Hanks G, Cherny N *et al.* (eds). *Oxford Textbook of Palliative Medicine*, 3rd edn. Oxford: Oxford University Press, 2005: 300.

* 12. Mental Capacity Act. UK, 2005: section 9.

* 13. Randall F, Downie RS. Autonomy, dignity, respect and the patient-centred approach. In: *The philosophy of palliative care: critique and reconstruction.* Oxford: Oxford University Press, 2006: 61–2.

14. Mental Capacity Act. UK, 2005: section 24–6.

* 15. Chan K, Sham M, Tse D, Thorsen A. In: Doyle D, Hanks G, Cherny N *et al.* (eds). *Oxford textbook of palliative medicine*, 3rd edn. Oxford: Oxford University Press, 2005: 612.

16. Thomas Aquinas. *Summa theologiae XVII*, 1274. Cambridge: Blackfriars, 1970: 1a2ae Q6, article 3, 15–16.

17. Randall F, Downie RS. Control of symptoms and prolongation of life. In: *The philosophy of palliative care: critique and reconstruction.* Oxford: Oxford University Press, 2006: 107–17.

PART II

DRUG THERAPIES FOR CANCER PAIN

10   Clinical pharmacology: principles of analgesic drug management   103
     Stephan A Schug and Kirsten Auret

11   Clinical pharmacology and therapeutics: nonopioids   123
     Victor Pace

12   Clinical pharmacology of opioids: basic pharmacology   151
     Sangeeta R Mehendale and Chun-Su Yuan

13   Clinical pharmacology of opioids: opioid switching and genetic basis for variability in opioid sensitivity   168
     Columba Quigley, Joy Ross, and Julia Riley

14   Clinical pharmacology of opioids: adverse effects of opioids   179
     Juan Manuel Núñez Olarte

15   Clinical pharmacology and therapeutics: drugs for neuropathic pain in cancer   200
     Carina Saxby and Michael Bennett

16   Control of procedure–related pain   213
     Iain Lawrie and Colin Campbell

Clinical pharmacology: principles of analgesic drug management

STEPHAN A SCHUG AND KIRSTEN AURET

Introduction	104	Evaluation of the WHO cancer pain guidelines	115
Clinical pharmacology	104	Other clinical guidelines for the treatment of cancer pain	116
Principles of the WHO cancer pain relief guidelines	108	References	117

KEY LEARNING POINTS

- Successful management of cancer pain requires a holistic approach to care, with an appreciation of the overall symptom burden and the psychosocial, emotional, and spiritual stresses upon patients.
- The goal of cancer pain treatment is to provide pain relief while maintaining freedom of choice and minimizing adverse effects.
- Good cancer pain management should enable patients to have a good quality of life, to function at an acceptable level, to tolerate diagnostic and therapeutic procedures, and to die relatively painlessly.
- Cancer pain treatment needs to begin with a careful evaluation and assessment of the patient, including a detailed history and a thorough examination leading to a pain diagnosis.
- Cancer pain treatment requires an explanation to the patient and his significant others and combines pharmacological, interventional, and psychological approaches.
- Analgesic drug management is often complex and requires detailed knowledge and understanding of the pharmacodynamics and pharmacokinetics of the medicines used.
- Such an approach requires an understanding of the effects of long-term exposure to analgesic compounds such as tolerance, physical dependence, and addiction.
- In addition, changes in extreme age groups and with deteriorating organ function need to be considered.

- The principles of analgesic drug management should follow established clinical guidelines.
- The use of guidelines for cancer pain management has been subjected to randomized trials, which have shown that guideline-based clinical decision-making improves pain outcomes in cancer patients.
- The most widely used guidelines are those promoted by the World Health Organization (WHO) for more than 20 years.
- The WHO guidelines promote an approach commonly summarized in five key points:
  - by the mouth;
  - by the clock;
  - by the ladder;
  - for the individual; and
  - attention to detail.
- The efficacy of the WHO guidelines has been demonstrated in multiple case series performed in multiple settings leading to adequate analgesia in 70–90 percent of patients treated accordingly.
- However, the WHO guidelines have been criticized as they have never been subjected to controlled trials, the gold standard of evidence-based medicine.
- A critical discussion has focused in particular on the use of weak opioids in step 2 of the ladder.
- Overall, the WHO guidelines have stood the test of time and have proven to be a simple, but thereby effective,

tool to improve pain control for the individual cancer patient, but also for large patient populations.
- Despite the simplicity and logical principles of these guidelines, their implementation has proven difficult for multiple reasons.
- Such reasons include absence of national policies on cancer pain relief and palliative care, lack of financial resources and healthcare delivery systems, and legal restrictions on the use and availability of opioids.
- Underutilization of opioids is due to the misconception that increased medical use will increase illicit drug traffic.

- Unfounded "opiophobia" continues to be a major problem, not only among politicians and government officials but also in healthcare professionals, patients, and their relatives.
- Here, the WHO guidelines are not only a valuable tool for clinical practice, but also for policy change.
- The concepts of the guidelines create an awareness of the appropriate use of opioids for pain management and thereby permit healthcare professionals worldwide to obtain the opioids their patients need.

INTRODUCTION

Prescribing well for cancer pain treatment requires knowledge of clinical pharmacology of the medications used and the principles of their use, and also assumes an understanding of cancer pain itself.

The latter requires knowledge of issues such as pain classification by pain type or cause, the epidemiology of cancer pain, and importantly the concept of "total pain" and suffering.[1, 2, 3] Successful management of cancer pain requires a holistic approach to care, with an appreciation of the overall symptom burden and the psychosocial, emotional, and spiritual stresses upon patients. The goal of cancer pain treatment is to provide pain relief while maintaining freedom of choice and minimizing adverse effects, thereby enabling patients to have a good quality of life, to function at an acceptable level, to tolerate diagnostic and therapeutic procedures, and to die relatively painlessly.[4, 5] These general considerations are covered in other parts of this volume.

Successful analgesic drug therapy in the cancer setting then needs to consider a number of issues:[6]

- methods of pain assessment;
- evaluation of the patient's goals and expectations of therapy;
- pharmacokinetic and pharmacodynamic properties of the medications under consideration;
- prescription following validated guidelines;
- evaluation of response to therapy; and
- assessment of lack of response to therapy.

The overall treatment plan needs to be seen as a dynamic process, which is responsive to the underlying progressive disease and might require multiple treatment interventions over time. This chapter will focus on general issues of clinical pharmacology relevant to cancer pain treatment and the principles of cancer pain treatment by use of analgesic drugs. They were outlined in the WHO's treatment guidelines,[7] first published in "Cancer Pain Relief"[8] in 1986 and updated in a second edition in 1996.[9]

Although systemic pharmacotherapy is the mainstay of these guidelines, control of cancer pain should also include consideration of:

- a straight forward explanation of the cause(s) of pain and the various treatment options available;[10, 11, 12, 13]
- potential modification of the underlying pathological process;[14, 15, 16, 17, 18]
- elevation of the pain threshold;
- the role of interruption, destruction, or stimulation of pain pathways; and
- modification of lifestyle.

The WHO treatment guidelines emphasize this very clearly, when stating "relief of psychological, social, and spiritual problems is paramount. Attempting to relieve pain without addressing the patient's nonphysical concerns is likely to lead to frustration and failure."[9]

CLINICAL PHARMACOLOGY

Therapy of cancer pain usually involves quite sophisticated pharmacotherapy with combinations of potent drugs. Such use of medication requires a profound knowledge of pharmacological principles and detailed familiarity with the clinical pharmacological properties of the medications used. One purpose of this chapter is to summarize general pharmacological knowledge relevant to the management of cancer pain, while Chapter 11, Clinical pharmacology and therapeutics: nonopioids; Chapter 12, Clinical pharmacology of opioids: basic pharmacology; Chapter 13, Clinical pharmacology of opioids: opioid switching and genetic basis for variability in opioid sensitivity; Chapter 14, Clinical pharmacology of opioids: adverse effects of opioids; Chapter 15, Clinical pharmacology and therapeutics: drugs for neuropathic pain in cancer will provide specific pharmacological information on the classes of drugs used to treat cancer pain.

Pharmacodynamic principles

EFFECTS ON RECEPTORS

Many drugs such as opioids act on receptors. Activity at receptors is based on the theory that receptors are specific membrane-bound proteins that interact selectively with extracellular substances to initiate biochemical events within the cell. These substances may be endogenous, such as neurotransmitters, or exogenous, such as drugs.

Drugs have two separate attributes at receptor sites, affinity and efficacy. Affinity is the tendency or ability to bind to a receptor to produce a stable complex. A drug with high affinity binds to a receptor more strongly than one with lower affinity. Fentanyl, for example, has a higher affinity for opioid receptors than morphine.

Efficacy, or intrinsic activity, is the ability of the drug, once bound, to produce a certain effect. Efficacy can range from no effect to a potential maximum effect for that particular receptor. A partial agonist may be more potent than a full agonist at the lower end of the effect range, however, even at maximal doses, a partial agonist cannot reach the full effect of an agonist. The partial agonist is displaying a ceiling effect that does not occur with a full agonist, where the maximum dose is limited not by lack of effect, but by adverse effects.

Based on these properties, drugs that bind to receptors can exhibit pure agonist activity, antagonist activity, or act as partial agonists or agonist–antagonists.

- An agonist acts at a receptor to initiate changes in cell function. Traditionally, an agonist produces the normal biological response of the cell.
- A partial agonist binds to the receptor, but causes less response than a full agonist; it has a lower efficacy. However, it may have a higher affinity for the receptor, and act as a competitive antagonist in the presence of a full agonist. A typical example would be the partial agonist, buprenorphine, which has a greater affinity for opioid receptors than morphine.
- An agonist–antagonist acts as an antagonist at certain receptors and an agonist or partial agonist at others. Pentazocine is a typical example, as it acts as μ receptor antagonist, but exerts its opioid effect by agonist activity at the κ receptor.
- Antagonists occupy the receptor but have no biological activity. A competitive antagonist such as naloxone binds reversibly to the receptor and can displace and is displaced by the agonist. A noncompetitive antagonist binds irreversibly to the receptor.

Of practical importance is finally the potency of a drug, i.e. its ability to produce a certain effect; in other words, the relative dose required to achieve an effect. Beside affinity and efficacy, a drug's absorption, distribution, metabolism, and excretion influence potency. However, potency is not a measure of efficacy as defined above.

Dose–response curves describe the relationships between the dose of a drug and the subsequent response (**Figure 10.1**). Curves are characterized by their position on the x-axis (potency), maximal height (efficacy), and slope (number of receptors that must be bound to produce a response).

EFFECTS OF LONG-TERM EXPOSURE

Tolerance describes a pharmacological phenomenon, where higher doses of a drug are required to produce the same effect or the same dose has decreasing efficacy.[19] Tolerance is a biological effect due to prior exposure to a drug and this exposure drives the diminution in effect.

Acquired tolerance can be acute or chronic. Acute tolerance (tachyphylaxis) is a phenomenon that typically occurs within minutes.

Pharmacokinetic tolerance refers to changes in distribution or metabolism of a drug, such that concentrations of the drug are reduced in the plasma and at the effect site. A common cause would be an increase in the rate of metabolism of a drug, by hepatic enzyme induction, and therefore lessening of effect by more rapid removal of the drug from the circulation.

Pharmacodynamic tolerance occurs at a receptor level in the system acted on by the drug.

Learned tolerance is a reduction in the effects of a drug due to learned compensatory mechanisms. For example, behavioral tolerance is involved in learning how to function in a mild state of intoxication or conditioned tolerance when environmental cues are constantly paired with drug administration.

Cross-tolerance occurs when repeated doses of a drug in a given category confer tolerance to that drug and to other drugs in similar structural and mechanistic categories.[19]

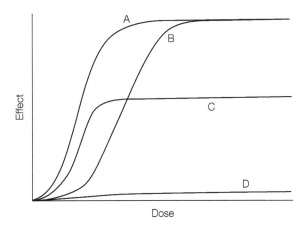

Figure 10.1 Dose–response curves for hypothetical opioids (A and B are full agonists and A is more potent than B, C is a partial agonist and D an antagonist).

Tolerance to opioids is predominantly pharmacodynamic, receptor selective and reversible.[20, 21] Opioid tolerance is characterized by a shortened duration and decreased intensity of analgesia, euphoria, and central nervous system (CNS) depressant effects and a significant elevation in the potentially lethal dose.[19]

Fear of tolerance to analgesic effects and escalating dose requirements limit the prescribing of opioids for cancer pain. Physicians feel that if they give too much too soon they will cause severe side effects or run out of analgesic options when the pain gets "really bad!"

However, despite all the publicity and animal studies, clinical evidence has shown that true analgesic tolerance to opioids in patients with pain is extremely rare. Patients with cancer can be maintained on a steady level of opioids for prolonged periods.[22, 23, 24][IV] It is useful to remember that a decline in analgesic effect has a differential diagnosis, with true tolerance being only one of the diagnoses.[25] The main reason for a reduced analgesic effect in such patients, however, is increased nociceptive input.[22, 26, 27][IV] If dose requirements increase and pain is no longer controlled, the patient should be carefully evaluated for disease progression. Other causes of decreasing analgesic effect are more likely to be psychological, with increasing anxiety, depression, change in cognitive state, or conditioned pain behavior.

In both animals and humans, cross-tolerance to opioids occurs and has been shown to be incomplete due to selective tolerance at different subpopulations of opioid receptors.[21] Cross-tolerance has an important role in patients who have their pain controlled by opioid agonists, particularly when considering opioid rotation.[28] Patients whose pain is poorly controlled with escalating doses of morphine and who are experiencing unbearable adverse effects can be rotated to an opioid that may provide a more tolerable balance between analgesia and side effects, although the evidence for this is largely anecdotal.[29][V]

Physical dependence is a physiological state that develops as a result of the adaptation produced by a resetting of homeostatic mechanisms in response to repeated drug use. It is a predictable effect that can be seen in both animals and humans and is characterized by the appearance of signs and symptoms of withdrawal syndrome after sudden dose reduction or discontinuation of a drug on which a patient is physically dependent. It can also be precipitated by administration of an antagonist.

Withdrawal symptoms are typical for a given category of drugs and they tend to be the opposite of the original effects of the medication. The symptoms are due to removal of the drug of dependence; such effects can be observed with many drugs and are not limited to CNS effects. Examples are rebound tachycardia after β-blocker withdrawal[30] and rebound hypertension after clonidine withdrawal.[31] On a CNS level, hyperarousal of the CNS by readaptation to absence of the drug occurs, for example

after antidepressant use.[32] Chronic agonist use can also increase sensitivity to even weak antagonists such as agonist–antagonists;[33] use of complete antagonists in patients on opioids precipitate severe withdrawal, possibly after only one or two doses of an agonist.[34]

The time to onset, duration, and severity of withdrawal symptoms after opioid use depends on the pharmacokinetics of the drug of dependence. Physical dependence probably starts after the first dose and symptoms will become noticeable after one to two weeks of exposure.[22] When reducing or discontinuing chronic opioid therapy, a tapering schedule is recommended. Prevention of withdrawal symptoms can be managed by decreasing the dose by 25 percent each day.[35][V] This rule can be used to titrate down to a lower dose or to eventually discontinue a drug when pain relief has been achieved by other means such as radiotherapy or surgery. Physical dependence is no significant clinical problem in cancer pain treatment.[22][V]

Addiction, also called psychological dependence, is the most complex of these terms; it is distinct from physical dependence and tolerance.[36] It is used to describe a pattern of drug use characterized by a continued craving for the drug, leading to an overwhelming involvement with the use and procurement of the drug. There is continued use of the substance despite knowledge and evidence that it causes physical and, or psychological harm.

Substance dependence is the alternative term used by the American Psychiatric Association (APA) in DSM-IV.[37] Criteria for substance dependence according to the APA are a maladaptive pattern of substance use, leading to clinically significant impairment or distress, as manifested by three or more of the symptoms of dependence, occurring at any time in the same 12-month period.

This diagnostic system requires further investigation to specify if with physiological dependence (evidence of tolerance or withdrawal) or without physiological dependence (no evidence of tolerance or withdrawal). Obviously neither tolerance nor withdrawal is necessary or sufficient for a diagnosis of substance dependence. It is extremely important to realize that patients with cancer pain may develop tolerance to prescribed opioids and show signs of withdrawal without any evidence of compulsive use. These patients may well be physically and therapeutically dependent on opioids, but they are not addicted.

Fears of inducing psychological addiction by appropriate pain therapy have been unfounded. Widespread clinical experience in supervised pain management programs has found that when strong opioids are used for the treatment of pain, psychological dependence is a very rare occurrence.[38, 39] In cancer pain patients treated with strong opioids, two surveys independently found an incidence of addiction of 0.2 percent.[22, 40]

The risk of inappropriate or criminal drug diversion has also been found to be low. In a number of countries the use of opioids has increased significantly to combat a high cancer pain problem, without a significant increase in diversion to illicit users, demonstrating that with reasonable regulation of opioid distribution, increase in clinical use is not linked to a rise in abuse problems.[41, 42, 43]

Therapeutic dependence is another important term here. When specific pharmacological therapy is needed to control or cure a disease process or a symptom of that disease, the patient is essentially dependent on it, for example antibiotics for sepsis, insulin for insulin-dependent diabetics, and opioids for patients with pain.[35] Some patients with good pain control may seem to be obsessed with ensuring an adequate and regular supply of medication. This is not necessarily indicative of addiction but an understandable fear of running out of analgesia, not having enough to deal with breakthrough pain, or fear of withdrawal symptoms. The term pseudoaddiction, defined as an iatrogenic syndrome due to poorly managed and uncontrolled pain, has been used here.[44] It is characterized by behavioral changes very similar to those of drug addiction. The patient endures and complains of constant pain, which is at best only partially relieved. Drug seeking behavior, such as obtaining medication from multiple sources, repeated episodes of prescription loss, and requests for early refills from health workers for larger or more frequent doses of opioids, are often met with mistrust and, all too frequently, refusal. This can lead to a spiral of increasing demands and "clock watching," with anger and distrust on all sides.[19] It is vitally important that this disastrous failure of care is recognized and avoided. Failure to do so can lead to lengthy periods of unacceptable pain for a patient and years of resentment and stress for their families.

Pharmacokinetic principles

Knowledge of the disposition of drugs in the body is essential to prescribe correct doses and achieve the desired therapeutic effect, in this case, analgesia.

TERMINOLOGY

Most of the following definitions are applicable to all oral analgesic drugs, the most common form of drug administration for patients with cancer pain.

- Absorption is the extent to which the intact drug is absorbed from the gut lumen into the portal circulation. It is expressed as a fraction of the dose, which is absorbed from the gut. Factors affecting absorption are dissolution of the drug, gastric emptying rate, intestinal motility, drug interactions in the lumen, and passage through the gut wall.
- First pass clearance is the extent to which the drug is removed by the liver in its first pass in the portal blood through the liver to the systemic circulation. Changes in hepatic extraction are due to changes in microsomal enzyme activity and liver blood flow.

- Bioavailability (F) is the fraction of the dose that reaches the systemic circulation intact and is available at the effect site. Bioavailability depends on the fraction of drug absorbed and how much escapes first pass metabolism in the liver. The route of administration obviously has a significant effect on bioavailability. The intravenous (i.v.) route has a bioavailability of 100 percent. Most opioids are well absorbed from the gut, but undergo substantial first pass metabolism; for example the bioavailability of oral morphine varies from 15 to 35 percent.

$$\text{Bioavailability} = \text{absorption}$$
$$\times \text{ fraction escaping first pass metabolism}$$

- Volume of distribution (V_d) is the pharmacokinetic parameter used to determine the loading dose of a drug. It is an imaginary volume, relating the total amount of drug in the body to the plasma concentration of the drug.

$$V_d = \text{total amount of drug in the body}/$$
$$\text{plasma concentration of drug}$$

Opioids commonly have an initial V_d of 20–50 L, but after some time the drugs will distribute from more vascularized regions to fat tissues, thereby increasing the initial V_d to a steady state V_d of 150–250 L.
- Clearance (Cl) describes the efficiency of irreversible elimination of a drug from the body, by excretion or metabolism. It is defined as the volume of blood cleared of the drug in time. Total body clearance is the sum of the clearances of all the organs, e.g. liver, kidney, lung, etc. For example, almost all opioids are extensively metabolized in the liver and clearance is then approximately equal to hepatic blood flow. For systemic, chronically administered opioids which have reached steady state, changes in hepatic blood flow can cause major effects on the steady state concentrations of these highly extracted drugs.
- Elimination half-life ($t_{1/2}$) is the time taken for the amount of drug in the body to fall by half, for most opioids it is in the range of several hours. Clearance and volume of distribution determine half-life:

$$t_{1/2\beta} = \frac{V_d \times \ln 2}{Cl}$$

- Half-life is important in determining the duration of action after a single dose, the time required to reach steady state and the dosing interval with chronic dosing. It takes five half-lives to reach steady state, and the dosing interval required to avoid excessive fluctuations in plasma concentration is in the range of one half-life. It also takes approximately five half-lives to completely remove a drug from the body.

CALCULATING A DOSING REGIMEN OF A DRUG

When designing a dosing regimen, it is important to remember the loading dose. Without one, it could take five half-lives to achieve an adequate therapeutic effect. Morphine, for example, has a $t_{1\backslash 2\beta}$ of one to four hours, so that a poor dosing regimen could result in a 5–20 hour wait for adequate pain relief.

The values used here are approximate only, and vary considerably between patients.

For an intravenous infusion and intermittent bolus dosing the formula is:

$$\text{Loading dose} = \text{effective plasma concentration} \times V_d$$

As mentioned above, there are differences between the initial V_d and the steady state V_d, and these must be accounted for. As an example, the initial V_d of morphine is 25 L. If the required plasma concentration is 0.05 mg/L, then the initial bolus is $25 \times 0.05 = 1.25$ mg. If the V_d at steady state reaches 250 L, then the above initial loading dose needs to be followed by a loading infusion over an hour of $(250–25) \times 0.05 = 11.25$ mg.

Subsequent to this loading dose, there needs to be a dose calculated to maintain the target concentration over time:

$$\text{Maintenance dose} = \text{target plasma concentration} \times \text{Cl}$$

Returning to the above example, the clearance of morphine is approximately 1 L/min, so the hourly maintenance dose is $0.05 \times 60 = 3$ mg.

For oral administration, the same principles apply with two differences. The slower absorption of an oral dose means less fluctuation of plasma concentration between doses. Sustained release and transdermal formulations show an even better concentration/time profile, approaching that of a continuous infusion. Further on, the dose reaching the effect compartment is affected by the bioavailability, so that at steady state the calculation is:

$$\text{Oral maintenance dose rate}$$
$$= \text{target plasma concentration} \times \text{Cl}/F$$

FACTORS INFLUENCING PHARMACOKINETICS

Renal and hepatic disease can alter the pharmacokinetic parameters of analgesic drugs with clinical consequences.

The liver is the main site of metabolism for many analgesic drugs, including most opioids, and alterations in hepatic function may be expected to have an effect on drug clearance.[45] For example, liver blood flow, enzyme activity, and protein binding all influence opioid clearance. Severe hepatic cirrhosis can cause alterations in blood flow due to intra- and extra-hepatic shunting. Alcoholic cirrhosis and acute hepatitis, which affect the pericentral regions, impair oxidative metabolism. Diseases affecting the periportal regions have little effect on drug metabolism. The conjugating enzymes are only affected in end stage liver disease. Low albumin levels due to malnutrition, renal, or hepatic disease can lead to decreased protein binding and hence increase the response to drugs which are proteinbound.

Chronic liver disease can also cause a large increase in the bioavailability of oral opioids, and caution must be used with dosing regimens.[46] The rate of clearance is decreased, and in conjunction with the rise in bioavailability can lead to increased intensity and duration of action of opioids at relatively low doses.[47]

Renal disease can alter the pharmacokinetics, but also the pharmacodynamics of many drugs; the effects on cancer pain management have been reviewed recently.[48] The severity of renal dysfunction and the pharmacokinetics of a specific drug will determine the influence renal disease has on its elimination. Mild renal impairment (glomerular filtration rate > 2.4 L/hr or creatinine clearance > 50–90 mL/min) has little effect on drug kinetics and usually requires no consideration in prescribing analgesics.[49] However, when prescribing large doses of drugs in palliative care, caution may be required even in mild renal impairment. In more severe impairment, depending on the estimated reduction in creatinine clearance, many drugs are administered in smaller amounts and less frequently; this approach applies to medications that are primarily cleared by the kidney.[50] However, renal disease can also alter the kinetics of drugs that are not renally cleared;[51] drug absorption can be slowed secondary to prolonged gastric emptying time and increased gastric pH and reduced protein levels and altered pH-dependent protein binding may affect drug distribution. Drugs metabolized in the liver by oxidation or conjugation may have reduced hepatic clearance in renal impairment. When dialysis is used for control of symptoms in renal failure, drug removal and clearance is dependent on a number of factors including drug characteristics, type of dialysis, and equipment used.[52] Patients on dialysis will need adjustment of their pain relief medications to ensure adequate maintenance of analgesia and avoidance of toxicity.

Neither hepatic nor renal impairment is a contraindication to the use of opioids for cancer pain. Monitoring is needed and awareness of the potential need to reduce doses, increase dosing intervals, or switch to alternative opioids or routes of administration.

PRINCIPLES OF THE WHO CANCER PAIN RELIEF GUIDELINES

The WHO guidelines have become the internationally accepted standard for the principles governing treatment of cancer pain,[7] focusing on oral analgesic use as the mainstay of therapy;[8, 9] the detailed key principles of this approach are listed in **Box 10.1**. Access to these guidelines is listed in **Table 10.1**.

Their application has been studied in over 30,000 patients demonstrating their usefulness, efficacy, and low rates of complications.[54, 55, 56, 57, 58][IV]

They are commonly summarized in five key points:

1. by the mouth;
2. by the clock;
3. by the ladder;
4. for the individual; and
5. attention to detail.

By the mouth – the oral route

The oral route of analgesic therapy is preferred as it is simple, acceptable, and relatively cheap.[59, 60][V] Most analgesics, including opioids, have clinically useful oral bioavailability. Oral therapy requires little medical intervention and therefore the patient is independent of infrastructure and personnel. Further, there is no requirement for needles or syringes to dispose of, or risk of needle-stick injury to the administrator.

The delayed absorption after oral administration prolongs the duration of action of most drugs, giving further benefits. However, in the setting of acute (e.g. incident pain) the later peak time with oral administration may convey disadvantages and alternative routes of administration might be more appropriate. Other indications for a change of route of analgesic delivery (e.g. sublingual, parenteral, rectal, topical, or spinal) include:[61][V]

- vomiting;
- impaired swallow;
- gastrointestinal obstruction;
- malabsorption; and
- coma.

Simple failure of the oral therapy used, however, is usually not an indication to change the route of administration, but to reevaluate the pain diagnosis and treatment plan.[62][V]

Box 10.1 Key principles of the WHO method of cancer pain relief

- Cancer pain can, and should, be treated.
- Evaluation and treatment of cancer pain are best achieved by a team approach.
- The first steps are to take a detailed history, and to examine the patient carefully, to determine if the pain is:
  - caused by the cancer, related to the cancer, caused by anticancer treatment, or caused by another disorder;
  - part of a specific syndrome;
  - nociceptive, neuropathic, or mixed nociceptive and neuropathic.
- Treatment begins with an explanation and combines physical and psychological approaches, using both nondrug and drug treatments.
- It is useful to have a sequence of specific aims, such as to:
  - increase the hours of pain-free sleep;
  - relieve the pain when the patient is at rest;
  - relieve pain when the patient is standing or active.
- Drugs alone usually give adequate relief from pain caused by cancer, provided that the right drug is administered in the right dose at the right time intervals.
- "By mouth": the oral route is the preferred route for analgesics, including morphine.
- "By the clock": for persistent pain, drugs should be taken at regular time intervals and not "as needed".
- "By the ladder":
  - Unless the patient is in severe pain, begin by prescribing a nonopioid drug and adjust the dose, if necessary, to the maximum recommended dose.
  - If or when the nonopioid no longer adequately relieves the pain, an opioid drug should be prescribed in addition to the nonopioid.
  - If or when the nonopioid for mild to moderate pain (e.g. codeine) no longer adequately relieves the pain, it should be replaced by an opioid for moderate to severe pain (e.g. morphine).
- "For the individual": the right dose of an analgesic is the dose that relieves the pain. The dose of oral morphine may range from as little as 5 mg to more than 1000 mg.
- Adjuvant drugs should be prescribed as indicated.
- For neuropathic pain, a tricyclic antidepressant or an anticonvulsant is the analgesic of choice.
- "Attention to detail": it is essential to monitor the patient's response to the treatment to ensure that the patient obtains maximum benefit with as few adverse effects as possible.

Table 10.1 Availability of the WHO guidelines.

Language	Web address
English	http://whqlibdoc.who.int/publications/9241544821.pdf
Spanish	http://whqlibdoc.who.int/publications/9243544829.pdf
French	http://whqlibdoc.who.int/publications/9242544825.pdf
Information about ordering print editions from WHO and other publishers in all other languages	www.whocancerpain.wisc.edu/eng/Poster2002/cpr96.html

Reprinted with permission from *Cancer Pain Relief*, 2nd edn. Geneva: World Health Organization 1996.[9]

OTHER ROUTES OF DRUG ADMINISTRATION

Although the oral route for analgesia in cancer pain is the most common, up to 70 percent of patients with cancer related pain require an alternative route of opioid administration before death.[63, 64] It is therefore important to be familiar with the other routes of analgesic administration. There are differences in bioavailability when the route of administration is changed and dose adjustment is necessary to avoid under- or overdosing. The ideal technique for switching routes of administration remains individual titration; published dose ratios are only average approximations.

Recent advancements in the formulation of transdermal delivery systems have made such skin patches a viable alternative to oral drug administration. Transdermal delivery avoids the problem of first pass metabolism; lipid soluble, low molecular weight drugs are more appropriate for this route. Absorption is slow, and whilst therapeutic levels can be maintained for many days, this is an unsuitable route for rapid pain control. Compliance is usually good. Fentanyl and buprenorphine are available in patch form for transdermal administration, providing an alternative to oral opioids with a long duration of action.[65][II] Iontophoretic transdermal on-demand administration of fentanyl, recently developed for post-operative pain control,[66] might become a transdermal rescue analgesia system in the future.

If a change of route of administration from the oral one is indicated, then the rectal[67] or subcutaneous route[68] have been preferred due to ease, comfort, acceptability, and availability. [V]

The rectal route is cheap and requires no specialized skills, however, absorption is often variable and local irritation can occur. The rectal veins drain to both the hepatic portal vein and the inferior vena cava, thus some first pass metabolism is avoided. However, the variability of drainage makes uptake unpredictable. It has been shown that analgesia is of more rapid onset and longer duration than that achieved via the oral route.[67, 69][II] Morphine is well absorbed rectally and many others opioids and nonopioids can be given per rectum.[70][III] Morphine is available as both immediate-release and controlled-release suppositories and enemas. Alternatively, controlled-release morphine tablets may be used as suppositories.[71][II] Doses should be equivalent to oral dosage, but may show greater variability. This route should not be used in patients with diarrhea or fecal incontinence. Immunosuppressed patients are at risk of localized infection. Administration of opioids via colostomy has been shown not to be useful, probably due to comparatively poor vascularity.

The availability of simple portable syringe pumps has made continuous subcutaneous morphine administration easy and acceptable for the patient who is unable to take oral medication.[72][III] It avoids repeated injections and is relatively cheap, requiring little medical input for administration. Changing from enteral to parenteral administration requires adjustment, usually reduction of dose and frequent reassessment to take into account bioavailability differences resulting from lack of first-pass effect with the parenteral route.[73, 74] Subcutaneous bioavailability may be more than 90 percent for most drugs, but depends on the solubility of the drug, cardiovascular conditions, peripheral perfusion, the injection site, and physical exercise. Drugs with a short half-life reach steady state more quickly. Other parenteral routes play only a minor role in cancer pain treatment. The intravenous route produces rapid onset, short-lived analgesia, but is difficult to maintain at home. However, it is very useful for swift control of severe pain in the hospital setting; intermittent boluses, continuous infusions, and patient controlled analgesia are the usual options. Intramuscular administration is painful and carries the risk of tissue damage and infection. Subsequent absorption depends on local blood flow and body habitus. Absorption is therefore unpredictable and this route is not generally recommended.

If a patient is unable to ingest medication but has normal gastrointestinal function, the nasogastric tube is an alternative.[75] This is more invasive than oral medication, but useful for those patients who are receiving enteral feeding, then it is more suitable for administration of analgesics long term than the rectal route. Liquid preparations are the preferred choice as they can be administered unaltered and do not clog the tube.

Immediate release tablets can be dissolved or crushed. This method is unsuitable for most sustained release formulations, sublingual or buccal preparations and enteric-coated tablets. Morphine sulfate elixir and immediate release tablets are suitable to give by this route and are compatible with many different enteral formulas.[75][V]

Transmucosal drug administration by the sublingual or buccal route avoids hepatic first pass metabolism as the blood vessels in the area drain directly into the superior vena cava. Absorption is best for those drugs which are highly lipid soluble and potent, and which have a high proportion unionized in the alkaline medium of the mouth. Therefore, morphine has only 18 percent absorption by this route compared with fentanyl (51 percent), methadone (34 percent), and buprenorphine (55 percent).[76] A sublingual preparation of buprenorphine[77] is widely available; transmucosal fentanyl, absorbed through the buccal surfaces, is an effective rescue analgesia with a rapid onset.[78][I]

While the ladder focuses on the pharmacologic approach to cancer pain management, interventional therapies should be considered concurrently with the use of the ladder and may sometimes be appropriate for patients with pain of any intensity. It is therefore not appropriate to regard interventional techniques as a final fourth step of the ladder.[53] Such interventional techniques include epidural or intrathecal opioid administration or neurolytic blocks undertaken only after failure of systemic analgesics.[79][V] Each technique has advantages and disadvantages. However, they all require expertise, specialized equipment, and are invasive. These forms of treatment should only be necessary for 5–10 percent of patients when following the WHO analgesic guidelines.[14, 54, 55, 56, 80][IV]

By the clock – regular around the clock medication

Chronic pain, as occurs in patients with cancer, requires preventative therapy on a regular basis, thus avoiding recurrences of pain with unnecessary suffering and the potential development of chronic pain behavior.[81, 82] Analgesic drugs should therefore be given regularly in high enough doses to suppress pain continuously.[83] The dose intervals should be guided by the pharmacokinetics of the drugs utilized, with each successive dose given before the preceding one has worn off. This enables the plasma concentrations to reach a relative steady state without unnecessary troughs. Slow or sustained release preparations should be prescribed whenever available, as their use extends dosing intervals and stabilizes plasma concentrations.[84, 85][II]

The timing of medications should suit the patient's daily activities and consider their day–night rhythm and schedules.[86][II] It is useful to provide a medication plan

with the timing in writing to avoid confusion in patients and caregivers.

As well as regular medications to control pain, patients should also be provided with analgesic therapy to use "as required" or "PRN" for breakthrough or incident pain. This is also referred to as rescue analgesia. Not surprisingly, demands for rescue medications are reduced and analgesia improved when analgesic medications are provided regularly rather than just on demand.[87][II]

By the ladder – sequential use of analgesic medication

A basic principle of pain management in cancer patients is to begin treatment with less potent analgesics and to progress in response to more severe or increasing pain intensity with the use of more potent medications, while using adjuvant and coanalgesic drugs as appropriate. The WHO has suggested the simple model of an "analgesic ladder" to provide a framework for this approach to oral pharmacotherapy for cancer pain (**Figure 10.2**).[7, 8, 9]

Analgesics are selected according to increasing pain intensity in a sequential approach: inadequate pain relief at one level results in a step up to the next level instead of changing to another drug on the same level. In parallel, it encourages the combined use of nonopioid and opioid analgesics with adjuvant or coanalgesic drugs. The latter group are medications that are not conventionally regarded as analgesics, but have pain-relieving properties in defined conditions (e.g. steroids for pain from liver capsule distension).[88] The ladder is useful in the titration process of initiating therapy, as well as in adapting established plans in response to progressive disease.[56]

STEP ONE: USE OF NONOPIOIDS

The first step on the ladder is for control of pain of mild to moderate intensity with the use of simple nonopioids;[89] the efficacy of this step has been documented.[90][I] Examples within this group include paracetamol,[90, 91] dipyrone,[92] traditional nonsteroidal anti-inflammatory drugs (NSAID),[90, 93, 94] and the newer COX-2 inhibitors.[94] They are prescribed in established doses and frequency. In contrast to opioids, nonopioids do show a ceiling effect to their analgesic action, and therefore a further increase of their dose beyond maximum established guidelines will not result in improved analgesia. Therefore, inadequate pain control by their use at maximum doses makes a move up the ladder necessary, if appropriate adjuvant therapy is already being used and cannot be improved.[89][IV]

The benefits gained from the first step should be continued, however, even as stronger analgesia is required.[90, 91][I] The combination of NSAIDs and a strong opioid, with or without paracetamol, has been

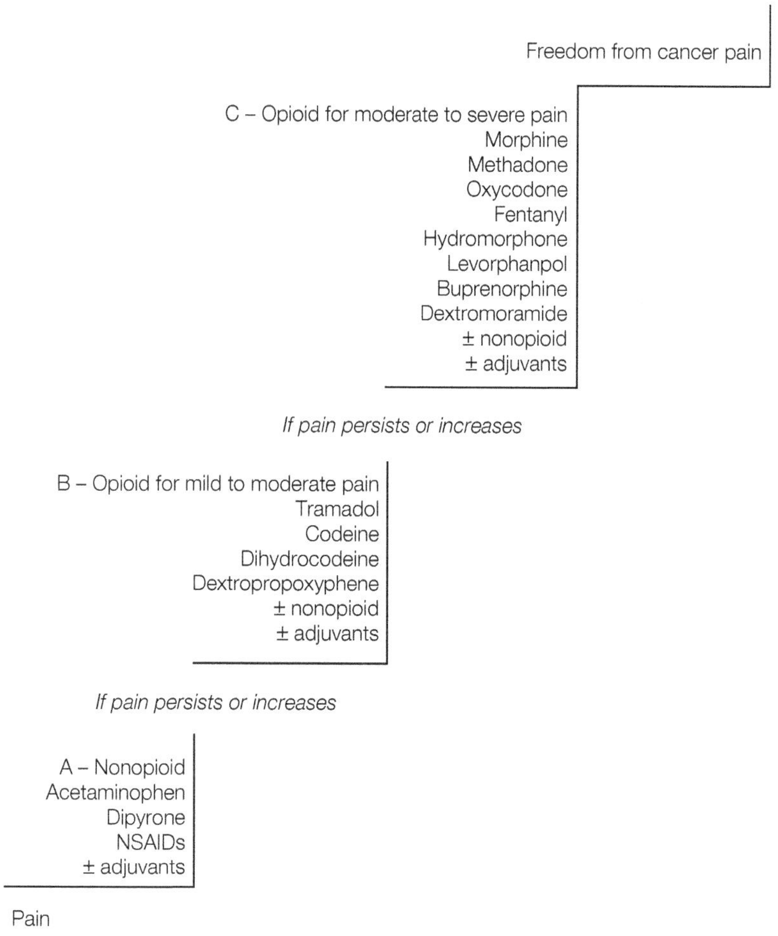

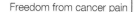

Freedom from cancer pain

C – Opioid for moderate to severe pain
Morphine
Methadone
Oxycodone
Fentanyl
Hydromorphone
Levorphanpol
Buprenorphine
Dextromoramide
± nonopioid
± adjuvants

If pain persists or increases

B – Opioid for mild to moderate pain
Tramadol
Codeine
Dihydrocodeine
Dextropropoxyphene
± nonopioid
± adjuvants

If pain persists or increases

A – Nonopioid
Acetaminophen
Dipyrone
NSAIDs
± adjuvants

Pain

Figure 10.2 The WHO analgesic ladder. For adjuvants, see Chapter 15, Clinical pharmacology and therapeutics: drugs for neuropathic pain in cancer.

demonstrated to enhance analgesia and patient satisfaction with therapy and decrease opioid use without an increase in side effects.[90, 91, 95, 96, 97][I]

STEP TWO: USE OF WEAK OPIOIDS

The next step of the ladder involves the addition of a weak opioid without discontinuation of the nonopioid. Examples of drugs within this category include codeine phosphate,[98, 99] dextropropoxyphene,[100, 101] dihydrocodeine,[102, 103] and tramadol.[104, 105, 106]

However, a discussion on the validity of step two has been initiated, as a meta-analysis showed that the combination of NSAIDs and weak opioids produces little improvement in analgesia, with an increased incidence of toxicity.[107][I] This second step is currently the subject of a wide-ranging discussion with its use being questioned in terms of its pharmacological validity (e.g. low doses of a strong opioid given as an alternative in step two), its efficacy,[101, 107, 108] its only "didactic" nature,[109, 110] and its concession to morphine-related fears ("opiophobia").[111, 112, 113] However, limited data in cancer pain patients suggest a role for weak opioids.[100, 114][III]

In more detail, in most countries, weak opioids are nonscheduled drugs, making them convenient and easy to prescribe for the physician, and at the same time more readily available and more acceptable to patients, the general public, and government authorities. Introduction of a weak opioid might facilitate patient acceptance and compliance, while there is often also a much lower barrier among medical practitioners to prescribe these drugs. It is important to realize that neither of these reasons is a pharmacological one, but rather the result of inappropriate education and societal pressures.[113] In this context it is important to note that there are still countries in which strong opioids are unavailable or their availability is severely restricted by legislation;[42] in these countries weak opioids are often the only option to treat cancer pain requiring more than nonopioid use.

Tramadol might be a different issue here; it is listed as a step two opioid, although it is better described as an atypical centrally acting analgesic because its mechanism of action combines opioid and monaminergic properties.[115] The analgesic efficacy of this compound in cancer pain[104][III], its specific effect on neuropathic pain[116][I], and its superior adverse effect profile in comparison to conventional opioids[117, 118][III] makes it an interesting different step between the nonopioids and the strong opioids, although its efficacy can blur the boundaries between steps two and three.[114]

STEP THREE: USE OF STRONG OPIOIDS

When the first two steps fail, a weak opioid is replaced with a strong opioid, again without abandoning the nonopioids and adjuvants if possible; a strong opioid should be immediately started in the setting of initial presentation with severe cancer pain. Over 50 percent of patients with pain and advanced cancer will require treatment with strong opioids at some stage of their illness.[22] While the effective and safe use of opioids does require the consideration of several factors (previous opioid exposure, severity and nature of pain, age of patient, extent of disease, and concurrent disease[9]) this step-up process is shown to be safe and effective.[119] Further increases in pain are then counteracted with increasing doses of strong opioid.

Morphine is the gold standard strong opioid of choice as recommended by the WHO[8,9] and the European Association for Palliative Care.[60] Wide clinical experience has been gained in its use and acceptable analgesia can be achieved in over 80 percent by using morphine in combination with a nonopioid analgesic.[22] The Cochrane Database of Systemic Reviews collated 45 published randomized clinical trials involving oral morphine for cancer pain. These trials only include 3061 participants but clearly demonstrate oral morphine to be an effective analgesic in this setting.[120][I] Adverse effects were common but only resulted in 4 percent of patients discontinuing therapy due to their severity. Morphine has no clinically significant ceiling effect to analgesia, allowing large variation in the doses used to achieve pain relief.[60] It is the only strong opioid placed on the WHO essential medications list.[121]

There are, however, some limitations to morphine therapy including the accumulation of active metabolites in renal impairment, lack of complete response in some pain types (particularly neuropathic pain),[60] and large interindividual variability in morphine pharmacokinetics requiring careful titration against pain relief.[73,122]

A number of other strong oral opioids are therefore also available for choice at step three if indicated by the clinical scenario. These include methadone,[123,124] oxycodone,[125] and hydromorphone.[126] Fentanyl[127] and buprenorphine[128] are also available in sustained release topical delivery systems (patches).[65] Due to accumulation of neurotoxic metabolites, particularly in renal impairment, and its short duration of action, pethidine is not recommended for the treatment of chronic cancer pain if alternatives are available.[9,129][V]

Fears of side effects such as respiratory depression, tolerance, and physical dependence and psychological dependence have led to worldwide underutilization of step three opioids in the management of cancer pain.[130,131] Pain acts as a stimulant to counteract any initial respiratory centre depression,[132] while the CNS rapidly becomes tolerant to the effects of opioids over time. Therefore, respiratory depression due to opioid treatment of cancer pain almost never occurs: fear of this is an inappropriate reason to underutilize opioids.[133] The exception to this is the sudden relief of pain by other procedures (e.g. neurolysis) or spinal cord compression when high doses of opioids, suddenly not counterbalanced by pain, can lead to respiratory depression.[133,134][V]

Because of the common occurrence of nausea and constipation with the use of strong opioids it is advisable to initiate therapy in combination with a regular antiemetic and laxative.[135][V] Nausea often subsides as treatment continues over a few weeks, but treatment for constipation needs to be both continued and aggressive.[136,137][IV] Sedation also occurs commonly with initial and increasing doses of opioids but will usually subside within a week of stable dosing.[138] However, if sedation or nausea is persistent, rotating to another opioid may be useful, as cross-tolerance between strong opioids is often incomplete.[139][V] Cognitive impairment does occur in patients who are initiated on opioid treatment or who undergo a significant increase in opioid dosage, but this effect lasts no longer than a week and patients on stable doses of opioid have no gross change in cognitive abilities.[138] However, comparisons between patients on stable doses of opioids to patients not on opioid or healthy volunteers have found small, but statistically significant differences in cognitive abilities.[140,141,142][III] Other less frequent side effects of strong opioids are pruritus, urinary retention, and sweating.[143]

USE OF ADJUVANTS

At any step, additional adjuvants and coanalgesic drugs should be added as appropriate for the individual patient and pain diagnosis.[8,9]

Examples of coanalgesic drugs used here include, in particular, medications for the treatment of neuropathic pain. Here, membrane stabilizers such as the anticonvulsants,[144] class I antiarrhythmics,[145] and tricyclic antidepressants[146] are used. Other coanalgesics include bisphosphonates[147] and steroids.[148] These drugs provide an alternative for patients who are unable to be treated with conventional analgesics alone without encountering unacceptable toxicity.[6,149,150,151][IV] The recognition that not all pain responds completely to classical analgesics is important as adjuvants may be required by up to 90 percent of patients at death.[80] However, as these medications have a significant risk of side effects, most should be reserved until the more traditional methods are failing to treat specific pain types.[81]

Many other groups of drugs may be used to treat the adverse effects of analgesics, to enhance pain relief and to treat concomitant psychological disturbances such as insomnia, anxiety, and depression.[9] Laxatives are essential to chronic opioid therapy.[137] Antiemetics should be prescribed regularly on commencement of an opioid and their use reviewed at one week. Anxiolytics such as the benzodiazepines, psychotropic drugs, and major tranquilizers have no specific analgesic effects and lead to increased sedation, so their use should be restricted to those patients requiring assistance with sleep, anxiety, depression, and muscle spasm. [V]

It is recommended that only one agent from each group be used at one time. When one drug fails to provide pain relief, a representative of the next step should be used rather than switching within a group of drugs with similar efficacy and potency.[9] However, if one drug results in unacceptable side effects, then it should be replaced by another agent from the same step. There is most discussion about this strategy in terms of opioid rotation,[28, 139, 152] particularly if morphine causes hyperalgesia[153] or neuro-excitatory effects, presumably by retention of the metabolite, morphine-3-glucuronide.[154]

"RESCUE" ANALGESICS

A short-acting opioid, such as immediate-release morphine, should be available to all cancer patients taking controlled-release preparations to treat pain not covered by their regular medications. This is referred to as "breakthrough pain."[155, 156, 157] "Incident pain," where pain is due to activity, is best managed with rescue analgesia prior to planned movement. Pain during periods of inactivity can be covered by the controlled-release preparation – an increase in this dose will generally only result in sedation while resting.[158, 159][V] Requirement for rescue doses for breakthrough pain just prior to the next dose of controlled-release medication often indicates progressing disease or inadequate regular dosing. Reassessment of the pain and increased doses of controlled-release preparation, guided by the amount of rescue analgesia used, will usually be required.[160][V]

For the individual

Pain is by definition "a sensory and emotional experience" and "always subjective."[161] Any analgesic regime must therefore be adapted to the individual patient, the intensity and cause of the pain, and the nature of the disease. Although the analgesic ladder gives the impression of a standardized approach to the problem of cancer pain, the stepwise should be seen more as a guideline to the development of an individualized treatment plan.

There is no "right" medication and/or dose for every patient. In particular, with regard to opioids, the correct dose is the one that treats this patient's pain. It is best found by individual dose titration until a patient is comfortable. As an example of the individual variability

of opioid response, the dose range quoted by the WHO for oral morphine is 5–1000 mg every four hours,[9] confirmed by a study.[162]

Setting realistic and obtainable aims of analgesic therapy clarifies the titration process. It is important to be aware of the patient's own priorities and expectations. A night's sleep without pain may be an appropriate first goal to negotiate. Subsequently, most patients will also be able to become pain-free at rest, while many ultimately achieve pain-free activity.[163] Aiming for a goal that is too high initially can result in early failure, thereby frustrating the patient and possibly undermining trust in the treating physician.

The starting dose of strong opioids recommended for the titration process depends on a number of patient factors including age, disease, concurrent morbidities, and previous exposure to opioids. In general, titration should be performed only with immediate-release and not with controlled-release preparations, as their long half-life makes titration more difficult and protracted.[119, 164, 165] During the titration process of the background analgesia, patients must have free access to additional rescue medication. The utilization pattern of the rescue medication gives an indication for the adequacy of the background analgesia and provides a good guide for any changes required.

Clinical practice suggests that if a starting opioid dose provides good analgesia, but with excessive sedation, then the subsequent dose should be 50 percent lower. If, on the initial dose, pain relief is inadequate after 24 hours, then doses should be increased, based on rescue drug used, but a typical increase would be by 50 percent, with frequent reevaluation at least at 48 and 72 hours. [V]

Medication needs to be continued throughout the night, therefore doses may need to be increased to cover the period of sleep, until a longer acting drug such as controlled-release morphine is used.

Attention to detail

The analgesic regime ought to be written out in full for the patient and caregivers. The reason for use, timing of doses, and possible side effects with their relevant treatments should be listed for each medication prescribed.[81] Patients should be encouraged to maintain a diary of pain intensity, analgesia, and adverse events; thus, daily fluctuations in symptom control can be monitored and treated accordingly.

Frequent reassessment ensures that correct diagnoses are made and that goals are being reached. The adequacy of the management plan should be assessed by discussion with the patient in terms of the original goals of therapy, function, and quality of life; review of the number of rescue doses required per day; recording pain severity and excluding significant side effects. If treatment is not providing adequate pain relief then the analgesic regime or the original diagnoses should be reviewed, remembering that a patient may have more than one source of pain. Patient review must also be frequent enough to detect and manage side effects, while continuing to tailor the analgesic regime. Modification of the analgesic prescription may be required on average every two weeks.[14] [V] There is often a need to change therapy due to the nature of changing disease: either progression of malignancy, imminent death, or response to disease-modifying treatment such as chemotherapy or radiotherapy.

EVALUATION OF THE WHO CANCER PAIN GUIDELINES

Difficulties with implementing the WHO cancer pain guidelines

Pain is the most common symptom in over 70 percent of patients with advanced cancer,[166, 167] and opioids are the mainstay of pain management.[8, 9] Some patients with cancer would rather die than experience unrelieved, escalating, severe pain.[168] However, many cancer patients with pain are consistently undertreated, enduring an unnecessary, living hell of uncontrolled pain.[112, 169, 170, 171]

The reasons for this are multiple, including absence of national policies on cancer pain relief and palliative care, lack of financial resources and healthcare delivery systems, and legal restrictions on the use and availability of opioids due to the misconception that increased medical use will increase illicit drug traffic. There is a lack of awareness on the part of health workers that cancer pain can and should be relieved, and concern that medical use of opioids will produce dependence and drug abuse.

Many physicians and nursing staff underprescribe and underadminister opioid analgesia for moderate to severe pain through fear and ignorance; fear of tolerance and addiction,[169, 171] and of escalating dose requirements and adverse effects, and ignorance of the pharmacokinetics and pharmacodynamics of opioids and the meaning and mechanisms of tolerance, physical dependence and substance abuse.[172, 173] One reason is the "dual pharmacology" of opioids, i.e. the significant differences between opioid laboratory pharmacology (in experimental animals, healthy volunteers, addicts) and opioid clinical pharmacology (in pain patients).[174] These differences are mainly dependent on the absence or presence of pain and lead to inappropriate fear of adverse effects such as respiratory depression, tolerance, physical dependence, and psychological addiction; e.g. not understanding the difference between physical dependence and psychological addiction influences drug dispensing by pharmacists.[175] However, even with the correct knowledge and attitude, behavior changes do not occur necessarily: one-third of nurses, who in 94 percent approved the use of opioids for patient comfort, stated that they would administer the least possible opioid prescribed and nearly half of them

would encourage the patient to have a nonopioid instead of an opioid.[176]

Patients also fear opioids, the stigma attached to their use, loss of control over their disease, and the potential for addiction. Patients and their families also fear that opioids are being used as a kind of surreptitious euthanasia.[177, 178] Particularly at risk of physician opiophobia and poor pain control are patients in perceived "minority" groups[179] and those whose first language is not that of their health workers, and of the pain assessment tools available, such as the Brief Pain Inventory (BPI).[180, 181] The Single Convention on Narcotic Drugs stated in 1961 that "the medical use of narcotic drugs continues to be indispensable for the relief of pain" and "addiction to narcotic drugs constitutes a serious evil."[182] Unfortunately, whilst paying lip service to the first statement, health workers and legislative authorities still seem to have an irrational attachment to the idea that the use of opioids causes addiction. This opiophobia is widespread and persistent, possibly as common today as when discussed over 20 years ago.[112, 169]

Therefore, the WHO analgesic ladder remains not only a valuable tool for clinical practice, but also for policy change. Its concepts create an awareness of the appropriate use of opioids for pain management and thereby permit healthcare professionals to obtain the opioids their patients need. Internationally, it continues to be difficult to provide pain control to cancer patients due to inadequate local access to opioid analgesics. Healthcare professionals, patient representatives, and government authorities must collaborate to develop laws and policies that permit ready access of patients to opioids worldwide.[42]

Efficacy of the WHO cancer pain guidelines

The WHO cancer pain guidelines are the internationally accepted standard for the treatment of cancer pain. In treatment programs for large numbers of cancer patients with previously intractable pain over long periods of time, following the WHO guidelines has decreased pain intensity to none to moderate for 80–90 percent of the treatment period providing adequate analgesia in 70–90 percent of patients.[6, 14, 53, 54, 55, 56, 57] [IV] Utilization of the guidelines has been shown to result in rapid improvement in pain relief; usually giving adequate analgesia within one week.[56, 80] [IV] A validation study following over 2000 patients treated according to WHO guidelines confirmed their effectiveness prospectively.[57] [III]

However, a systematic review of eight studies evaluating the effectiveness of the WHO ladder concludes that these provide insufficient evidence to confidently assess the effectiveness of the WHO analgesic ladder for the management of cancer pain.[183] [I] There were relevant limitations with all of the studies, including all being case series with no control groups and none providing information on the conditions in which pain was assessed. These authors conclude that "until results from carefully designed controlled trials are available, it would be inappropriate to judge the performance of clinicians, programs, and institutions or to design policies based on such evidence."

This is in line with a study showing that immediate use of strong opioids in cancer pain might be superior to following WHO guidelines; patients started on strong opioids had significantly better pain relief than patients treated according to WHO guidelines, required significantly fewer changes in therapy, and reported greater satisfaction with treatment.[24][II]

The oral route of therapy promoted in the WHO ladder is possible in over 80 percent of the treatment time.[57] Oral treatment continues to be effective even in the last days of life,[55, 80][IV] where at the time of death 50–70 percent of patients may be pain-free and less than 5 percent may have severe pain.[80, 184] This is much lower than the worldwide estimate that 25 percent of patients suffer unnecessarily from severe pain at the time of death. Also, up to 80 percent of patients managed according to the guidelines may be able to maintain communication, orientation, and consciousness during the last 24 hours of life.[80]

The judicious use of coanalgesics and other adjuvant drugs in approximately 90 percent of cases means that serious side effects are rare. Overall, side effects are unlikely to lead to a change of regime, with the WHO guidelines providing a safe and effective means for treatment of cancer pain.[14, 57, 80][IV]

Apparent failure of the WHO guidelines

If treatment based on these principles does not appear to be successful, inadequacy of dose or dosing interval, inappropriateness of the prescribed route, or the need to step up the ladder should be excluded. Before abandoning the principles expressed in the guidelines, the following scenarios should also be considered:

- There has been inadequate assessment of the pain and its meaning to the patient. Has a neuropathic component been missed? Have adjuvant medications been utilized appropriately?
- The patient's lifestyle and levels of activity result in high levels of incident pain. Modification of lifestyle may be required.
- The pain is exacerbated by other factors such as depression, anger, hopelessness, or anxiety. This has been termed "opioid irrelevant pain" and should encourage the practitioner to reflect on the broader context of suffering.[2, 3] Psychiatric or psychological intervention may be useful here.
- Other medical problems are occurring. These may include infection, hypercalcemia of malignancy,

constipation, pressure sores, or complications of the tumor location such as pathological fracture or spinal cord compression.

If a patient remains poorly responsive to therapy, the available options include attempts to increase the therapeutic window by aggressively controlling the dose-limiting side effects of medications (e.g. use of psychostimulants to reduce opioid-induced somnolence);[185, 186][V] rotating strong opioids to achieve a better balance of analgesia and toxicity;[28, 29, 79, 133, 139, 152, 187][IV] investigation of disease-modifying treatments such as chemotherapy, radiotherapy, antibiotics, or hormonal manipulation; maximization of adjuvant and coanalgesic effects; and offering a trial of a more aggressive intervention. The latter may include surgery, spinal analgesia,[188] and nerve blocks[189] or stimulation.

The WHO treatment guidelines have often been criticized as being too simplistic. However, they were designed to enable healthcare professionals in many settings and countries to control cancer pain; therefore they had to follow simple concepts. These concepts should not distract from the fact that cancer pain relief works best when patients receive individual attention and close monitoring; this is emphasized by the points "for the individual" and "attention to detail."[53]

OTHER CLINICAL GUIDELINES FOR THE TREATMENT OF CANCER PAIN

There are now a number of clinical guidelines available that expand on the principles of cancer pain management and provide expert consensus where supporting evidence is lacking. Examples available online are listed in **Table 10.2**.

As shown for the WHO guidelines, such clinical guidelines offer a number of benefits.[190] Their application reduces variation in the clinical management of cancer pain, while improving the basis and quality of clinical decision making. To healthcare professionals they offer clarification of the proven benefit of analgesic approaches by documenting the quality of the supporting evidence. Following such guidelines does not only improve the outcome of an individual patient, but has also a positive impact on large patient populations. Clinical guidelines have a political impact, too, as they increase awareness of the burden of cancer pain as well as increase consumer demand for better pain relief. Last, but not least, such guidelines provide criteria to rate compliance with best pain management practices and permit identification of research gaps.

However, clinical guidelines have been criticized for a number of reasons.[190] They are claimed to ignore the needs of individual patients and their specific circumstances and to be ineffective in complex clinical cases because they oversimplify treatment options. Their didactic approach appears to make clinical judgment

Table 10.2 Other clinical guidelines on cancer pain management available online.

Guidelines	Web address
National Comprehensive Cancer Network (NCCN) Practice Guidelines for Adult Cancer Pain. Version 2. NCCN. 2005. United States of America.	www.nccn.org/professionals/physician_gls/PDF/pain.pdf
National Health and Medical Research Council. Acute Pain Management: Scientific Evidence. Australia and New Zealand College of Anaesthetists. 2005. Australia.	www.nhmrc.gov.au/publications/files_/cp104.pdf
American Pain Society (APS) Guidelines for the Management of Cancer Pain in Adults and Children. APS. 2005. United States of America.	www.ampainsoc.org/pub/cancer.htm
National Institutes of Health (NIH) Symptom Management in Cancer: Pain, Depression and Fatigue. NIH Consensus Statement online. 2002. United States of America.	http://consensus.nih.gov/2002/2002CancerPainDepressionFatiguesos022.html.htm
European Association for Palliative Care: Morphine and Alternative Opioids for Cancer Pain: the EAPC Recommendations. Expert Working Group of the Research Network of the EAPC. 2001. Europe.	www.eapcnet.org/publications/eapcpub.asp#BJC
Scottish Intercollegiate Guidelines Network (SIGN) Control of Pain in Patients with Cancer: a National Clinical Guideline. SIGN. 2000. Scotland.	www.sign.ac.uk/guidelines/fulltext/44/index.html

dispensable and too many guidelines with different levels of evidence can contribute to information overload of clinicians.

Recent research has shown that guideline-based clinical decision-making improves pain outcomes in cancer patients.[191, 192][II]

REFERENCES

1. Woodruff R. *Cancer pain*, 2nd edn. Heidelberg, Victoria: Asperula, 1999.
2. Cassell E. The nature of suffering and the goals of medicine. *New England Journal of Medicine*. 1982; **306**: 639–45.
3. Saunders C. *The management of terminal illness*. London: Edward Arnold, 1967.
4. Skaer TL. Management of pain in the cancer patient. *Clinical Therapeutics*. 1993; **15**: 638–49.
5. Hammack J, Loprinzi C. Use of orally administered opioids for cancer-related pain [review]. *Mayo Clinic Proceedings*. 1994; **69**: 384–90.
6. Portenoy R. Pharmacologic management of cancer pain. *Seminars in Oncology*. 1995; **22**: 112–20.
7. Meldrum M. The ladder and the clock: cancer pain and public policy at the end of the twentieth century. *Journal of Pain and Symptom Management*. 2005; **29**: 41–54.
8. World Health Organization. *Cancer pain management*. WHO Technical Report Series. Geneva: WHO, 1986.
* 9. World Health Organization. *Cancer pain relief. With a guide to opioid availability*, 2nd edn. Geneva: WHO, 1996.
10. Hillier R. Control of pain in terminal cancer. *British Medical Bulletin*. 1990; **46**: 279–91.
11. Blanchard CG, Ruckdeschel JC. Psychosocial aspects of cancer in adults: implications for teaching medical students. *Journal of Cancer Education*. 1986; **1**: 237–48.
12. Gadow S. An ethical case for patient self-determination. *Seminars in Oncology Nursing*. 1989; **5**: 99–101.
13. Levenson BS. A multidimensional approach to the treatment of pain in the oncology patient. *Frontiers of Radiation Therapy and Oncology*. 1980; **15**: 138–41.
14. Grond S, Zech D, Lynch J et al. Validation of the World Health Organization guidelines for pain relief in head and neck cancer. A prospective study. *Annals of Otology, Rhinology, and Laryngology*. 1993; **102**: 342–8.
15. Donato V, Montagna A, Musio D, Cellini N. Radiotherapy in the symptomatic treatment of the oncological patients. *Anticancer Research*. 1999; **19**: 3375–82.
16. Ramirez AJ, Towlson KE, Leaning MS et al. Do patients with advanced breast cancer benefit from chemotherapy? *British Journal of Cancer*. 1998; **78**: 1488–94.
17. Fourneau I, Broos P. Pathologic fractures due to metastatic disease. A retrospective study of 160 surgically treated fractures. *Acta Chirurgica Belgica*. 1998; **98**: 255–60.
18. Weigel B, Maghsudi M, Neumann C et al. Surgical management of symptomatic spinal metastases. Postoperative outcome and quality of life. *Spine*. 1999; **24**: 2240–6.
19. Collett BJ. Opioid tolerance: the clinical perspective. *British Journal of Anaesthesia*. 1998; **81**: 58–68.
20. Portenoy RK. Opioid tolerance and responsiveness: research findings and clinical observations. In: Gebhart GF, Hammond DL, Jensen TS (eds). *Proceedings of the 7th World Congress on Pain, Progress in Pain Research and Management*. Seattle: IASP Press, 1994: 595–619.
21. Stevens CW, Yaksh TL. Studies of morphine and D-ala2-D-leu5-enkephalin (DADLE) cross-tolerance after continuous

intrathecal infusion in the rat. *Anesthesiology.* 1992; **76**: 596–603.

* 22. Schug SA, Zech D, Grond S *et al.* A long-term survey of morphine in cancer pain patients. *Journal of Pain and Symptom Management.* 1992; **7**: 259–66.

23. Brescia FJ, Portenoy RK, Ryan M *et al.* Pain, opioid use, and survival in hospitalized patients with advanced cancer. *Journal of Clinical Oncology.* 1992; **10**: 149–55.

24. Marinangeli F, Ciccozzi A, Leonardis M *et al.* Use of strong opioids in advanced cancer pain: a randomized trial. *Journal of Pain and Symptom Management.* 2004; **27**: 409–16.

25. Portenoy RK. Tolerance to opioid analgesics: Clinical aspects. *Cancer Surveys.* 1994; **21**: 49–65.

26. Kanner RM, Foley KM. Patterns of narcotic drug use in a cancer pain clinic. *Annals of the New York Academy of Sciences.* 1981; **362**: 161–72.

27. Foley KM. Controversies in cancer pain. Medical perspectives. *Cancer.* 1989; **63**: 2257–65.

28. Mercadante S. Opioid rotation for cancer pain: rationale and clinical aspects. *Cancer.* 1999; **86**: 1856–66.

* 29. Quigley C. Opioid switching to improve pain relief and drug tolerability. *Cochrane Dataase of Systematic Reviews.* 2004; **CD004847**.

30. Miller RR, Olson HG, Amsterdam EA, Mason DT. Propranolol-withdrawal rebound phenomenon. Exacerbation of coronary events after abrupt cessation of antianginal therapy. *New England Journal of Medicine.* 1975; **293**: 416–8.

31. Neusy AJ, Lowenstein J. Blood pressure and blood pressure variability following withdrawal of propranolol and clonidine. *Journal of Clinical Pharmacology.* 1989; **29**: 18–24.

32. Warner CH, Bobo W, Warner C *et al.* Antidepressant discontinuation syndrome. *American Family Physician.* 2006; **74**: 449–56.

33. Kreek MJ, Koob GF. Drug dependence: stress and dysregulation of brain reward pathways. *Drug and Alcohol Dependence.* 1998; **51**: 23–47.

34. Manfredi PL, Ribeiro S, Chandler SW, Payne R. Inappropriate use of naloxone in cancer patients with pain. *Journal of Pain and Symptom Management.* 1996; **11**: 131–4.

* 35. Hanks GWC, Cherny N. Opioid analgesic therapy. In: Doyle D (ed.). *Oxford textbook of palliative medicine,* 2nd edn. Oxford: Oxford University Press, 1998: 331–54.

36. Savage SR. Assessment for addiction in pain-treatment settings. *Clinical Journal of Pain.* 2002; **18**: S28–38.

37. Anonymous. *Diagnostic and Statistical Manual of Mental Disorders, Text Revision (DSM-IV-TR®),* 4th edn. Arlington: American Psychiatric Association, 2000: 992.

38. Porter J, Jick H. Addiction rare in patients treated with narcotics. *New England Journal of Medicine.* 1980; **302**: 123.

* 39. Chapman CR, Hill HF. Prolonged morphine self-administration and addiction liability. Evaluation of two

theories in a bone marrow transplant unit. *Cancer.* 1989; **63**: 1636–44.

40. Sun WZ, Chen TL, Fan SZ *et al.* Can cancer pain attenuate the physical dependence on chronic long-term morphine treatment? *Journal of the Formosan Medical Association.* 1992; **91**: 513–20.

41. Joranson D. Availability of opioids for cancer pain: recent trends, assessment of system barriers, new World Health Organization guidelines, and the risk of diversion. *Journal of Pain and Symptom Management.* 1993; **8**: 353–60.

* 42. Joranson DE, Ryan KM, Gilson AM, Dahl JL. Trends in medical use and abuse of opioid analgesics. *Journal of the American Medical Association.* 2000; **283**: 1710–4.

43. Costa e Silva JA. Evidence-based analysis of the worldwide abuse of licit and illicit drugs. *Human Psychopharmacology.* 2002; **17**: 131–40.

* 44. Weissman DE, Haddox JD. Opioid pseudoaddiction – an iatrogenic syndrome. *Pain.* 1989; **36**: 363–6.

45. Secor JW, Schenker S. Drug metabolism in patients with liver disease. *Advances in Internal Medicine.* 1987; **32**: 379–405.

46. Sawe J. High-dose morphine and methadone in cancer patients. Clinical pharmacokinetic considerations of oral treatment. *Clinical Pharmacokinetics.* 1986; **11**: 87–106.

47. Neal EA, Meffin PJ, Gregory PB, Blaschke TF. Enhanced bioavailability and decreased clearance of analgesics in patients with cirrhosis. *Gastroenterology.* 1979; **77**: 96–102.

* 48. Schug SA, Morgan J. Treatment of cancer pain: special considerations in patients with renal disease. *American Journal of Cancer.* 2004; **3**: 247–56.

49. Fillastre JP, Singlas E. Pharmacokinetics of newer drugs in patients with renal impairment. *Clinical Pharmacokinetics.* 1991; **20**: 293–310.

50. Lam YW, Banerji S, Hatfield C, Talbert RL. Principles of drug administration in renal insufficiency. *Clinical Pharmacokinetics.* 1997; **32**: 30–57.

51. Touchette MA, Slaughter RL. The effect of renal failure on hepatic drug clearance. *DICP.* 1991; **25**: 1214–24.

52. Reetze-Bonorden P, Bohler J, Keller E. Drug dosage in patients during continuous renal replacement therapy. *Clinical Pharmacokinetics.* 1993; **24**: 362–79.

* 53. World Health Organization. *Cancer pain relief and palliative care,* 2nd edn. Geneva: WHO, 1996: 63.

54. Takeda F. Results of field testing in Japan of the WHO Draft Interim Guidelines on relief of cancer pain. *Pain Clinic.* 1986; **1**: 83–9.

55. Ventafridda V, Tamburini M, Caraceni A *et al.* A validation study of the WHO method for cancer pain relief. *Cancer.* 1987; **59**: 850–6.

* 56. Schug SA, Zech D, Doerr U. Cancer pain management according to WHO Analgesic Guidelines. *Journal of Pain and Symptom Management.* 1990; **5**: 27–32.

* 57. Zech D, Grond S, Lynch J *et al.* Validation of the World Health Organization Guidelines for cancer pain relief: a 10-year prospective study. *Pain.* 1995; **63**: 65–76.

58. Stjernsward J, Colleau S, Ventafridda V. The World Health Organization cancer pain and palliative car program. Past, present and future. *Journal of Pain and Symptom Management*. 1996; **12**: 65–72.

59. Walsh TD. Oral morphine in chronic cancer pain. *Pain*. 1984; **18**: 1–11.

60. Hanks GW, Conno F, Cherny N *et al*. Morphine and alternative opioids in cancer pain: the EAPC recommendations. *British Journal of Cancer*. 2001; **84**: 587–93.

61. Mercadante SG. When oral morphine fails in cancer pain: the role of the alternative routes. *American Journal of Hospice and Palliative Care*. 1998; **15**: 333–42.

62. Glare P. Problems with opiates in cancer pain: parenteral opioids. *Supportive Care in Care Cancer*. 1997; **5**: 445–50.

63. Coyle N, Adelhardt J, Foley KM, Portenoy RK. Character of terminal illness in the advanced cancer patient: pain and other symptoms during the last four weeks of life. *Journal of Pain and Symptom Management*. 1990; **5**: 83–93.

64. Cherny NJ, Chang V, Frager G *et al*. Opioid pharmacotherapy in the management of cancer pain: a survey of strategies used by pain physicians for the selection of analgesic drugs and routes of administration. *Cancer*. 1995; **76**: 1283–93.

65. Skaer TL. Transdermal opioids for cancer pain. *Health and Quality of Life Outcomes*. 2006; **4**: 24.

66. Chelly JE. An iontophoretic, fentanyl HCl patient-controlled transdermal system for acute postoperative pain management. *Expert Opinion on Pharmacotherapy*. 2005; **6**: 1205–14.

67. DeConno F, Ripamonti C, Saita L *et al*. Role of rectal route in treating cancer pain: a randomised crossover clinical trial of oral versus rectal morphine administration in opioid-naive cancer patients with pain. *Journal of Clinical Oncology*. 1995; **13**: 1004–08.

68. Moulin DE, Johnson NG, Murray-Parsons N *et al*. Subcutaneous narcotic infusions for cancer pain: treatment outcome and guidelines for use. *Canadian Medical Association Journal*. 1992; **146**: 891–7.

69. Ripamonti C, Bruera E. Rectal, buccal, and sublingual narcotics for the management of cancer pain. *Journal of Palliative Care*. 1991; **7**: 30–5.

70. Breda M, Bianchi M, Ripamonti C *et al*. Plasma morphine and morphine-6-glucuronide patterns in cancer patients after oral, subcutaneous, sublabial and rectal short-term administration. *International Journal of Clinical Pharmacology Research*. 1991; **11**: 93–7.

71. Wilkinson TJ, Robinson BA, Begg EJ *et al*. Pharmacokinetics and efficacy of rectal versus oral sustained-release morphine in cancer patients. *Cancer Chemotherapy and Pharmacology*. 1992; **31**: 251–4.

72. Nelson KA, Glare PA, Walsh D, Groh ES. A prospective, within-patient, crossover study of continuous intravenous and subcutaneous morphine for chronic cancer pain. *Journal of Pain and Symptom Management*. 1997; **13**: 262–7.

73. Glare PA, Walsh TD. Clinical pharmacokinetics of morphine. *Therapeutic Drug Monitoring*. 1991; **13**: 1–23.

74. Hanks GW, de Conno F, Ripamonti V *et al*. Morphine in cancer pain: modes of administration. *British Medical Journal*. 1996; **312**: 823–6.

* 75. Gilbar PJ. A guide to enteral drug administration in palliative care. *Journal of Pain and Symptom Management*. 1999; **17**: 197–207.

76. Weinberg DS, Inturrisi CE, Reidenberg B *et al*. Sublingual absorption of selected opioid analgesics. *Clinical Pharmacology and Therapeutics*. 1988; **44**: 335–42.

77. Davis MP. Buprenorphine in cancer pain. *Supportive Care in Cancer*. 2005; **13**: 878–87.

* 78. Zeppetella G, Ribeiro MD. Opioids for the management of breakthrough (episodic) pain in cancer patients. *Cochrane Database of Systematic Reviews*. 2006; **CD004311**.

79. Portenoy RK. Managing cancer pain poorly responsive to systemic opioid therapy. *Oncology (Williston Park)*. 1999; **13**: 25–9.

80. Grond S, Zech D, Schug SA *et al*. Validation of the World Health Organization guidelines for cancer pain relief during the last days and hours of life. *Journal of Pain and Symptom Management*. 1991; **6**: 411–22.

* 81. Schug SA, Dunlop R, Zech D. Pharmacological management of cancer pain. *Drugs*. 1992; **43**: 44–53.

82. Moote C. The prevention of postoperative pain. *Canadian Journal of Anaesthesia*. 1994; **41**: 527–33.

83. Tuttle C. Drug management of pain in cancer patients. *Canadian Medical Association Journal*. 1985; **132**: 121–34.

84. Smith K, Broomhead A, Kerr R *et al*. Comparison of a once-a-day sustained-release morphine formulation with standard oral morphine treatment for cancer pain. *Journal of Pain and Symptom Management*. 1997; **14**: 63–73.

85. Arkinstall WW, Goughnour BR, White JA, Stewart JH. Control of severe pain with sustained-release morphine tablets voral morphine solution. *Canadian Medical Association Journal*. 1989; **140**: 653–7, 61.

86. Goughnour BR, Arkinstall WW, Stewart JH. Analgesic response to single and multiple doses of controlled-release morphine tablets and morphine oral solution in cancer patients. *Cancer*. 1989; **63**: 2294–7.

87. McCormack J, Warriner C, Levine M, Glick N. A Comparison of regularly dosed oral morphine and on-demand intramuscular morphine in the treatment of postsurgical pain. *Canadian Journal of Anaesthesiology*. 1993; **40**: 819–24.

88. Foley K. The treatment of cancer pain. *The New England Journal of Medicine*. 1985; **313**: 84–95.

89. Grond S, Zech D, Schug SA *et al*. The importance of non-opioid analgesics for cancer pain relief according to the guidelines of the World Health Organization. *International Journal of Clinical Pharmacology Research*. 1991; **11**: 253–60.

* 90. McNicol E, Strassels SA, Goudas L *et al*. NSAIDS or paracetamol, alone or combined with opioids, for cancer pain. *Cochrane Database of Systematic Reviews*. 2005; **CD005180**.

* 91. Stockler M, Vardy J, Pillai A, Warr D. Acetaminophen (paracetamol) improves pain and well-being in people with advanced cancer already receiving a strong opioid regimen: a randomized, double-blind, placebo-controlled cross-over trial. *Journal of Clinical Oncology.* 2004; **22**: 3389–94.

92. Rodriguez M, Barutell C, Rull M *et al.* Efficacy and tolerance of oral dipyrone versus oral morphine for cancer pain. *European Journal of Cancer.* 1994; **5**: 584–7.

93. Ventafridda V, De Conno F, Panerai AE *et al.* Non-steroidal anti-inflammatory drugs as the first step in cancer pain therapy: double-blind, within-patient study comparing nine drugs. *Journal of International Medical Research.* 1990; **18**: 21–9.

* 94. Jenkins CA, Bruera E. Nonsteroidal anti-inflammatory drugs as adjuvant analgesics in cancer patients. *Palliative Medicine.* 1999; **13**: 183–96.

95. Stambaugh J, Drew J. The combination of ibuprofen and oxycodone/acetaminophen in the management of chronic cancer pain. *Clinical Pharmacology and Therapeutics.* 1988; **44**: 665–9.

96. Weingart W, Sorkness C, Earhart R. Analgesia with oral narcotics and added ibuprofen in cancer patients. *Clinical Pharmacy.* 1985; **4**: 53–8.

97. Mercadante S, Sapio M, Caligara M *et al.* Opioid sparing effect of Diclofenac in cancer pain. *Journal of Pain and Symptom Management.* 1997; **14**: 15–20.

98. Dhaliwal HS, Sloan P, Arkinstall WW *et al.* Randomized evaluation of controlled-release codeine and placebo in chronic cancer pain. *Journal of Pain and Symptom Management.* 1995; **10**: 612–23.

99. Jochimsen PR, Noyes Jr R. Appraisal of codeine as an analgesic in older patients. *Journal of the American Geriatrics Society.* 1978; **26**: 521–3.

100. Mercadante S, Salvaggio L, Dardanoni G *et al.* Dextropropoxyphene versus morphine in opioid-naive cancer patients with pain. *Journal of Pain and Symptom Management.* 1998; **15**: 76–81.

101. Li Wan Po A, Zhang WY. Systematic overview of co-proxamol to assess analgesic effects of addition of dextropropoxyphene to paracetamol. *British Medical Journal.* 1997; **315**: 1565–71.

102. Jurna I, Komen W, Baldauf J, Fleischer W. Analgesia by dihydrocodeine is not due to formation of dihydromorphine: evidence from nociceptive activity in rat thalamus. *Journal of Pharmacology and Experimental Therapeutics.* 1997; **281**: 1164–70.

103. Klepstad P, Kaasa S, Cherny N *et al.* Pain and pain treatments in European palliative care units. A cross sectional survey from the European Association for Palliative Care Research Network. *Palliative Medicine.* 2005; **19**: 477–84.

104. Petzke F, Radbruch L, Sabatowski R *et al.* Slow-release tramadol for treatment of chronic malignant pain – an open multicenter trial. *Supportive Care in Cancer.* 2001; **9**: 48–54.

105. Wilder-Smith CH, Schimke J, Osterwalder B, Senn HJ. Oral tramadol, a mu-opioid agonist and monoamine reuptake-blocker, and morphine for strong cancer-related pain. *Annals of Oncology.* 1994; **5**: 141–6.

106. Grond S, Zech D, Lynch J *et al.* Tramadol – A weak opioid for relief of cancer pain. *Pain Clinic.* 1992; **5**: 241–7.

*107. Eisenberg E, Berkey C, Carr D *et al.* Efficacy and safety of non-steroidal antiinflammatory drugs for cancer pain: a meta-analysis. *Journal of Clinical Oncology.* 1994; **12**: 2756–65.

108. Furlan AD, Sandoval JA, Mailis-Gagnon A, Tunks E. Opioids for chronic noncancer pain: a meta-analysis of effectiveness and side effects. *Canadian Medical Association Journal.* 2006; **174**: 1589–94.

109. Freynhagen R, Zenz M, Strumpf M. WHO step II-clinical reality or a didactic instrument? *Schmerz.* 1994; **8**: 210–15.

*110. Grond S, Meuser T. Weak opioids – An educational substitute for morphine? *Current Opinion in Anaesthesiology.* 1998; **11**: 559–65.

111. Zenz M, Willweber-Strumpf A. Opiophobia and cancer pain in Europe. *Lancet.* 1993; **341**: 1075–6.

*112. Morgan JP. American opiophobia: Customary underutilization of opioid analgesics. *Advances in Alcohol and Substance Abuse.* 1985; **5**: 163–73.

113. Weinstein SM, Laux LF, Thornby JI *et al.* Medical students' attitudes toward pain and the use of opioid analgesics: implications for changing medical school curriculum. *Southern Medical Journal.* 2000; **93**: 472–8.

114. Grond S, Radbruch L, Meuser T *et al.* High-dose tramadol in comparison to low-dose morphine for cancer pain relief. *Journal of Pain and Symptom Management.* 1999; **18**: 174–9.

115. Raffa RB, Friderichs E, Reimann W *et al.* Opioid and nonopioid components independently contribute to the mechanism of action of tramadol, an 'atypical' opioid analgesic. *Journal of Pharmacology and Experimental Therapeutics.* 1992; **260**: 275–85.

116. Duhmke RM, Cornblath DD, Hollingshead JR. Tramadol for neuropathic pain. *Cochrane Database of Systematic Reviews.* 2004; **CD003726.**

*117. Radbruch L, Grond S, Lehmann KA. A risk-benefit assessment of tramadol in the management of pain. *Drug Safety.* 1996; **15**: 8–29.

118. Sacerdote P, Bianchi M, Gaspani L *et al.* The effects of tramadol and morphine on immune responses and pain after surgery in cancer patients. *Anesthesia and Analgesia.* 2000; **90**: 1411–14.

119. Klepstad P, Kaasa S, Borchgrevink PC. Start of oral morphine to cancer patients: effective serum morphine concentrations and contribution from morphine-6-glucuronide to the analgesia produced by morphine. *European Journal of Clinical Pharmacology.* 2000; **55**: 713–19.

*120. Wiffen PJ, Edwards JE, Barden J, McQuay HJ. Oral morphine for cancer pain. *Cochrane Database of Systematic Reviews.* 2003; **CD003868.**

121. World Health Organization. Essential Medicines. WHO Model List. Last updated: revised March 2005; cited 03 Oct, 2006. Available from: www.who.int/medicines/publications/essentialmedicines/en/.

122. Gourlay GK, Cherry DA, Cousins MJ. A comparative study of the efficacy and pharmacokinetics of oral methadone and morphine in the treatment of severe pain in patients with cancer. *Pain*. 1986; **25**: 297–312.

*123. Nicholson AB. Methadone for cancer pain. *Cochrane Database of Systematic Reviews*. 2004; **CD003971**.

124. Bruera E, Palmer JL, Bosnjak S et al. Methadone versus morphine as a first-line strong opioid for cancer pain: a randomized, double-blind study. *Journal of Clinical Oncology*. 2004; **22**: 185–92.

125. Reid CM, Martin RM, Sterne JA et al. Oxycodone for cancer-related pain: meta-analysis of randomized controlled trials. *Archives of Internal Medicine*. 2006; **166**: 837–43.

126. Murray A, Hagen NA. Hydromorphone. *Journal of Pain and Symptom Management*. 2005; **29**: S57–66.

127. Mystakidou K, Parpa E, Tsilika E et al. Pain management of cancer patients with transdermal fentanyl: a study of 1828 step I, II, & III transfers. *Journal of Pain*. 2004; **5**: 119–32.

*128. Sittl R. Transdermal buprenorphine in cancer pain and palliative care. *Palliative Medicine*. 2006; **20**: s25–30.

129. Latta KS, Ginsberg B, Barkin RL. Meperidine: a critical review. *American Journal of Therapeutics*. 2002; **9**: 53–68.

130. Venegas G, Ripamonti C, Sbanotto A, Conno FD. Side effects of morphine administration in cancer pain. *Cancer Nursing*. 1998; **21**: 289–97.

131. Walsh TD. Prevention of opioid side effects. *Journal of Pain and Symptom Management*. 1990; **5**: 362–7.

132. Hanks GW, Twycross RG. Pain, the physiological antagonist of opioid analgesics. *Lancet*. 1984; **1**: 1477–8.

133. Ravenscroft P, Schneider J. Bedside perspectives on the use of opioids: transferring results of clinical research into practice. *Clinical and Experimental Pharmacology and Physiology*. 2000; **27**: 529–32.

134. Quevedo F, Walsh D. Morphine-induced ventilatory failure after spinal cord compression. *Journal of Pain and Symptom Management*. 1999; **18**: 140–2.

135. Curtis EB, Walsh TD. Prescribing practices of a palliative care service. *Journal of Pain and Symptom Management*. 1993; **8**: 312–6.

136. Lazarus H, Fitzmartin R, Goldenheim P. A multi-investigator clinical evaluation of oral controlled-release morphine (MS Contin tablets) administered to cancer patients. *Hospice Journal*. 1990; **6**: 1–15.

*137. Mancini I, Bruera E. Constipation in advanced cancer patients. *Supportive Care in Cancer*. 1998; **6**: 356–64.

138. Bruera E, Macmillan K, Hanson J, MacDonald RN. The cognitive effects of the administration of narcotic analgesics in patients with cancer pain. *Pain*. 1989; **39**: 13–6.

139. de Stoutz ND, Bruera E, Suarez-Almazor M. Opioid rotation for toxicity reduction in terminal cancer patients. *Journal of Pain and Symptom Management*. 1995; **10**: 378–84.

140. Vainio A, Ollila J, Matikainen E et al. Driving ability in cancer patients receiving long-term morphine analgesia. *Lancet*. 1995; **346**: 667–70.

141. Banning A, Sjogren P. Cerebral effects of long-term oral opioids in cancer patients measured by continuous reaction time. *Clinical Journal of Pain*. 1990; **6**: 91–5.

142. Banning A, Sjogren P, Kaiser F. Reaction time in cancer patients receiving peripherally acting analgesics alone or in combination with opioids. *Acta Anaesthesiologica Scandinavica*. 1992; **36**: 480–2.

143. Schug S, Zech D, Grond S et al. A long-term survey of morphine in cancer pain patients. *Journal of Pain and Symptom Management*. 1992; **7**: 259–66.

*144. Wiffen P, Collins S, McQuay H et al. Anticonvulsant drugs for acute and chronic pain. *Cochrane Database of Systematic Reviews*. 2005; **CD001133**.

*145. Challapalli V, Tremont-Lukats I, McNicol E et al. Systemic administration of local anesthetic agents to relieve neuropathic pain. *Cochrane Database of Systematic Reviews*. 2005; **CD003345**.

*146. Saarto T, Wiffen P. Antidepressants for neuropathic pain. *Cochrane Database of Systematic Reviews*. 2005; **CD005454**.

*147. Body JJ. Bisphosphonates for malignancy-related bone disease: current status, future developments. *Supportive Care in Cancer*. 2006; **14**: 408–18.

148. Hanks GW, Trueman T, Twycross RG. Corticosteroids in terminal cancer — a prospective analysis of current practice. *Postgraduate Medical Journal*. 1983; **59**: 702–6.

149. Kopf A. [Co-analgesics in the treatment of chronic pain]. *Therapeutische Umschau*. 1999; **56**: 441–5.

150. Mancini I, Body JJ. [Treatment of cancer pain: the role of co-analgesics]. *Revue Medicale de Bruxelles*. 1998; **19**: A319–22.

151. Rouveix B, Bauwens MC, Giroud JP. [Treatment of different types of pain]. *Bulletin de l'Academie Nationale Medecine*. 1999; **183**: 889–901.

*152. Bruera E, Pereira J, Watanabe S et al. Opioid rotation in patients with cancer pain. A retrospective comparison of dose ratios between methadone, hydromorphone, and morphine. *Cancer*. 1996; **78**: 852–7.

153. Sjogren P, Jensen NH, Jensen TS. Disappearance of morphine-induced hyperalgesia after discontinuing or substituting morphine with other opioid agonists. *Pain*. 1994; **59**: 313–6.

154. Smith MT. Neuroexcitatory effects of morphine and hydromorphone: evidence implicating the 3-glucuronide metabolites. *Clinical and Experimental Pharmacology and Physiology*. 2000; **27**: 524–8.

*155. Caraceni A, Martini C, Zecca E et al. Breakthrough pain characteristics and syndromes in patients with cancer pain. An international survey. *Palliative Medicine*. 2004; **18**: 177–83.

156. Simmonds MA. Management of breakthrough pain due to cancer. *Oncology (Huntingt)*. 1999; **13**: 1103–08; discussion 10, 13–14.

157. Patt RB, Ellison NM. Breakthrough pain in cancer patients: characteristics, prevalence, and treatment. *Oncology (Huntingt)*. 1998; **12**: 1035–46; discussion 49–52.

158. Rogers AG. How to manage incident pain. *Journal of Pain and Symptom Management*. 1987; **2**: 99.

159. McQuay HJ, Jadad AR. Incident pain. *Cancer Surveys*. 1994; **21**: 17–24.

160. Portenoy R, Hagen N. Breakthrough pain: definition, prevalence and characteristics. *Pain*. 1990; **41**: 273–81.

161. International Association for the Study of Pain. Pain terms. *Pain*. 1979; **6**: 249.

162. Boisvert M, Cohen SR. Opioid use in advanced malignant disease: why do different centers use vastly different doses? A plea for standardized reporting. *Journal of Pain and Symptom Management*. 1995; **10**: 632–8.

163. Twycross R. Medical treatment of cancer pain. *Bulletin on Cancer*. 1980; **67**: 209–16.

164. Klepstad P, Borchgrevink PC, Kaasa S. Effects on cancer patients' health-related quality of life after the start of morphine therapy. *Journal of Pain and Symptom Management*. 2000; **20**: 19–26.

165. Brooks I, De Jager R, Blumenreich M *et al*. Principles of cancer pain management. Use of long-acting oral morphine. *Journal of Family Practice*. 1989; **28**: 275–80.

166. Cleeland CS, Gonin R, Hatfield AK *et al*. Pain and its treatment in outpatients with metastatic cancer. *New England Journal of Medicine*. 1994; **330**: 592–6.

167. Bonica JJ. *The Management of Pain*, 2nd edn. Vol. 1. Philadelphia: Lea and Febiger Press, 1990.

168. Sullivan M, Rapp S, Fitzgibbon D, Chapman CR. Pain and the choice to hasten death in patients with painful metastatic cancer. *Journal of Palliative Care*. 1997; **13**: 18–28.

169. Marks RM, Sachar EJ. Undertreatment of medical inpatients with narcotic analgesics. *Annals of Internal Medicine*. 1973; **78**: 173–81.

170. Janjan N, Payne R, Gillis T *et al*. Presenting symptoms in patients referred to a multidisciplinary clinic for bone metastases. *Journal of Pain and Symptom Management*. 1998; **16**: 171–8.

171. Lander J. Fallacies and phobias about addiction and pain. *British Journal of Addiction*. 1990; **85**: 803–9.

172. Kaasalainen V, Vainio A, Ali-Melkkila T. Developments in the treatment of cancer pain in Finland: the third nationwide survey. *Pain*. 1997; **70**: 175–83.

173. Mercadante S, Salvaggio L. Cancer pain knowledge in Southern Italy: data from a postgraduate refresher course. *Journal of Pain and Symptom Management*. 1996; **11**: 108–15.

174. McQuay HJ. Opioids in pain management. *Lancet*. 1999; **353**: 2229–32.

175. Joranson DE, Gilson AM. Pharmacists' knowledge of and attitudes toward opioid pain medications in relation to federal and state policies. *Journal of the American Pharmaceutical Association*. 2001; **41**: 213–20.

176. Edwards HE, Nash RE, Najman JM *et al*. Determinants of nurses' intention to administer opioids for pain relief. *Nursing and Health Sciences*. 2001; **3**: 149–59.

177. Gaylin W, Kass LR, Pellegrino ED, Siegler M. 'Doctors must not kill'. *Journal of the American Medical Association*. 1988; **259**: 2139–40.

178. Wall PD. The generation of yet another myth on the use of narcotics. *Pain*. 1997; **73**: 121–2.

179. Cleeland CS, Gonin R, Baez L *et al*. Pain and treatment of pain in minority patients with cancer. The Eastern Cooperative Oncology Group Minority Outpatient Pain Study. *Annals of Internal Medicine*. 1997; **127**: 813–6.

180. Saxena A, Mendoza T, Cleeland CS. The assessment of cancer pain in North India: The validation of the hindi brief pain inventory – BPI-H. *Journal of Pain and Symptom Management*. 1999; **17**: 27–41.

181. Uki J, Mendoza T, Cleeland CS *et al*. A brief cancer pain assessment tool in Japanese: the utility of the Japanese Brief Pain Inventory – BPI-J. *Journal of Pain and Symptom Management*. 1998; **16**: 364–73.

182. United Nations. Single Convention on Narcotic Drugs. *United Nations, Treaty Series*. 1961; **520**: 151.

183. Jadad A, Browman G. The WHO analgesic ladder for cancer pain management. Stepping up the quality of its evaluation. *Journal of the American Medical Association*. 1995; **274**: 1870–3.

184. Lichter I, Hunt E. The last 48 hours of life. *Journal of Palliative Care*. 1990; **6**: 7–15.

185. Rozans M, Dreisbach A, Lertora J, Kahn M. Palliative uses of methylphenidate in patients with cancer: a review. *Journal of Clinical Oncology*. 2002; **20**: 335–9.

186. Dalal S, Melzack R. Potentiation of opioid analgesia by psychostimulant drugs: a review. *Journal of Pain and Symptom Management*. 1998; **16**: 245–53.

187. Thomsen AB, Becker N, Eriksen J. Opioid rotation in chronic non-malignant pain patients. A retrospective study. *Acta Anaesthesiologica Scandinavica*. 1999; **43**: 918–23.

188. Wang JK. Intrathecal morphine for intractable pain secondary to cancer of pelvic organs. *Pain*. 1985; **21**: 99–102.

189. Lynch J, Zech D, Grond S. The role of intrathecal neurolysis in the treatment of cancer-related perianal and perineal pain. *Palliative Medicine*. 1992; **6**: 140–5.

190. Field MJ, Lohr KN. *Clinical practice guidelines: directions for a new program*. Institute of Medicine. Washington DC: National Academy Press, 1990.

191. Cleeland CS, Portenoy RK, Rue M *et al*. Does an oral analgesic protocol improve pain control for patients with cancer? An intergroup study coordinated by the Eastern Cooperative Oncology Group. *Annals of Oncology*. 2005; **16**: 972–80.

192. Du Pen SL, Du Pen AR, Polissar N *et al*. Implementing guidelines for cancer pain management: results of a randomized controlled clinical trial. *Journal of Clinical Oncology*. 1999; **17**: 361–70.

Clinical pharmacology and therapeutics: nonopioids

VICTOR PACE

Introduction	124	Nonsteroidal anti-inflammatory drugs	126
Paracetamol (acetaminophen)	124	The future	138
Dipyrone	125	General conclusions	138
Nefopam	126	References	138

KEY LEARNING POINTS

PARACETAMOL

- No good evidence of effectiveness in cancer pain.
- Central mechanism, precise nature unclear.
- Chronic use increases risk of chronic renal failure.
- Controversy over risk of gastrointestinal bleeding.

DIPYRONE AND NEFOPAM

- Complex pharmacology, not yet fully elucidated.
- Risk of agranulocytosis with dipyrone is small, but increases with prolonged use or higher doses, limiting usefulness in cancer pain.
- The dearth of cancer pain studies with nefopam makes it difficult to produce recommendations for use.

NONSTEROIDAL ANTI-INFLAMMATORY DRUG BASIC PHARMACOLOGY

- Nonsteroidal anti-inflammatory drugs (NSAIDs) inhibit prostaglandin production from arachidonic acid. Alternative routes produce leukotrienes and lipoxins.
- Both cyclooxygenase (COX)-1 and COX-2 occur constitutively, although COX-1 predominates, and both are necessary for inflammation and in pain pathways.
- Myriad variations in COX structure (splice variants, single nucleotide polymorphisms (SNPs)) mean great individual variability in effects.
- Not all NSAID effects are COX-mediated.

CLASSIFICATION OF NSAIDS

- The chemical classification of NSAIDs is singularly useless in guiding clinical use.

- NSAIDs are classified into nonselective, COX-2 selective, and COX-2 highly selective (COX-2 inhibitors).
- Ranking by COX-2 selectivities ignores other key pharmacokinetic factors.

CLINICAL USE IN CANCER PAIN

- NSAIDs are better than placebo for cancer pain.
- A poor evidence-base makes it impossible to settle questions such as superiority of one NSAID over another, whether NSAIDs are opioid sparing, or effectiveness in metastatic bone pain.

GASTROPATHY

- Erosions occur rapidly but mucosal adaptation usually occurs within a week.
- NSAID-induced dyspepsia is not a marker for peptic ulcer.
- Prevalence of peptic ulceration from NSAIDs is falling, but serious complications may be increasing.
- In the UK, NSAID gastropathy may be responsible for 200 deaths a month.

BOWEL, RENAL, AND THROMBOTIC RISK

- NSAID-induced small bowel damage may be as important as peptic ulceration. It causes anaemia, protein losing enteropathy, acute bleeding, perforation, or bowel obstruction.
- Reactivation of inflammatory bowel disease, perforation, or colonic bleeding can also occur.

- Avoid NSAIDs in conditions of low effective circulating volume to reduce the risk of acute renal failure.
- COX-2 inhibitors and NSAIDs (apart from naproxen) carry increased risks of thrombotic events, perhaps

heart failure and hypertension. COX-2 inhibitors should be avoided, and nonselective NSAIDs used with caution, in patients with cardiovascular risk factors.

INTRODUCTION

Although strong opioids remain the mainstay of pain control in advanced cancer, other analgesics are often used instead of or in conjunction with these drugs. They include the World Health Organization (WHO) Ladder Step I drugs, particularly paracetamol; nonsteroidal anti-inflammatory drugs (NSAIDs), the main subject of this chapter; and a small number of other drugs which we shall briefly review.

PARACETAMOL (ACETAMINOPHEN)

In the 1880s in Germany, the staff of Professor Kussmaul (of Kussmaul breathing fame) accidentally gave acetanilide to a patient with worms, and serendipitously discovered its antipyretic and analgesic properties. Phenacetin was synthesized from acetanilide by Bayer a few years later, and paracetamol was developed from phenacetin in 1893.[1] Fears of hematological toxicity restricted paracetamol use until the 1940s. Only in 1953 did Sterling-Winthrop market it as an alternative to aspirin.

The average UK adult consumed 12 tablets of paracetamol in the year 2000, down from 21 in 1998 due to competition from over-the-counter ibuprofen.[2] This popularity reflects its safety profile. Paracetamol was well tolerated for a year in osteoarthritis.[3][II] Its analgesic effect is dose-related.[4] It is synergistic with NSAIDs in experimental,[5] dental,[6][II] and chronic pains;[7][II] with tramadol in acute pain;[8][II] and with opioids in postoperative pain, but without reducing opioid-related adverse effects in the latter setting.[9][I] A Cochrane review of trials comparing paracetamol with NSAIDs in rheumatoid arthritis found insufficient data for firm conclusions, but patients and investigators preferred the NSAID.[10] In another Cochrane review, NSAIDs delivered better analgesia, global assessment scores, and functional gains in osteoarthritis patients than paracetamol, with no safety difference. However, the median trial length was six weeks.[11][I]

Doubts remain as to whether paracetamol improves analgesia in cancer pain,[12] despite extensive use as a WHO Step I analgesic ladder drug.[13] A Cochrane cancer pain review found insufficient evidence of its effectiveness.[14]

Mechanism of action

Paracetamol is analgesic and antipyretic but lacks anti-inflammatory and antiplatelet activity at antipyretic doses. Although it inhibits both cyclooxygenase (COX)-1 and COX-2 with low sensitivities,[15] its behavior varies widely among different tissues. It inhibits prostaglandin synthesis in brain, spleen, kidney, and lung but not in platelets and stomach mucosa.[15]

A number of putative mechanisms for paracetamol's activity have been proposed.

- Paracetamol inhibits COX *in vivo* when levels of arachidonic acid are low, when prostaglandin synthesis is mediated mainly by COX-2, even in cells possessing both COX isoforms.[16] Paracetamol may inhibit COX-2 pathways proceeding at low rates but not in inflammation, where COX-2 activity is ramped up.[17]
- Paracetamol works centrally, probably inhibiting descending serotonergic pathways.[17] (Recent work suggests other roles for serotonergic pathways in paracetamol analgesia.[18]) However, it lacks a peripheral effect. To explain this it has been hypothesized that a different type of COX, exquisitely sensitive to paracetamol, exists in the central nervous system (CNS) and vascular epithelium.[19] In 2002, Chandrasekharan *et al.*[20] identified COX-3, a splice variant of COX-1 (hence also called COX-1b), as the site of action of paracetamol. There are doubts about the human relevance of this work, carried out on canine COX-3.[21] Many feel the name COX-3 should only be used if a totally different COX, encoded by a separate gene, is discovered.[21] It is improbable that Chandrasekharan's "COX-3" has important physiological functions. This was confirmed when recently demonstrated multiple COX-1 splice variants in the human appeared unlikely to be the paracetamol targets.[22]
- Paracetamol may reduce the active, oxidized form of cyclooxygenase, rendering it inactive.[23] This indirect effect on COX function is inhibited by cellular peroxides, explaining why paracetamol has little effect on inflamed tissue or platelets but significant effect in central and peripheral nervous tissue and endothelial cells.[19, 24] Paracetamol inhibits COX, but not at the same molecular site that NSAIDs do (confusingly called the COX-active site), but at a distinct peroxidise (POX)-active site, in which the final reduction from unstable prostaglandin G_2 (PGG_2) to PGH_2 takes place (see **Figure 11.1**).[25]

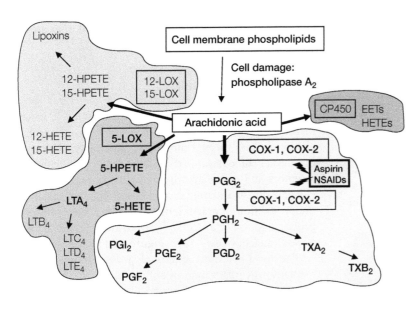

Figure 11.1 Arachidonic acid metabolism and prostaglandin synthesis. COX, cyclooxygenase; CP450, cytochrome CP450; LOX, lipoxygenase; LT, leukotriene; HETE, hydroxyeicosatetraenoic acid; HPETE, hydroperoxieicosatetraenoic acid; PG, prostaglandin; TX, thromboxane.

- The differential activity of paracetamol in different cells may be explained by the production of different active metabolites, or different inactivation patterns in different tissues.[19]
- Recently it has been shown that an analgesic metabolite of paracetamol, AM404, activates vanilloid and cannabinoid receptors and may explain the activity of paracetamol on COX-1 and 2.[26] The relevance of this to analgesic activity and to humans is unknown.
- Paracetamol inhibits NO-synthase in mouse spinal cord.[27]

Adverse effects

Paracetamol overdosage is the most common cause of acute hepatic failure.[28] Otherwise paracetamol is remarkably safe, with some exceptions.

RENAL FAILURE

Overdosage can be associated with acute renal failure,[29] usually reversible without dialysis.[30] Chronic renal failure from all causes is increased 2.5-fold in frequent paracetamol users, correlated to cumulative lifetime dose and average dose taken.[31] The risk was significant for diabetic nephropathy, vasculitis, and renal failure associated with systemic disease.

GASTROINTESTINAL BLEEDS WITH PARACETAMOL

Some epidemiological surveys suggest that paracetamol carries an increased risk of gastrointestinal (GI) bleeding.[32] Garcia-Rodriguez and Hernandez-Diaz,[33] in a case–control study, found a relative risk (RR) of 3.6 (95 percent CI 2.6–5.1) in users of 2 g daily or more, though little risk with lower doses; and RR 13.2 (95 percent CI

9.2–18.9) if using 2 g or more daily in conjunction with an NSAID.[33][III] Rahme *et al.*[34] found that elderly patients receiving paracetamol tended to be older, iller, and more at risk of GI complications than those prescribed NSAIDs. After accounting for this, those prescribed more than 2.6 g paracetamol per day ran a higher risk of dyspepsia, but risk of ulcer or hospitalization for GI events was much less elevated.[34] However, a meta-analysis of three case–control studies,[35][III] and a survey of over-the-counter medication,[36] showed no increased GI bleeding risk for paracetamol. Although case fatality rates were similar, patients on paracetamol with GI bleeds had shorter hospitalizations and less surgery than similar patients on ibuprofen, despite having more risk factors.[37]

DIPYRONE

Dipyrone (metimazole) is a pyrazolone analgesic and antipyretic, banned or restricted in some countries, but popular in some European and developing countries. It enjoyed a minor resurgence in Germany after rofecoxib was withdrawn.[38] The restrictions arise from an association with agranulocytosis. The risk is small (0.56 per million population per year), disappears ten days after stopping dipyrone, but increases with continued use.[39] Earlier, much higher risk estimates of 1 in 1439 prescriptions[40] have been criticized for methodological failings.[41]

In cancer pain

Two grams eight-hourly are superior to 10 mg oral morphine four-hourly,[42][II] but 500 mg t.d.s. were less effective than an NSAID.[43][III] Despite use in childhood cancer pain,[44] the increased risk of agranulocytosis with prolonged use and higher doses limits its role in malignancy.

NEFOPAM

Nefopam is a nonopioid analgesic, related to orphenadrine and diphenhydramine. It acts centrally and peripherally, with an unknown mechanism of action distinct from that of NSAIDs or opioids. It has an effect on α-2 receptors,[45] demonstrates noncompetitive N-methyl-D-aspartic acid (NMDA) receptor antagonism,[46] inhibits reuptake of noradrenaline, serotonin (via descending pathways[47]), and dopamine[48] and has sympathomimetic and anticholinergic actions. Nefopam does not cause respiratory depression. Some accumulation occurs in moderate or severe renal or hepatic failure. It should be avoided in patients with histories of fits or on monoamine oxidase inhibitors.

Animal[49] and postoperative[50, 51] studies suggest an opioid sparing effect. The few studies in cancer pain are either uncontrolled,[52] small randomized controlled trials (RCTs), or RCTs with large numbers of dropouts due to inefficacy and adverse effects.[53] No firm conclusions can be drawn from these data.

NONSTEROIDAL ANTI-INFLAMMATORY DRUGS

NSAID are used extensively.

- Thirty million people worldwide take NSAIDs daily.[54]
- US doctors wrote 111 million NSAID prescriptions in one year.[55]
- US patients buy 30 billion over-the-counter NSAID tablets annually.[56]
- In some US states, more than 40 percent of over-65s are prescribed NSAIDs.[57]
- From the introduction of COX-2 inhibitors in 1998 to 2003, NSAID prescribing in the USA rose by 67.7 percent.[58] By 2002 coxibs had become the seventh most prescribed drugs in that country, used widely even in low risk patients.[59, 60]
- A sharp decline in use followed the withdrawal of rofecoxib in September 2004.[38]
- COX-2 inhibitor use in high cardiovascular risk patients has also declined.[61]

NSAIDs are very widely prescribed in cancer pain and in palliative care because they:

- are effective across many different pains;[62][II], [63][V], [64][V]
- are inexpensive and easily accessible;
- can be given orally, rectally, topically, by injection, and as skin patches;[65, 66, 67]
- have an effect on pyrexia,[68] postradiotherapy mucositis,[69][II], [62][II] and even, for nonselective NSAIDs,[70, 71][III] urge incontinence.

Using one multivalent drug in patients already facing polypharmacy is an attractive option. However, recent developments necessitate a reevaluation of the use of NSAIDs in cancer pain.

Mechanisms of action

NSAIDs inhibit prostaglandin synthase (COX).[72] In cell membranes, arachidonic acid is esterified to glycerol in phospholipids. Various molecules (glutamate, serotonin, histamine, bradykinin, etc.) bind to cell membrane receptors and deacylate cell membrane phospholipid, for example during inflammation. Phospholipase A_2 catalyses the production of arachidonic acid, which then produces prostaglandins (via COX)[73] leukotrienes (via lipoxygenase) and lipoxins[74] (see **Figure 11.1**).

The most relevant actions of prostaglandins are the mediation of inflammation and pain, gastric protection, maintenance of renal perfusion in low volume states, and modulating thrombosis.

COX-1 AND COX-2

In the early 1990s, it became clear that there were two isoforms of COX.[75] Early findings suggested that COX-1 performed a constitutive, housekeeping role in health, such as providing gastric mucosal protection; while COX-2 was inducible only in inflammation. Selectively suppressing COX-2 would therefore reduce the harm and pain of inflammation without impairing useful prostaglandin activities. This led to the development of selective (e.g. meloxicam) and then highly selective (e.g. rofecoxib) COX-2 inhibitors.

This differentiation between COX isoforms has turned out to be a gross oversimplification.

- COX-1 is produced by a gene on chromosome 9. While responsible for most prostaglandin roles in health, it does play important roles in inflammation, participating in the production of proinflammatory prostaglandins, and being itself induced at inflammatory sites. COX-1 deficient mice mount a reduced inflammatory response. Furthermore, the gastroprotective role is not a pure COX-1 function. Mice deficient in gastric mucosal COX-1 are not more prone to peptic ulceration.[76] In rats, a highly selective COX-1 inhibitor only produces gastric ulcers when a COX-2 inhibitor is added.[77]
- COX-2, secreted by a gene on chromosome 1, is capable of fast induction in the presence of inflammation, dehydration, or trauma, and can be upregulated by cytokines, growth factors, and tumor promoters. COX-2 activity initially leads to production of the proinflammatory PGE_2 and PGI_2; later it induces production of the anti-inflammatory PGD_2. COX-2 inhibition can slow down healing:[78] both peptic ulcer healing[79, 80] and bone repair[81, 82] require COX-2. Although mainly inducible, COX-2 is

constitutive in the brain, renal cortex, stomach, uterus, cartilage, and bone. Since many tumors over-express COX-2, COX-2 inhibitors have a number of antitumor properties.

SPLICE VARIANTS AND SINGLE NUCLEOTIDE POLYMORPHISMS

Significant interindividual variation exists in the response of patients with rheumatoid arthritis to different NSAIDs,[83, 84, 85] partly due to pharmacogenetic factors. Small disparities between molecules of the same COX isoform, and variability in gene expression, sometimes produce real differences in activity.[86] For example, genetic differences may determine the cardiovascular risk of COX-2 inhibitors and therefore individual usage for cancer prevention.[87] Genes contain active areas, or exons, separated by "punctuation" areas called introns which do not themselves code for protein production. Variation in exon splicing results in molecules with somewhat different properties. Several splice variants of COX have been described. The most well-known example is so-called COX-3. Even altering a single nucleotide in the gene sequence can have far-reaching consequences. The NCBI single nucleotide polymorphisms (SNP) website[88] listed 409 reported human COX SNPs, including 137 COX-2 SNPs, in December 2007.

OTHER CAUSES OF INTERINDIVIDUAL VARIABILITY OF RESPONSE TO NSAIDS

All NSAIDs inhibit prostaglandin synthesis and hence inflammation. However, there is little relationship between the anti-inflammatory capacity of NSAIDs and their effectiveness as analgesics.[89] Non-COX mediated effects must therefore also play important therapeutic roles for individual NSAIDs.[90] NSAIDs modulate wind-up and central sensitization through prostaglandin mechanisms, but have other, nonprostaglandin, central effects. They influence leukocyte function and the release of inflammatory mediators via inhibition of leukotriene-induced neutrophil chemotaxis, altered cell to cell

adhesion and reduced superoxide formation.[91] Other mechanisms include the L-arginine-nitric oxide (L-arginine-NO) pathway, and effects on endogenous opiate and serotonergic pathways.[92] Thus there is tremendous scope for interpatient variability of response in therapeutic and adverse effect profiles of NSAIDs. With so many modulating influences as well as pharmacogenetic differences, precise targeting of individual NSAIDs for individual patients may remain elusive for years.

Classification of NSAIDs

Most NSAIDs are nonselective, inhibiting both COX-1 and COX-2. NSAIDs belong to various chemical families (Table 11.1), but one must not read too much into such a classification, for example in deciding how to proceed if one NSAID has failed in a particular patient. NSAIDs are very diverse drugs, whose only link is their ability to inhibit prostaglandin synthesis,[91] and this may not be their most important analgesic activity in many situations. Furthermore, the ability of an NSAID to inhibit prostaglandin production does not necessarily correlate with its analgesic activity.[89]

Preferential COX-2 inhibitors inhibit COX-2 more than COX-1, but COX-1 inhibition is still clinically significant, especially at high doses. The reported COX-2 inhibition of a drug depends upon the assay method used: meloxicam is 3–77 times as selective for COX-2 as COX-1, and nimesulide 5–16 times. Etodolac and nabumetone are also usually classified as preferential COX-2 inhibitors.

Highly selective COX-2 inhibitors (usually called COX-2 inhibitors) inhibit COX-2 much more than COX-1, so that at clinical doses COX-1 inhibition remains insignificant. They include rofecoxib, celecoxib, valdecoxib (and parecoxib, its injectable prodrug), etoricoxib, and lumiracoxib. Rofecoxib and valdecoxib have been withdrawn, as has lumiracoxib in Australia, New Zealand, Canada, and the European Union (it had never obtained US FDA approval).

Attempts have been made to rank COX-2 inhibitors by their COX-2 selectivity,[93] using the whole blood assay, chosen by consensus,[94] to harmonize different studies.

Table 11.1 Chemical classification of NSAIDs.

Class	Examples
Salicylic acid derivatives	Aspirin, choline magnesium trisilicate, diflunisal
Indole and indene acetic acids	Indometacin, sulindac, etodolac
Heteroaryl acetic acids	Tolmetin, diclofenac, ketorolac
Arylpropionic acids	Ibuprofen, naproxen, flurbiprofen, ketoprofen
Anthranilic acids (fenamates)	Oxicams: piroxicam, tenoxicam, meloxicam
	Pyrazolidinediones: phenylbutazone
Alkanones	Nabumetone
Coxibs	Rofecoxib, celecoxib, valdecoxib, etoricoxib, lumiracoxib

The utility of such a classification is dubious. The whole blood assay varies in its ability to predict *in vivo* activity for different NSAIDs.[95] Some selective COX-2 inhibition occurs through a two-phase process distinct from the one-step nonselective COX inhibition, rendering the test unreliable.[96] Above all, pharmacokinetic factors predominate over *in vivo* selectivities in real-life situations.[97]

Clinical use of NSAIDs in cancer pain

The usefulness of NSAIDs in cancer pain has been examined in three systematic reviews;[14, 98, 99] as the evidence bar has been raised, they have drawn progressively fewer firm conclusions. McNicol *et al.*[100][I] reviewed 42 trials involving 3084 patients. Study heterogeneity precluded meta-analysis. They concluded that:

- NSAIDs give better analgesia than placebo for cancer pain;
- data were insufficient to label any NSAID as superior;
- no conclusions can yet be drawn on possible synergism between opioids and NSAIDs.

Of the 42 studies in this systematic review, 11 were single dose, 16 lasted a week or longer, and none followed patients for more than 12 weeks. Extrapolation from such short-term work to long-term clinical use is clearly unsafe. There is a desperate need for medium- and long-term studies to guide clinical practice.

NSAIDS IN METASTATIC BONE PAIN

Work in the early 1970s showing that prostaglandins play an important role in metastatic bone destruction[101, 102, 103] led to a belief that NSAIDs are particularly effective in metastatic bone pain. Early, sketchy case reports appeared to support this contention.[104, 105] However, the very few RCTs in this area have been small and of limited power and quality. Some, including an unpublished report quoted in Pace[106] have shown no effect, a statistically insignificant trend towards effectiveness,[107, 108] or limited evidence of a dose–response;[109, 110] a few suggested a reduction in opioid requirement.[111] In his recent systematic review, McNicol felt unable to conclude whether NSAIDs had an effect in bone pain due to a combination of insufficient data and study heterogeneity.

Adverse effects of NSAIDs

With so many uses, and with up to 3 percent of the population of developed countries disabled by rheumatological conditions,[112] NSAIDs are widely used. However, an increasing appreciation of their risks (**Table 11.2**) has now tempered this enthusiasm.

Gastrointestinal risk

GASTRIC EROSIONS AND DYSPEPSIA

Gastric mucosal ultrastructural changes occur within minutes of ingesting a NSAID, and erosions within hours.[113, 114] Erosions are present in around 50 percent of patients on NSAIDs. The initial damage may[115] or may not[116, 117, 118][III] be influenced by the presence of *Helicobacter pylori*, which may predispose to duodenal but not gastric erosions.[119][II] Mucosal adaptation usually occurs within a week,[120, 121] but is slower in the presence of *H. pylori*, smokers, older patients,[122] or higher NSAID doses.[123][IV] COX-2 inhibitors (see below) produce fewer erosions in the first week.[124]

Table 11.2 Risks of NSAID use.

System	Risks	
GIT	Esophagitis	Ulceration, bleeding, stricture
	Gastric erosions, gastritis	Relapse of inflammatory bowel disease
	Peptic ulceration, increase in PU complications	Complications of diverticular disease
	Small bowel inflammation, bleeding, stricture	Hepatitis, liver failure, cholestasis
	Colitis, proctitis	
Thrombotic	Myocardial infarction	Stroke
Renal	Salt and water retention	Exacerbation of hypertension
	Nephrotic syndrome	Chronic renal failure from analgesic nephropathy
	Acute renal failure	
Marrow	Agranulocytosis	Thrombocytopenia
	Hemolytic anemia	Aplastic anemia
Skin	Rashes	Erythema multiforme
	Stevens–Johnson	Photosensitivity
Respiratory	Exacerbated asthma	Eosinophilic lung infiltrates
CNS	Headaches	Depression
	Memory loss	Cognitive dysfunction

Dyspepsia occurs in 10–60 percent of NSAID users, leading to drug discontinuation in 5–15 percent of rheumatoid arthritis patients.[125][II] A meta-analysis showed that dyspepsia, defined as epigastric discomfort, was 36 percent more common in NSAID users.[126][I] Its presence is not predictive of peptic ulceration,[127][V] but dyspeptic patients may be more likely to bleed if taking NSAIDs.[128]

PEPTIC ULCERATION

This is the main GI risk of NSAID use. The relative risk compared to unexposed patients is 5–6 for gastric ulcer (GU) development.[129] The generally accepted relative risk for duodenal ulcer (DU) is only 1.1, but a recent population-based nested case–control study from the UK suggested it was as high as 3.1 (95 percent C.I. 2.3–4.2).[130][III] On mini-dose aspirin, 48 percent of asymptomatic patients had endoscopic ulcers or erosions.[131]

Ulceration is unpleasant and disruptive but it is perforation, bleeding, and gastric outlet obstruction that cause deaths. There may be no warning signs: in 58–81 percent, serious complications are the first sign of the presence of ulceration.[125, 132]

TRENDS IN PEPTIC ULCERATION

While the overall risk for uncomplicated ulcer (GU, DU) has declined worldwide, the number of patients presenting with serious ulcer complications has been steady or even increased.[133, 134] A survey in Dusseldorf[135] suggests that prevalence of bleeding peptic ulcers has not fallen, but that they occur in older patients, and more of them are attributable to NSAIDs than in the past. This may mean that more NSAIDs are being prescribed to higher risk patients. There has also been a reported increase in aggressive *H. pylori*-negative ulcers in patients *not* taking NSAIDs.[136, 137] Confusingly, a study spanning eight US centers and 5500 patients on the ARAMIS database of rheumatoid arthritis patients, has shown that hospitalizations for perforation, bleeding, or gastric outlet obstruction declined by 67 percent between 1990 and 2000 after increasing for ten years. The authors attribute 24 percent of this decline to lower NSAID doses, 18 percent to protein-pump inhibitors (PPIs), and 14 percent to availability of safer NSAIDs.[138] Changing prescribing behavior clearly influences NSAID mortality and morbidity. Yet prescribing patterns are remarkably resistant to the evidence and the presence of protocols and guidelines.[139, 140, 141] Indeed, there is recent evidence of low utilization of gastroprotection in the presence of significant risk.[142, 143, 144]

ABSOLUTE PEPTIC ULCER RISK OF NSAIDS

Singh[145] estimated 107,000 hospitalizations and 16,500 deaths occur a year in the USA from NSAID GI complications, based on ARAMIS data. These figures have been labeled conservative in a paper coauthored by Singh himself,[146] but "probably an overestimate" in expert evidence given by Dr Byron Cryer to the FDA in 2005.[147] A study of epidemiological surveys suggested much lower figures of over 32,000 hospitalizations and 3200 deaths a year in the USA from NSAID-induced GI bleeding.[148] A population-based epidemiological study of district hospitals covering 80 percent of the target population in Spain found 15.3 attributable deaths/100,000 NSAID or aspirin users. The authors concluded that up to one-third of all NSAID/aspirin deaths could be due to low-dose aspirin use.[149]

In the UK, figures projected from emergency admissions to two district hospitals with a catchment area of 500,000 suggested there are 12,000 emergency admissions and 2230 hospital deaths plus 330 deaths in the community annually from NSAID gastropathy.[150] Tramer et al.[151][I] analyzed data from RCTs, cohort studies, case–control studies, case series, and case reports for 11,040 patients with bleeding or perforation. They concluded that one patient in every 1220 treated for two months or longer with NSAIDs dies as a result. They extrapolate this to 2000 deaths a year for the UK.

Upper GI catastrophes carry a higher mortality if the subject is on NSAIDs.[152] Patients on NSAIDs who perforated were 1.6 times as likely to die in the first 30 days as patients not on NSAIDs. Worryingly, the mortality rate was similar for COX-2 inhibitors.[153] A US survey of epidemiological surveys in the 1990s found a dose-related relative risk for upper GI bleeding of 4–6 for prescribed and 2 for over-the-counter NSAIDs.[148] It found that NSAIDs accounted for 34 percent of all GI bleeds in the USA. Singh,[154] using ARAMIS data, also concluded over-the-counter NSAIDs were risky (RR 3–4 for serious complications, versus 6–7 for prescription NSAIDs.

ASPIRIN

A meta-analysis of 24 RCTs calculated that using low-dose aspirin (50–162.5 mg daily) for an average of 28 months increases the risk of a GI bleed against placebo 1.6-fold. GI bleeding risk from aspirin is not dose-related; enteric-coated tablets do not reduce the risk.[155][I] In a recent prospective study of 991 patients on low-dose aspirin, the annual risk of a bleed was 1.5 percent, but no fatalities were reported over a two-year follow-up. Forty-five percent of bleeds occurred within four months of starting aspirin.[156] In some patients GI risk may outweigh the cardiovascular benefit.[157] Loke et al.[158] suggest a way of calculating low-dose aspirin risks and benefits for particular individuals.

Mechanisms of GI damage by NSAIDs

The stomach is continuously bathed in acid of pH 1–4, and yet the delicate mucosa remains undamaged. The most important gastroprotective mechanism is the thin mucus layer which buffers stomach acid to a neutral pH by the time it comes into contact with gastric mucosa, but a number of prostaglandin-dependent mechanisms exist.[159] Prostaglandin inhibition by NSAID increases injury and counters healing by reducing:

- epithelial mucus production;
- bicarbonate secretion;
- mucosal blood flow;
- epithelial proliferation;
- mucosal resistance to injury.

Almost all nonselective NSAIDs are weakly acidic and unionized in the acid environment of the stomach lumen. However, once inside the gastric epithelial cells they ionize and are then trapped and accumulate there (ion trapping).[160] The sum total of all these effects is ulceration.

Several lines of evidence suggest the COX theory is not the full explanation of NSAID gastric damage.[161, 162] COX-1 deficient mice do not develop spontaneous gastric ulceration,[163] nor does use of a potent COX-1 inhibitor cause ulceration until a COX-2 inhibitor is added. In fact, COX-1 deficient mice appear more resistant to indometacin (indomethacin)-induced ulceration.[76, 164] Reducing gastric prostaglandins by 90 percent by using parenteral NSAIDs does not induce gastric damage. Animal data suggest that some NSAIDs (sulindac, aspirin, ibuprofen) cause gastric damage far more if the drug is given via the stomach, but others (indometacin, diclofenac, ketoprofen) cause toxicity even if they are administered parenterally. All these latter drugs are secreted into bile by enterohepatic transport. Ligating the bile duct prevents ulceration in these cases,[165] and the ulcerative potential of a drug correlates highly significantly with the percentage of its secretion into bile. In man, although prostaglandin levels remain very low, the gastric mucosa adapts to indometacin or aspirin within four weeks. Low-dose aspirin or intravenous aspirin inhibits prostaglandins significantly but cause relatively little gastric damage. Coxibs cause significantly less ulceration; they all happen to be nonacidic, except lumiracoxib, unlike nonselective NSAIDs, which are all acids apart from the much safer nabumetone. All this evidence suggests that other mechanisms must complement COX inhibition.

The topical theory[166] suggests that phosphatidylcholine and other zwitterionic phospholipids in gastric mucus and bile help protect mucosa from hydrochloric acid and bile salts. Acidic NSAIDs given orally combine with these molecules and neutralize their effect, also explaining why enterohepatic recirculation could have a significant effect. There is recent evidence of changes in mucin in reactive gastropathy from NSAIDs or bile reflux.[167]

Risk reduction strategies

Risk reduction strategies are shown in **Box 11.1**.

Box 11.1 Managing the peptic risk of NSAIDs

Identify risk factors (Tables 11.3, 11.4, 11.5, and 11.6)

If a patient has any risk factors for gastropathy:

- Is there any alternative to NSAID (e.g. increased opioid dose, radiotherapy, nerve block)?
- Can risk factors be altered (e.g. changing antidepressant, reviewing need for ongoing anticoagulation)?
- The weighting of each factor can be assessed from the table.
- The presence of multiple risk factors makes the prescription of NSAIDs even less desirable.

Choose the safest NSAID possible

- See **Table 11.7** for gastroduodenal safety. Only use the less safe NSAIDs in exceptional cases.

Use the lowest effective dose

- High doses or concurrent multiple NSAIDs increase risk significantly. Giving less than the effective dose exposes the patient to risk without benefit. Is the patient on over-the-counter NSAIDs?

Use prophylaxis with nonselective NSAIDs in advanced cancer patients

- Give misoprostol or a PPI, or if neither is possible, a high dose H2 blocker. In particularly high risk cases, consider using a COX-2 inhibitor or nabumetone plus prophylaxis.

Consider a COX-2 inhibitor

- Weigh up the reduced risk of gastropathy with COX-2 inhibitors against any increase in cardiovascular risk. Many nonselective inhibitors also carry thrombotic risks.
- Review the effectiveness of the NSAID on an ongoing basis.
- STOP IT if there is no clear continuing benefit.

RISK FACTORS

For risk factors, see **Tables 11.3, 11.4, 11.5, and 11.6**.

Table 11.3 Age and sex as risk factors for NSAID-associated complications.

Risk factor		Complication studied	Relative risk (95% confidence intervals)	Study type and source
Age			Odds ratio	
	≤35 years	Endoscopic ulcers	20.3 (2.7–151.7)	Meta-analysis[168]
	36–45		5.7 (1.7–19.0)	
	46–55		7.7 (3.1–19.1)	
	56–65		10.9 (5.0–23.5)	
	66–75		6.5 (3.6–11.7)	
	>75		4.3 (1.6–11.6)	
	<65	Serious complications	1.65 (1.08–2.53)	Meta-analysis[169]
	>60		5.52 (4.63–6.60)	
	60–75	Peptic ulcer complications	3.5 (1.8–7.1)	Case–control study[170]
	>75		8.9 (4.3–18.3)	
Sex	Male	Peptic ulcer complications	1.7 (1.0–3.0)	Case control study[170]
	Male	Serious GI complications	2.4 (1.85–3.11)	Meta-analysis[169]
	Female		2.32 (1.91–2.82)	
	Male	Upper GI bleeding	2.8	Cohort study[171]
	Female		2.3	

Table 11.4 Peptic ulcer and NSAID characteristics as risk factors for NSAID-associated complications.

Risk factor		Complication studied	Relative risk (95% confidence intervals)	Study type and source
Peptic ulcer history				
Previous peptic ulcer		Bleeding risk	3.8 (2.6–4.9)	Case–control study[172]
		Peptic ulcer complications	2.5 (1.2–5.1)	Case–control study[170]
Prior history of complicated peptic ulcer		Serious complications	4.76 (4.05–5.59)	Meta-analysis[169]
Previous ulcer bleed		Bleeding or perforation	13.5 (10.3–17.7)	Case–control study[173]
NSAID factors				
Length of time on NSAIDs	<1 month	Serious complications	8.00 (6.37–10.06)	Meta-analysis[169]
	1–3 months		3.31 (2.27–4.82)	
	>3 months		1.92 (1.19–3.13)	
Dose	Low dose NSAID	Bleeding or perforation	2.6 (1.8–3.8)	Case–control study[173]
	High dose NSAID		7.0 (5.2–9.6)	
	High dose	Bleeding or perforation	5.8	Nested case–control study[174]
	Medium dose		4.2	
	Low dose		2.9	
	Low to medium daily dose	Symptomatic ulcer	2.6 (2.0–3.5)	Nested case–control study[130]
	High daily dose		4.9 (3.8–6.5)	
Multiple NSAIDs		Bleeding or perforation	9.0	Nested case–control study[174]

Which NSAIDs are safer?

Table 11.7 stratifies NSAIDs according to their upper GI risk in long-term use. Langman[181] claims substantial risk reductions from using ibuprofen as the NSAID of choice or using only low-dose aspirin, although others find no relationship between aspirin dose and risk.[155][I] A population-based case–control study by Hippisley-Cox et al.[182][III] showed that naproxen, diclofenac, rofecoxib, aspirin, and ibuprofen all carried significant risks of

Table 11.5 Concomitant medication use as risk factors for NSAID-associated complications.

Risk factor		Complication studied	Relative risk (95% confidence intervals)	Study type and source
Low dose aspirin	Alone + NSAID	Upper gastrointestinal bleeding (UGIB)	SIR 2.6 (1.8–3.50) SIR 5.6 (4.4–7.0)	Cohort study[171]
Oral anticoagulants		Bleeding risk	SIR 8.0 (2.1–20.4)	Cohort study[175]
		Bleeding risk	NS NSAID OR 1.9 (1.4–3.7) Celecoxib OR, 1.7 (1.2–3.6) Rofecoxib OR, 2.4 (1.7–3.6)	Nested case-control study[176]
		Bleeding risk	OR 7. 8 (2.8–21.5)	Case–control study[172]
Corticosteroids		Serious complications	1.83 (1.20–2.78)	Meta-analysis[169]
		Bleeding risk	2.7 (1.3–4.5)	Case–control study[172]
		Peptic ulcer complications	2.0 (0.8–4.6)	Case–control study[170]
SSRI		Serious upper GI event	4.19 (3.30–5.31)	Case–control study[175]
		New prescription of peptic ulcer drugs	SIR 12.4 (3.2–48.0)	Cohort study[177]
		Upper GI bleeding	12.2 (7.1–19.5)	Population-based cohort study[170]

NS NSAID, nonselective NSAID; SIR, standard incidence rate ratio.

Table 11.6 Concomitant conditions as risk factors for NSAID-induced peptic ulceration.

Risk factor	Complication studied	Relative risk (95% confidence intervals)	Study type and source
Treatment of heart failure	Bleeding risk	5.9 (2.3–13.1)	Case–control study[172]
Treatment for diabetes	Bleeding risk	3.1 (1.2–4.3)	
Current smoking	Bleeding risk	1.6 (1.2–2.0)	
	Peptic ulcer complications	1.6 (0.9–2.7)	Case–control study[170]
Alcohol use	Peptic ulcer complications	1.8 (0.9–3.6)	

Table 11.7 Stratified risk of gastrointestinal events from NSAIDs.

Risk level	References			
	173	178[a]	179[b]	180[c]
High	Azapropazone Piroxicam	Azapropazone Ketoprofen	Azapropazone Tolmetin Ketoprofen Piroxicam	Azapropazone
Medium	Indometacin Ketoprofen	Indometacin Naproxen Piroxicam	Indometacin Naproxen Sulindac Aspirin	Piroxicam Indometacin Ketoprofen Diclofenac Naproxen Ibuprofen
Low	Diclofenac Naproxen Ibuprofen	Diclofenac Ibuprofen	Diclofenac Ibuprofen	

[a]Risks are dose dependent for each drug.
[b]Higher doses of ibuprofen carry risks equivalent to naproxen/indometacin.
[c]Piroxicam comes close to being high risk.

gastropathy, unlike celecoxib. Prophylactic gastroprotection removed the risk except for diclofenac.

NABUMETONE

Nabumetone is missing from these drug comparisons, yet has an impressive safety profile. Given over 12 weeks, it produced fewer endoscopic ulcers than ibuprofen, and no more than ibuprofen plus misoprostol 200 µg q.d.s.[183][II] It was significantly less ulcerogenic than naproxen over five years and better tolerated.[184][II] In a meta-analysis of 13 studies with 49,500 patients, it produced 10–36 times fewer GI adverse events than comparator NSAIDs.[185][I] A six-week RCT revealed more patients satisfied with the analgesia from 12.5 mg of rofecoxib a day than 1 g of nabumetone daily, but the rofecoxib group suffered more overall and serious gastrointestinal adverse effects.[186][II] A population-based cohort study indicated that Arthrotec (diclofenac plus misoprostol) produced marginally fewer hospitalizations for GI problems, although the lower confidence interval was 1.0; there was no difference in admissions for GI bleeding.[187][III] However, nabumetone was safer than naproxen or diclofenac plus misoprostol given separately (presumably the misoprostol was often not taken). An extensive review of nabumetone is available.[161]

A number of factors may explain nabumetone's safety profile. Unlike other non-specific NSAIDs, but like all COX-2 inhibitors apart from lumiracoxib, it is a non-acidic drug. This may diminish any topical effect or ion trapping. It is a prodrug, undergoing extensive first pass metabolism to the active 6-methoxy, 2-naphtylactic acid (6-MNA), which does not undergo enterohepatic circulation, fitting well with the topical theory. Finally, nabumetone is somewhat COX-2 selective.

COX-2 INHIBITORS

The VIGOR trial showed that using rofecoxib instead of a nonselective NSAID reduced the risk of a symptomatic ulcer, GI bleed or perforation by 54 percent; the risk of gastric outlet obstruction, perforation, or major GI bleed by 57 percent; and the risk of a major bleed by 62 percent. One serious complication would be averted per 41 patients treated for one year.[188][II] In an industry sponsored review of 20 RCTs, Watson et al.[189] found that rofecoxib had a relative risk of 0.36 against nonselective NSAIDs, consistent over two years. Moore et al.,[190][I] using detailed company clinical trial reports, showed that celecoxib carried a third of the risk of comparator nonselective NSAIDs of producing symptomatic ulcers or gastrointestinal bleeding. A COX-2 inhibitor reduces risk of ulcer complications as much as giving a nonselective NSAID plus a PPI.[191, 192][II]

Low-dose aspirin reduces the GI benefits of COX-2 inhibitors to the level of nonselective NSAIDs according to some data.[193, 194][II] If this is the case, if an NSAID must be used with aspirin, one should choose cheaper nonselective agents. Fortunately, concomitant lansoprazole or misoprostol may substantially reduce this risk.[195] However, animal[196] and human trial data[197][III] also suggest that low-dose aspirin loses its antithrombotic effect when used with COX-2 inhibitors. Disturbingly, epidemiological work indicates the same might happen when nonselective NSAIDs are used with low-dose aspirin.[197][III] However a recent review concluded that it is still advantageous both from the gastrointestinal and thrombotic point of view to choose a COX-2 inhibitor as the anti-inflammatory when aspirin needs to be used concomitantly.[198]

PROPHYLAXIS FOR PEPTIC ULCERATION

A number of prophylactic measures are available,[199][I] (see **Box 11.2**).

Option 1: Reduce acid level in the stomach

Prophylactic H2 blockers (e.g. ranitidine) at conventional doses are discouraged because they only reduce the already marginal prevalence of NSAID-related duodenal ulcers.[199, 200, 201, 202][I] However, high-dose famotidine provides useful prophylaxis.[203] A Cochrane review concluded that double dose H2 blockers reduced the risk of endoscopic gastric and duodenal ulcers.[199][I]

The mainstay of acid reduction for prophylaxis remains the PPIs. They are very significantly better than placebo,[204, 205][II] and decidedly superior to H2 blockers.[206, 207, 208][II] Their tolerability is good and they are the best choice for healing ulcers while continuing NSAIDs, even at six months of use, as well as preventing ulcer relapse in this setting.[207, 209, 210][II] On the other hand, while a reduction in serious peptic ulcer complications with PPIs has been demonstrated in epidemiological studies,[211][III] this has not as yet been backed up by large randomized controlled trials.

Option 2: Replace the missing prostaglandin

Misoprostol, a synthetic PGE₁ analog, replaces the gastric prostaglandin inhibited by NSAIDs. After rapid absorption it is de-esterified to its pharmacologically active acid. It is unclear whether its antisecretory effect, reducing gastric acid production, or its mucosal protective effect predominates in man.

In a large trial misoprostol reduced life-threatening NSAID peptic complications by 40 percent.[212][II] This is the holy grail of mucosal protection; similar convincing evidence of a reduction in perforation and bleeding episodes exists for the COX-2 inhibitors, but not for PPIs. This protective effect was established using misoprostol 200 µg q.d.s. However a significant number of patients do not tolerate misoprostol because of diarrhea, abdominal cramps, or other adverse effects. Graham et al.[213][II]

Box 11.2 Weighing up the choices for ulcer prophylaxis

- Avoid H2 blockers at normal doses and sucralfate.
- Double-dose H2 blockers have some prophylactic value.
- Only misoprostol and COX-2 inhibitors have been clearly shown in large controlled trials to reduce the risk of perforation or bleeding on NSAIDs, the one end point that really matters. There is epidemiological evidence that the same may be true for PPIs, but the level of confidence that this is the case is not yet as high.
- The risk to the stomach from COX-2 inhibitors is similar to using a nonselective NSAID plus PPI.
- Many, perhaps all, COX-2 inhibitors, as well as some nonselective NSAIDs, carry appreciable thrombotic risks.
- Ulcers are less common with COX-2 inhibitors, but may be more liable to perforate or bleed in long-term use, as the COX-2 inhibitor may inhibit their healing, though evidence is conflicting.
- PPIs are better tolerated than misoprostol.
- PPIs are superior to misoprostol in producing long-term healing in patients continuing to take NSAIDs. They also prevent ulcer relapse in this situation.

Advice:

- Use H2 blockers or a PPI for dyspepsia
- Use misoprostol or a PPI for prophylaxis; a high dose H2 blocker may be used if neither is an option. You may consider a COX-2 inhibitor if cardiovascular risk is low.
- Use a PPI in patients who need to continue their NSAIDs.

showed that misoprostol was superior to lansoprazole at preventing NSAID-induced ulcers, but when the number of patients stopping the misoprostol due to adverse effects was taken into account, the results of the two drugs were equivalent. In patients with established GI bleeding, adding misoprostol to intravenous PPIs does not improve outcome.[214][II]

OTHER APPROACHES

Prophylactic sucralfate is very significantly inferior to misoprostol[215] and should be avoided.

Interest in the role of nitric oxide-donating NSAIDs in reducing peptic ulceration has existed for a number of years (see below under Enteropathy). Lanas *et al.*,[216] in a case–control study, showed that nitrovasodilators reduced the risk of upper GI bleeding with NSAIDs. An Italian epidemiological study[32] reached the same conclusion.

In reading the literature, one must always keep in mind that the mere presence of ulcers is relatively unimportant. Most ulcers are silent and heal without ever being noticed. The possible rise in serious complications despite falling ulcer prevalence reminds us just how poor ulcers are as a proxy measure. The essential endpoint is the number and type of life-threatening complications. Papers examining only endoscopic or even symptomatic ulceration are less satisfactory.

Small bowel toxicity

The small bowel is finally yielding to routine clinical investigation, especially through capsule endoscopy. A swallowed 2.7 cm capsule passes through the bowel by peristalsis, taking two photographs per second and transmitting them wirelessly for clinicians to review the computer-analyzed images.[217] More specialized techniques such as enteroscopy and permeability studies are also available.

ENTEROPATHY

Bjarnason *et al.*[218] showed many years ago that NSAIDs increase small bowel permeability, blood and protein loss,[219] and produce multiple, concentric diaphragm-like strictures that "can reduce the lumen to a pinhead."[220] Animal studies also showed deficient anastomotic healing.[221] We now know that small bowel damage is more common than gastric ulceration.[222] It can lead to:

- chronic anemia;
- protein losing enteropathy;
- hemorrhage;
- perforation;
- bowel obstruction.

Adebayo and Bjarnason[222] suggest that intestinal bleeding is likely to be as significant as that from the stomach, and that many deaths ascribed to peptic ulceration arise from bowel perforation. Maiden[223] found macroscopic ulceration in 68 percent of healthy volunteers on two weeks of sustained release diclofenac. Small bowel injury was detected by capsule endoscopy in 71 percent of a small sample of healthy patients on NSAIDs for at least three months as against 10 percent of controls; a quarter, but none of the controls, had more serious lesions.[224]

PATHOPHYSIOLOGY AND MANAGEMENT

Both COX-1 and COX-2 inhibition are required for initial small bowel lesions,[225] compounded by the topical effect of medication.[226] Mitochondrial damage and a break-down of intercellular integrity result,[227] together with neutrophil activation by intraluminal bacteria.[228, 229] Drugs which undergo enterohepatic recirculation are more enterotoxic,[230, 231, 232] while the presence of bile appears to be as important as the drug itself, at least in rats,[233] where addition of ursodeoxycholic acid reduces small bowel toxicity.[234] Rapid ulcer healing would greatly reduce long-term effects; it has been suggested that COX-2 is important early on in intestinal ulcer healing and COX-1 later.[235]

MANAGEMENT

Patients on NSAIDs with gastroscopy-negative anemia should have their bowel investigated. COX-2 inhibitors and drugs with no enterohepatic recirculation are probably less toxic to the small bowel than nonselective inhibitors. Sulfasalazine and metronidazole are suggested treatment options for patients who need to continue their NSAIDs.[236][V]

Large bowel toxicity

Small bowel damage can extend into the cecum.[237] The large bowel is also liable to perforation and diverticular bleeding. NSAIDs can reactivate inflammatory bowel disease, perhaps particularly ulcerative colitis.[238] This may need inhibition of both COX isoforms to occur.[239][III]

NSAIDs and the kidneys

NSAIDs cause a number of potentially serious renal problems (**Figure 11.2** and **Table 11.2**).

FLUID AND SALT RETENTION, HYPERTENSION

This may worsen heart failure.[240] Both nonselective NSAIDs[241, 242][I] and COX-2 inhibitors[243, 244][I] can cause hypertension, although the meta-analyses come to discrepant conclusions as to which nonselective drugs are riskier. For most patients blood pressure rise is minor but sometimes it is clinically significant.

NEPHROTIC SYNDROME

Nonselective NSAIDs[245] and COX-2 inhibitors[246] can induce the nephrotic syndrome, often via membranous or minimal change glomerulonephritis.[247]

CHRONIC RENAL FAILURE

Perneger *et al.*,[248][III] in a case–control study, found the risk of end-stage renal failure to be related to current dose

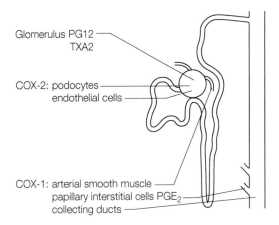

Figure 11.2 Localization of prostaglandins and COX in the nephron. COX-1, cyclooxygenase-1; COX-2, cyclooxygenase-2; PGE$_2$, prostaglandin E$_2$; PGI$_2$, prostacyclin; TXA$_2$, thromboxane.

and cumulative dose of NSAIDs consumed (odds ratio 8.8 for patients who had taken 5000 NSAID tablets or more in their lifetime). There was no increased risk for aspirin consumption. On the other hand, classical analgesic nephropathy, with its characteristic pathological changes, has all but disappeared since phenacetin use was banned,[249] which exculpates NSAIDs as causation. Proving cause and effect in these epidemiological studies is difficult – for example proving that extra analgesic consumption antedated the onset of renal disease rather than simply being a response to increased symptoms from this. A detailed review of studies, published in 1998, found strong evidence of causality for phenacetin, but not for paracetamol or NSAIDs.[250] Thus, the results must be considered as suggestive rather than conclusive.

ACUTE RENAL FAILURE

Acute renal failure (ARF) can result from NSAIDs, particularly when there is an effective reduced circulation volume (see **Box 11.3**). The vasculature of the kidney is controlled by a balance between vasoconstrictor angiotensin II and norepinephrine and vasodilator prostaglandins. Renal COX-2 is constitutive, and in health only small amounts of prostaglandin are secreted. In serious fluid loss, such as hemorrhage, the kidneys are involved in the generalized vasoconstriction which only spares heart and brain. This induces a massive outpouring of renal prostaglandin, and thus renal vasodilatation, preserving renal circulation. NSAIDs block this compensatory response and precipitate acute renal failure. COX-2 metabolites have also been implicated in renin release.[251] ARF was ascribed to NSAIDs in 22 percent of patients on a medical renal failure unit in one series,[252] [V] but only in 1.6 percent of patients in a similar series which discounted other interactive risk factors.[253][V] Case–control studies suggest relative risks of 1.58 to 3.2,[254, 255][III] with the risk increasing with higher doses,

Box 11.3 Effective low circulating volume states where NSAID use may precipitate acute renal failure

Symptoms:

- blood loss;
- severe diarrhea or vomiting;
- dehydration;
- diuretics;
- heart failure;
- cirrhosis;
- nephrotic syndrome;
- severe ascites.

concurrent use of diuretics or calcium channel blockers. Griffin et al.[256] estimated that there would be 25 excess hospitalizations associated with renal failure per 10,000 years of NSAID use.

In palliative care, acute prerenal failure from NSAIDs is not uncommon. Fortunately it is usually reversible if the NSAID is stopped,[257] although rehydration and occasionally dialysis may be needed.[258] Avoidance of NSAIDs in low volume states (**Box 11.3**) should go a long way in minimizing this problem.

Some series also now show NSAIDs to be the most common cause of immunological acute interstitial nephritis, another cause of acute renal failure.[259] These cases present with oliguria, arthralgia, fever, and a skin rash, sometimes with a moderate proteinuria and eosinophilia.[260] Recovery may be slower, more patients require dialysis, and renal damage is more often permanent (**Figure 11.3**).

Cardiovascular and thrombotic risk

The last few years have seen a dawning appreciation that many, perhaps most, NSAIDs (not just COX-2 inhibitors) can cause myocardial infarction and stroke.

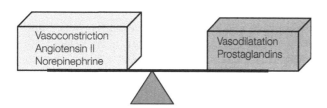

Figure 11.3 Mechanisms responsible for acute renal failure in NSAIDs. In low effective circulating volume conditions, PG levels increase when renal vasoconstrictors are produced, locally opposing renal vasoconstriction (autocoids!), hence preserving kidney function.

MECHANISM

In health, a balance is kept between the endothelial- and vascular smooth muscle-generated, antithrombotic, PGI_2 (prostacyclin) and the platelet-derived, prothrombotic, TXA_2 (thromboxane). Prostacyclin synthesis is mediated by both COX-1 and COX-2. On the other hand, only COX-1 mediates thromboxane synthesis. Nonselective inhibitors therefore inhibit both the prothrombotic and antithrombotic prostaglandins; but COX-2 inhibitors inhibit only prostacyclin production, leaving prothrombotic forces unopposed (**Figure 11.4**).[261]

This explains the increased thrombotic risk of COX-2 inhibitors. It is less clear why many nonselective NSAIDs also carry a thrombotic risk. Relatively high COX-2 selectivity could explain the prothrombotic tendency of diclofenac but not that of indometacin. Meloxicam carries a moderately elevated risk;[262, 263][III] if due to predominant COX-2 inhibition this should reduce with higher doses, as COX-1 inhibition becomes more relevant. Celecoxib, whose in vitro COX-2 selectivity is roughly in line with diclofenac, may undermine this hypothesis (but see below under Individual NSAIDs). It is entirely plausible, of course, that non-COX mechanisms might contribute with individual drugs. Indeed, experimental data suggest that at least some of the thrombotic activity of rofecoxib may be independent of the active cyclooxygenase site.[23]

EPIDEMIOLOGY

Two substantial, complementary, recent meta-analyses of thrombotic events following use of COX-2 and non-selective NSAIDs[264, 265][I] have reached broadly similar conclusions as a third meta-analysis, confining itself to epidemiological studies of nonselective NSAIDs.[266][III] Kearney et al.'s study[265] of RCTs calculated there would be three (95 percent CI 1–5) excess vascular events and three (95 percent CI 1–4) excess myocardial infarctions per 1000 person years of coxib use, but no excess number of strokes. The excess in cardiovascular deaths was one (95 percent CI 0–2) per 1000 patient years. Morbidity and mortality may of course be yet higher in prothrombotic malignancies. This meta-analysis could not confirm a dose-related increase in risk with any COX-2 inhibitor, though for celecoxib there was a nonstatistically significant trend. From controlled observational studies, McGettigan and Henry[264] were able to rank the different NSAIDs and COX-2 inhibitors for risk of serious vascular events. **Table 11.8** compares outcomes of the three studies.

Kearney et al.[265] found no significant overall difference in cardiovascular events between users of COX-2 inhibitors and those of nonselective NSAIDs. However, comparing only trials involving COX-2 inhibitors versus naproxen, there was a highly significant excess of cardiovascular events as well as a two-fold increase in

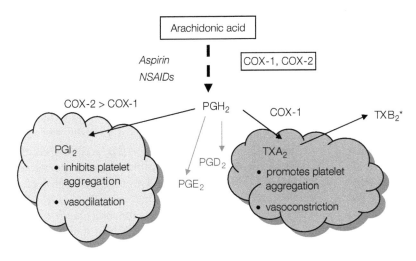

Figure 11.4 Mechanism of COX-2 mediated thrombosis. *, Urinary marker of TXA_2. COX, cyclooxygenase; PG, prostaglandin; TX, thromboxane.

Table 11.8 Thrombotic potential of NSAIDs and COX-2 inhibitors from three meta-analyses, ranked according to risk in McGettigan's study.

Drug	Relative risk serious cardiovascular events (95% C.I.) McGettigan and Henry[264]	Relative risk myocardial infarction (95% C.I.) Singh et al.[266]	Relative risk any vascular event (95% C.I.) Kearney et al.[265]
Rofecoxib >25 mg daily	2.19 (1.64–2.91)		
Diclofenac	1.40 (1.16–1.70)	1.38 (1.22–1.57)	1.63 (1.12–2.37)
Rofecoxib ≤25 mg daily	1.33 (1.00–1.79)		
Indometacin	1.30 (1.07–1.60)		
Meloxicam	1.25 (1.00–1.55)		
Any/other NSAID	1.10 (1.00–1.21)		
Ibuprofen	1.07 (0.97–1.18)	1.11 (1.06–1.17)	1.51 (0.96–2.37)
Piroxicam	1.06 (0.70–1.59)		
Celecoxib	1.06 (0.91–1.23)		
Naproxen	0.97 (0.87–1.07)	0.99 (0.88–1.11)	0.92 (0.67–1.26)

myocardial infarction risk in the COX-2 inhibitor group, although stroke risk was the same. Oddly, COX-2 inhibitors carried the same risk of vascular events or myocardial infarction as non-naproxen NSAIDs, but a significantly lower risk of stroke.

INDIVIDUAL NSAIDS

Rofecoxib carries a dose-related cardiovascular risk.[264][III] Despite Merck's continued insistence that risk only increases after 18 months of use,[267, 268, 269] substantial evidence indicates that it is elevated early on.[262, 264, 270, 271, 272] Meta-analysis of epidemiological studies,[264][III] and of RCTs,[273][I] found no increased cardiovascular risk from celecoxib, in contrast to Kearney's review of RCTs,[265][I] which found celecoxib to be as risky as rofecoxib. However, more recent trial and survey results showed an increased risk[274, 275][III] especially in the presence of previous myocardial infarction.[276, 277][III] Despite an early

negative meta-analysis,[278] valdecoxib was withdrawn in 2005 due to severe dermatological reactions, but also after the FDA had expressed disquiet about early toxicity,[279] a lack of adequate cardiovascular safety data, and a lack of demonstrated advantages over other NSAIDs. A recent survey ascribed it the highest risk of myocardial infarction,[275][III] (rofecoxib surprisingly came out as the lowest risk). Data for etoricoxib are limited but suggest moderate thrombogenicity.[280][I] The TARGET study suggests that lumiracoxib carries similar risks to naproxen or ibuprofen, irrespective of aspirin use.[281][II] A trade-sponsored meta-analysis confirms low risk,[282][I] but powerful data are still scarce.

NONSELECTIVE INHIBITORS

Diclofenac is relatively highly thrombogenic (almost comparable to rofecoxib).[197, 264, 275, 276, 283, 284, 285][III] Naproxen may carry low risk[266, 283, 286][III] (the latter study carries very broad confidence intervals for all drugs). The risk with ibuprofen is slightly elevated, while indometacin is moderately thrombogenic.[264][III] There are insufficient data to draw meaningful conclusions regarding nabumetone; for example a Finnish case–control study suggests a relative risk of 1.26 but has wide, unsafe 95 percent confidence intervals (0.59–2.69).[262][III]

A very recent publication by Pfizer using data modeling suggests that GI benefits still outweigh cardiovascular risk for celecoxib.[287] The validity of these findings needs to be confirmed. However the American Heart Association recently advised that, whenever possible, NSAIDs should not be used in patients with risk factors or a history of ischemic heart disease; that if needed, non-selective NSAIDs should be used first line, followed by preferential COX-2 inhibitors; COX-2 inhibitors should only be used if other approaches have failed.[288]

THE FUTURE

A number of novel safer alternative to NSAIDs are being explored.

CINODs (NO-NSAIDs)

The vasodilator nitric oxide protects gastric mucosal blood flow and mucus and bicarbonate production, counteracting suppression by COX inhibitors.[289] It also reduces neutrophil adherence to endothelial surfaces, enhancing its anti-inflammatory role.[290] CINODs (COX inhibitors and NO donors) were developed in the 1990s by adding a nitric oxide-donating moiety to NSAID molecules (producing, for example, NO-naproxen, now called naproxcinod, NO-aspirin, NO-indometacin, and NO-ibuprofen).[291] Despite a potency and range of activity equaling conventional NSAIDs,[292] they have no deleterious effect on blood pressure.[293] CINODs are anti-inflammatory and antipyretic in animals[294] but cause less gastric toxicity than conventional NSAIDs.[295] Human volunteer trials confirmed limited gastropathy and showed no increase in intestinal permeability after 12 days use.[296] Astra Zeneca bought rights to a number of CINODs from NiCOX, the originator company. However, phase II trial results did not meet Astra Zeneca's targets,[297] as gastroduodenal toxicity was no better than with naproxen,[298][II] and this led it to resell rights to two NO-NSAIDs to NiCOX.[299] A number of NO-NSAIDs are in phase III trials and there are hopes of submitting the drugs for approval by 2009.[300]

LOX-COX inhibitors

When NSAIDs block COX, arachidonic acid degradation is shunted mainly into the production of leukotrienes via lipoxygenase (LOX) (**Figure 11.1**). Leukotrienes attract neutrophils to inflammatory sites, causing the release of proteolytic enzymes, toxic oxygen radicals, chemokines and cytokines, inducing inflammation.[301] They also probably reduce gastric mucosal blood flow, potentiating mucosal damage. Agents which block COX-1, COX-2, and LOX (LOX-COX inhibitors),[302] theoretically and experimentally are less gastrotoxic[303, 304, 305] and nephrotoxic than nonselective NSAIDs, and have antithrombotic, analgesic, anti-inflammatory, antihyperalgesic, antipyretic, antiasthmatic, and even chondroprotective properties.[306] Indeed, licofelone, the first LOX-COX inhibitor, interfered with platelet function *in vitro* more than acetylsalicylic acid did.[307] In rabbits, it also reduced neointimal formation and inflammation.[308] Early human trials confirm low gastric toxicity.[309]

Phospholipase-A_2 inhibitors

Phospholipase-A_2 (PLA$_2$) hydrolyzes cell membrane phospholipids to arachidonic acid and lyso-phospholipids. PLA$_2$ inhibitors were discovered a hundred years ago in insect and snake venoms. Much more recently their role as potent anti-inflammatories is being elucidated. They inhibit all eicosanoid production (prostaglandins, leukotrienes, thromboxanes, endoperoxides, and lipoxins) from arachidonic acid.[310] There are many PLA$_2$ inhibitor isoforms with complex and diverse roles.[311] This complexity has so far prevented their development into useful anti-inflammatory agents.[312]

GENERAL CONCLUSIONS

NSAID use has diminished as knowledge of their adverse effects, especially GI, renal, and cardiovascular, has developed. Despite this, they still have an important place in cancer pain. Their continued use needs to be informed by an awareness of risk factors and protective strategies. Recognition of these problems has led to some exciting new concepts which might usher in an era of increased safety for these versatile drugs.

REFERENCES

1. Ellis F. Paracetamol. London: Royal Society of Chemistry. Last updated 2002; cited January 3, 2007. Available from: http://www.chemsoc.org/pdf/LearnNet/rsc/paracetamol.pdf.

2. How many people use retail analgesics? Bandolier [serial on the Internet]. 2002; 106: Available from: http://www.jr2.ox.ac.uk/bandolier/band106/b106-6.html.

3. Temple AR, Benson GD, Zinsenheim JR, Schweinle JE. Multicenter, randomized, double-blind, active-controlled,

parallel-group trial of the long-term (6-12 months) safety of acetaminophen in adult patients with osteoarthritis. *Clinical Therapeutics*. 2006; **28**: 222–35.

4. McQuay HJ, Moore RA. Dose-response in direct comparisons of different doses of aspirin, ibuprofen and paracetamol (acetaminophen) in analgesic studies. *British Journal of Clinical Pharmacology*. 2007; **63**: 271–8.

5. Miranda HF, Puig MM, Prietoa JC, Pinardia G. Synergism between paracetamol and nonsteroidal anti-inflammatory drugs in experimental acute pain. *Pain*. 2006; **121**: 22–8.

6. Haglund B, von Bultzingslowen I. Combining paracetamol with a selective cyclooxygenase-2 inhibitor for acute pain relief after third molar surgery: a randomized, double-blind, placebo-controlled study. *European Journal of Oral Sciences*. 2006; **114**: 293–301.

7. Seideman P. Additive effect of combined naproxen and paracetamol in rheumatoid arthritis. *British Journal of Rheumatology*. 1993; **32**: 1077–82.

8. Fricke Jr JR, Hewitt DJ, Jordan DM et al. A double-blind placebo-controlled comparison of tramadol/acetaminophen and tramadol in patients with postoperative dental pain. *Pain*. 2004; **109**: 250–7.

9. Remy C, Marret E, Bonnet F. Effects of acetaminophen on morphine side-effects and consumption after major surgery: meta-analysis of randomized controlled trials. *British Journal of Anaesthesia*. 2005; **94**: 505–13.

∗ 10. Wienecke T, Gøtzsche PC. Paracetamol versus nonsteroidal anti-inflammatory drugs for rheumatoid arthritis. *Cochrane Database of Systematic Reviews*. 2004; **CD003789**.

∗ 11. Towheed TE, Judd MJ, Hochberg MC, Wells G. Acetaminophen for osteoarthritis. *Cochrane Database of Systematic Reviews*. 2003; **CD004257**.

12. Hardy J, Reymond E, Charles M. Acetaminophen in cancer pain. *Journal of Clinical Oncology*. 2005; **23**: 1586; author reply 186–7.

13. Grond S, Zech D, Schug SA et al. The importance of non-opioid analgesics for cancer pain relief according to the guidelines of the World Health Organization. *International Journal of Clinical Pharmacology Research*. 1991; **11**: 253–60.

∗ 14. McNicol E, Strassels SA, Goudas L et al. NSAIDS or paracetamol, alone or combined with opioids, for cancer pain. *Cochrane Database of Systematic Reviews*. 2005; **CD005180**.

∗ 15. Botting RM. Mechanism of action of acetaminophen: is there a cyclooxygenase 3? *Clinical Infectious Diseases*. 2000; **31**: S202–10.

16. Kis B, Snipes JA, Simandle SA, Busija DW. Acetaminophen-sensitive prostaglandin production in rat cerebral endothelial cells. *American Journal of Physiology. Regulatory, Integrative and Comparative Physiology*. 2004; **288**: R897–902.

∗ 17. Graham GG, Scott KF. Mechanism of action of paracetamol. *American Journal of Therapeutics*. 2005; **12**: 46–55.

18. Bonnefont J, Daulhac L, Etienne M et al. Acetaminophen recruits spinal p42/p44 MAPKs and GH/IGF-1 receptors to produce analgesia via the serotonergic system. *Molecular Pharmacology*. 2007; **71**: 407–15.

∗ 19. Aronoff DM, Oates JA, Boutaud O. New insights into the mechanism of action of acetaminophen: Its clinical pharmacologic characteristics reflect its inhibition of the two prostaglandin H2 synthases. *Clinical Pharmacology and Therapeutics*. 2006; **79**: 9–19.

20. Chandrasekharan NV, Dai H, Roos KL et al. COX-3, a cyclooxygenase-1 variant inhibited by acetaminophen and other analgesic/antipyretic drugs: cloning, structure, and expression. *Proceedings of the National Academy of Sciences of the United States of America*. 2002; **99**: 13926–31.

21. Kis B, Snipes JA, Busija DW. Acetaminophen and the cyclooxygenase-3 puzzle: sorting out facts, fictions, and uncertainties. *Journal of Pharmacology and Experimental Therapeutics*. 2005; **315**: 1–7.

22. Qin N, Zhang SP, Reitz TL et al. Cloning, expression, and functional characterization of human cyclooxygenase-1 splicing variants: evidence for intron 1 retention. *Journal of Pharmacology and Experimental Therapeutics*. 2005; **315**: 1298–305.

∗ 23. Lucas R, Warner TD, Vojnovic I, Mitchell JA. Cellular mechanisms of acetaminophen: role of cyclo-oxygenase. *Faseb Journal*. 2005; **19**: 635–7.

24. Boutaud O, Aronoff DM, Richardson JH et al. Determinants of the cellular specificity of acetaminophen as an inhibitor of prostaglandin H(2) synthases. *Proceedings of the National Academy of Sciences of the United States of America*. 2002; **99**: 7130–5.

25. Aronoff DM, Boutaud O, Marnett LJ, Oates JA. Inhibition of prostaglandin H2 synthases by salicylate is dependent on the oxidative state of the enzymes. *Journal of Pharmacology and Experimental Therapeutics*. 2003; **304**: 589–95.

26. Hogestatt ED, Jonsson BA, Ermund A et al. Conversion of acetaminophen to the bioactive N-acylphenolamine AM404 via fatty acid amide hydrolase-dependent arachidonic acid conjugation in the nervous system. *Journal of Biological Chemistry*. 2005; **280**: 31405–12.

27. Godfrey L, Bailey I, Toms NJ et al. Paracetamol inhibits nitric oxide synthesis in murine spinal cord slices. *European Journal of Pharmacology*. 2007; **562**: 68–71.

28. Perkins JD. Acetaminophen sets records in the United States: Number 1 analgesic and number 1 cause of acute liver failure. *Liver Transplantation*. 2006; **12**: 682–3.

29. Mour G, Feinfeld DA, Caraccio T, McGuigan M. Acute renal dysfunction in acetaminophen poisoning. *Renal Failure*. 2005; **27**: 381–3.

30. von Mach MA, Hermanns-Clausen M, Koch I et al. Experiences of a poison center network with renal insufficiency in acetaminophen overdose: an analysis of 17 cases. *Clinical Toxicology*. 2005; **43**: 31–7.

* 31. Fored CM, Ejerblad E, Lindblad P et al. Acetaminophen, aspirin, and chronic renal failure. New England Journal of Medicine. 2001; 345: 1801–08.

32. Gallerani M, Simonato M, Manfredini R et al. Risk of hospitalization for upper gastrointestinal tract bleeding. Journal of Clinical Epidemiology. 2004; 57: 103–10.

33. Garcia-Rodriguez LA, Hernandez-Diaz S. Relative risk of upper gastrointestinal complications among users of acetaminophen and nonsteroidal anti-inflammatory drugs. Epidemiology. 2001; 12: 570–6.

34. Rahme E, Pettitt D, LeLorier J. Determinants and sequelae associated with utilization of acetaminophen versus traditional nonsteroidal antiinflammatory drugs in an elderly population. Arthritis and Rheumism. 2002; 46: 3046–54.

35. Lewis SC, Langman MJ, Laporte JR et al. Dose-response relationships between individual nonaspirin nonsteroidal anti-inflammatory drugs (NANSAIDs) and serious upper gastrointestinal bleeding: a meta-analysis based on individual patient data. British Journal of Clinical Pharmacology. 2002; 54: 320–6.

36. Blot WJ, McLaughlin JK. Over the counter non-steroidal anti-inflammatory drugs and risk of gastrointestinal bleeding. Journal of Epidemiology and Biostatistics. 2000; 5: 137–42.

37. Blot WJ, Fischer T, Nielsen GL et al. Outcome of upper gastro-intestinal bleeding and use of ibuprofen versus paracetamol. Pharmacy World and Science. 2004; 26: 319–23.

38. Schussel K, Schulz M. Prescribing of COX-2 inhibitors in Germany after safety warnings and market withdrawals. Die Pharmazie. 2006; 61: 878–86.

39. Ibanez L, Vidal X, Ballarin E, Laporte J. Agranulocytosis associated with dipyrone (metamizol). European Journal of Clinical Pharmacology. 2005; 60: 821–9.

40. Hedenmalm K, Spigset O. Agranulocytosis and other blood dyscrasias associated with dipyrone (metamizole). European Journal of Clinical Pharmacology. 2002; 58: 265–74.

* 41. Edwards JE, McQuay HJ. Dipyrone and agranulocytosis: what is the risk? Lancet. 2002; 360: 1438.

42. Rodriguez M, Barutell C, Rull M et al. Efficacy and tolerance of oral dipyrone versus oral morphine for cancer pain. European Journal of Cancer. 1994; 30A: 584–7.

43. Yalcin S, Gullu IH, Tekuzman G et al. A comparison of two nonsteroidal antiinflammatory drugs (diflunisal versus dipyrone) in the treatment of moderate to severe cancer pain: a randomized crossover study. American Journal of Clinical Oncology. 1998; 21: 185–8.

44. Zernikow B, Smale H, Michel E et al. Paediatric cancer pain management using the WHO analgesic ladder – results of a prospective analysis from 2265 treatment days during a quality improvement study. European Journal of Pain. 2006; 10: 587–95.

45. Girard P, Coppe MC, Verniers D et al. Role of catecholamines and serotonin receptor subtypes in nefopam-induced antinociception. Pharmacological Research. 2006; 54: 195–202.

46. Novelli A, Diaz-Trelles R, Groppetti A, Fernandez-Sanchez MT. Nefopam inhibits calcium influx, cGMP formation, and NMDA receptor-dependent neurotoxicity following activation of voltage sensitive calcium channels. Amino Acids. 2005; 28: 183–91.

47. Hunskaar S, Fasmer OB, Broch OJ, Hole K. Involvement of central serotonergic pathways in nefopam-induced antinociception. European Journal of Pharmacology. 1987; 12;138: 77–82.

48. Rosland JH, Hole K. The effect of nefopam and its enantiomers on the uptake of 5-hydroxytryptamine, noradrenaline and dopamine in crude rat brain synaptosomal preparations. Journal of Pharmacy and Pharmacology. 1990; 42: 437–8.

49. Girard P, Pansart Y, Gillardin JM. Nefopam potentiates morphine antinociception in allodynia and hyperalgesia in the rat. Pharmacology, Biochemistry, and Behavior. 2004; 77: 695–703.

50. Beloeil H, Delage N, Negre I et al. The median effective dose of nefopam and morphine administered intravenously for postoperative pain after minor surgery: a prospective randomized double-blinded isobolographic study of their analgesic action. Anesthesia and Analgesia. 2004; 98: 395–400.

51. Tramoni G, Viale JP, Cazals C, Bhageerutty K. Morphine-sparing effect of nefopam by continuous intravenous injection after abdominal surgery by laparotomy. European Journal of Anaesthesiology. 2003; 20: 990–2.

52. Schietzel M. [Analgesia with mild side effects]. Fortschritte der Medizin. 1977; 95: 2743–6.

53. Minotti V, Patoia L, Roila F et al. Double-blind evaluation of analgesic efficacy of orally administered diclofenac, nefopam, and acetylsalicylic acid (ASA) plus codeine in chronic cancer pain. Pain. 1989; 36: 177–83.

54. Astra-Zeneca International Press Office. Nexium receives FDA approval for risk reduction of NSAID-associated stomach ulcers. Available from: http://www.astrazeneca.com/pressrelease/3979.aspx.

55. Laine L. Approaches to nonsteroidal anti-inflammatory drug use in the high-risk patient. Gastroenterology. 2001; 120: 594–606.

56. Green GA. Understanding NSAIDs: from aspirin to COX-2. Clinical Cornerstone. 2001; 3: 50–60.

57. Griffin MR. Epidemiology of nonsteroidal anti-inflammatory drug-associated gastrointestinal injury. American Journal of Medicine. 1998; 104: 23S–9S; discussion 41S–2S.

58. Ansani N, Fedutes B, Vogt M, et al. Rheumatologic medication utilization in 2003: Prescribing trends and retail sales costs. American College of Rheumatology Annual Scientific Meeting. San Antonio, Texas. American College of Rheumatology; 2004. Presentation Number: 45, 2004.

59. Solomon DH, Schneeweiss S, Glynn RJ et al. Determinants of selective cyclooxygenase-2 inhibitor prescribing: are

patient or physician characteristics more important? *American Journal of Medicine*. 2003; **115**: 715–20.

60. Landsberg PG, Pillans PI, Radford JM. Evaluation of cyclooxygenase 2 inhibitor use in patients admitted to a large teaching hospital. *Internal Medicine Journal*. 2003; **33**: 225–8.

61. Thiebaud P, Patel BV, Nichol MB. Impact of rofecoxib withdrawal on cyclooxygenase-2 utilization among patients with and without cardiovascular risk. *Value in Health*. 2006; **9**: 361–8.

62. Epstein JB, Silverman Jr S, Paggiarino DA *et al.* Benzydamine HCl for prophylaxis of radiation-induced oral mucositis: results from a multicenter, randomized, double-blind, placebo-controlled clinical trial. *Cancer*. 2001; **92**: 875–85.

63. Mercadante S, Casuccio A, Agnello A *et al.* Analgesic effects of nonsteroidal anti-inflammatory drugs in cancer pain due to somatic or visceral mechanisms. *Journal of Pain and Symptom Management*. 1999; **17**: 351–6.

64. Blackwell N, Bangham L, Hughes M *et al.* Treatment of resistant pain in hypertrophic pulmonary arthropathy with ketorolac. *Thorax*. 1993; **48**: 401.

65. Martens M. Efficacy and tolerability of a topical NSAID patch (local action transcutaneous flurbiprofen) and oral diclofenac in the treatment of soft-tissue rheumatism. *Clinical Rheumatology*. 1997; **16**: 25–31.

66. Hatori M, Kokubun S. Clinical evaluation of indomethacin-containing patches for osteoarthritis and extremity trauma. *Current Medical Research and Opinion*. 1997; **13**: 511–15.

67. Devi K, Paranjothy KL. Pharmacokinetic profile of a new matrix-type transdermal delivery system: diclofenac diethyl ammonium patch. *Drug Development and Industrial Pharmacy*. 1999; **25**: 695–700.

68. Simmons DL, Wagner D, Westover K. Nonsteroidal anti-inflammatory drugs, acetaminophen, cyclooxygenase 2, and fever. *Clinical Infectious Diseases*. 2000; **31**: S211–8.

69. Pillsbury 3rd HC, Webster WP, Rosenman J. Prostaglandin inhibitor and radiotherapy in advanced head and neck cancers. *Archives of Otolaryngology – Head and Neck Surgery*. 1986; **112**: 552–3.

70. Wibberley A, McCafferty GP, Evans C *et al.* Dual, but not selective, COX-1 and COX-2 inhibitors, attenuate acetic acid-evoked bladder irritation in the anaesthetised female cat. *British Journal of Pharmacology*. 2006; **148**: 154–61.

71. Cardozo LD, Stanton SL, Robinson H, Hole D. Evaluation of flurbiprofen in detrusor instability. *British Medical Journal*. 1980; **280**: 281–2.

∗ 72. Vane JR. Inhibition of prostaglandin synthesis as a mechanism of action for aspirin-like drugs. *Nature: New Biology*. 1971; **231**: 232–5.

73. Kozak KR, Crews BC, Morrow JD *et al.* Metabolism of the endocannabinoids, 2-arachidonylglycerol and anandamide, into prostaglandin, thromboxane, and prostacyclin glycerol esters and ethanolamides. *Journal of Biological Chemistry*. 2002; **277**: 44877–85.

74. Parkinson JF. Lipoxin and synthetic lipoxin analogs: an overview of anti-inflammatory functions and new concepts in immunomodulation. *Inflammation and Allergy Drug Targets*. 2006; **5**: 91–106.

75. Simmons DL, Botting RM, Hla T. Cyclooxygenase isozymes: the biology of prostaglandin synthesis and inhibition. *Pharmacological Reviews*. 2004; **56**: 387–437.

76. Loftin CD, Tiano HF, Langenbach R. Phenotypes of the COX-deficient mice indicate physiological and pathophysiological roles for COX-1 and COX-2. *Prostaglandins and Other Lipid Mediators*. 2002; **68–69**: 177–85.

77. Wallace JL, McKnight W, Reuter BK, Vergnolle N. NSAID-induced gastric damage in rats: requirement for inhibition of both cyclooxygenase 1 and 2. *Gastroenterology*. 2000; **119**: 706–14.

78. Peskar BM. Role of cyclooxygenase isoforms in gastric mucosal defense and ulcer healing. *Inflammopharmacology*. 2005; **13**: 15–26.

79. Kapoor M, Shaw O, Appleton I. Possible anti-inflammatory role of COX-2-derived prostaglandins: implications for inflammation research. *Current Opinion in Investigational Drugs*. 2005; **6**: 461–6.

80. Halter F, Tarnawski AS, Schmassmann A, Peskar BM. Cyclooxygenase 2-implications on maintenance of gastric mucosal integrity and ulcer healing: controversial issues and perspectives. *Gut*. 2001; **49**: 443–53.

81. Gerstenfeld LC, Einhorn TA. COX inhibitors and their effects on bone healing. *Expert Opinion on Drug Safety*. 2004; **3**: 131–6.

82. Simon AM, Manigrasso MB, O'Connor JP. Cyclo-oxygenase 2 function is essential for bone fracture healing. *Journal of Bone and Mineral Research*. 2002; **17**: 963–76.

83. Huskisson EC, Woolf DL, Balme HW *et al.* Four new anti-inflammatory drugs: responses and variations. *British Medical Journal*. 1976; **1**: 1048–9.

84. Furst DE. Are there differences among nonsteroidal antiinflammatory drugs? Comparing acetylated salicylates, nonacetylated salicylates, and nonacetylated nonsteroidal antiinflammatory drugs. *Arthritis and Rheumatism*. 1994; **37**: 1–9.

85. Brooks PM, Dougan MA, Mugford S, Meffin E. Comparative effectiveness of 5 analgesics in patients with rheumatoid arthritis and osteoarthritis. *Journal of Rheumatology*. 1982; **9**: 723–6.

86. Lee YS, Kim H, Wu TX *et al.* Genetically mediated interindividual variation in analgesic responses to cyclooxygenase inhibitory drugs. *Clinical Pharmacology and Therapeutics*. 2006; **79**: 407–18.

87. Ulrich CM, Bigler J, Potter JD. Non-steroidal anti-inflammatory drugs for cancer prevention: promise, perils and pharmacogenetics. Nature Reviews. *Cancer*. 2006; **6**: 130–40.

88. NCBI dbSNP. NCBI; 2007. Updated 2007; cited June 21, 2007. Available from: http://www.ncbi.nlm.nih.gov/sites/entrez?db=Snp&TabCmd=Limits.

∗ 89. McCormack K, Brune K. Dissociation between the antinociceptive and anti-inflammatory effects of the nonsteroidal anti-inflammatory drugs. A survey of their analgesic efficacy. *Drugs*. 1991; **41**: 533–47.

90. Tegeder I, Pfeilschifter J, Geisslinger G. Cyclooxygenase-independent actions of cyclooxygenase inhibitors. *FASEB Journal*. 2001; **15**: 2057–72.

91. McCormack K. The spinal actions of nonsteroidal anti-inflammatory drugs and the dissociation between their anti-inflammatory and analgesic effects. *Drugs*. 1994; **47**: 28–45. discussion 6–7.

92. Diaz-Reval MI, Ventura-Martinez R, Deciga-Campos M *et al*. Evidence for a central mechanism of action of S-(+)-ketoprofen. *European Journal of Pharmacology*. 2004; **483**: 241–8.

93. Warner TD, Giuliano F, Vojnovic I *et al*. Nonsteroid drug selectivities for cyclo-oxygenase-1 rather than cyclo-oxygenase-2 are associated with human gastrointestinal toxicity: a full in vitro analysis. *Proceedings of the National Academy of Sciences of the United States of America*. 1999; **96**: 7563–8.

94. Brooks P, Emery P, Evans JF *et al*. Interpreting the clinical significance of the differential inhibition of cyclooxygenase-1 and cyclooxygenase-2. *Rheumatology (Oxford, England)*. 1999; **38**: 779–88.

95. Blain H, Boileau C, Lapicque F *et al*. Limitation of the in vitro whole blood assay for predicting the COX selectivity of NSAIDs in clinical use. *British Journal of Clinical Pharmacology*. 2002; **53**: 255–65.

96. Verburg KM, Maziasz TJ, Weiner E *et al*. Cox-2-specific inhibitors: definition of a new therapeutic concept. *American Journal of Therapeutics*. 2001; **8**: 49–64.

97. Brune K, Hinz B. Selective cyclooxygenase-2 inhibitors: similarities and differences. *Scandinavian Journal of Rheumatology*. 2004; **33**: 1–6.

98. Eisenberg E, Berkey CS, Carr DB *et al*. Efficacy and safety of nonsteroidal antiinflammatory drugs for cancer pain: a meta-analysis. *Journal of Clinical Oncology*. 1994; **12**: 2756–65.

99. Goudas LM, PhD, Carr DBM, Bloch RM, *et al*. Management of Cancer Pain. Rockville, MD 20852: Agency for Healthcare Research and Quality; October 2001 Contract No.: Document Number.

∗100. McNicol E, Strassels S, Goudas L *et al*. Nonsteroidal anti-inflammatory drugs, alone or combined with opioids, for cancer pain: a systematic review. *Journal of Clinical Oncology*. 2004; **22**: 1975–92.

101. Klein DC, Raisz LG. Prostaglandins: stimulation of bone resorption in tissue culture. *Endocrinology*. 1970; **86**: 1436–40.

102. Tashjian Jr AH, Voelkel EF, Levine L, Goldhaber P. Evidence that the bone resorption-stimulating factor produced by mouse fibrosarcoma cells is prostaglandin E 2. A new model for the hypercalcemia of cancer. *Journal of Experimental Medicine*. 1972; **136**: 1329–43.

103. Powles TJ, Clark SA, Easty DM *et al*. The inhibition by aspirin and indomethacin of osteolytic tumor deposits and hypercalcaemia in rats with Walker tumour, and its possible application to human breast cancer. *British Journal of Cancer*. 1973; **28**: 316–21.

104. Stoll BA. Indomethacin in breast cancer. *Lancet*. 1973; **2**: 384.

105. Brodie GN. Letter: Indomethacin and bone pain. *Lancet*. 1974; **1**: 1160.

106. Pace V. Use of nonsteroidal anti-inflammatory drugs in cancer. *Palliative Medicine*. 1995; **9**: 273–86.

107. Lomen PL, Samal BA, Lamborn KR *et al*. Flurbiprofen for the treatment of bone pain in patients with metastatic breast cancer. *American Journal of Medicine*. 1986; **80**: 83–7.

108. Johnson JR, Miller AJ. The efficacy of choline magnesium trisalicylate (CMT) in the management of metastatic bone pain: a pilot study. *Palliative Medicine*. 1994; **8**: 129–35.

109. Levick S, Jacobs C, Loukas DF *et al*. Naproxen sodium in treatment of bone pain due to metastatic cancer. *Pain*. 1988; **35**: 253–8.

110. Sacchetti G, Camera P, Rossi AP *et al*. Injectable ketoprofen vs. acetylsalicylic acid for the relief of severe cancer pain: a double-blind, crossover trial. *Drug Intelligence and Clinical Pharmacy*. 1984; **18**: 403–06.

111. Stambaugh Jr JE, Drew J. The combination of ibuprofen and oxycodone/acetaminophen in the management of chronic cancer pain. *Clinical Pharmacology and Therapeutics*. 1988; **44**: 665–9.

112. Kean WF, Buchanan WW. The use of NSAIDs in rheumatic disorders 2005: a global perspective. *Inflammopharmacology*. 2005; **13**: 343–70.

113. Graham DY, Smith JL. Aspirin and the stomach. *Annals of Internal Medicine*. 1986; **104**: 390–8.

114. O'Laughlin JC, Hoftiezer JW, Ivey KJ. Effect of aspirin on the human stomach in normals: endoscopic comparison of damage produced one hour, 24 hours, and 2 weeks after administration. *Scandinavian Journal of Gastroenterology. Supplement*. 1981; **67**: 211–4.

115. Taha AS, Sturrock RD, Russell RI. Mucosal erosions in longterm non-steroidal anti-inflammatory drug users: predisposition to ulceration and relation to Helicobacter pylori. *Gut*. 1995; **36**: 334–6.

116. Hawkey CJ, Naesdal J, Wilson I *et al*. Relative contribution of mucosal injury and Helicobacter pylori in the development of gastroduodenal lesions in patients taking non-steroidal anti-inflammatory drugs. *Gut*. 2002; **51**: 336–43.

117. Lanza FL, Evans DG, Graham DY. Effect of Helicobacter pylori infection on the severity of gastroduodenal mucosal injury after the acute administration of naproxen or aspirin to normal volunteers. *American Journal of Gastroenterology*. 1991; **86**: 735–7.

118. Laine L, Cominelli F, Sloane R *et al*. Interaction of NSAIDs and Helicobacter pylori on gastrointestinal injury and prostaglandin production: a controlled double-blind trial. *Alimentary Pharmacology and Therapeutics*. 1995; **9**: 127–35.

119. Rybar I, Masaryk P, Mateicka F et al. Nonsteroidal antiinflammatory drug-induced mucosal lesions of the upper gastrointestinal tract and their relationship to Helicobacter pylori. *International Journal of Clinical Pharmacology Research.* 2001; **21**: 119–25.

120. Graham DY, Smith JL, Dobbs SM. Gastric adaptation occurs with aspirin administration in man. *Digestive Diseases and Sciences.* 1983; **28**: 1–6.

121. Yeomans ND, Skeljo MV. Repair and healing of established gastric mucosal injury. *Journal of Clinical Gastroenterology.* 1991; **13**: S37–41.

122. Lipscomb GR, Campbell F, Rees WD. The influence of age, gender, Helicobacter pylori and smoking on gastric mucosal adaptation to non-steroidal anti-inflammatory drugs. *Alimentary Pharmacology and Therapeutics.* 1997; **11**: 907–12.

123. Olivero JJ, Graham DY. Gastric adaptation to nonsteroidal anti-inflammatory drugs in man. *Scandinavian Journal of Gastroenterology.* 1992; **193**: 53–8.

124. Moberly JB, Harris SI, Riff DS et al. A randomized, double-blind, one-week study comparing effects of a novel COX-2 inhibitor and naproxen on the gastric mucosa. *Digestive Diseases and Sciences.* 2007; **52**: 442–50.

125. Singh G, Ramey DR, Morfeld D et al. Gastrointestinal tract complications of nonsteroidal anti-inflammatory drug treatment in rheumatoid arthritis. A prospective observational cohort study. *Archives of Internal Medicine.* 1996; **156**: 1530–6.

126. Straus WL, Ofman JJ, MacLean C et al. Do NSAIDs cause dyspepsia? a meta-analysis evaluating alternative dyspepsia definitions. *American Journal of Gastroenterology.* 2002; **97**: 1951–8.

127. Larkai EN, Smith JL, Lidsky MD, Graham DY. Gastroduodenal mucosa and dyspeptic symptoms in arthritic patients during chronic nonsteroidal anti-inflammatory drug use. *American Journal of Gastroenterology.* 1987; **82**: 1153–8.

128. Kurata JH, Nogawa AN, Noritake D. NSAIDs increase risk of gastrointestinal bleeding in primary care patients with dyspepsia. *Journal of Family Practice.* 1997; **45**: 227–35.

129. Fries JF, Williams CA, Bloch DA, Michel BA. Nonsteroidal anti-inflammatory drug-associated gastropathy: incidence and risk factor models. *American Journal of Medicine.* 1991; **91**: 213–22.

130. Garcia Rodriguez LA, Hernandez-Diaz S. Risk of uncomplicated peptic ulcer among users of aspirin and nonaspirin nonsteroidal antiinflammatory drugs. *American Journal of Epidemiology.* 2004; **159**: 23–31.

131. Niv Y, Battler A, Abuksis G et al. Endoscopy in asymptomatic minidose aspirin consumers. *Digestive Diseases and Sciences.* 2005; **50**: 78–80.

132. Armstrong CP, Blower AL. Non-steroidal anti-inflammatory drugs and life threatening complications of peptic ulceration. *Gut.* 1987; **28**: 527–32.

*133. Kurata JH, Corboy ED. Current peptic ulcer time trends. An epidemiological profile. *Journal of Clinical Gastroenterology.* 1988; **10**: 259–68.

134. Post PN, Kuipers EJ, Meijer GA. Declining incidence of peptic ulcer but not of its complications: a nation-wide study in The Netherlands. *Alimentary Pharmacology and Therapeutics.* 2006; **23**: 1587–93.

135. Ohmann C, Imhof M, Ruppert C et al. Time-trends in the epidemiology of peptic ulcer bleeding. *Scandinavian Journal of Gastroenterology.* 2005; **40**: 914–20.

136. Howden CW, Leontiadis GI. Current indications for acid suppressants in Helicobacter pylori-negative ulcer disease. *Best Practice and Research.* 2001; **15**: 401–12.

137. Hung LC, Ching JY, Sung JJ et al. Long-term outcome of Helicobacter pylori-negative idiopathic bleeding ulcers: a prospective cohort study. *Gastroenterology.* 2005; **128**: 1845–50.

138. Fries JF, Murtagh KN, Bennett M et al. The rise and decline of nonsteroidal antiinflammatory drug-associated gastropathy in rheumatoid arthritis. *Arthritis and Rheumatism.* 2004; **50**: 2433–40.

139. van Dijk KN, ter Huurne K, de Vries CS et al. Prescribing of gastroprotective drugs among elderly NSAID users in The Netherlands. *Pharmacy World and Science.* 2002; **24**: 100–03.

140. Watson M, Gunnell D, Peters T et al. Guidelines and educational outreach visits from community pharmacists to improve prescribing in general practice: a randomised controlled trial. *Journal of Health Services Research and Policy.* 2001; **6**: 207–13.

141. Aguas M, Pons M, Barrera N et al. Prevention of non-steroidal antiinflammatory drugs-induced gastropathy: follow up of protocol adherence. *Revista Española de Enfermedades Digestivas.* 2002; **94**: 679–86.

142. Vonkeman HE, Fernandes RW, van de Laar MA. Under-utilization of gastroprotective drugs in patients with NSAID-related ulcers. *International Journal of Clinical Pharmacology and Therapeutics.* 2007; **45**: 281–8.

143. van Leen MW, van der Eijk I, Schols JM. Prevention of NSAID gastropathy in elderly patients. An observational study in general practice and nursing homes. *Age and Ageing.* 2007; **36**: 414–8.

144. Lanas A, Ferrandez A. Inappropriate prevention of NSAID-induced gastrointestinal events among long-term users in the elderly. *Drugs and Aging.* 2007; **24**: 121–31.

*145. Singh G. Recent considerations in nonsteroidal anti-inflammatory drug gastropathy. *American Journal of Medicine.* 1998; **105**: 31S–8S.

146. Wolfe MM, Lichtenstein DR, Singh G. Gastrointestinal toxicity of nonsteroidal antiinflammatory drugs. *New England Journal of Medicine.* 1999; **340**: 1888–99.

*147. FDA. Joint meeting of the Arthritis Advisory Committee and the Drug Safety and Risk Management Advisory Committee of the Food and Drug Administration.: Center for Drug Evaluation and Research. February 16–18, 2005.

148. Tarone RE, Blot WJ, McLaughlin JK. Nonselective nonaspirin nonsteroidal anti-inflammatory drugs and gastrointestinal bleeding: relative and absolute risk estimates from recent epidemiologic studies. *American Journal of Therapeutics.* 2004; **11**: 17–25.

149. Lanas A, Perez-Aisa MA, Feu F et al. A nationwide study of mortality associated with hospital admission due to severe gastrointestinal events and those associated with nonsteroidal antiinflammatory drug use. *American Journal of Gastroenterology.* 2005; **100**: 1685–93.

150. Blower AL, Brooks A, Fenn GC et al. Emergency admissions for upper gastrointestinal disease and their relation to NSAID use. *Alimentary Pharmacology and Therapeutics.* 1997; **11**: 283–91.

*151. Tramer MR, Moore RA, Reynolds DJ, McQuay HJ. Quantitative estimation of rare adverse events which follow a biological progression: a new model applied to chronic NSAID use. *Pain.* 2000; **85**: 169–82.

152. Vreeburg EM, de Bruijne HW, Snel P et al. Previous use of non-steroidal anti-inflammatory drugs and anticoagulants: the influence on clinical outcome of bleeding gastroduodenal ulcers. *European Journal of Gastroenterology and Hepatology.* 1997; **9**: 41–4.

153. Thomsen RW, Riis A, Munk EM et al. 30-Day mortality after peptic ulcer perforation among users of newer selective Cox-2 inhibitors and traditional NSAIDs: A population-based study. *American Journal of Gastroenterology.* 2006; **101**: 2704–10.

154. Singh G. Gastrointestinal complications of prescription and over-the-counter nonsteroidal anti-inflammatory drugs: a view from the ARAMIS database. Arthritis, Rheumatism, and Aging Medical Information System. *American Journal of Therapeutics.* 2000; **7**: 115–21.

155. Derry S, Loke YK. Risk of gastrointestinal haemorrhage with long term use of aspirin: meta-analysis. *British Medical Journal (Clinical research ed.).* 2000; **321**: 1183–7.

156. Ng W, Wong WM, Chen WH et al. Incidence and predictors of upper gastrointestinal bleeding in patients receiving low-dose aspirin for secondary prevention of cardiovascular events in patients with coronary artery disease. *World Journal of Gastroenterology.* 2006; **12**: 2923–7.

157. Hernandez-Diaz S, Garcia Rodriguez LA. Cardioprotective aspirin users and their excess risk of upper gastrointestinal complications. *BMC Medicine [electronic resource].* 2006; **4**: 22.

*158. Loke YK, Bell A, Derry S. Aspirin for the prevention of cardiovascular disease: calculating benefit and harm in the individual patient. *British Journal of Clinical Pharmacology.* 2003; **55**: 282–7.

159. Arakawa T, Higuchi K, Fukuda T et al. Prostaglandins in the stomach: an update. *Journal of Clinical Gastroenterology.* 1998; **27**: S1–11.

160. Ellis GA, Blake DR. Why are non-steroidal anti-inflammatory drugs so variable in their efficacy? A description of ion trapping. *Annals of the Rheumatic Diseases.* 1993; **52**: 241–3.

*161. Hedner T, Samulesson O, Wahrborg P et al. Nabumetone: therapeutic use and safety profile in the management of osteoarthritis and rheumatoid arthritis. *Drugs.* 2004; **64**: 2315–43. discussion 44–5.

162. Bjarnason I, Takeuchi K, Simpson R. NSAIDs: the emperor's new dogma? *Gut.* 2003; **52**: 1376–8.

163. Fiorucci S, Antonelli E, Morelli A. Mechanism of non-steroidal anti-inflammatory drug-gastropathy. *Digestive and Liver Disease.* 2001; **33**: S35–43.

164. Langenbach R, Loftin CD, Lee C, Tiano H. Cyclooxygenase-deficient mice. A summary of their characteristics and susceptibilities to inflammation and carcinogenesis. *Annals of the New York Academy of Sciences.* 1999; **889**: 52–61.

165. Hemmati M, Abtahi F, Farrokhsiar M, Djahanguiri B. Prevention of restraint and indomethacin-induced gastric ulceration by bile duct or pylorus ligation in rats. *Digestion.* 1974; **10**: 108–12.

*166. Giraud MN, Motta C, Romero JJ. Interaction of indomethacin and naproxen with gastric surface-active phospholipids: a possible mechanism for the gastric toxicity of nonsteroidal anti-inflammatory drugs (NSAIDs). *Biochemical Pharmacology.* 1999; **57**: 247–54.

167. Mino-Kenudson M, Tomita S, Lauwers GY. Mucin expression in reactive gastropathy: an immunohistochemical analysis. *Archives of Pathology and Laboratory Medicine.* 2007; **131**: 86–90.

168. Boers M, Tangelder MJ, van Ingen H et al. The rate of NSAID-induced endoscopic ulcers increases linearly but not exponentially with age: a pooled analysis of 12 randomised trials. *Annals of the Rheumatic Diseases.* 2007; **66**: 417–8.

169. Gabriel SE, Jaakkimainen L, Bombardier C. Risk for serious gastrointestinal complications related to use of nonsteroidal anti-inflammatory drugs. A meta-analysis. *Annals of Internal Medicine.* 1991; **115**: 787–96.

170. Hansen JM, Hallas J, Lauritsen JM, Bytzer P. Non-steroidal anti-inflammatory drugs and ulcer complications: a risk factor analysis for clinical decision-making. *Scandinavian Journal of Gastroenterology.* 1996; **31**: 126–30.

171. Sorensen HT, Mellemkjaer L, Blot WJ et al. Risk of upper gastrointestinal bleeding associated with use of low-dose aspirin. *American Journal of Gastroenterology.* 2000; **95**: 2218–24.

172. Weil J, Langman MJ, Wainwright P et al. Peptic ulcer bleeding: accessory risk factors and interactions with non-steroidal anti-inflammatory drugs. *Gut.* 2000; **46**: 27–31.

173. Garcia Rodriguez LA, Jick H. Risk of upper gastrointestinal bleeding and perforation associated with individual non-steroidal anti-inflammatory drugs. *Lancet.* 1994; **343**: 769–72.

174. Gutthann SP, Garcia Rodriguez LA, Raiford DS. Individual nonsteroidal antiinflammatory drugs and other risk factors for upper gastrointestinal bleeding and perforation. *Epidemiology (Cambridge, Mass.).* 1997; **8**: 18–24.

175. Johnsen SP, Sorensen HT, Mellemkjoer L et al. Hospitalisation for upper gastrointestinal bleeding associated with use of oral anticoagulants. *Thrombosis and Haemostasis.* 2001; **86**: 563–8.

176. Battistella M, Mamdami MM, Juurlink DN et al. Risk of upper gastrointestinal hemorrhage in warfarin users

treated with nonselective NSAIDs or COX-2 inhibitors. *Archives of Internal Medicine.* 2005; **165**: 189–92.

177. de Jong JC, van den Berg PB, Tobi H, de Jong-van den Berg LT. Combined use of SSRIs and NSAIDs increases the risk of gastrointestinal adverse effects. *British Journal of Clinical Pharmacology.* 2003; **55**: 591–5.

178. Langman MJ, Weil J, Wainwright P *et al.* Risks of bleeding peptic ulcer associated with individual non-steroidal anti-inflammatory drugs. *Lancet.* 1994; **343**: 1075–8.

179. Henry D, Lim LL, Garcia Rodriguez LA *et al.* Variability in risk of gastrointestinal complications with individual non-steroidal anti-inflammatory drugs: results of a collaborative meta-analysis. *British Medical Journal (Clinical research ed.).* 1996; **312**: 1563–6.

180. MCA/CSM. Non-steroidal anti-inflammatory drugs (NSAIDs) and gastrointestinal (GI) safety. *Current Problems in Pharmacovigilance.* 2002; **28**: 5–6.

181. Langman M. Population impact of strategies designed to reduce peptic ulcer risks associated with NSAID use. *International Journal of Clinical Practice.* 2003; **135**: 38–42.

182. Hippisley-Cox J, Coupland C, Logan R. Risk of adverse gastrointestinal outcomes in patients taking cyclo-oxygenase-2 inhibitors or conventional non-steroidal anti-inflammatory drugs: population based nested case-control analysis. *British Medical Journal (Clinical research ed.).* 2005; **331**: 1310–6.

183. Roth SH, Tindall EA, Jain AK *et al.* A controlled study comparing the effects of nabumetone, ibuprofen, and ibuprofen plus misoprostol on the upper gastrointestinal tract mucosa. *Archives of Internal Medicine.* 1993; **153**: 2565–71.

184. Roth SH, Bennett R, Caldron P *et al.* A long-term endoscopic evaluation of patients with arthritis treated with nabumetone vs naproxen. *Journal of Rheumatology.* 1994; **21**: 1118–23.

*185. Huang JQ, Sridhar S, Hunt RH. Gastrointestinal safety profile of nabumetone: a meta-analysis. *American Journal of Medicine.* 1999; **107**: 55S–61S. discussion S–4S.

186. Weaver AL, Messner RP, Storms WW *et al.* Treatment of patients with osteoarthritis with rofecoxib compared with nabumetone. *Journal of Clinical Rheumatology.* 2006; **12**: 17–25.

187. Ashworth NL, Peloso PM, Muhajarine N, Stang M. Risk of hospitalization with peptic ulcer disease or gastrointestinal hemorrhage associated with nabumetone, Arthrotec, diclofenac, and naproxen in a population based cohort study. *Journal of Rheumatology.* 2005; **32**: 2212–7.

*188. Bombardier C, Laine L, Reicin A *et al.* Comparison of upper gastrointestinal toxicity of rofecoxib and naproxen in patients with rheumatoid arthritis. VIGOR Study Group. *New England Journal of Medicine.* 2000; **343**: 1520–8.

189. Watson DJ, Yu Q, Bolognese JA *et al.* The upper gastrointestinal safety of rofecoxib vs. NSAIDs: an updated combined analysis. *Current Medical Research and Opinion.* 2004; **20**: 1539–48.

*190. Moore RA, Derry S, Makinson GT, McQuay HJ. Tolerability and adverse events in clinical trials of celecoxib in osteoarthritis and rheumatoid arthritis: systematic review and meta-analysis of information from company clinical trial reports. *Arthritis Research and Therapy.* 2005; **7**: R644–65.

191. Chan FK, Hung LC, Suen BY *et al.* Celecoxib versus diclofenac plus omeprazole in high-risk arthritis patients: results of a randomized double-blind trial. *Gastroenterology.* 2004; **127**: 1038–43.

192. Lai KC, Chu KM, Hui WM *et al.* Celecoxib compared with lansoprazole and naproxen to prevent gastrointestinal ulcer complications. *American Journal of Medicine.* 2005; **118**: 1271–8.

*193. Silverstein FE, Faich G, Goldstein JL *et al.* Gastrointestinal toxicity with celecoxib vs nonsteroidal anti-inflammatory drugs for osteoarthritis and rheumatoid arthritis: the CLASS study: A randomized controlled trial. Celecoxib Long-term Arthritis Safety Study. *Journal of the American Medical Association.* 2000; **284**: 1247–55.

194. Lanas A, Garcia-Rodriguez LA, Arroyo MT *et al.* Risk of upper gastrointestinal ulcer bleeding associated with selective COX-2 inhibitors, traditional non-aspirin NSAIDs, aspirin, and combinations. *Gut.* 2006; **55**: 1731–8.

195. Goldstein JL, Huang B, Amer F, Christopoulos NG. Ulcer recurrence in high-risk patients receiving nonsteroidalanti-inflammatory drugs plus low-dose aspirin: results of a post HOC subanalysis. *Clinical Therapeutics.* 2004; **26**: 1637–43.

196. Umar A, Boisseau M, Yusup A *et al.* Interactions between aspirin and COX-2 inhibitors or NSAIDs in a rat thrombosis model. *Fundamental and Clinical Pharmacology.* 2004; **18**: 559–63.

197. Hippisley-Cox J, Coupland C. Risk of myocardial infarction in patients taking cyclo-oxygenase-2 inhibitors or conventional non-steroidal anti-inflammatory drugs: population based nested case-control analysis. *British Medical Journal (Clinical research ed.).* 2005; **330**: 1366.

198. Strand V. Are COX-2 inhibitors preferable to non-selective non-steroidal anti-inflammatory drugs in patients with risk of cardiovascular events taking low-dose aspirin? *Lancet.* 2007; **370**: 2138–51.

*199. Rostom A, Dube C, Wells G *et al.* Prevention of NSAID-induced gastroduodenal ulcers. *Cochrane Database of Systematic Reviews.* 2002; **CD002296**.

200. Robinson M, Mills RJ, Euler AR. Ranitidine prevents duodenal ulcers associated with non-steroidal anti-inflammatory drug therapy. *Alimentary Pharmacology and Therapeutics.* 1991; **5**: 143–50.

201. Ehsanullah RS, Page MC, Tildesley G, Wood JR. Prevention of gastroduodenal damage induced by non-steroidal anti-inflammatory drugs: controlled trial of ranitidine. *British Medical Journal (Clinical research ed.).* 1988; **297**: 1017–21.

202. Robinson MG, Griffin Jr JW, Bowers J *et al.* Effect of ranitidine on gastroduodenal mucosal damage induced by

nonsteroidal antiinflammatory drugs. *Digestive Diseases and Sciences*. 1989; **34**: 424–8.

203. Taha AS, Hudson N, Hawkey CJ *et al*. Famotidine for the prevention of gastric and duodenal ulcers caused by nonsteroidal antiinflammatory drugs. *New England Journal of Medicine*. 1996; **334**: 1435–9.

204. Ekstrom P, Carling L, Wetterhus S *et al*. Prevention of peptic ulcer and dyspeptic symptoms with omeprazole in patients receiving continuous non-steroidal anti-inflammatory drug therapy. A Nordic multicentre study. *Scandinavian Journal of Gastroenterology*. 1996; **31**: 753–8.

205. Cullen D, Bardhan KD, Eisner M *et al*. Primary gastroduodenal prophylaxis with omeprazole for non-steroidal anti-inflammatory drug users. *Alimentary Pharmacology and Therapeutics*. 1998; **12**: 135–40.

206. Agrawal NM, Campbell DR, Safdi MA *et al*. Superiority of lansoprazole vs ranitidine in healing nonsteroidal anti-inflammatory drug-associated gastric ulcers: results of a double-blind, randomized, multicenter study. NSAID-Associated Gastric Ulcer Study Group. *Archives of Internal Medicine*. 2000; **160**: 1455–61.

207. Goldstein JL, Johanson JF, Suchower LJ, Brown KA. Healing of gastric ulcers with esomeprazole versus ranitidine in patients who continued to receive NSAID therapy: a randomized trial. *American Journal of Gastroenterology*. 2005; **100**: 2650–7.

208. Yeomans ND, Svedberg LE, Naesdal J. Is ranitidine therapy sufficient for healing peptic ulcers associated with non-steroidal anti-inflammatory drug use? *International Journal of Clinical Practice*. 2006; **60**: 1401–7.

209. Hawkey CJ, Karrasch JA, Szczepanski L *et al*. Omeprazole compared with misoprostol for ulcers associated with nonsteroidal antiinflammatory drugs. Omeprazole versus Misoprostol for NSAID-induced Ulcer Management (OMNIUM) Study Group. *New England Journal of Medicine*. 1998; **338**: 727–34.

210. Lai KC, Lam SK, Chu KM *et al*. Lansoprazole reduces ulcer relapse after eradication of Helicobacter pylori in nonsteroidal anti-inflammatory drug users – a randomized trial. *Alimentary Pharmacology and Therapeutics*. 2003; **18**: 829–36.

211. Vonkeman HE, Fernandes RW, Van der Palen J *et al*. Proton-pump inhibitors are associated with a reduced risk for bleeding and perforated gastroduodenal ulcers attributable to non-steroidal anti-inflammatory drugs: a nested case-control study. *Arthritis Research and Therapy*. 2007; **9**: R52.

*212. Silverstein FE, Graham DY, Senior JR *et al*. Misoprostol reduces serious gastrointestinal complications in patients with rheumatoid arthritis receiving nonsteroidal anti-inflammatory drugs. A randomized, double-blind, placebo-controlled trial. *Annals of Internal Medicine*. 1995; **123**: 241–9.

*213. Graham DY, Agrawal NM, Campbell DR *et al*. Ulcer prevention in long-term users of nonsteroidal anti-inflammatory drugs: results of a double-blind, randomized,

multicenter, active- and placebo-controlled study of misoprostol vs lansoprazole. *Archives of Internal Medicine*. 2002; **162**: 169–75.

214. Yilmaz S, Bayan K, Dursun M *et al*. Does adding misoprostol to standard intravenous proton pump inhibitor protocol improve the outcome of aspirin/NSAID-induced upper gastrointestinal bleeding? a randomized prospective study. *Digestive Diseases and Sciences*. 2007; **52**: 110–8.

215. Agrawal NM, Roth S, Graham DY *et al*. Misoprostol compared with sucralfate in the prevention of nonsteroidal anti-inflammatory drug-induced gastric ulcer. A randomized, controlled trial. *Annals of Internal Medicine*. 1991; **115**: 195–200.

216. Lanas A, Bajador E, Serrano P *et al*. Nitrovasodilators, low-dose aspirin, other nonsteroidal antiinflammatory drugs, and the risk of upper gastrointestinal bleeding. *New England Journal of Medicine*. 2000; **343**: 834–9.

217. Qvigstad G, Hatlen-Rebhan P, Brenna E, Waldum HL. Capsule endoscopy in clinical routine in patients with suspected disease of the small intestine: a 2-year prospective study. *Scandinavian Journal of Gastroenterology*. 2006; **41**: 614–8.

218. Bjarnason I, Zanelli G, Prouse P *et al*. Effect of non-steroidal anti-inflammatory drugs on the human small intestine. *Drugs*. 1986; **32**: 35–41.

219. Bjarnason I, Zanelli G, Prouse P *et al*. Blood and protein loss via small-intestinal inflammation induced by non-steroidal anti-inflammatory drugs. *Lancet*. 1987; **2**: 711–4.

220. Bjarnason I, Price AB, Zanelli G *et al*. Clinicopathological features of nonsteroidal antiinflammatory drug-induced small intestinal strictures. *Gastroenterology*. 1988; **94**: 1070–4.

221. de Sousa JB, Soares EG, Aprilli F. Effects of diclofenac sodium on intestinal anastomotic healing. Experimental study on the small intestine of rabbits. *Diseases of the Colon and Rectum*. 1991; **34**: 613–7.

*222. Adebayo D, Bjarnason I. Is non-steroidal anti-inflammaory drug (NSAID) enteropathy clinically more important than NSAID gastropathy? *Postgraduate Medical Journal*. 2006; **82**: 186–91.

*223. Maiden L, Thjodleifsson B, Theodors A *et al*. A quantitative analysis of NSAID-induced small bowel pathology by capsule enteroscopy. *Gastroenterology*. 2005; **128**: 1172–8.

224. Graham DY, Opekun AR, Willingham FF, Qureshi WA. Visible small-intestinal mucosal injury in chronic NSAID users. *Clinical Gastroenterology and Hepatology*. 2005; **3**: 55–9.

225. Tanaka A, Hase S, Miyazawa T, Takeuchi K. Up-regulation of cyclooxygenase-2 by inhibition of cyclooxygenase-1: a key to nonsteroidal anti-inflammatory drug-induced intestinal damage. *Journal of Pharmacology and Experimental Therapeutics*. 2002; **300**: 754–61.

226. Hotz-Behofsits CM, Walley MJ, Simpson R, Bjarnason IT. COX-1, COX-2 and the topical effect in NSAID-induced enteropathy. *Inflammopharmacology*. 2003; **11**: 363–70.

227. Fortun PJ, Hawkey CJ. Nonsteroidal antiinflammatory drugs and the small intestine. *Current Opinion in Gastroenterology.* 2005; **21**: 169–75.

228. Hagiwara M, Kataoka K, Arimochi H *et al.* Role of unbalanced growth of gram-negative bacteria in ileal ulcer formation in rats treated with a nonsteroidal anti-inflammatory drug. *Journal of Medical Investigation.* 2004; **51**: 43–51.

229. Dalby AB, Frank DN, St Amand AL *et al.* Culture-independent analysis of indomethacin-induced alterations in the rat gastrointestinal microbiota. *Applied and Environmental Microbiology.* 2006; **72**: 6707–15.

230. Bjarnason I, Fehilly B, Smethurst P *et al.* Importance of local versus systemic effects of non-steroidal anti-inflammatory drugs in increasing small intestinal permeability in man. *Gut.* 1991; **32**: 275–7.

231. Reuter BK, Davies NM, Wallace JL. Nonsteroidal anti-inflammatory drug enteropathy in rats: role of permeability, bacteria, and enterohepatic circulation. *Gastroenterology.* 1997; **112**: 109–17.

232. Beck WS, Schneider HT, Dietzel K *et al.* Gastrointestinal ulcerations induced by anti-inflammatory drugs in rats. Physicochemical and biochemical factors involved. *Archives of Toxicology.* 1990; **64**: 210–7.

233. Jacob M, Foster R, Sigthorsson G *et al.* Role of bile in pathogenesis of indomethacin-induced enteropathy. *Archives of Toxicology.* 2007; **81**: 291–8.

234. Lloyd-Still JD, Beno DW, Uhing MR *et al.* Ursodeoxycholic acid ameliorates ibuprofen-induced enteropathy in the rat. *Journal of Pediatric Gastroenterology and Nutrition.* 2001; **32**: 270–3.

235. Hatazawa R, Ohno R, Tanigami M *et al.* Roles of endogenous prostaglandins and cyclooxygenase isozymes in healing of indomethacin-induced small intestinal lesions in rats. *Journal of Pharmacology and Experimental Therapeutics.* 2006; **318**: 691–9.

*236. Fortun PJ, Hawkey CJ. Nonsteroidal antiinflammatory drugs and the small intestine. *Current Opinion in Gastroenterology.* 2007; **23**: 134–41.

237. Haque S, Haswell JE, Dreznick JT, West AB. A cecal diaphragm associated with the use of nonsteroidal anti-inflammatory drugs. *Journal of Clinical Gastroenterology.* 1992; **15**: 332–5.

238. Hawkey CJ. NSAIDs, coxibs, and the intestine. *Journal of Cardiovascular Pharmacology.* 2006; **47**: S72–5.

239. Takeuchi K, Smale S, Premchand P *et al.* Prevalence and mechanism of nonsteroidal anti-inflammatory drug-induced clinical relapse in patients with inflammatory bowel disease. *Clinical Gastroenterology and Hepatology.* 2006; **4**: 196–202.

240. Manfredini R, Ricci L, Giganti M *et al.* An uncommon case of fluid retention simulating a congestive heart failure after aspirin consumption. *American Journal of the Medical Sciences.* 2000; **320**: 72–4.

241. Pope JE, Anderson JJ, Felson DT. A meta-analysis of the effects of nonsteroidal anti-inflammatory drugs on blood pressure. *Archives of Internal Medicine.* 1993; **153**: 477–84.

242. Johnson AG, Nguyen TV, Day RO. Do nonsteroidal anti-inflammatory drugs affect blood pressure? A meta-analysis. *Annals of Internal Medicine.* 1994; **121**: 289–300.

243. Krum H, Aw TJ, Liew D, Haas S. Blood pressure effects of COX-2 inhibitors. *Journal of Cardiovascular Pharmacology.* 2006; **47**: S43–8.

244. Aw TJ, Haas SJ, Liew D, Krum H. Meta-analysis of cyclooxygenase-2 inhibitors and their effects on blood pressure. *Archives of Internal Medicine.* 2005; **165**: 490–6.

245. Schwartzman M, D'Agati V. Spontaneous relapse of naproxen-related nephrotic syndrome. *American Journal of Medicine.* 1987; **82**: 329–32.

246. AlperJr AB, Meleg-Smith S, Krane NK. Nephrotic syndrome and interstitial nephritis associated with celecoxib. *American Journal of Kidney Diseases.* 2002; **40**: 1086–90.

247. Radford Jr MG, Holley KE, Grande JP *et al.* Reversible membranous nephropathy associated with the use of nonsteroidal anti-inflammatory drugs. *Journal of the American Medical Association.* 1996; **276**: 466–9.

248. Perneger TV, Whelton PK, Klag MJ. Risk of kidney failure associated with the use of acetaminophen, aspirin, and nonsteroidal antiinflammatory drugs. *New England Journal of Medicine.* 1994; **331**: 1675–9.

249. Mihatsch MJ, Khanlari B, Brunner FP. Obituary to analgesic nephropathy – an autopsy study. *Nephrology, Dialysis, Transplantation.* 2006; **21**: 3139–45.

*250. Delzell E, Shapiro S. A review of epidemiologic studies of nonnarcotic analgesics and chronic renal disease. *Medicine (Baltimore).* 1998; **77**: 102–21.

*251. Harris RC. COX-2 and the kidney. *Journal of Cardiovascular Pharmacology.* 2006; **47**: S37–42.

252. Baraldi A, Ballestri M, Rapana R *et al.* Acute renal failure of medical type in an elderly population. *Nephrology, Dialysis, Transplantation.* 1998; **13**: 25–9.

253. Horackova M, Charvat J, Hasa J *et al.* Life-threatening renal failure caused by vasomotor nephropathy associated with nonsteroidal anti-inflammatory drugs. *International Journal of Clinical Pharmacology Research.* 2004; **24**: 117–22.

254. Evans JM, McGregor E, McMahon AD *et al.* Non-steroidal anti-inflammatory drugs and hospitalization for acute renal failure. *Quarterly Journal of Medicine.* 1995; **88**: 551–7.

255. Huerta C, Castellsague J, Varas-Lorenzo C, Garcia Rodriguez LA. Nonsteroidal anti-inflammatory drugs and risk of ARF in the general population. *American Journal of Kidney Diseases.* 2005; **45**: 531–9.

256. Griffin MR, Yared A, Ray WA. Nonsteroidal antiinflammatory drugs and acute renal failure in elderly persons. *American Journal of Epidemiology.* 2000; **151**: 488–96.

257. Ulinski T, Guigonis V, Dunan O, Bensman A. Acute renal failure after treatment with non-steroidal

anti-inflammatory drugs. *European Journal of Pediatrics.* 2004; **163**: 148–50.

258. Esteve JB, Launay-Vacher V, Brocheriou I *et al.* COX-2 inhibitors and acute interstitial nephritis: case report and review of the literature. *Clinical Nephrology.* 2005; **63**: 385–9.

259. Schwarz A, Krause PH, Kunzendorf U *et al.* The outcome of acute interstitial nephritis: risk factors for the transition from acute to chronic interstitial nephritis. *Clinical Nephrology.* 2000; **54**: 179–90.

260. Clarkson MR, Giblin L, O'Connell FP *et al.* Acute interstitial nephritis: clinical features and response to corticosteroid therapy. *Nephrology, Dialysis, Transplantation.* 2004; **19**: 2778–83.

261. Catella-Lawson F. Vascular biology of thrombosis: platelet-vessel wall interactions and aspirin effects. *Neurology.* 2001; **57**: S5–7.

262. Helin-Salmivaara A, Virtanen A, Vesalainen R *et al.* NSAID use and the risk of hospitalization for first myocardial infarction in the general population: a nationwide case-control study from Finland. *European Heart Journal.* 2006; **27**: 1657–63.

263. Huang WF, Hsiao FY, Tsai YW *et al.* Cardiovascular events associated with long-term use of celecoxib, rofecoxib and meloxicam in Taiwan: an observational study. *Drug Safety.* 2006; **29**: 261–72.

*264. McGettigan P, Henry D. Cardiovascular risk and inhibition of cyclooxygenase: a systematic review of the observational studies of selective and nonselective inhibitors of cyclooxygenase 2. *Journal of the American Medical Association.* 2006; **296**: 1633–44.

*265. Kearney PM, Baigent C, Godwin J *et al.* Do selective cyclo-oxygenase-2 inhibitors and traditional non-steroidal anti-inflammatory drugs increase the risk of atherothrombosis? Meta-analysis of randomised trials. *British Medical Journal (Clinical research ed.).* 2006; **332**: 1302–8.

*266. Singh G, Wu O, Langhorne P, Madhok R. Risk of acute myocardial infarction with non-selective non-steroidal anti-inflammatory drugs: a meta-analysis. *Arthritis Research and Therapy.* 2006; **8**: R153.

267. Merck & Co I. Response to Article by Juni *et al.* Published in The Lancet on Nov. 5. Lancet. 2004 Last updated: 5 Nov 2004; cited January 2008. Available from: www.merck.com/statement_2004_1105/lancet.pdf.

268. Merck & Co I. An open letter from Merck. Whitehouse Station, NJ; 2006. Updated 26 June 2006; cited 29 Dec 2006. Available from: www.merck.com/newsroom/vioxx/pdf/Open_Letter_Concerning_VIOXX_June_26_2006.pdf.

*269. Bresalier RS, Sandler RS, Quan H *et al.* Cardiovascular events associated with rofecoxib in a colorectal adenoma chemoprevention trial. *New England Journal of Medicine.* 2005; **17**: 1092–102.

270. Solomon DH, Avorn J, Sturmer T *et al.* Cardiovascular outcomes in new users of coxibs and nonsteroidal antiinflammatory drugs: high-risk subgroups and time course of risk. *Arthritis and Rheumatism.* 2006; **54**: 1378–89.

271. Velentgas P, West W, Cannuscio CC, Watson DJ, Walker AM. Cardiovascular risk of selective cyclooxygenase-2 inhibitors and other non-aspirin non-steroidal anti-inflammatory medications. *Pharmacoepidemiology and Drug Safety.* 2006; **15**: 641–52.

*272. Lagakos SW. Time-to-event analyses for long-term treatments – the APPROVe trial. *New England Journal of Medicine.* 2006; **355**: 113–7.

*273. White WB, West CR, Borer JS *et al.* Risk of cardiovascular events in patients receiving celecoxib: a meta-analysis of randomized clinical trials. *American Journal of Cardiology.* 2007; **99**: 91–8.

274. Motsko SP, Rascati KL, Busti AJ *et al.* Temporal relationship between use of NSAIDs, including selective COX-2 inhibitors, and cardiovascular risk. *Drug Safety.* 2006; **29**: 621–32.

275. Andersohn F, Suissa S, Garbe E. Use of first- and second-generation cyclooxygenase-2-selective nonsteroidal antiinflammatory drugs and risk of acute myocardial infarction. *Circulation.* 2006; **113**: 1950–7.

276. Gislason GH, Jacobsen S, Rasmussen JN *et al.* Risk of death or reinfarction associated with the use of selective cyclooxygenase-2 inhibitors and nonselective nonsteroidal antiinflammatory drugs after acute myocardial infarction. *Circulation.* 2006; **113**: 2906–13.

277. Brophy J, Levesques L, Zhang B. The coronary risk of cyclooxygenase-2 (cox-2) inhibitors in subjects with a previous myocardial infarction. *Heart.* 2007; **93**: 189–94.

278. White WB, Strand V, Roberts R, Whelton A. Effects of the cyclooxygenase-2 specific inhibitor valdecoxib versus nonsteroidal antiinflammatory agents and placebo on cardiovascular thrombotic events in patients with arthritis. *American Journal of Therapeutics.* 2004; **11**: 244–50.

279. Nussmeier NA, Whelton AA, Brown MT *et al.* Complications of the COX-2 inhibitors parecoxib and valdecoxib after cardiac surgery. *New England Journal of Medicine.* 2005; **352**: 1081–91.

280. Aldington S, Shirtcliffe P, Weatherall M, Beasley R. Systematic review and meta-analysis of the risk of major cardiovascular events with etoricoxib therapy. *New Zealand Medical Journal.* 2005; **118**: U1684.

281. Farkouh ME, Kirshner H, Harrington RA *et al.* Comparison of lumiracoxib with naproxen and ibuprofen in the Therapeutic Arthritis Research and Gastrointestinal Event Trial (TARGET), cardiovascular outcomes: randomised controlled trial. *Lancet.* 2004; **364**: 675–84.

282. Matchaba P, Gitton X, Krammer G *et al.* Cardiovascular safety of lumiracoxib: a meta-analysis of all randomized controlled trials > or = 1 week and up to 1 year in duration of patients with osteoarthritis and rheumatoid arthritis. *Clinical Therapeutics.* 2005; **27**: 1196–214.

283. Schneeweiss S, Solomon DH, Wang PS *et al.* Simultaneous assessment of short-term gastrointestinal benefits and cardiovascular risks of selective cyclooxygenase 2 inhibitors and nonselective nonsteroidal antiinflammatory

drugs: an instrumental variable analysis. *Arthritis and Rheumatism.* 2006; **54**: 3390–8.

284. Garcia Rodriguez L, Gonzalez-Perez A. Long-term use of non-steroidal anti-inflammatory drugs and the risk of myocardial infarction in the general population. *BMC Medicine.* 2005; **3**: 17.

285. Rahme E, Nedjar H. Risks and benefits of COX-2 inhibitors vs non-selective NSAIDs: does their cardiovascular risk exceed their gastrointestinal benefit? A retrospective cohort study. *Rheumatology (Oxford, England).* 2007; **46**: 435–8.

286. Hernandez-Diaz S, Varas-Lorenzo C, Garcia Rodriguez LA. Non-steroidal antiinflammatory drugs and the risk of acute myocardial infarction. *Basic and Clinical Pharmacology and Toxicology.* 2006; **98**: 266–74.

287. Varas-Lorenzo C, Maguire A, Castellsague J, Perez-Gutthann S. Quantitative assessment of the gastrointestinal and cardiovascular risk-benefit of celecoxib compared to individual NSAIDs at the population level. *Pharmacoepidemiology and Drug Safety.* 2007; **16**: 366–76.

*288. Antman EM, Bennett JS, Daugherty A *et al.* Use of nonsteroidal antiinflammatory drugs: an update for clinicians: a scientific statement from the American Heart Association. *Circulation.* 2007; **115**: 1634–42.

289. Walley M, Hotz-Behofsits C, Simpson R, Bjarnason I. Nitric oxide: potential role for reducing gastro-enteropathy. *Inflammopharmacology.* 2003; **11**: 429–36.

290. Provost P, Lam JY, Lacoste L *et al.* Endothelium-derived nitric oxide attenuates neutrophil adhesion to endothelium under arterial flow conditions. *Arteriosclerosis and Thrombosis.* 1994; **14**: 331–5.

291. Cirino G, Wheeler-Jones CP, Wallace JL *et al.* Inhibition of inducible nitric oxide synthase expression by novel nonsteroidal anti-inflammatory derivatives with gastrointestinal-sparing properties. *British Journal of Pharmacology.* 1996; **117**: 1421–6.

292. Schnitzer TJ, Kivitz AJ, Lipetz RS *et al.* Comparison of the COX-inhibiting nitric oxide donor AZD3582 and rofecoxib in treating the signs and symptoms of osteoarthritis of the knee. *Arthritis and Rheumatism.* 2005; **53**: 827–37.

293. Muscara MN, Wallace JL. COX-inhibiting nitric oxide donors (CINODs): potential benefits on cardiovascular and renal function. *Cardiovascular and Hematological Agents in Medicinal Chemistry.* 2006; **4**: 155–64.

294. Hoogstraate J, Andersson LI, Berge OG *et al.* COX-inhibiting nitric oxide donors (CINODs) – a new paradigm in the treatment of pain and inflammation. *Inflammopharmacology.* 2003; **11**: 423–8.

295. Whittle BJ. Nitric oxide and the gut injury induced by non-steroidal anti-inflammatory drugs. *Inflammopharmacology.* 2003; **11**: 415–22.

296. Hawkey CJ, Jones JI, Atherton CT *et al.* Gastrointestinal safety of AZD3582, a cyclooxygenase inhibiting nitric oxide donor: proof of concept study in humans. *Gut.* 2003; **52**: 1537–42.

297. Astra-Zeneca Press Office. ASTRAZENECA research update on AZD3582. 2003. Updated 2003; cited June 29, 2007. Available from: http://www.astrazeneca.com/pressrelease/476.aspx.

*298. Lohmander LS, McKeith D, Svensson O *et al.* A randomised, placebo controlled, comparative trial of the gastrointestinal safety and efficacy of AZD3582 versus naproxen in osteoarthritis. *Annals of the Rheumatic Diseases.* 2005; **64**: 449–56.

299. Astra Zeneca. Annual Report and Form 20-F Information 2003. London: Astra Zeneca; 2005 Contract No.: Document Number. Available from: www.astrazeneca.com/article/503063.aspx.

*300. Anonymous. Naproxcinod: AZD 3582, HCT 3012, naproxen nitroxybutylester, nitronaproxen, NO-naproxen. *Drugs in R&D.* 2007; **8**: 255–8.

301. Fiorucci S, Distrutti E, Mencarelli A *et al.* Evidence that 5-lipoxygenase and acetylated cyclooxygenase 2-derived eicosanoids regulate leukocyte-endothelial adherence in response to aspirin. *British Journal of Pharmacology.* 2003; **139**: 1351–9.

302. Moreau M, Daminet S, Martel-Pelletier J *et al.* Superiority of the gastroduodenal safety profile of licofelone over rofecoxib, a COX-2 selective inhibitor, in dogs. *Journal of veterinary pharmacology and therapeutics.* 2005; **28**: 81–6.

303. Fischer L, Hornig M, Pergola C *et al.* The molecular mechanism of the inhibition by licofelone of the biosynthesis of 5-lipoxygenase products. *British Journal of Pharmacology.* 2007; **152**: 471–80.

304. Singh VP, Patil CS, Kulkarni SK. Anti-inflammatory effect of licofelone against various inflammatory challenges. *Fundamental and Clinical Pharmacology.* 2006; **20**: 65–71.

*305. Kulkarni SK, Singh VP. Licofelone – a novel analgesic and anti-inflammatory agent. *Current Topics in Medicinal Chemistry.* 2007; **7**: 251–63.

306. Lajeunesse D, Martel Pelletier J, Fernandes JC *et al.* Treatment with licofelone prevents abnormal subchondral bone cell metabolism in experimental dog osteoarthritis. *Annals of the Rheumatic Diseases.* 2004; **63**: 78–83.

307. Hernandez MR, Tonda R, Pedreno J *et al.* Effects on primary haemostasis of an anti-inflammatory agent with 5-lipoxygenase and cyclooxygenase inhibitory activity. *Journal of Cardiovascular Medicine (Hagerstown, Md.).* 2006; **7**: 859–65.

308. Vidal C, Gomez-Hernandez A, Sanchez-Galan E *et al.* Licofelone, a balanced inhibitor of cyclooxygenase and 5-lipoxygenase, reduces inflammation in a rabbit model of atherosclerosis. *Journal of Pharmacology and Experimental Therapeutics.* 2007; **320**: 108–16.

309. Bias P, Buchner A, Klesser B, Laufer S. The gastrointestinal tolerability of the LOX/COX inhibitor, licofelone, is similar to placebo and superior to naproxen therapy in healthy volunteers: results from a randomized, controlled trial. *American Journal of Gastroenterology.* 2004; **99**: 611–8.

310. Meyer MC, Rastogi P, Beckett CS, McHowat J. Phospholipase A2 inhibitors as potential anti-inflammatory agents. *Current Pharmaceutical Design.* 2005; **11**: 1301–12.

311. Narendra Sharath Chandra JN, Ponnappa KC, Sadashiva CT *et al.* Chemistry and structural evaluation of different phospholipase A2 inhibitors in arachidonic acid pathway mediated inflammation and snake venom toxicity. *Current Topics in Medicinal Chemistry.* 2007; **7**: 787–800.

312. Yedgar S, Cohen Y, Shoseyov D. Control of phospholipase A2 activities for the treatment of inflammatory conditions. *Biochimica et Biophysica Acta.* 2006; **1761**: 1373–82.

Clinical pharmacology of opioids: basic pharmacology

SANGEETA R MEHENDALE AND CHUN-SU YUAN

Introduction	151	Adverse effects of opioids	156
Opioid receptors	152	Therapeutic use of opioids in cancer	157
Endogenous opioids	153	Summary	163
Classification of opioid compounds used for analgesia	153	References	163
Pharmacological effects of opioids	154		

KEY LEARNING POINTS

- Opioids mediate pharmacological actions through three principal types of receptors.
- Most clinically used opioid analgesics are mu-receptor agonists.
- Moderate to severe cancer pain is effectively treated with strong opioid agonists.

- Availability of opioid compounds exhibiting a range of pharmacokinetic and pharmacodynamic properties enables customizing analgesia for a spectrum of cancer pain presentations.

INTRODUCTION

Pain in cancer is a cause of significant suffering contributing to reduced functional ability, depression, and anxiety.[1, 2] The causes of cancer-related pain are diverse and could be classified as those that occur from tumor growth directly (e.g. tissue infiltration), from treatment (e.g. surgery, chemotherapy, or radiotherapy), from conditions associated with disability of cancer (herpes, pressure sores), and from causes unrelated to cancer or cancer treatment. In the 1980s, it was estimated that more than 25 percent of the patients suffering from cancer died without pain relief.[3] Considering the psychological and social consequences from untreated cancer pain,[1] the alarming proportion of patients with unrelieved pain has

been deemed unacceptable. Today, with the advances in the understanding of pain management, it is possible to significantly alleviate pain and suffering with an improvement in patients' quality of life. To this effect, the World Health Organization (WHO) has established recommendations for management of cancer pain using various analgesics, in a stepladder fashion, with opioids forming the mainstay of treatment of moderate to severe pain.[4] Institution of the WHO guidelines has resulted in a considerable improvement in cancer pain management.

There are, however, several obstacles to achieving satisfactory relief of cancer pain with opioids. Although many potent opioid drugs are available, often the doses of opioid drugs that are necessary to control pain adequately also cause unacceptable adverse effects.[5] The fear of severe adverse effects of opioids, such as respiratory depression, tolerance, and addiction, although demonstrated to be unfounded,[6, 7, 8] further adds to the underutilization of these potent analgesics. Some of the issues that compromise the adequacy of pain relief in cancer patients are significant interpatient variability in responsiveness to opioids, occurrence of breakthrough pain, type of pain with neuropathic pain being harder to treat, change in the character and intensity of pain due to progression of disease, and psychological status affecting the perception of pain.[5, 7, 9]

Optimizing opioid regimen to provide adequate analgesia with minimal adverse effects requires an understanding of the pharmacokinetic and pharmacodynamic properties of opioid compounds.[5] This chapter focuses on the basic pharmacology of opioid compounds from the perspective of cancer pain management.

OPIOID RECEPTORS

Opioids mediate their pharmacological actions through opioid receptors. There are three principal types of opioid receptors, mu (OP3/MOR/OPRM), delta (OP1/DOR/OPRD), and kappa (OP2/KOR/OPRK). The cDNAs of the three major opioid receptors have been cloned, sequenced, and appear to encode highly similar proteins with a primary structure typical for G protein-coupled membrane receptors. In general, mu and delta receptors appear to be structurally more similar to each other as compared to kappa receptors.[10] Most clinically used opioids are relatively selective for mu receptors. Although other opioid receptors such as orphanin (ORL-1) have been described in the past decade, their roles in opioid physiology and in mediating analgesia are still being defined.[11, 12]

Receptor-specific actions

The major pharmacological actions for each receptor type are enumerated. Mu receptor stimulation causes supraspinal and spinal analgesia, slowed respiration, nausea, inhibition of gastrointestinal transit, increased feeding, and increased sedation. Delta receptor stimulation results in similar effects as mu receptor stimulation such as supraspinal and spinal analgesia, nausea, slowed gastrointestinal transit, and increased feeding. Delta receptors also modulate the activity of mu receptors.[13, 14, 15, 16] Kappa-receptor stimulation, apart from causing analgesia, slowed gastrointestinal transit, increased feeding, increased sedation, and diuresis, also results in psychotomimetic effects. Although the common response to opioid receptor activation (agonist binding) for all three receptors is analgesia, the mu receptor appears to be principally responsible for this effect.[17, 18]

Apart from the beneficial effect of analgesia, some of the aforementioned effects of opioid-receptor stimulation are undesirable. Newer, experimental opioid compounds with affinity to more than one receptor type are being developed with the goal of optimizing analgesia while minimizing adverse effects, for example, a compound that is a partial agonist to both the mu and the kappa receptors, can potentially produce additive analgesia without the adverse addictive and dysphoric effects.[19] Similarly, complementary delta-receptor activation may result in modulation of the mu-mediated response to produce greater analgesia and reduced addictive effect.[20] Using delta agonists along with mu agonists results in enhancement of analgesic potency, while using delta antagonists with mu agonists results in reduced tolerance and physical dependence.[13, 14, 15, 16] Coexistence of mu and delta receptors as complexes or presence of both receptor types in single neurons in the pain-modulating pathways suggests that endogenous opioids may operate similarly.[21, 22]

Subtypes

Subtypes of receptors have been described within each receptor type such as mu-1, -2, -3; delta-1, -2; and kappa-1, -2, -3.[23, 24, 25, 26] Although pharmacological studies suggest that opioid receptor subtypes may exist, molecular cloning has demonstrated only one, not multiple, cDNA clones for each type of opioid receptor. A proposed theory is that receptor subtypes are formed by alternative splicing of the RNA[23, 27, 28, 29] from the single gene, by oligomerization of receptor proteins[30] or by other mechanisms.[31] Since most opioid analgesics used clinically are mu agonists, the mu-receptor subtypes have been researched extensively. Discovery of the multiple mu opioid receptor subtypes may help explain the wide range of analgesic response elicited by opioid drugs.[26, 27]

Distribution

Each major receptor type has a unique anatomical distribution in the brain, spinal cord, and the periphery, suggesting that there may be distinct functions associated with these receptors.[32] All three receptors are found throughout the nervous system, in somatic and visceral sensory neurons, spinal cord projections and interneurons, midbrain, and cortex. Apart from the central nervous system, the opioid receptors are also found on the peripheral nerves and on other tissues such as leukocytes, the gastrointestinal tract, and the cardiovascular system.[33, 34, 35, 36]

Action on pain pathway

Analgesic effects of opioids are exerted by their ability to directly inhibit the ascending transmission of the nociceptive impulses from the dorsal horn in the spinal cord[37] and by activating the pain control pathway that begins in the midbrain and descends to the spinal cord. All the three major types of opioid receptors are found in high concentrations in the dorsal horn of the spinal cord. Receptors are also found on the primary afferents that relay pain sensation to the spinal cord. Opioid agonists inhibit release of neurotransmitters from the primary afferents and directly inhibit pain transmission. Thus a direct analgesic effect of opioids is exerted in the spinal cord. Opioids also produce analgesia by acting on supraspinal receptor sites located in the pain-modulating descending pathways including the rostral ventromedial medulla (RVM), the locus ceruleus (LC), and the mid-brain periaqueductal gray (PAG) area.[38]

Signal transduction

All three receptors, i.e. mu, delta, and kappa, are coupled via pertussis toxin-sensitive GTP binding proteins. The opioid agonist binding leads to receptor activation, which triggers cascading events through GTP binding proteins. Adenylyl cyclase activity is inhibited which reduces cAMP-mediated effects. The activation of inwardly rectifying K^+ channels results in removal of intracellular K^+ leading to a hyperpolarized neuronal cell membrane. In addition, Ca^{2+} entry into the neuron is limited by suppression of voltage-gated calcium channels. The hyperpolarized cell membrane and the limited intracellular Ca^{2+} availability both inhibit neurotransmitter release, thereby inhibiting pain sensation.[37] Other second messengers, such as mitogen-activated protein kinases and phospholipase C, are also involved in opioid-mediated signal transduction.[37] It is now known, however, that the aforementioned events represent only a simplistic view of a highly complicated, signal transduction, which remains to be deciphered in its entirety.[39]

ENDOGENOUS OPIOIDS

Opioid peptides are endogenously produced predominantly in the central nervous system and the spinal cord.[37] The three distinct families of peptides, endorphins, enkephalins, and dynorphins, are natural agonist ligands for opioid receptors mu, delta, and kappa, respectively (**Table 12.1**).[35] Each family of opioid peptides is derived from a distinct precursor molecule, with pro-opiomelanocortin, proenkephalin, and prodynorphin being precursors of endorphins, enkephalins, and dynorphins, respectively. Of the relatively newly discovered endogenous opioid-related peptides, endomorphin-1 and -2 are selective, potent mu-receptor agonists that demonstrate a significant degree of analgesic activity.[42, 43] Endomorphin-1 at equianalgesic doses appears to cause less severe respiratory depression compared with other mu agonists,[43] suggesting that it may act on specific mu receptor subtypes.[44] Another notable endogenous peptide orphanin NQ/nociceptin, a ligand to receptor

Table 12.1 Binding characteristics of endogenous peptides.[10, 37, 40, 41]

Peptides	mu	Delta	kappa
Beta-endorphin	+++	+++	+
[Leu5]enkephalin	++	+++	
[Met5]enkephalin	++	+++	
Dynorphin A	+	++	++
Dynorphin B	+	+	+++
Alpha-neoendorphin	+	+	+++
Beta-neoendorphin		+	+++
Endomorphin-1	+++	+	
Endomorphin-2	+++	++	
Orphanin/nociceptin	(binds ORL-1 receptor)		

ORL-1, plays a complex role in producing analgesia and is being investigated.[45]

CLASSIFICATION OF OPIOID COMPOUNDS USED FOR ANALGESIA

The term opioid refers to opium-related compounds and is broadly used to describe all chemical compounds, including natural, semisynthetic, and synthetic, which act on opioid receptors. The most commonly clinically used opioid, morphine, is a naturally occurring alkaloid purified from opium, a substance obtained from poppy seeds.

Pure agonists

Opioids that bind to the receptor to produce a potent biological response are described as pure agonists.

- Alkaloids (also semisynthetic alkaloids):
  - phenanthrene derivatives: morphine, hydromorphone, oxymorphone, oxycodone, hydrocodone, heroin.
- Synthetic opioids:
  - phenylpiperidine derivatives: fentanyl and congeners, pethidine (meperidine);
  - diphenylheptanes: methadone and its congeners;
  - morphinans: levorphanol.

Partial agonists

Compounds in this class bind to the receptor with great affinity; however, the stimulated response is not as potent as that with a pure agonist. In fact, if administered with a pure agonist, such a chemical acts as a competitive antagonist that blocks the effect of a pure agonist.

- Semi-synthetic alkaloids:
  - phenanthrene derivatives: codeine, dihydrocodeine.
- Synthetic opioids:
  - diphenylheptanes: dextropropoxyphene;
  - other: tramadol (also exerts analgesic effect by inhibition of monoamine reuptake).[46]

Agonist–antagonists

The existence of different types of opioid receptors, i.e. the mu, delta, and kappa receptors, makes the concept of an agonist–antagonist possible. These compounds are agonists to one type of opioid receptor, while an antagonist to another type. As an example, drugs in this class antagonize mu receptors, but act as agonists at kappa receptors.

- Semisynthetic:
  - phenanthrene derivatives: nalbuphine;
  - thebaine derivatives: buprenorphine.
- Synthetic:
  - benzomorphan derivatives: pentazocine, dezocine;
  - morphinan derivatives: butorphanol.

Pure antagonists

Compounds in this category bind to opioid receptors, but do not produce biological activity. Currently, antagonists in clinical use are:

- synthetic chemicals:
  - permeable to the blood–brain barrier: naloxone, naltrexone, nalmefene (derived from chemical modification of oxymorphone);
  - impermeable to the blood–brain barrier: methylnaltrexone bromide, alvimopan[47, 48] (these compounds antagonize only the peripheral effects of opioids, while preserving centrally mediated analgesia).

PHARMACOLOGICAL EFFECTS OF OPIOIDS

This section describes the general pharmacological effects of opioids.[37] For the most part, the effects produced by the most commonly used opioid, morphine, are described.

Central nervous system

ANALGESIA

Opioids induce analgesia while maintaining consciousness and without affecting other sensations. Opioids reduce both the sensory and the affective components of pain. When administered for analgesia in therapeutic doses, other affective responses to pain also improve, with the subject experiencing less discomfort and distress. The other important effects associated with analgesia are euphoria and drowsiness. The clinical effect of morphine is distinct in the presence and absence of pain. In individuals without pain, opioid administration sometimes results in dysphoria and an unpleasant feeling associated with nausea and vomiting, drowsiness, and reduced physical and mental activity. A continuous dull aching pain is more easily treated with morphine. However, with higher doses, sharp, intermittent pain, such as that experienced in a colic, may also be treated (however, morphine itself may induce colic). Although all three opioid receptors, mu, delta, and kappa, mediate the analgesic action, the mu receptor agonists are more commonly available for use in a clinical setting.

Since the analgesic action of opioids is mediated by receptors present in the central nervous system, the drugs need to permeate the blood–brain barrier. Morphine and most clinically used opioids act predominantly on mu-opioid receptors and do cross the blood–brain barrier. Delta-opioid agonists are also potent analgesics, however, most need to be administered intraspinally to allow access to the sites within central nervous system. Chemical modifications to delta-opioid agonists have resulted in improved blood–brain barrier permeability.[49, 50] An added incentive to further develop delta agonists as analgesic agents for clinical use is their reduced dependence potential compared to mu-receptor agonists.[51]

AFFECTIVE CHANGES

Effects such as euphoria, tranquility, and other mood alterations are stimulated by morphine. Dysphoria may be experienced when opioids are used in the absence of pain. Dysphoria is also observed with kappa-opioid agonists.

SEDATION

Drowsiness and reduced mentation are common effects of opioids. Morphine disrupts the REM (rapid eye movement) and the non-REM components of sleep. The sedative effect is more pronounced in the elderly than in the younger individuals. There is no associated amnesia.

RESPIRATORY SYSTEM

The direct effect of morphine and morphine-like drugs on the brainstem respiratory centers results in respiratory depression. The reduced respiration is characterized by reduced rate and tidal volume. The mechanism is reduced responsiveness of respiratory centers to accumulating carbon dioxide. Respiratory depression occurs rapidly when more lipophilic opioids are administered.[37] This being said, respiratory depression is not often observed with therapeutic doses of morphine and may be observed with clinical conditions, such as renal dysfunction, that allow accumulation of active metabolites.[7]

COUGH

Morphine and related compounds act on the cough center in the medulla to depress cough. The cough-suppressive activity is independent of the respiratory depression produced by opioids. The effect of cough suppression is greatest with compounds such as codeine and a dextrorotatory compound of levorphanol (dextromethorphan).

NAUSEA AND VOMITING

Morphine stimulates receptors in the chemoreceptor trigger zone in the area postrema of the medulla. The symptoms are very obvious in ambulatory patients with nausea seen in 40 percent and vomiting in 15 percent of patients. Morphine increases vestibular sensitivity and explains the higher incidence of these symptoms in ambulatory patients. Morphine and other opioids may stimulate increased feeding at lower doses than those used for analgesia consistent with the stimulating effect of endogenous opioids on feeding.[52]

MIOSIS

Morphine and other opioids produce the classic pinpoint pupils by an excitatory action on the parasympathetic nerve innervating the pupil. Tolerance does not develop to this pharmacological effect. Morphine lowers intraocular tension both in normal and glaucomatous eyes.

NEUROENDOCRINE EFFECTS

Morphine inhibits release of gonadotropin-releasing hormone, corticotropin-releasing factor, thus decreasing circulating levels of luteinizing hormone (LH), follicle-stimulating hormone (FSH), adrenocorticotropic hormone (ACTH), and beta-endorphin, which in turn results in reduced formation of testosterone and cortisol. Mu-agonists stimulate release of prolactin, probably via dopaminergic mechanism. Antidiuretic hormone (ADH) release is also stimulated. However, chronic use of mu-agonists results in tolerance to these effects and therefore may not be bothersome in cancer patients being chronically treated with opioids.

INCREASED MUSCULAR TONE

An increased tone in the large truncal muscles and other alterations in muscular activity are observed with opioid treatment. This effect appears to be mediated through the central nervous system. Rapid parenteral administration of highly lipid-soluble agents, such as fentanyl, is known to cause an increased muscular rigidity and a reduction in thoracic compliance.[37, 53]

Cardiovascular system

Morphine produces vasodilation, reduced peripheral resistance, and reduced sensitivity of baroreflex. This results in orthostatic hypotension. These effects may be partly mediated by the released histamine and possible depression of the vasomotor center. However, the response of histamine release may not be observed consistently.[54]

Gastrointestinal system

STOMACH

Although the direct effect of morphine on parietal cells is stimulation of acid secretion, in an organism, morphine treatment causes decreased acid secretion mediated through increased secretion of somatostatin and a reduced secretion of acetylcholine.[55] Morphine also causes increased gastric retention and decreased gastric motility.

SMALL INTESTINE

Morphine increases the resting tone of the intestinal smooth muscle. The nonpropulsive contractions are also increased. Morphine reduces biliary, pancreatic, and intestinal secretions.

LARGE INTESTINE

Similar to small intestine, morphine increases the nonpropulsive contractions and decreases the propulsive peristaltic waves leading to increased transit time in the gut. These effects then lead to constipation.

BILIARY TRACT

Morphine causes constriction of sphincter of Oddi and an increased pressure in the common bile duct.

Renal system

Mu agonists in high doses reduce urine formation by reducing renal plasma flow caused by reduced blood pressure. Increased tone of bladder and ureteral muscle is also observed. This pharmacological action may lead to urinary retention. Kappa agonists on the other hand appear to cause a diuretic effect. The action of opioids on renal function is complex as opioids also stimulate release of ADH.[56]

Skin

Morphine in therapeutic doses causes cutaneous vasodilation, especially in the face, neck, and the upper thorax. The sweating and pruritus associated with systemic morphine administration is partly attributable to the accompanying histamine release. Pruritus is a more common occurrence with intraspinal opioid administration compared to that with systemic administration.

Immune system

Overall, the effects of morphine and opioids on the immune system may be described as suppressive. Not all opioids cause immunosuppression.[57, 58, 59] The mechanism of this action is not very clear and may be mediated by the effects of morphine on the sympathetic nervous system and the hypothalamopituitary axis. Although administering opioids to cancer patients may seem harmful due to the effects on immunity, it is the untreated pain that may actually cause more immunosuppression.[60] It is also important to note that immunosuppression is more of an issue with acute administration rather than chronic administration, probably due to tolerance to the effect.[57]

ADVERSE EFFECTS OF OPIOIDS

The common adverse effects of opioids include constipation, sedation, nausea, vomiting, dry mouth, and myoclonus. Other less frequent adverse effects, nevertheless bothersome, include symptoms like delirium, confusion, weakness, flushing, sweating, urinary hesitancy, disturbed sleep, hyperalgesia, and dysphoria.[37, 61] The pathophysiology and the management of several of these effects are discussed in detail in Chapter 14, Clinical pharmacology of opioids: adverse effects of opioids.

Specific adverse effects with long-term opioid use are tolerance, physical dependence, and addiction. Fear of experiencing these adverse effects, in both the healthcare workers and the patients, often leads to undertreatment of malignant pain.[62] Approaching the management of cancer pain with the knowledge of the clinical relevance and implications of these effects will result in optimal use of opioids and prevent unnecessary pain and suffering.

Tolerance

Tolerance is a commonly observed physiological effect associated with prolonged opioid use. It is defined as a state of adaptation in which exposure to opioids induce changes that result in a diminution of one or more of the medication's effects over time.[63] Tolerance is thus characterized by a shortened duration of action, a higher-dose requirement for the same intensity of a pharmacologic effect, and a significant increase in the lethal dose.[64]

The degree of tolerance differs for different pharmacological effects of morphine and may suggest involvement of different mu-receptor subtypes.[25, 65] Tolerance develops to effects such as analgesia, respiratory depression, nausea, vomiting, antidiuresis, sedation, and euphoria, while it does not develop to effects such as constipation and miosis.[65] Tolerance to respiratory depression develops rapidly and also is reversed rapidly. Patients who have been medicated with opioids on a chronic basis almost never experience respiratory depression.[7] Tolerance to the analgesic effect of a mu-receptor agonist is encountered occasionally in spite of escalating the agonist dose. Switching treatment to a different mu-receptor agonist in such a situation is shown to restore analgesia even at lower doses, suggesting that tolerance between various mu-receptor agonists is incomplete. The phenomenon of incomplete cross-tolerance may be explained by the binding of various mu-receptor agonists only to specific mu-receptor subtypes.[25, 26, 27, 65]

Mechanisms such as mu receptor down-regulation, cAMP system up-regulation, and uncoupling of mu receptor with the second messenger systems have been proposed to lead to opioid tolerance.[66, 67] Other mechanisms, such as activation of delta receptor and N-methyl-D-aspartic acid (NMDA) receptor, and nitric oxide release, also induce opioid tolerance.[20, 68]

Development of tolerance to analgesia has not been described as a major problem with chronic opioid use in cancer patients.[8, 69] Very often, adequate analgesia is maintained over prolonged periods without a significant change in dose. Some of the more common causes that result in inadequate analgesic effects of an established opioid dose include disease progression and psychological causes, rather than tolerance development.[64] If, however, tolerance is determined to be the cause of inadequate analgesia, it should be managed by either increasing the opioid dose or by changing to a different opioid (opioid switching).

Physical dependence

Physical dependence due to repeated opioid use is defined as a state of adaptation that is manifested as a withdrawal syndrome that can be produced by abrupt cessation, rapid dose reduction, decreasing blood level of the opioids, and/or administration of an antagonist.[63] The withdrawal syndrome is characterized by increased pain sensitivity, irritability, dysphoria, anxiety, and insomnia. The mechanism of this phenomenon is not clearly understood, but may be mediated by a rebound increase in cyclic AMP and increased activity of adenyly cyclase.[70]

In cancer patients who achieve pain relief by other nonpharmacological modalities and eventually reduce or discontinue opioids, the dose can be systematically reduced gradually to prevent experience of withdrawal symptoms.[71] A supervised management of the opioid discontinuation should preclude the phenomenon of withdrawal. Physical dependence should be of little concern in terminal cancer patients. Thus, the concern of developing opioid dependence should not interfere with opioid use for analgesia in cancer patients.

Addiction

Addiction is defined as a primary, chronic, neurobiologic disease, with genetic, psychosocial, and environmental factors influencing its development and manifestations. Addiction to opioids results from chronic opioid use and is characterized by one or more of the following: impaired control over medication use, compulsive use, continued use despite harm, and craving.[63] Addiction appears to be mediated by pathological mechanisms distinct from those of tolerance and dependence, which are physiological effects. Addiction in cancer patients being chronically treated with opioids is extremely rare, reported to be between 0 to 8 percent, and the fear of opioid addiction should not impede opioid use for cancer pain relief.[8, 72]

THERAPEUTIC USE OF OPIOIDS IN CANCER

Mild to moderate pain

As per the recommendations by the WHO, weaker opioids (step 2) such as codeine, dihydrocodeine, dextropropoxyphene, and tramadol, are used in combination with nonopioid analgesics for mild to moderate pain.

CODEINE

Codeine is a naturally found alkaloid of opium with mu-receptor affinity, although the agonistic activity is significantly lower than morphine. Codeine also acts as an agonist at the delta and kappa receptors.

Pharmacokinetics

Codeine is metabolized in the liver by cytochrome P450 enzyme CYP2D6, with 6–15 percent being biotransformed to morphine.[37] When administered orally at 30–60 mg, the duration of analgesic action is four to six hours. The plasma half-life is short at two to four hours. Thus, using codeine for analgesia requires consuming it three to four times times a day.

Pharmacodynamics

The analgesic activity of codeine is dependent on its biotransformation to morphine. Genetic polymorphisms for the metabolizing enzyme, CYP2D6, results in inability to produce analgesic effect with codeine and is seen in 10 percent of the Caucasian population.[73] Codeine also has antitussive activity, which may involve distinct receptors that bind codeine itself.

Side effects

Codeine commonly produces side effects such as constipation, nausea, vomiting, and drowsiness. Other less common effects such as tachycardia, hypotension, lightheadedness, and urinary retention are also observed. In therapeutic doses, it is less likely to produce adverse effects compared to morphine, however.

Routes of administration/formulations

Codeine is available as oral medication in combination with ibuprofen and paracetamol (acetaminophen).

Use in cancer pain

Codeine is used only for mild cancer pain as its analgesic action on mu receptors is significantly weaker than that of morphine.[37]

TRAMADOL

Tramadol is a synthetic analog of codeine, a weak mu-receptor agonist (affinity 1/6000 that of morphine), and a weaker agonist for delta and kappa receptor. It is distinct from other mu-receptor agonists in that it also inhibits the reuptake of serotonin and norepinephrine, thereby enhancing the activity of descending inhibitory pain pathway and inhibiting transmission of painful stimuli in the dorsal horn of spinal cord.[46] Thus, tramadol-induced analgesia is not completely reversible by naloxone.

Pharmacokinetics

Tramadol is 68 percent bioavailable after oral administration.[74] It is metabolized by the liver and mostly excreted by the kidney. Similar to codeine, cytochrome P450 enzyme CYP2D6 enzyme is required for the biotransformation of tramadol to its active metabolite M1(O-desmethyltramadol).[75] The duration of analgesia is about six hours. The elimination half-life is six hours, which increases with hepatic and renal insufficiency.

Pharmacodynamics

Tramadol produces mild analgesia, as it is a partial agonist. The O-demethylated metabolite, M1, is two to four times potent as the parent drug.[37, 76]

Side effects

Commonly observed side effects with tramadol use are nausea, vomiting, dizziness, dry mouth, sedation, headache, and orthostatic hypotension. Respiratory depression occurs less frequently than that experienced with equianalgesic morphine dose, except when administered in renal failure. Also, constipation is less than that seen with equianalgesic dose of codeine. Tramadol can cause seizures, especially in patients with predisposing conditions.

Routes of administration/formulations

Tramadol is available as capsules, soluble tablets, suppositories, and intramuscular and intravenous injections in the USA. The usual oral dose is 50–100 mg per four to six hours in adults. The maximum recommended daily dose is 400 mg. Extended release formulations are also available in USA and some European countries.[77, 78]

Use in cancer pain

Tramadol is used in step 2 of the analgesic ladder treating only mild–moderate pain. It is sometimes effective in treating severe pain.[77, 79] Tramadol forms an alternative for patients who experience bothersome side effects of opioids, such as sedation and constipation.[77] Additionally, it is determined to have minimum physical dependence and abuse potential compared to other opioids.[80] It is also useful in treating neuropathic pain.[81]

Moderate to severe pain

According to the WHO guidelines, strong opioids (step 3) are used to treat pain of high intensity, which does not respond to nonopioid or weak opioid drugs or their combinations.

MORPHINE

Morphine is considered the prototype opioid drug to which other opioid drugs are compared and is the most commonly used opioid. It is a naturally occurring alkaloid extracted from poppy seeds. Morphine is a potent mu-receptor agonist with low kappa-receptor binding and extremely low delta-receptor binding.[37]

Pharmacokinetics

Morphine is readily absorbed from the gastrointestinal tract. The bioavailability of morphine after oral administration is approximately 25 percent due to its high first-pass metabolism. The onset of analgesic activity after an oral administration is observed at one hour, with the duration of action at four to five hours. The onset of action after a parenteral administration is observed by 15–30 minutes, while the peak effect is observed at 45–90 minutes. The elimination half-life of morphine is 1.7–4.5 hours with normal renal function. Morphine does not permeate the blood–brain barrier easily, due to its hydrophilicity, its presence in an ionized form at a physiological pH, and its protein binding. However, to achieve an analgesic effect, an adequate cerebrospinal fluid (CSF) morphine concentration must be reached. Thus, slower transport across the blood–brain barrier may be responsible for the delay in action observed even with a parenteral morphine administration. When administered intrathecally, delayed side effects may be observed because morphine, unlike some highly lipophilic opioid compounds, is not absorbed locally in the nervous tissue. The delayed effects of morphine on supraspinal respiratory centers may be observed even 24 hours following intrathecal administration.

Morphine is metabolized in the liver and in the extrahepatic tissues like the kidneys mainly through glucuronization. About 75–85 percent of morphine is converted to morphine-3-glucuronide and about 5–10 percent is converted to morphine-6-glucuronide. Morphine is rapidly conjugated as suggested by a ten-fold increase in morphine conjugates compared to the unchanged compound within 90 minutes of administration. Other metabolites are by-products of N-demethylation and N-dealkylation. The glucuronide metabolites are predominantly excreted by kidneys and therefore may accumulate in patients with renal disease and may have prolonged adverse effects.[82] About 10 percent of metabolites are excreted in the feces. Of the two major pharmacologically active metabolites, morphine-6-glucuronide produces agonist effects at mu receptors.[83] Morphine-3-glucuronide, on the other hand, antagonizes morphine action and produces hyperalgesia and central nervous system excitability.

Pharmacodynamics

Morphine is effective against both visceral and somatic pain, unlike other nonopioid analgesics that affect only somatic pain. In humans, morphine produces analgesia, euphoria, sedation, and mental clouding. Morphine (and other analgesic opioids) not only reduces the pain sensation, but also changes the affective response to pain, whereby the anxiety and fear of pain is reduced. This may elevate the threshold of pain and increase patients' ability to tolerate pain. When administered in the absence of pain, morphine causes dysphoria instead of euphoria (see Pharmacological effects of opioids). Morphine-6-glucuronide, which is a potent analgesic metabolite of morphine also contributes to the analgesia.

Side effects

The common adverse effects with morphine use are nausea, vomiting, constipation, and sedation.[37] Other effects, such as dryness of mouth and myoclonus, have also been reported to be common.[84] Adverse effects associated with chronic opioid use such as tolerance, physical dependence, and addiction may be observed in cancer patients. These effects can be managed effectively, however, and the concern of developing them should not prevent adequate opioid use in cancer pain.

Routes of administration/formulations

Therapeutically used morphine is available as a sulfate, a tartarate, and a hydrochloride. It is available for both oral and parenteral use. Oral preparations are available as an elixir, immediate-release tablets, controlled-release tablets, and controlled release suspensions. Parenteral preparations are available for intravenous, intramuscular, subcutaneous, epidural, and intrathecal use.

Use in cancer pain

Morphine has been considered a gold standard in the treatment of cancer pain. Oral morphine has been described as an appropriate first choice for management of moderate to severe cancer pain.[85] Use of morphine has been associated with satisfactory analgesia in cancer patients over 80 percent of the time.[8] Not surprisingly, most clinical studies testing newer opioids in cancer pain compare the efficacy to that of morphine. Newer formulations of morphine that allow less frequent dosing, compared to immediate-release morphine preparations that have to be administered three to four times a day, have had a significant impact on improving effective analgesia and patient adherence.[86, 87, 88] Oral administration is relatively inexpensive and easy to titrate and several long-acting oral morphine formulations are available. The dose should be titrated individually based on adequate analgesia since there is a large interpersonal variability in morphine pharmacokinetics.[89] Unlike nociceptive pain, morphine is not very effective in neuropathic pain, which results from damage to neural tissue. Morphine therapy can be initiated as the prescribed minimum dose and titrated upwards without concern of a ceiling effect, while monitoring adverse effects.

BUPRENORPHINE

Buprenorphine is a low-molecular-weight, lipophilic, semisynthetic agonist–antagonist. Its lipid solubility is very high compared to morphine due to its two nonpolar side chains. It has a high affinity for mu receptors, but a mixed activity at the kappa-receptor subtypes.[90, 91]

Pharmacokinetics

When administered orally, a low bioavailability (<20 percent) of buprenorphine is demonstrated due to strong first-pass effect.[92] Therefore, although absorbed well, it is not the preferred route of administration. Bioavailability with the sublingual route is 30–55 percent. With intranasal administration the bioavailability was found to be 70–90 percent in an animal model; however, the intranasal formulations are not available for clinical use as yet.[93] Use of a buprenorphine transdermal patch is emerging as a preferred route of administration,[94, 95] since the transdermal route significantly improves biovailability. Buprenorphine exhibits a high volume of distribution because of high lipid solubility. It easily crosses the blood–brain barrier. It is metabolized in the liver and intestinal wall by dealkylation followed by glucuronization. The dealkylation produces an active metabolite, norbuprenorphine.[92] About 70 percent of the buprenorphine is excreted via bile and the rest is excreted via kidneys. Duration of effect is six to nine hours due to slow receptor dissociation of the drug.

Pharmacodynamics

This partial agonist has 25–30 times stronger affinity towards mu receptors than that of morphine.[92] The high affinity to mu receptor, but a submaximal analgesic response compared to morphine, makes buprenorphine a partial agonist. Buprenorphine produces the same pharmacological effects as morphine and include analgesia, euphoria, respiratory depression, and dependence. While buprenorphine is an antagonist at the kappa-2 receptor, which reduces dysphoria, it is an agonist at the kappa-1 and kappa-3 receptor, which further potentiates analgesia.[91, 96] Buprenorphine has only a weak affinity for delta receptors and may cause a reduced "high" feeling.[96]

Side effects

The most common systemic adverse drug reactions observed are nausea, dizziness, vomiting, constipation, and tiredness.[94] Buprenorphine causes less constipation, respiratory depression, tolerance, and dependence compared to morphine, but more dizziness, nausea, and vomiting.[92]

Routes of administration/formulations

Buprenorphine is available for sublingual, intravenous, intramuscular, epidural, and transdermal use.

Use in cancer pain

Buprenorphine plays an important role in cancer patients unable to take oral medication. Buprenorphine clinically tested as a transdermal patch has been shown to be highly efficacious in cancer patients with moderate to severe pain and pain unresponsive to nonopioid analgesics.[94, 95, 97] Opioid switching from weak opioids or low doses of step 3 opioids to transdermal buprenorphine did not precipitate withdrawal symptoms or did not antagonize pain relief.[95] The important pharmacodynamic issue for chronic treatment of pain with opioids is development of tolerance. In a long-term clinical study, a low incidence of tolerance was observed with use of buprenorphine patches.[97] Analgesia with the patch in the same study was rated as at least satisfactory by 90 percent of patients and was assessed as user friendly by 94.6 percent of patients. Transdermal buprenorphine was also well tolerated. When switching of opioids is indicated to improve pain relief or reduce adverse events, equipotency dosage ratios for morphine to buprenorphine may be used.[95] Transdermal buprenorphine has superior safety with respect to respiratory depression, immunological, and renal effects compared with standard WHO step-3 opioids, which makes it highly suitable for treating moderate-to-severe pain in cancer patients.[95]

FENTANYL

Fentanyl is a highly lipid-soluble, low-molecular-weight, synthetic mu-receptor agonist of the phenylpiperidine class and is 100 times as potent as morphine. The congener drugs, such as sufentanil and alfentanil, have a similar spectrum of pharmacodynamics and pharmacokinetics.

Pharmacokinetics

Following intravenous fentanyl administration, a rapid onset of action within five minutes (rapidly crosses the blood–brain barrier) is seen with the duration of effect at one to two hours and elimination half-life of 3–12 hours. Since fentanyl is a highly lipophilic drug, when administered intrathecally, it is absorbed in the local neural tissue producing localized and segmental analgesia.[37] Fentanyl undergoes hepatic metabolism to form inactive metabolites that are excreted by the kidneys.

Pharmacodynamics

The analgesic effects of fentanyl and other similar drugs are analogous to those of morphine, although are significantly more potent. (Fentanyl is 100 times as potent and sufentanil is 1000 times as potent as morphine.)

Side effects

Nausea, vomiting, and itching are observed as with other mu agonists. Muscular rigidity is seen when administered as an intravenous bolus. Respiratory depression is also a common side effect. Delayed respiratory depression occurs, however, only with prolonged infusions or larger doses.

Routes of administration/formulations

Fentanyl may be administered through an intravenous, intrathecal, epidural, transdermal, or transmucosal (oral mucosa) route.

Use in cancer pain

The more commonly used routes for chronic cancer pain are transdermal, epidural, and intrathecal, while that for breakthrough and incident cancer pain is a transmucosal route.[89, 98, 99, 100] Since commonly available analgesics are not effective in relieving breakthrough pain rapidly, the oral transmucosal fentanyl citrate (OTFC) or fentanyl buccal tablet (FBT) are ideal for producing a rapid analgesic effect (within 5–15 minutes) and have been demonstrated to be very safe and effective.[89, 98, 99] The transdermal fentanyl patch used for chronic pain is also well-tolerated, safe, and efficacious.[89, 98]

METHADONE

Methadone is a lipophilic long-acting synthetic mu-receptor agonist and also an NMDA-receptor antagonist.[101]

Pharmacokinetics

Methadone is well absorbed from the gastrointestinal tract and reaches peak concentration in the plasma by four hours.[37] In contrast to morphine it has high bioavailability after oral administration at approximately 75 percent.[102] About 90 percent of methadone is bound to plasma proteins, which results in low hepatic extraction. Peak concentrations in the brain are observed within one to two hours of parenteral administration, which coincide with the analgesic effect. The drug undergoes biotransformation in the liver by a process of N-demethylation and forms inactive metabolites.[37] Methadone continues to accumulate in the tissues with repeated administration due to its high protein binding and its long terminal half-life of 15–55 hours.[37, 103]

Pharmacodynamics

Methadone has excellent analgesic properties. It shows consistent analgesic effects with tolerance developing relatively slowly compared to that with morphine. Methadone shows incomplete cross-tolerance to other mu agonists. A prolonged miotic and respiratory depression activity is seen after a single dose even at 24 hours.

Side effects

Overall adverse effects are similar to those observed with morphine treatment.[104] Adverse effects seen with long-term administration are excessive sweating, lymphocytosis, and increased concentration of prolactin, albumin, and globulins.[37]

Routes of administration/formulations

Methadone is available for oral, rectal, and parenteral administration.

Use in cancer pain

Methadone is not different from morphine as a first line of treatment, with methadone and morphine showing similar analgesia and similar spectrum of adverse effects.[104, 105] Methadone is commonly used for switching from other opioids with encouraging results.[61, 106, 107, 108] Methadone shows a significant interpersonal variability in the pharmacokinetics and the pharmacokinetic–pharmacodynamic relationship of the drug.[109] The treatment with methadone should therefore be initiated with smaller doses and titrated against the analgesic requirement. In addition, accumulation of the drug due to high protein binding and long half-life may cause delayed severe adverse effects. The drug should therefore be used under the supervision of experienced clinicians. Methadone may also be useful in treating neuropathic pain.[110, 111]

OXYCODONE

Oxycodone is a strong opioid belonging to the phenanthrene group of drugs and possesses morphine-like analgesic potency.

Pharmacokinetics

The drug has a good bioavailability compared to morphine at 50–70 percent. Its half-life is two to three hours and the duration of action is four to five hours. The drug is demethylated in the liver to form oxymorphone, which is the active metabolite, and is catalyzed by the enzyme P450-2D6.[112]

Pharmacodynamics

The analgesic effect of oxycodone is comparable to morphine. Other actions of oxycodone are also similar to a typical mu agonist. When used spinally, oxycodone is significantly less potent compared to morphine.

Side effects

The side effects are similar to those seen with other strong mu-opioid agonists.

Routes of administration/formulations

Oxycodone may be administered orally, rectally, subcutaneously, or parenterally. An oral controlled release formulation allows twice daily dosing which is more acceptable than the four times daily dose to maintain analgesia.

Use in cancer pain

Oxycodone is considered as potent as morphine for treating moderate to severe cancer-related pain.[113, 114] Higher bioavailability compared to morphine may be an advantage for oral opioid treatment of chronic cancer pain.[112, 115]

OXYMORPHONE

Oxymorphone is a semisynthetic mu opioid agonist. It is more lipid-soluble than morphine, but has a much lower lipid solubility compared to fentanyl.

Pharmacokinetics

After an oral dose, only 10 percent of the drug is bioavailable. Protein binding of oxymorphone is 20–40 percent. The half-life is seven to nine hours, which is longer than that of morphine. Oxymorphone undergoes extensive hepatic and intestinal metabolism via glucuronization and reduction of keto-group.[116] The reduced metabolite 6-OH-oxymorphone may have analgesic activity as well.[116]

Pharmacodynamics

Oxymorphone produces similar pharmacological effects as other mu agonists. It binds delta receptor with significantly higher affinity than morphine.[117] The affinity for mu and delta receptor is advantageous as the analgesic actions are potentiated.[117] It is approximately eight-fold more potent than morphine on intramuscular administration.[118]

Side effects

Overall, the side effects are similar to those seen with other mu-opioid receptor agonists.

Routes of administration/formulations

Oral tablets are available as sustained-release and immediate-release formulations. Formulations are also available for subcutaneous, intravenous, and rectal use.

Use in cancer pain

When evaluated for moderate to severe pain, extended release preparation of oxymorphone showed similar efficacy and side effects spectrum as that with controlled release (CR) morphine or CR oxycodone. However, the extended release oxymorphone-treated group needed less treatment for breakthrough pain.[119]

HYDROMORPHONE

Hydromorphone is a pure opioid agonist, which is more potent than morphine.

Pharmacokinetics

Hydromorphone is very lipid soluble, with a half-life of 1.5–3 hours and a duration of action of three to four hours.[64]

Pharmacodynamics

The pharmacological effects are similar to morphine and other mu agonists.

Side effects

The adverse effects with hydromorphone are similar to those of morphine.

Routes of administration/formulations

Hydromorphone is available for oral, rectal, subcutaneous, intravenous, intramuscular, and spinal administration.

Use in cancer pain

Hydromorphone is a potent alternative to morphine. A slow release preparation is more convenient to use and has potency similar to the immediate-release preparation.[64]

LEVORPHANOL

Levorphanol is a strong opioid and is the only commercially available morphinan agonist.

Pharmacokinetics

Levorphanol has a long half-life (12–16 hours), but a short duration of action (four to six hours).[120] It is a useful alternative to morphine, but must be used cautiously to prevent accumulation. Similar to morphine, levorphanol undergoes glucuronidization in the liver, and the glucuronidated products are excreted in the kidney.

Pharmacodynamics

The strong analgesia produced by levorphanol is mediated via its interactions with mu-, delta-, and kappa-opioid receptors. Levorphanol may act through other mechanisms, such as NMDA receptor antagonism and inhibition of reuptake of norepinephrine and serotonin.[121, 122]

Side effect

Accumulation of the drug with repeated dosing may cause excessive sedation.

Routes of administration/formulations

Levorphanol can be given orally, intravenously, and subcutaneously.

Use in cancer pain

It is considered a step 3 opioid by the WHO and has a greater potency than morphine. Levorphanol represents a useful medication for patients who are unable to tolerate morphine and methadone.[123] Levorphanol also demonstrates efficacy in treating neuropathic pain.[124]

PETHIDINE

Pethidine is a phenylpiperidine derivative and is a mu agonist and also an agonist at kappa receptors. In addition, it possesses local anesthetic activity and atropine-like activity.[125]

Pharmacokinetics

It has a relatively short elimination half-life of two to four hours and duration of action of two to three hours. It is metabolized in the liver to norpethidine and is excreted by the kidneys.

Pharmacodynamics

It is 1/10th as potent as morphine. The metabolite is half as potent as the parent drug as an analgesic.[125]

Side effects

Accumulation of the metabolite, pethidine, especially in renal impairment, causes central nervous system excitability, muscle fasciculations, involuntary movements, and seizures.

Routes of administration/formulations

Pethidine is available for oral and parenteral use.

Use in cancer pain

Due to toxicity of the metabolites, this drug should not be used for chronic cancer pain since safer alternatives are available. Intrathecal administration of pethidine has been used in cases of intractable cancer pain in advanced stages of the disease.[126, 127] The toxicity due to metabolite accumulation is also seen with intrathecal use.

Mixed agonists–antagonists

Opioids in this group – pentazocine, nalbuphine, butorphanol – are agonists at kappa receptors, but are weak antagonists at mu receptors. These drugs show a range of analgesic efficacy with pentazocine producing weak analgesia similar to paracetamol, nalbuphine being as potent as morphine, while butorphanol with analgesic efficacy significantly higher than that of morphine.[128] When these drugs are administered to patients being treated with mu-agonist opioids, the analgesic effects are reversed and withdrawal symptoms are induced.[37, 128, 129] Additionally, the psychomimetic adverse effects due to kappa agonistic activity and the ceiling effect for analgesia make them unsuitable for use in cancer pain. Therefore, these drugs are not commonly used for the treatment of cancer pain.

Opioid antagonists

The primary indication for use of opioid antagonists in cancer patients is for reversing opioid-induced adverse effects.

NALOXONE

Naloxone is a competitive opioid antagonist at mu, delta, and kappa receptors. It is the drug of choice to reverse acute adverse effects of opioids, such as respiratory depression. Since the bioavailability of naloxone is very poor due to high first-pass metabolism, it is administered subcutaneously or intramuscularly. It is a short-acting compound (one to two hours); therefore, repeated injections may be required to reverse the adverse effect. Using higher doses for reversing opioid adverse effects may precipitate withdrawal and reversal of analgesia. Therefore, in adults, lower titration doses of 0.04–0.08 mg intravenously should be used initially.

NALTREXONE

Naltrexone is a long-acting antagonist at mu, delta, and kappa receptors. Its half-life is four to ten hours. It is available as an oral preparation and is commonly used to treat opioid abuse.

NALMEFENE

Nalmefene is also a long-acting antagonist with a half-life of eight to eleven hours. The duration of action is eight hours.[130] The long-acting antagonists should not be used in cancer patients as they may precipitate withdrawal and pain.

Newer antagonist compounds

Newer opioid antagonists are designed such that they cannot permeate the blood–brain barrier and thus reverse only the peripheral opioid effects, while retaining the central analgesic effects of opioids. These compounds, methylnaltrexone and alvimopan, are being investigated for use in reversing opioid-induced constipation.[131, 132]

SUMMARY

Opioid analgesics exhibit a wide range of pharmacokinetic and pharmacodynamic characteristics and are available in several controlled-release formulations. Thus, choosing an appropriate opioid for managing various presentations of cancer pain is definitely possible. A constant assessment of the balance between opioid-induced analgesia and the accompanying adverse effects should be conducted to ensure proper use of opioids.

REFERENCES

1. Wool MS, Mor V. A multidimensional model for understanding cancer pain. *Cancer Investigation*. 2005; **23**: 727–34.
2. NIH State-of-the-Science Statement on Symptom Management in Cancer. Pain, depression, and fatigue. *NIH Consensus and State-of-the-Science Statements*. 2002; **19**: 1–29.
3. Foley KM. The treatment of cancer pain. *New England Journal of Medicine*. 1985; **313**: 84–95.
4. World Health Organization. *Cancer pain relief*, 2nd edn. Geneva: World Health Organization, 1996.
* 5. Mercadante S, Portenoy RK. Opioid poorly-responsive cancer pain. Part 3. Clinical strategies to improve opioid responsiveness. *Journal of Pain and Symptom Management*. 2001; **21**: 338–54.

6. Hanks GW, Twycross RG, Lloyd JW. Unexpected complication of successful nerve block. Morphine induced respiratory depression precipitated by removal of severe pain. *Anaesthesia*. 1981; **36**: 37–9.
7. Ravenscroft P, Schneider J. Bedside perspectives on the use of opioids: transferring results of clinical research into practice. *Clinical and Experimental Pharmacology and Physiology*. 2000; **27**: 529–32.
8. Schug SA, Zech D, Grond S *et al*. A long-term survey of morphine in cancer pain patients. *Journal of Pain and Symptom Management*. 1992; **7**: 259–66.
* 9. Mercadante S, Portenoy RK. Opioid poorly-responsive cancer pain. Part 1: clinical considerations. *Journal of Pain and Symptom Management*. 2001; **21**: 144–50.
10. Mansour A, Hoversten MT, Taylor LP *et al*. The cloned mu, delta and kappa receptors and their endogenous ligands: evidence for two opioid peptide recognition cores. *Brain Research*. 1995; **700**: 89–98.
11. Reinscheid RK, Nothacker HP, Bourson A *et al*. Orphanin FQ: a neuropeptide that activates an opioid-like G protein-coupled receptor. *Science*. 1995; **270**: 792–4.
12. Meunier JC. Nociceptin/orphanin FQ and the opioid receptor-like ORL1 receptor. *European Journal of Pharmacology*. 1997; **340**: 1–15.
13. Horan P, Tallarida RJ, Haaseth RC *et al*. Antinociceptive interactions of opioid delta receptor agonists with morphine in mice: supra- and sub-additivity. *Life Sciences*. 1992; **50**: 1535–41.
14. He L, Lee NM. Delta opioid receptor enhancement of mu opioid receptor-induced antinociception in spinal cord. *Journal of Pharmacology and Experimental Therapeutics*. 1998; **285**: 1181–6.
15. Kest B, Lee CE, McLemore GL, Inturrisi CE. An antisense oligodeoxynucleotide to the delta opioid receptor (DOR-1) inhibits morphine tolerance and acute dependence in mice. *Brain Research Bulletin*. 1996; **39**: 185–8.
16. Abdelhamid EE, Sultana M, Portoghese PS, Takemori AE. Selective blockage of delta opioid receptors prevents the development of morphine tolerance and dependence in mice. *Journal of Pharmacology and Experimental Therapeutics*. 1991; **258**: 299–303.
17. Kieffer BL, Gaveriaux-Ruff C. Exploring the opioid system by gene knockout. *Progress in Neurobiology*. 2002; **66**: 285–306.
* 18. Uhl GR, Sora I, Wang Z. The mu opiate receptor as a candidate gene for pain: polymorphisms, variations in expression, nociception, and opiate responses. *Proceedings of the National Academy of Sciences of the United States of America*. 1999; **96**: 7752–5.
19. Park HS, Lee HY, Kim YH *et al*. A highly selective kappa-opioid receptor agonist with low addictive potential and dependence liability. *Bioorganic and Medicinal Chemistry Letters*. 2006; **16**: 3609–13.
20. Ananthan S. Opioid ligands with mixed mu/delta opioid receptor interactions: an emerging approach to novel analgesics. *The AAPS Journal*. 2006; **8**: E118–25.

21. Egan TM, North RA. Both mu and delta opiate receptors exist on the same neuron. *Science.* 1981; **214**: 923–4.

22. Gomes I, Jordan BA, Gupta A *et al.* Heterodimerization of mu and delta opioid receptors: A role in opiate synergy. *Journal of Neuroscience.* 2000; **20**: RC110.

23. Cadet P. Mu opiate receptor subtypes. *Medical Science Monitor.* 2004; **10**: MS28–32.

24. Kaczor A, Matosiuk D. Non-peptide opioid receptor ligands – recent advances. Part I: agonists. *Current Medicinal Chemistry.* 2002; **9**: 1567–89.

25. Pasternak GW. Incomplete cross tolerance and multiple mu opioid peptide receptors. *Trends in Pharmacological Sciences.* 2001; **22**: 67–70.

* 26. Pasternak GW. Molecular biology of opioid analgesia. *Journal of Pain and Symptom Management.* 2005; **29**: S2–9.

27. Pan YX. Diversity and complexity of the mu opioid receptor gene: alternative pre-mRNA splicing and promoters. *DNA Cell Biology.* 2005; **24**: 736–50.

* 28. Pan L, Xu J, Yu R *et al.* Identification and characterization of six new alternatively spliced variants of the human mu opioid receptor gene, Oprm. *Neuroscience.* 2005; **133**: 209–20.

29. Rossi GC, Pan YX, Brown GP, Pasternak GW. Antisense mapping the MOR-1 opioid receptor: evidence for alternative splicing and a novel morphine-6 beta-glucuronide receptor. *FEBS Letters.* 1995; **369**: 192–6.

30. Jordan BA, Cvejic S, Devi LA. Opioids and their complicated receptor complexes. *Neuropsychopharmacology.* 2000; **23**: S5–18.

* 31. Zaki PA, Bilsky EJ, Vanderah TW *et al.* Opioid receptor types and subtypes: the delta receptor as a model. *Annual Review of Pharmacology and Toxicology.* 1996; **36**: 379–401.

32. Holden JE, Jeong Y, Forrest JM. The endogenous opioid system and clinical pain management. *AACN Clinical Issues.* 2005; **16**: 291–301.

33. Rittner HL, Machelska H, Stein C. Leukocytes in the regulation of pain and analgesia. *Journal of Leukocyte Biology.* 2005; **78**: 1215–22.

34. Pepe S, van den Brink OW, Lakatta EG, Xiao RP. Cross-talk of opioid peptide receptor and beta-adrenergic receptor signalling in the heart. *Cardiovascular Research.* 2004; **63**: 414–22.

35. Kromer W. Endogenous opioids, the enteric nervous system and gut motility. *Digestive Diseases.* 1990; **8**: 361–73.

36. Sharp BM. Multiple opioid receptors on immune cells modulate intracellular signaling. *Brain, Behavior, and Immunity.* 2006; **20**: 9–14.

37. Gutstein HB, Akil H. Opioid analgesics. In: Hardman JG, Limbird LE (eds). *Goodman and Gilman's the pharmacological basis of therapeutics,* 10th edn. New York: McGraw-Hill, 2001: 569–619.

38. Pert A, Yaksh T. Sites of morphine induced analgesia in the primate brain: relation to pain pathways. *Brain Research.* 1974; **80**: 135–40.

* 39. Law PY, Wong YH, Loh HH. Molecular mechanisms and regulation of opioid receptor signaling. *Annual Review of Pharmacology and Toxicology.* 2000; **40**: 389–430.

40. Jinsmaa Y, Fujita Y, Shiotani K *et al.* Differentiation of opioid receptor preference by [Dmt1]endomorphin-2-mediated antinociception in the mouse. *European Journal of Pharmacology.* 2005; **509**: 37–42.

41. Jinsmaa Y, Marczak E, Fujita Y *et al.* Potent *in vivo* antinociception and opioid receptor preference of the novel analogue [Dmt(1)]endomorphin-1. *Pharmacology, Biochemistry, and Behavior.* 2006; **84**: 252–8.

42. Horvath G. Endomorphin-1 and endomorphin-2: pharmacology of the selective endogenous mu-opioid receptor agonists. *Pharmacology and Therapeutics.* 2000; **88**: 437–63.

43. Zadina JE. Isolation and distribution of endomorphins in the central nervous system. *Japanese Journal of Pharmacology.* 2002; **89**: 203–08.

* 44. Pasternak GW. Multiple opiate receptors: deja vu all over again. *Neuropharmacology.* 2004; **47** (Suppl. 1): 312–23.

45. Meunier JC. Utilizing functional genomics to identify new pain treatments: the example of nociceptin. *American Journal of Pharmacogenomics.* 2003; **3**: 117–30.

46. Raffa RB, Friderichs E, Reimann W *et al.* Opioid and nonopioid components independently contribute to the mechanism of action of tramadol, an 'atypical' opioid analgesic. *Journal of Pharmacology and Experimental Therapeutics.* 1992; **260**: 275–85.

47. Yuan CS, Israel RJ. Methylnaltrexone, a novel peripheral opioid receptor antagonist for the treatment of opioid side effects. *Expert Opinion on Investigational Drugs.* 2006; **15**: 541–52.

48. Liu SS, Hodgson PS, Carpenter RL, Fricke Jr JR. ADL 8-2698, a trans-3,4-dimethyl-4-(3-hydroxyphenyl) piperidine, prevents gastrointestinal effects of intravenous morphine without affecting analgesia. *Clinical Pharmacology and Therapeutics.* 2001; **69**: 66–71.

49. Egleton RD, Mitchell SA, Huber JD *et al.* Improved bioavailability to the brain of glycosylated Met-enkephalin analogs. *Brain Research.* 2000; **881**: 37–46.

50. Elmagbari NO, Egleton RD, Palian MM *et al.* Antinociceptive structure-activity studies with enkephalin-based opioid glycopeptides. *Journal of Pharmacology and Experimental Therapeutics.* 2004; **311**: 290–7.

51. Bilsky EJ, Egleton RD, Mitchell SA *et al.* Enkephalin glycopeptide analogues produce analgesia with reduced dependence liability. *Journal of Medicinal Chemistry.* 2000; **43**: 2586–90.

52. Sanger DJ, McCarthy PS. Increased food and water intake produced in rats by opiate receptor agonists. *Psychopharmacology.* 1981; **74**: 217–20.

53. Mercadante S. Pathophysiology and treatment of opioid-related myoclonus in cancer patients. *Pain.* 1998; **74**: 5–9.

54. Rosow CE, Moss J, Philbin DM, Savarese JJ. Histamine release during morphine and fentanyl anesthesia. *Anesthesiology.* 1982; **56**: 93–6.

55. Kromer W. Endogenous and exogenous opioids in the control of gastrointestinal motility and secretion. *Pharmacological Reviews.* 1988; **40**: 121–62.

∗ 56. Mercadante S, Arcuri E. Opioids and renal function. *Journal of Pain.* 2004; **5**: 2–19.

57. Martucci C, Panerai AE, Sacerdote P. Chronic fentanyl or buprenorphine infusion in the mouse: similar analgesic profile but different effects on immune responses. *Pain.* 2004; **110**: 385–92.

58. Sacerdote P. Opioids and the immune system. *Palliative Medicine.* 2006; **20** (Suppl. 1): s9–15.

59. Sacerdote P, Bianchi M, Gaspani L et al. The effects of tramadol and morphine on immune responses and pain after surgery in cancer patients. *Anesthesia and Analgesia.* 2000; **90**: 1411–14.

60. Page GG, Ben-Eliyahu S. The immune-suppressive nature of pain. *Seminars in Oncology Nursing.* 1997; **13**: 10–15.

61. Mancini I, Lossignol DA, Body JJ. Opioid switch to oral methadone in cancer pain. *Current Opinion in Oncology.* 2000; **12**: 308–13.

∗ 62. Bennett DS, Carr DB. Opiophobia as a barrier to the treatment of pain. *Journal of Pain and Palliative Care Pharmacotherapy.* 2002; **16**: 105–09.

63. American Academy of Pain Medicine, American Pain Society, American Society of Addiction Medicine. *Definitions related to the use of opioids for the treatment of pain.* Glenview, IL: American Academy of Pain Medicine, American Pain Society, American Society of Addiction Medicine, 2001.

64. Schug SA, Cardwell HMD. Clinical pharmacology-including tolerance. In: Sykes N, Fallon MT, Patt RB (eds). *Clinical pain management: cancer pain.* London: Arnold Publishers, 2003: 33–62.

65. Ling GS, Paul D, Simantov R, Pasternak GW. Differential development of acute tolerance to analgesia, respiratory depression, gastrointestinal transit and hormone release in a morphine infusion model. *Life Sciences.* 1989; **45**: 1627–36.

66. Christie MJ, Williams JT, North RA. Cellular mechanisms of opioid tolerance: studies in single brain neurons. *Molecular Pharmacology.* 1987; **32**: 633–8.

67. Bagley EE, Chieng BC, Christie MJ, Connor M. Opioid tolerance in periaqueductal gray neurons isolated from mice chronically treated with morphine. *British Journal of Pharmacology.* 2005; **146**: 68–76.

68. Raith K, Hochhaus G. Drugs used in the treatment of opioid tolerance and physical dependence: a review. *International Journal of Clinical Pharmacology and Therapeutics.* 2004; **42**: 191–203.

69. Brescia FJ, Portenoy RK, Ryan M et al. Pain, opioid use, and survival in hospitalized patients with advanced cancer. *Journal of Clinical Oncology.* 1992; **10**: 149–55.

70. Bailey CP, Connor M. Opioids: cellular mechanisms of tolerance and physical dependence. *Current Opinion in Pharmacology.* 2005; **5**: 60–8.

71. O'Brien CP. Drug addiction and drug abuse. In: Hardman JG, Limbird LE (eds). *Goodman and Gilman's the pharmacological basis of therapeutics.* New York: McGraw-Hill, 2001: 621–42.

∗ 72. Hojsted J, Sjogren P. Addiction to opioids in chronic pain patients: A literature review. *European Journal of Pain.* 2007; **11**: 490–518.

73. Sindrup SH, Brosen K. The pharmacogenetics of codeine hypoalgesia. *Pharmacogenetics.* 1995; **5**: 335–46.

74. Lintz W, Barth H, Osterloh G, Schmidt-Bothelt E. Bioavailability of enteral tramadol formulations. 1st communication: capsules. *Arzneimittel Forschung.* 1986; **36**: 1278–83.

75. Poulsen L, Arendt-Nielsen L, Brosen K, Sindrup SH. The hypoalgesic effect of tramadol in relation to CYP2D6. *Clinical Pharmacology and Therapeutics.* 1996; **60**: 636–44.

76. Gillen C, Haurand M, Kobelt DJ, Wnendt S. Affinity, potency and efficacy of tramadol and its metabolites at the cloned human mu-opioid receptor. *Naunyn-Schmiedeberg's Archives of Pharmacology.* 2000; **362**: 116–21.

∗ 77. Leppert W, Luczak J. The role of tramadol in cancer pain treatment – a review. *Supportive Care in Cancer.* 2005; **13**: 5–17.

78. Gana TJ, Pascual ML, Fleming RR et al. Extended-release tramadol in the treatment of osteoarthritis: a multicenter, randomized, double-blind, placebo-controlled clinical trial. *Current Medical Research and Opinion.* 2006; **22**: 1391–401.

79. Lewis KS, Han NH. Tramadol: a new centrally acting analgesic. *American Journal of Health-System Pharmacy.* 1997; **54**: 643–52.

80. Epstein DH, Preston KL, Jasinski DR. Abuse liability, behavioral pharmacology, and physical-dependence potential of opioids in humans and laboratory animals: lessons from tramadol. *Biological Psychology.* 2006; **73**: 90–9.

81. Sindrup SH, Andersen G, Madsen C et al. Tramadol relieves pain and allodynia in polyneuropathy: a randomised, double-blind, controlled trial. *Pain.* 1999; **83**: 85–90.

∗ 82. Davies G, Kingswood C, Street M. Pharmacokinetics of opioids in renal dysfunction. *Clinical Pharmacokinetics.* 1996; **31**: 410–22.

83. Vaughan CW, Connor M. In search of a role for the morphine metabolite morphine-3-glucuronide. *Anesthesia and Analgesia.* 2003; **97**: 311–12.

∗ 84. Glare P, Walsh D, Sheehan D. The adverse effects of morphine: a prospective survey of common symptoms during repeated dosing for chronic cancer pain. *American Journal of Hospice and Palliative Care.* 2006; **23**: 229–35.

∗ 85. Hanks GW, Conno F, Cherny N et al. Morphine and alternative opioids in cancer pain: the EAPC recommendations. *British Journal of Cancer.* 2001; **84**: 587–93.

∗ 86. Hagen NA, Thirlwell M, Eisenhoffer J et al. Efficacy, safety, and steady-state pharmacokinetics of once-a-day controlled-release morphine (MS Contin XL) in cancer pain. *Journal of Pain and Symptom Management.* 2005; **29**: 80–90.

87. Eisen SA, Miller DK, Woodward RS et al. The effect of prescribed daily dose frequency on patient medication compliance. Archives of Internal Medicine. 1990; 150: 1881–4.

88. Broomhead A, Kerr R, Tester W et al. Comparison of a once-a-day sustained-release morphine formulation with standard oral morphine treatment for cancer pain. Journal of Pain and Symptom Management. 1997; 14: 63–73.

89. Schug SA, Ritchie JE. Principles of oral analgesic therapy in cancer pain. In: Sykes N, Fallon MT, Patt RB (eds). Clinical pain management: cancer pain. London: Arnold Publishers, 2003: 123–41.

90. Rang HP, Dale MM, Ritter JM, Moore PK. Analgesic drugs. In: Rang HP, Dale MM, Ritter JM, Moore PK (eds). Pharmacology, 5th edn. New York: Churchill Livingstone, 2003: 562–93.

91. Pick CG, Peter Y, Schreiber S, Weizman R. Pharmacological characterization of buprenorphine, a mixed agonist-antagonist with kappa 3 analgesia. Brain Research. 1997; 744: 41–6.

* 92. Davis MP. Buprenorphine in cancer pain. Supportive Care in Cancer. 2005; 13: 878–87.

93. Lindhardt K, Ravn C, Gizurarson S, Bechgaard E. Intranasal absorption of buprenorphine – in vivo bioavailability study in sheep. International Journal of Pharmaceutics. 2000; 205: 159–63.

94. Likar R, Kayser H, Sittl R. Long-term management of chronic pain with transdermal buprenorphine: a multicenter, open-label, follow-up study in patients from three short-term clinical trials. Clinical Therapeutics. 2006; 28: 943–52.

95. Sittl R. Transdermal buprenorphine in cancer pain and palliative care. Palliative Medicine. 2006; 20 (Suppl. 1): s25–30.

96. Marquet P. Pharmacology of high-dose buprenorphin. In: Kintz P, Marquet P (eds). Buprenorphine therapy of opiate addiction. Totowa, NJ: Humana Press, 2002: 1–11.

97. Sittl R. Transdermal buprenorphine in the treatment of chronic pain. Expert Review of Neurotherapeutics. 2005; 5: 315–23.

98. Jeal W, Benfield P. Transdermal fentanyl. A review of its pharmacological properties and therapeutic efficacy in pain control. Drugs. 1997; 53: 109–38.

99. Portenoy RK, Taylor D, Messina J, Tremmel L. A randomized, placebo-controlled study of fentanyl buccal tablet for breakthrough pain in opioid-treated patients with cancer. Clinical Journal of Pain. 2006; 22: 805–11.

100. Darwish M, Kirby M, Robertson Jr P et al. Absolute and relative bioavailability of fentanyl buccal tablet and oral transmucosal fentanyl citrate. Journal of Clinical Pharmacology. 2007; 47: 343–50.

101. Ebert B, Andersen S, Krogsgaard-Larsen P. Ketobemidone, methadone and pethidine are non-competitive N-methyl-D-aspartate (NMDA) antagonists in the rat cortex and spinal cord. Neuroscience Letters. 1995; 187: 165–8.

102. Eap CB, Buclin T, Baumann P. Interindividual variability of the clinical pharmacokinetics of methadone: implications for the treatment of opioid dependence. Clinical Pharmacokinetics. 2002; 41: 1153–93.

103. Ripamonti C, Zecca E, Bruera E. An update on the clinical use of methadone for cancer pain. Pain. 1997; 70: 109–15.

*104. Nicholson AB. Methadone for cancer pain. Cochrane Database of Systematic Reviews. 2004; CD003971.

105. Bruera E, Palmer JL, Bosnjak S et al. Methadone versus morphine as a first-line strong opioid for cancer pain: a randomized, double-blind study. Journal of Clinical Oncology. 2004; 22: 185–92.

106. Mercadante S, Casuccio A, Fulfaro F et al. Switching from morphine to methadone to improve analgesia and tolerability in cancer patients: a prospective study. Journal of Clinical Oncology. 2001; 19: 2898–904.

107. Benitez-Rosario MA, Feria M, Salinas-Martin A et al. Opioid switching from transdermal fentanyl to oral methadone in patients with cancer pain. Cancer. 2004; 101: 2866–73.

108. Scholes CF, Gonty N, Trotman IF. Methadone titration in opioid-resistant cancer pain. European Journal of Cancer Care. 1999; 8: 26–9.

109. Inturrisi CE, Colburn WA, Kaiko RF et al. Pharmacokinetics and pharmacodynamics of methadone in patients with chronic pain. Clinical Pharmacology and Therapeutics. 1987; 41: 392–401.

110. Foley KM. Opioids and chronic neuropathic pain. New England Journal of Medicine. 2003; 348: 1279–81.

111. Bruera E, Neumann CM. Role of methadone in the management of pain in cancer patients. Oncology. 1999; 13: 1275–82.

*112. Kalso E. Oxycodone. Journal of Pain and Symptom Management. 2005; 29: S47–56.

113. Reid CM, Martin RM, Sterne JA et al. Oxycodone for cancer-related pain: meta-analysis of randomized controlled trials. Archives of Internal Medicine. 2006; 166: 837–43.

114. Heiskanen T, Kalso E. Controlled-release oxycodone and morphine in cancer related pain. Pain. 1997; 73: 37–45.

115. Kalso E, Vainio A. Hallucinations during morphine but not during oxycodone treatment. Lancet. 1988; 2: 912.

116. Adams MP, Ahdieh H. Single- and multiple-dose pharmacokinetic and dose-proportionality study of oxymorphone immediate-release tablets. Drugs in R&D. 2005; 6: 91–9.

117. Prommer E. Oxymorphone: a review. Supportive Care in Cancer. 2006; 14: 109–15.

118. Beaver WT, Wallenstein SL, Houde RW, Rogers A. Comparisons of the analgesic effects of oral and intramuscular oxymorphone and of intramuscular oxymorphone and morphine in patients with cancer. Journal of Clinical Pharmacology. 1977; 17: 186–98.

119. Sloan P, Slatkin N, Ahdieh H. Effectiveness and safety of oral extended-release oxymorphone for the treatment of cancer pain: a pilot study. Supportive Care in Cancer. 2005; 13: 57–65.

120. Dixon R, Crews T, Inturrisi C, Foley K. Levorphanol: pharmacokinetics and steady-state plasma concentrations

in patients with pain. *Research Communications in Chemical Pathology and Pharmacology.* 1983; **41**: 3–17.

121. Makin MK. Strong opioids for cancer pain. *Journal of the Royal Society of Medicine.* 2001; **94**: 17–21.

122. Stringer M, Makin MK, Miles J, Morley JS. D-morphine, but not L-morphine, has low micromolar affinity for the non-competitive N-methyl-D-aspartate site in rat forebrain. Possible clinical implications for the management of neuropathic pain. *Neuroscience Letters.* 2000; **295**: 21–4.

123. Inturrisi CE. Clinical pharmacology of opioids for pain. *Clinical Journal of Pain.* 2002; **18**: S3–13.

124. Prommer E. Levorphanol: the forgotten opioid. *Supportive Care in Cancer.* 2007; **15**: 259–64.

125. Stoelting RK, Hillier SC. Opioid agonists and antagonists. In: Stoelting RK, Hillier SC (eds). *Pharmacology and physiology in anesthetic practice*, 4th edn. Philadelphia, PA: Lippincott Williams and Wilkins, 2006: 87–126.

126. Vranken JH, van der Vegt MH, van Kan HJ, Kruis MR. Plasma concentrations of meperidine and normeperidine following continuous intrathecal meperidine in patients with neuropathic cancer pain. *Acta Anaesthesiologica Scandinavica.* 2005; **49**: 665–70.

127. Souter KJ, Davies JM, Loeser JD, Fitzgibbon DR. Continuous intrathecal meperidine for severe refractory cancer pain: a case report. *Clinical Journal of Pain.* 2005; **21**: 193–6.

128. Hoskin PJ, Hanks GW. Opioid agonist-antagonist drugs in acute and chronic pain states. *Drugs.* 1991; **41**: 326–44.

129. Lamas X, Farre M, Cami J. Acute effects of pentazocine, naloxone and morphine in opioid-dependent volunteers. *Journal of Pharmacology and Experimental Therapeutics.* 1994; **268**: 1485–92.

130. Wang DS, Sternbach G, Varon J. Nalmefene: a long-acting opioid antagonist. Clinical applications in emergency medicine. *Journal of Emergency Medicine.* 1998; **16**: 471–5.

131. Yuan CS. Clinical status of methylnaltrexone, a new agent to prevent and manage opioid-induced side effects. *Journal of Supportive Oncology.* 2004; **2**: 111–17; discussion 9-22.

132. Paulson DM, Kennedy DT, Donovick RA *et al.* Alvimopan: an oral, peripherally acting, mu-opioid receptor antagonist for the treatment of opioid-induced bowel dysfunction – a 21-day treatment-randomized clinical trial. *Journal of Pain.* 2005; **6**: 184–92.

13

Clinical pharmacology of opioids: opioid switching and genetic basis for variability in opioid sensitivity

COLUMBA QUIGLEY, JOY ROSS, AND JULIA RILEY

Background	168	Genetics	170
Opioid switching: clinical rationale	169	Summary	174
Opioid switching: evidence base	170	References	174
Interindividual variability in opioid response: scientific rationale	170		

KEY LEARNING POINTS

- Ten to thirty percent of patients with cancer-related pain do not achieve adequate analgesia with morphine.
- For these patients, a switch to an alternative opioid can improve pain control.
- Opioid switching is now an established therapeutic maneuver for this group of patients.

- There is little robust evidence to support the clinical superiority of one opioid over another.
- The clinical variability in opioid responsiveness may have a significant genetic component.
- Many potential candidate genes are currently under study.

BACKGROUND

For patients with cancer, pain is the symptom which is most feared. Since a third of the population will die from cancer, and of these 80 percent will experience severe pain in their final year of life, effective treatment of cancer-related pain remains a high priority and ongoing challenge in clinical practice.[1] Individuals with moderate to severe cancer-related pain require treatment with strong analgesics, namely opioids.

Advanced cancer patients often present with multiple pains affecting different anatomical sites. These pains may be of differing etiology and related to different underlying pathophysiological mechanisms.[2] In one prospective study of 2266 cancer patients, 30 percent of patients presented with one, 39 percent with two, and 31 percent with three or more distinct pain syndromes. Pain was classified as originating from nociceptors in bone in 35 percent, soft tissue in 45 percent, visceral structures in 33 percent, and nerve dysfunction in 34 percent of patients.[3] Opioids are used in the treatment of all these types of pain, with or without adjuvant analgesics. Adjuvant drugs are commonly used with opioids in the treatment of opioid-refractory neuropathic pain[4, 5, 6] or opioid-refractory malignant bone pain.[7, 8]

An important advance in promoting the principles of good pain control for cancer patients worldwide was the publication of the World Health Organization (WHO) analgesic ladder in 1982.[9] Whilst the recommendations for each step of the analgesic ladder have not been individually evaluated in randomized controlled trials (RCTs), the use of the analgesic ladder as a treatment strategy has been validated in the clinical setting with up to 88 percent of patients obtaining satisfactory relief from pain.[3, 10, 11] It is now widely accepted in clinical practice.

Whilst morphine is the opioid of choice for the treatment of moderate to severe cancer pain,[9] 10–30 percent of patients treated with oral morphine do not have successful outcomes, either because of intolerable adverse effects, inadequate analgesia, or a combination of both.[12] This is a significant problem. Patients who do not receive the desired analgesic effect or suffer intolerable side effects from morphine are often "switched" to alternative strong opioids. The decision to switch is predominately a clinical one, and the degree of pain control which is deemed acceptable to both the patient and/or clinician may vary for different patients. However, opioid switching, or changing from morphine to an alternative opioid, is a therapeutic maneuver that is gaining popularity in pain management as a method of improving analgesic response and/or reducing adverse side effects.[13, 14] This strategy can be confused with opioid rotation, which in some centers also includes patients simply switched to an alternative drug either to change route of administration or because of either patient or clinician preference.

OPIOID SWITCHING: CLINICAL RATIONALE

As an accepted therapeutic maneuver, the practice of opioid switching assumes that there is a true clinical difference between opioids. However, this assumption is not supported by robust clinical evidence. There is currently little evidence to support the use of one strong opioid over another. Caution needs to be exercised when extrapolating data from trials that have focused largely on acute or noncancer pain.[15, 16] Large RCTs have not been undertaken to directly compare opioids in cancer-related

pain, and smaller individual trials are underpowered to demonstrate superiority of one opioid over another.[17, 18, 19, 20, 21, 22] Therefore, the decision by both the WHO and the European Association for Palliative Care (EAPC) to recommend morphine as the opioid of choice is based largely on clinical expertise and pragmatic reasons such as the general availability of morphine sulphate worldwide, low cost, as well as considerable clinical experience in using this drug. **Table 13.1** lists some of the alternative strong opioids which are currently available.[23]

In theory, providing equianalgesic doses are used, all opioids should have equal analgesic potency. In practice, however, a wide variability in both dose conversion tables and in opioid response is reported. When converting from morphine to oxycodone a dose-ratio of oral morphine:oxycodone of 2:1 is frequently used. In a prospective trial evaluating opioid switching in 44 patients, the median dose-ratio of morphine:oxycodone was found to be 1.7.[24] However, the range in dose-ratio from individual patient data was 0.25 to 12.0, highlighting the fact that conversion tables are at best a guide and that doses need to be individualized. This problem, of accurately calculating doses when converting from one opioid to another, is accentuated with methadone which is stored in adipose tissue and, following oral administration, has a rapid distribution phase and slow elimination phase with slow transfer between adipose tissue and plasma resulting in a long half-life. A steady state is reached within two to ten days following repeated oral administration.[25, 26]

Even if all opioids are assumed to be equipotent providing appropriate dose-conversion ratios are used, there may be differences between opioids in terms of adverse effect profiles. Again, as for analgesic efficacy, evidence is lacking, with published trials underpowered to definitively demonstrate true difference between opioid tolerability.[17, 18, 19, 20, 21, 22] Evidence is particularly lacking in the cancer population as most studies have been

Table 13.1 Comparison of oral and transdermal strong opioids for the treatment of cancer-related pain.

Opioid	Major metabolite(s)	Polymorphic enzyme(s)	Receptor(s) to which drug binds	Potency ratio (compared to morphine)
Morphine	Morphine-3-glucuronide Morphine-6-glucuronide	UGT2B7 (UGT1A1)	μ-opioid	NA
Oxycodone	Oxymorphone Noroxycodone Noroxymorphone	CYP2D6 CYP3A4	μ and ? κ-opioid	1.5–2
Hydromorphone	Hydromorphone-3-glucuronide	UGT2B7	μ-opioid	7.5
Methadone	EDDP	CYP2B6 CYP3A4	μ and weak δ-opioid ? NMDA channel blocker	5–10
Fentanyl	Norfentanyl	CYP3A4 CYP3A5	μ-opioid	100–150 (transdermal)
Buprenorphine	Buprenorphine-glucuronide N-dealkylbuprenorphine Norbuprenorphine-glucuronide	CYP3A4	μ, δ, and κ-opioid	50–75 (transdermal)

EDDP, 2-ethylidene-1, 5-dimethyl-3, 3-diphenylpyrrolidine.

undertaken in nonmalignant pain. Opioid adverse-effect profiles may well be different in patients with advanced cancer who may be on multiple other drugs and who also may suffer comorbidities.

Lack of evidence does not necessarily exclude the possibility that different opioids have different adverse effect profiles. The studies have yet to be carried out to prove a real difference, both in terms of opioid analgesic efficacy and tolerability and patient interindividual variations.

OPIOID SWITCHING: EVIDENCE BASE

There is a paucity of robust clinical data available to support the practice of opioid switching. Two systematic reviews have been published. Both conclude that data are limited to open studies and small case series.[14, 27] No RCTs were located despite searching for all potential studies involving adults and children with either cancer or noncancer pain.[14] Published reports tend to be positive, with improvement in pain, and/or adverse effects when an alternative opioid is used. Less frequently, failure of opioid switching to improve symptoms has been reported.[28] In most reports of opioid switching, morphine tends to be the opioid of first choice.[14, 27] Methadone is the most frequently reported opioid of second choice. In the reports included in both reviews, a variety of confounding variables, such as pain mechanism (neuropathic versus nociceptive), change of route as well as drug, failure to exclude other potential causes of adverse effects, make it very difficult to draw definitive conclusions. **Table 13.2** lists prospective studies that have been published on opioid switching included in these reviews.

Since publication of the systematic reviews, there has been a further prospective study involving 186 palliative care patients.[24] The study investigated the effects, both in terms of analgesia and tolerability, of switching from morphine to an alternative opioid. "Responders" were those patients who had been on morphine for at least four weeks and had reported good pain relief with few side effects. "Nonresponders" or "switchers" either suffered intolerable morphine-related adverse effects or had uncontrolled pain. Forty-seven of the total population of 186 patients were in the switchers' group. These patients had an opioid switch to oxycodone and 37/47 (79 percent) of those who switched had a successful outcome with the alternative opioid.

INTERINDIVIDUAL VARIABILITY IN OPIOID RESPONSE: SCIENTIFIC RATIONALE

Individuals vary in their response to drugs for a variety of reasons. From a pharmacokinetic perspective, determinants include how a drug is absorbed, distributed, metabolized, and eliminated. Pharmacodynamic factors such as drug concentration at receptor site, absolute number as well as morphology of receptors, also play a role in determining how an individual responds to a drug. In addition, age, concomitant medication, comorbidity, and environmental factors influence drug handling. **Table 13.1** lists some of the alternative strong opioids available and includes their metabolite and receptor profiles.[23]

It has been demonstrated that interindividual variability in morphine response cannot be solely attributed to renal or liver function, age, cancer diagnosis, or gender.[47] Increasingly, the potential importance of genetic variability in opioid response has been reported in the literature.[48, 49, 50, 51] It now seems likely that although individual factors such as previous pain experience, age, and pain intensity have an impact on opioid sensitivity, much of the clinical variability seen in opioid responsiveness could have a significant genetic component.[52]

GENETICS

The genetic code, deoxyribonucleic acid (DNA), carries the complete genetic information of a cell and consists of thousands of genes. Each gene serves as a code or template for building a protein molecule, such as a receptor or an enzyme. Variation in the genetic code can alter protein expression and function. Given the broad spectrum of proteins involved in determining response to a drug, genetic variation in multiple genes could influence an individual's response to opioids.[53] When considering the mechanism(s) of opioid activity, a number of putative candidate genes can be identified which might influence interindividual variation in opioid activity or cause an individual to show a differential response to various opioids.

Candidate genes

DRUG TRANSPORTERS: P-GLYCOPROTEIN

The membrane bound drug transporter P-glycoprotein protects cells from toxic xenobiotics, limiting the uptake of compounds from the gastrointestinal tract and contributing to drug absorption and excretion via the liver, kidneys, and intestine.[54] It is also important in regulating the ability of drugs to cross the blood–brain barrier[55] and can actively pump drugs out of the central nervous system (CNS). P-glycoprotein knock-out mice have enhanced absorption and high CNS concentrations of P-glycoprotein substrates.[56, 57] Morphine has increased analgesic effect in P-glycoprotein knockout mice compared to wild-type mice[57] and antinociceptive effects of morphine are increased in wild-type rats that are pretreated with a P-glycoprotein inhibitor.[58] P-glycoprotein modulation of opioid CNS levels varies substantially between different opioids.[59] Other drugs can act as substrates for or inducers or inhibitors of P-glycoprotein. For example,

Table 13.2 Comparison of prospective studies of switching from one opioid to an alternative opioid.

Study	Switch or rotation	Opioids used	Patient group/Setting	Outcomes
Ashby et al.[29]	Switch for SE: Confusion 51%, drowsiness 31% N and V 39% (one rotation for route)	Various to various	n = 49 Palliative care unit	Confusion improved 18/25 (72%) N and V improved 13/19 (68%) Drowsiness improved 8/15 (53%)
Benitez-Rosario et al.[30]	Switch for uncontrolled pain: 41.1% Switch for neurotoxic SE: 58.9%	Transdermal fentanyl to p.o. methadone	n = 17 Palliative care unit	Switching fully effective in 80%; partially effective in 20% [Neuropathic pain not improved with switch] Delirium reversed in 80% Myoclonus reversed in 100%
Bruera et al.[31]	Switch for pain [NB. neuropathic (38%) and incident pain (46%)]	S.C. hydromorphone to p.o. or p.r. methadone	n = 37 Palliative care unit	Pain ↓ −VAS 51 ± 22 to 34 ± 21 p = 0.001 (One pt discontinued due to toxicity)
Cherny et al.[13]	Switch for pain and/or SE 71% Rotation others	Various to various	n = 100 Cancer center	Pain ↓ − 77% rated pain intensity 0–3 on discharge compared to 5 pts on admission
de Leon and Lema[32]	Switch for pain	Epidural morphine to epidural sufentanil	n = 20 Post-op, anesthetic unit	All improved with VAS <5
Gagnon et al.[33]	Switch for SE (21% change of route of oxycodone)	Morphine, hydromorphone or methadone to oxycodone	n = 63 Palliative care unit	Delirium improved 13/38 (35%) Nausea improved 1/3 (33%) Sedation improved 1/4 (25%)
Maddocks et al.[34]	Switch for delirium	Morphine to oxycodone/fentanyl	n = 19 Hospice	Delirium improved 9/13 (69%) No significant improvement in pain
McNamara[35]	Switch for SE	Morphine to fentanyl	n = 19	Pain control maintained following switch. Improvement in sleepiness and drowsiness Decreased dizziness Improved cognitive function
Mercadante et al.[36]	Switch for SE Drowsiness 88%	Morphine to methadone	n = 24 Palliative care unit	Clinical improvement in 19/24 (79%)
Mercadante et al.[37]	Switch for pain (20%) Pain and SE (64%) SE (16%)	Morphine to methadone	n = 50 Palliative care unit	Clinical improvement in 80%

(Continued over)

Table 13.2 Comparison of prospective studies of switching from one opioid to an alternative opioid (continued).

Study	Switch or rotation	Opioids used	Patient group/Setting	Outcomes
Mercadante et al.[38]	Pain SE	Morphine to methadone	n = 10	Clinical improvement in 90%
Mercadante et al.[39]	Poor pain control (n = 4) SE (n = 4) Poor pain control plus SE (n = 14)	Transdermal fentanyl to p.o. morphine (n = 24), or vice versa (n = 7)	n = 31 Palliative care unit	Clinical improvement in 80% (25/31)
Morita et al.[40]	Switch for morphine-induced delirium	Morphine to fentanyl	n = 21 Palliative care units	Clinical improvement in delirium in 18/20 patients
Moryl et al.[28]	Switch for pain and SE (54%) Sedation (15%) Rotation (31%)	Methadone to various	n = 13 Cancer center	Improvement in 1/13 (8%) 12/13 had ↑ SE ± pain on new opioid
Santiago-Palma et al.[41]	Switch for pain and SE Sedation (66%) Confusion (33%)	I.V. PCA fentanyl to i.v. PCA methadone	n = 18 Cancer center	Clinical improvement in 89% Pain ↓ VAS 8.1 to 3.2 p = 0.001. Sedation ↓ p = 0.001 Confusion improved in 5/6 (83%)
Sawe et al.[42]	Switch or rotation unclear	Various to methadone p.o.	n = 14 General hospital and oncology dept	Improvement in 11/14 (79%)
Scholes et al.[43] Slover[44]	Switch for pain (79%) and SE Switch for pain and SE	P.O. morphine to p.o. methadone Morphine or oxycodone to fentanyl (transdermal)	n = 33 n = 5 3 in hospital/2 outpatients	Clinical improvement in 78% Improved pain and SE (one pt dose limited by drowsiness)
Tse et al.[45]	Switch for pain and SE	Morphine to methadone	n = 37 Hospice	27 patients completed the study – Pain improved in 24/27 (88.9%) and SE improved in 88.6%
Walsh et al.[46] (abstract only)	Switch for pain and SE Neurotoxicity 50% Pain 35% N and V 15%	Various to various	n = 40 Palliative medicine unit	Improvement in 100%

i.v., intravenous; N and V, nausea and vomiting; PCA, patient controlled analgesia; p.o., oral; SE, side effect; VAS, visual analog score; ↑, increase; ↓, decrease.

cyclosporin inhibits the P-glycoprotein transporter resulting in increased fentanyl and morphine-induced analgesia.[57, 59] Interindividual variability in P-glycoprotein activity is well recognized and genetic variation in the multidrug resistance gene MDR-1, which encodes for P-glycoprotein, has been associated with resultant alterations in P-glycoprotein activity.[55, 60, 61, 62]

DRUG METABOLISM

There is no single common metabolic pathway for the metabolism of opioids. Codeine[63] and oxycodone[64] are metabolized by the CYP2D6 enzyme. Oral morphine and hydromorphone are primarily metabolized in the liver through the uridine-diphosphoglucuronosyltransferase (UGT) system.[65] Fentanyl[66] and methadone[67] are metabolized by the cytochrome P450 3A4 (CYP3A4) enzyme which is responsible for the complete or partial metabolism of 50 percent of all known drugs. Genetic variation in CYP2D6 results in poor metabolism of the opioid codeine to its active metabolite morphine.[63, 68] Similar studies have shown important pharmacogenetic influences in oxycodone[64] and morphine[69] metabolism with variable frequencies of polymorphic enzymes in different population groups.

A number of single nucleotide polymorphisms (SNPs) in the promoter region of UGT2B7 have been reported but their impact on enzyme function is debated.[70] In vitro studies demonstrate altered transcription factor binding to polymorphic regions, but these do not translate into altered promoter activity.[71] Whilst one clinical study showed that genetic variation in the promoter region correlated with serum morphine and morphine-6-glucuronide concentrations,[72] this was not confirmed in a subsequent larger study.[73] One functional SNP in exon 2 results in an amino acid substitution, histidine to tyrosine, at the proposed location of the substrate binding site.[71] However, Holthe et al.[74] found no relationship between this variant and morphine metabolism in patients with cancer.

The large range in the absolute values and ratios between morphine and its metabolites could be explained by the wide (up to ten-fold) variability in the expression of UGT2B7 mRNA in human liver biopsy samples.[75] Differences in gene expression can be due to alterations in DNA promoter and enhancer sequences which form recognition sites for regulatory DNA binding proteins (transcription factors).[76] Transcription of UGT2B7 is regulated by the transcription factor hepatic nuclear factor-1α (HNF1α).[75, 77] Coregulatory proteins, such as octamer transcription factor-1 (OCT1)[77] and dimerization cofactor of HNF1α (DCOH),[78] may also be important.

RECEPTORS: μ-OPIOID RECEPTOR

Morphine and other commonly used opioid analgesics act at the same target receptor, primarily the μ-opioid receptor.[79] In μ-opioid receptor knockout mice, spinal and supraspinal analgesic models show complete loss of both analgesic activity and virtually all other effects of morphine, including reinforcing properties and withdrawal symptoms.[80] Ligand binding studies show that morphine binds primarily to μ receptors but has weak affinity for κ and negligible affinity for δ receptors. Some analgesic activity would therefore be expected at κ receptors in μ-receptor knockout mice. However, this does not occur, suggesting permissiveness in functioning of κ receptors. Prototypical δ and κ agonists also function poorly without μ opioid receptors.

Data from mouse studies therefore suggest that μ-opioid receptors are necessary for morphine analgesia and that changes in μ-opioid receptor densities, potentially contributed to by allelic variants, can produce changes in nociceptive responses and effect opioid response.[80] Binding studies to post-mortem brain samples and in vivo positron emission tomography radioligand analyses suggest 30–50 percent or even larger ranges of individual human differences in μ-opioid receptor densities.[81]

Chaturvedi et al.[82] demonstrated decreased binding affinities of different opioids in mutated receptors lacking the N-terminal domain. The magnitude of this effect varied between drugs; the affinity of morphine, β-endorphin and DAMGO in binding to the mutated versus the wild-type receptor decreased three- to eight-fold, compared with methadone and fentanyl which decreased 20–60-fold. Studies by Wang et al.[83, 84] confirm minimal change in binding of morphine to mutated receptors lacking the N-terminal domain. In addition, mutation of charged amino acids in the transmembrane domains will selectively increase or decrease different agonist's affinity.[85]

Clinical studies which have assessed genetic variation and μ-opioid receptor function have focused on genetic variation in the μ-opioid receptor gene itself. Addiction studies have linked this with tolerance to or dependence on different opioids, and pain studies have considered both analgesic response and opioid-related side effects.

The most widely studied SNP in the μ-opioid receptor gene is the A118G nucleotide substitution which codes for the amino acid change asparagine (Asn) to aspartic acid (Asp). Addiction studies have published conflicting results. The mutant allele was found to be increased in both a Hispanic subgroup, protecting against drug abuse,[86] and a Caucasian population, protecting against alcohol abuse.[87] However, other studies found no association.[88, 89, 90] In pain studies, case reports have suggested that the mutant allele may decrease the potency of morphine or morphine-6-glucuronide in cancer patients.[88, 89, 90, 91, 92] A study in normal volunteers ($n = 11$) showed reduced pupil constriction in response to morphine-6-glucuronide, but not morphine in subjects carrying the G allele.[93] Klepstad et al.[94] found that cancer patients homozygous for the variant G allele needed more morphine to achieve pain control. Other studies show no association between this SNP and pain or analgesic response.[48, 95]

RECEPTOR SIGNALING

Once opioids bind to the receptor, a complex sequence of events is initiated resulting in G-protein activation and subsequent activation of second messenger signaling cascades. Ligand-induced signal transduction is then terminated; the receptor is phosphorylated and internalized into the cell. A number of studies have examined the ability of different opioids to induce G-protein activation (by measuring GTPγS binding), second messenger signaling (cAMP activation) and regulation of the number of surface μ opioid receptors (receptor internalization). Whilst studies measuring second messenger signaling show little variation between different ligands and their ability to inhibit cAMP,[96, 97] induction of receptor internalization varies significantly between ligands.[97] Fentanyl induced 66 percent, and morphine only 10 percent, of the maximal receptor internalization induced by etorphine. B-endorphin, etorphine, and DAMGO cause rapid receptor internalization; morphine, codeine, M6G,[98] and diamorphine cause minimal or no internalization; methadone[98] and fentanyl will cause internalization at higher doses.[78] This can be linked to the different abilities of opioids to induce phosphorylation of serine and threonine residues in the c-terminal tail of the receptor and the third intracellular loop.[99, 100, 101]

Conformations of different ligand/receptor complexes alter the accessibility of phosphorylation sites to various intracellular kinases and binding proteins. βarrestin2 is an important intracellular protein which regulates opioid receptor phosphorylation and internalization;[102] βarrestin2 knockout mice show increased and prolonged analgesia in response to morphine.[103] The βarrestin2 gene is on chromosome 17p13.2. It is 11 kb in length and has 15 exons. Mutation of serine and threonine residues in opioid receptors alters binding of βarrestin2 to the receptor[104] and mutation of various aa in βarrestin2 have been shown to alter its binding to clathrin.[105]

INTERACTION BETWEEN PAIN PATHWAYS

Response to a painful stimulus is regulated by interactions between multiple regions within the brain via different neurochemical pathways.[106] We know that alteration in mood, additional stressors, or distraction therapies can alter both an individual's perception of pain and their response to an analgesic. These processes can be linked to differential activity of areas in the brain and activation of different neuronal pathways.[107, 108, 109]

Catechol-O-methyltransferase (COMT) is one of the enzymes that metabolizes catecholamines. It is an important modulator of neurotransmitters in the brain.

Evidence supports interaction between dopaminergic and adrenergic pathways and opioid signaling pathways in the CNS. For example, chronic activation of dopaminergic neurones (via dopamine (D_2) receptors) reduces neuronal enkephalin peptides and produces a compensatory up-regulation in regional μ-opioid receptors.[110] Clinical studies have shown interindividual variation in pain perception and analgesic response, linked to genetic variation in the COMT gene.[111, 112]

SUMMARY

Cancer-related pain is highly prevalent, particularly in patients with advanced disease. Strong opioids are the mainstay of treatment of moderate to severe cancer pain. Morphine remains the opioid of first choice according to the WHO guidelines and EAPC recommendations. However, approximately 10–30 percent of patients do not achieve adequate pain control with morphine. This minority either experience lack of analgesic benefit or intolerable morphine related side effects which preclude dose escalation. For these patients, a switch to an alternative opioid has become standard clinical practice. Robust evidence to support this therapeutic maneuver has been lacking. Further studies, with larger numbers of patients, are needed to augment the evidence base for the practice of opioid switching. Why some patients fail to respond to morphine but appear to benefit from an alternative opioid is not fully understood. However, it appears that the explanation may have a significant genetic component. Further studies are ongoing, investigating potential candidate genes which may help our understanding of interindividual variability in opioid response and thereby maximize the potential for true individualization of analgesic therapy for patients with cancer-related pain.

REFERENCES

1. McGuire DB. Occurrence of cancer pain. *Journal of the National Cancer Institute. Monographs.* 2004; **32**: 51–5.
2. Portenoy RK, Lesage P. Management of cancer pain. *Lancet.* 1999; **353**: 1695–700.
3. Grond S, Zech D, Diefenbach C *et al.* Assessment of cancer pain: a prospective evaluation in 2266 cancer patients referred to a pain service. *Pain.* 1996; **64**: 107–14.
4. Dworkin RH, Backonja M, Rowbotham MC *et al.* Advances in neuropathic pain: diagnosis, mechanisms, and treatment recommendations. *Archives of Neurology.* 2003; **60**: 1524–34.
5. Dickenson AH, Suzuki R. Opioids in neuropathic pain: clues from animal studies. *European Journal of Pain.* 2005; **9**: 113–16.

6. Portenoy RK, Foley KM, Inturrisi CE. The nature of opioid responsiveness and its implications for neuropathic pain: new hypotheses derived from studies of opioid infusions. *Pain.* 1990; **43**: 273–86.

7. Thurlimann B, de Stoutz ND. Causes and treatment of bone pain of malignant origin. *Drugs.* 1996; **51**: 383–98.

* 8. Wong R, Wiffen PJ. Bisphosphonates for the relief of pain secondary to bone metastases. *Cochrane Database of Systematic Reviews.* 2002; **CD002068**.

* 9. World Health Organization. *Cancer pain relief.* 2nd edn. Geneva, Switzerland: World Health Organization, 1996.

10. Ventafridda V, Tamburini M, Caraceni A *et al.* A validation study of the WHO method for cancer pain relief. *Cancer.* 1987; **59**: 850–6.

11. Zech DF, Grond S, Lynch J *et al.* Validation of World Health Organization Guidelines for cancer pain relief: a 10-year prospective study. *Pain.* 1995; **63**: 65–76.

* 12. Cherny N, Ripamonti C, Pereira J *et al.* Strategies to manage the adverse effects of oral morphine: an evidence-based report. *Journal of Clinical Oncology.* 2001; **19**: 2542–54.

13. Cherny NJ, Chang V, Frager G *et al.* Opioid pharmacotherapy in the management of cancer pain: a survey of strategies used by pain physicians for the selection of analgesic drugs and routes of administration. *Cancer.* 1995; **76**: 1283–93.

* 14. Quigley C. Opioid switching to improve pain relief and drug tolerability. *Cochrane Database of Systematic Reviews.* 2004; **CD004847**.

15. Hale ME, Fleischmann R, Salzman R *et al.* Efficacy and safety of controlled-release versus immediate-release oxycodone: randomized, double-blind evaluation in patients with chronic back pain. *Clinical Journal of Pain.* 1999; **15**: 179–83.

16. Gimbel JS, Richards P, Portenoy JK. Controlled-release oxycodone for pain in diabetic neuropathy: a randomized controlled trial. *Neurology.* 2003; **60**: 927–34.

17. Payne R, Mathias SD, Pasta DJ *et al.* Quality of life and cancer pain: satisfaction and side effects with transdermal fentanyl versus oral morphine. *Journal of Clinical Oncology.* 1998; **16**: 1588–93.

18. Ahmedzai S, Brooks D. Transdermal fentanyl versus sustained-release oral morphine in cancer pain: preference, efficacy, and quality of life. The TTS-Fentanyl Comparative Trial Group. *Journal of Pain and Symptom Management.* 1997; **13**: 254–61.

19. Hunt R, Fazekas B, Thorne D, Brooksbank M. A comparison of subcutaneous morphine and fentanyl in hospice cancer patients. *Journal of Pain and Symptom Management.* 1999; **18**: 111–19.

20. Lauretti GR, Oliveira GM, Pereira NL. Comparison of sustained-release morphine with sustained-release oxycodone in advanced cancer patients. *British Journal of Cancer.* 2003; **89**: 2027–30.

21. Heiskanen T, Kalso E. Controlled-release oxycodone and morphine in cancer related pain. *Pain.* 1997; **73**: 37–45.

22. Bruera E, Belzile M, Pituskin E *et al.* Randomized, double-blind, cross-over trial comparing safety and efficacy of oral controlled-release oxycodone with controlled-release morphine in patients with cancer pain. *Journal of Clinical Oncology.* 1998; **16**: 3222–9.

23. Riley J, Ross JR, Gretton S *et al.* Opioids in palliative care. *European Journal of Palliative Care.* 2006; **13**: 230–3, **14**: 6–10.

24. Riley JL, Ross JR, Rutter D *et al.* No pain relief from morphine? Individual variation in sensitivity to morphine and the need to switch to an alternative opioid in cancer patients. *Supportive Care in Cancer.* 2006; **14**: 56–64.

25. Bruera E, Neumann CM. Role of methadone in the management of pain in cancer patients. *Oncology.* 1999; **13**: 1275–82; discussion 1285–8, 1291.

26. Fainsinger R, Schoeller T, Bruera E. Methadone in the management of cancer pain: a review. *Pain.* 1993; **52**: 137–47.

* 27. Mercadante S, Bruera E. Opioid switching: A systematic and critical review. *Cancer Treatment Reviews.* 2006; **32**: 304–15.

28. Moryl N, Santiago-Palma J, Kornick C *et al.* Pitfalls of opioid rotation: substituting another opioid for methadone in patients with cancer pain. *Pain.* 2002; **96**: 325–8.

29. Ashby MA, Martin P, Jackson KA. Opioid substitution to reduce adverse effects in cancer pain management. *Medical Journal of Australia.* 1999; **170**: 68–71.

30. Benitez-Rosario MA, Feria M, Salinas-Martin A *et al.* Opioid switching from transdermal fentanyl to oral methadone in patients with cancer pain. *Cancer.* 2004; **101**: 2866–73.

31. Bruera E, Watanabe S, Fainsinger RL *et al.* Custom-made capsules and suppositories of methadone for patients on high-dose opioids for cancer pain. *Pain.* 1995; **62**: 141–6.

32. de Leon-Casasola OA, Lema MJ. Epidural bupivacaine/sufentanil therapy for postoperative pain control in patients tolerant to opioid and unresponsive to epidural bupivacaine/morphine. *Anesthesiology.* 1994; **80**: 303–9.

33. Gagnon B, Bielech M, Watanabe S *et al.* The use of intermittent subcutaneous injections of oxycodone for opioid rotation in patients with cancer pain. *Supportive Care in Cancer.* 1999; **7**: 265–70.

34. Maddocks I, Somogyi A, Abbott F *et al.* Attenuation of morphine-induced delirium in palliative care by substitution with infusion of oxycodone. *European Journal of Anaesthesiology.* 1996; **12**: 182–9.

35. McNamara P. Opioid switching for morphine to transdermal fentanyl for toxicity reduction in palliative care. *Palliative Medicine.* 2002; **16**: 425–34.

36. Mercadante S, Casuccio A, Calderone L. Rapid switching from morphine to methadone in cancer patients with poor response to morphine. *Journal of Clinical Oncology.* 1999; **17**: 3307–12.

37. Mercadante S, Casuccio A, Fulfaro F *et al.* Switching from morphine to methadone to improve analgesia and tolerability in cancer patients: a prospective study. *Journal of Clinical Oncology.* 2001; **19**: 2898–904.

38. Mercadante S, Bianchi M, Villari P et al. Opioid plasma concentrations during switching from morphine to methadone: preliminary data. *Supportive Care in Cancer.* 2003; **11**: 326–31.

39. Mercadante S, Ferrera P, Villari P, Casuccio A. Rapid switching between transdermal fentanyl and methadone in cancer patients. *Journal of Clinical Oncology.* 2005; **23**: 5229–34.

40. Morita T, Takigawa C, Onishi H et al. Opioid rotation from morphine to fentanyl in delirious cancer patients: an open-label trial. *Journal of Pain and Symptom Management.* 2005; **30**: 96–103.

41. Santiago-Palma J, Khojainova N, Kornick C et al. Intravenous methadone in the management of chronic cancer pain: safe and effective starting doses when substituting methadone for fentanyl. *Cancer.* 2001; **92**: 1919–25.

42. Sawe J, Hansen J, Ginman C et al. Patient-controlled dose regimen of methadone for chronic cancer pain. *British Medical Journal (Clinical Research ed.).* 1981; **282**: 771–3.

43. Scholes C, Gonty N, Trotman L. Methadone titration in opioid-resistant cancer pain. *European Journal of Cancer Care.* 1999; **8**: 26–9.

44. Slover R. Transdermal fentanyl: clinical trial at the University of Colorado Health Sciences Center. *Journal of Pain and Symptom Management.* 1992; **7**: S45–7.

45. Tse DM, Sham MM, Ng DK, Ma HM. An ad libitum schedule for conversion of morphine to methadone in advanced cancer patients: an open uncontrolled prospective study in a Chinese population. *Palliative Medicine.* 2003; **17**: 206–11.

46. Walsh D, Mahmoud FA, Sarhill N et al. Parenteral opioid rotation in advanced cancer: a prospective study. Proceedings of ASCO, 38th Annual Meeting, Orlando, FL, May 18–21, 2002 (abs 1429).

47. Riley J, Ross JR, Rutter D et al. A retrospective study of the association between haematological and biochemical parameters and morphine intolerance in patients with cancer pain. *Palliative Medicine.* 2004; **18**: 19–24.

48. Ross JR, Rutter D, Welsh KI et al. Clinical response to morphine in cancer patients and variation in candidate genes. *Pharmacogenomics J.* 2005; **5**: 324–36.

49. Kim H, Neubert JK, San Miguel A et al. Genetic influence on variability in human acute experimental pain sensitivity associated with gender, ethnicity and psychological temperament. *Pain.* 2004; **109**: 488–96.

50. Mogil JS. The genetic mediation of individual differences in sensitivity to pain and its inhibition. *Proceedings of the National Academy of Sciences of the United States of America.* 1999; **96**: 7744–51.

51. Uhl GR, Sora I, Wang Z. The mu opiate receptor as a candidate gene for pain: polymorphisms, variations in expression, nociception, and opiate responses. *Proceedings of the National Academy of Sciences of the United States of America.* 1999; **96**: 7752–5.

52. Ikeda K, Ide S, Han W et al. How individual sensitivity to opiates can be predicted by gene analyses. *Trends in Pharmacological Sciences.* 2005; **26**: 311–17.

53. Roses AD. Pharmacogenetics and the practice of medicine. *Nature.* 2000; **405**: 857–65.

54. Thiebaut F, Tsuruo T, Hamada H et al. Cellular localization of the multidrug-resistance gene product P-glycoprotein in normal human tissues. *Proceedings of the National Academy of Sciences of the United States of America.* 1987; **84**: 7735–8.

55. Schinkel AH. The physiological function of drug-transporting P-glycoproteins. *Seminars in Cancer Biology.* 1997; **3**: 161–70.

56. Chiou WL, Chung SM, Wu TC. Potential role of P-glycoprotein in affecting hepatic metabolism of drugs. *Pharmaceutical Research.* 2000; **17**: 903–5.

57. Thompson SJ, Koszdin K, Bernards CM. Opiate-induced analgesia is increased and prolonged in mice lacking P-glycoprotein. *Anesthesiology.* 2000; **92**: 1392–9.

58. Letrent SP, Pollack GM, Brouwer KR, Brouwer KL. Effect of GF120918, a potent P-glycoprotein inhibitor, on morphine pharmacokinetics and pharmacodynamics in the rat. *Pharmaceutical Research.* 1998; **15**: 599–605.

59. Dagenais C, Graff CL, Pollack GM. Variable modulation of opioid brain uptake by P-glycoprotein in mice. *Biochemical Pharmacology.* 2004; **67**: 269–76.

60. Marzolini C, Paus E, Buclin T, Kim RB. Polymorphisms in human MDR1 (P-glycoprotein): recent advances and clinical relevance. *Clinical Pharmacology and Therapeutics.* 2004; **75**: 13–33.

61. Sakaeda T, Nakamura T, Okumura K. Pharmacogenetics of MDR1 and its impact on the pharmacokinetics and pharmacodynamics of drugs. *Pharmacogenomics.* 2003; **4**: 397–410.

62. Schwab M, Eichelbaum M, Fromm MF. Genetic polymorphisms of the human MDR1 drug transporter. *Annual Review of Pharmacology and Toxicology.* 2003; **43**: 285–307.

63. Sindrup SH, Brosen K. The pharmacogenetics of codeine hypoalgesia. *Pharmacogenetics.* 1995; **5**: 335–46.

64. Heiskanen T, Olkkola KT, Kalso E. Effects of blocking CYP2D6 on the pharmacokinetics and pharmacodynamics of oxycodone. *Clinical Pharmacology and Therapeutics.* 1998; **64**: 603–11.

65. Radominska-Pandya A, Czernik PJ, Little JM et al. Structural and functional studies of UDP-glucuronosyltransferases. *Drug Metabolism Reviews.* 1999; **31**: 817–99.

66. Chapman CR, Hill HF, Saeger L, Gavrin J. Profiles of opioid analgesia in humans after intravenous bolus administration: alfentanil, fentanyl and morphine compared on experimental pain. *Pain.* 1990; **43**: 47–55.

67. Iribarne C, Dreano Y, Bardou LG et al. Interaction of methadone with substrates of human hepatic cytochrome P450 3A4. *Toxicology.* 1997; **117**: 13–23.

68. Caraco Y, Sheller J, Wood AJ. Pharmacogenetic determination of the effects of codeine and prediction of drug interactions. *Journal of Pharmacology and Experimental Therapeutics.* 1996; **278**: 1165–74.

69. Lampe JW, Bigler J, Bush AC, Potter JD. Prevalence of polymorphisms in the human UDP-glucuronosyltransferase 2B family: UGT2B4(D458E), UGT2B7(H268Y), and UGT2B15(D85Y). *Cancer Epidemiology, Biomarkers and Prevention*. 2000; **9**: 329–33.

70. Duguay Y, Baar C, Skorpen F, Guillemette C. A novel functional polymorphism in the uridine diphosphate-glucuronosyltransferase 2B7 promoter with significant impact on promoter activity. *Clinical Pharmacology and Therapeutics*. 2004; **75**: 223–33.

71. Mackenzie PI, Gregory PA, Lewinsky RH *et al.* Polymorphic variations in the expression of the chemical detoxifying UDP glucuronosyltransferases. *Toxicology and Applied Pharmacology*. 2005; **207**: 77–83.

72. Sawyer MB, Innocenti F, Das S *et al.* A pharmacogenetic study of uridine diphosphate-glucuronosyltransferase 2B7 in patients receiving morphine. *Clinical Pharmacology and Therapeutics*. 2003; **73**: 566–74.

73. Holthe M, Rakvag TN, Klepstad P *et al.* Sequence variations in the UDP-glucuronosyltransferase 2B7 (UGT2B7) gene: identification of 10 novel single nucleotide polymorphisms (SNPs) and analysis of their relevance to morphine glucuronidation in cancer patients. *Pharmacogenomics Journal*. 2003; **3**: 17–26.

74. Holthe M, Klepstad P, Zahlsen K *et al.* Morphine glucuronide-to-morphine plasma ratios are unaffected by the UGT2B7 H268Y and UGT1A1*28 polymorphisms in cancer patients on chronic morphine therapy. *European Journal of Clinical Pharmacology*. 2002; **58**: 353–6.

75. Toide K, Takahashi Y, Yamazaki H *et al.* Hepatocyte nuclear factor-1alpha is a causal factor responsible for interindividual differences in the expression of UDP-glucuronosyltransferase 2B7 mRNA in human livers. *Drug Metabolism and Disposition*. 2002; **30**: 613–5.

76. Wendel B, Hoehe MR. The human mu opioid receptor gene: 5′ regulatory and intronic sequences. *Journal of Molecular Medicine*. 1998; **76**: 525–32.

77. Ishii Y, Hansen AJ, Mackenzie PI. Octamer transcription factor-1 enhances hepatic nuclear factor-1alpha-mediated activation of the human UDP glucuronosyltransferase 2B7 promoter. *Molecular Pharmacology*. 2000; **57**: 940–7.

78. Rhee KH, Stier G, Becker PB *et al.* The bifunctional protein DCoH modulates interactions of the homeodomain transcription factor HNF1 with nucleic acids. *Journal of Molecular Biology*. 1997; **265**: 20–9.

79. Keith DE, Anton B, Murray SR *et al.* mu-Opioid receptor internalization: opiate drugs have differential effects on a conserved endocytic mechanism in vitro and in the mammalian brain. *Molecular Pharmacology*. 1998; **53**: 377–84.

80. Clarke S, Kitchen I. Opioid analgesia: new information from gene knockout studies. *Current Opinion in Anaesthesiology*. 1999; **12**: 609–14.

81. Ravert HT, Bencherif B, Madar I, Frost JJ. PET imaging of opioid receptors in pain: progress and new directions. *Current Pharmaceutical Design*. 2004; **10**: 759–68.

82. Chaturvedi K, Shahrestanifar M, Howells RD. mu-Opioid receptor: role for the amino terminus as a determinant of ligand binding affinity. *Molecular Brain Research*. 2000; **76**: 64–72.

83. Surratt CK, Johnson PS, Moriwaki A *et al.* -mu opiate receptor. Charged transmembrane domain amino acids are critical for agonist recognition and intrinsic activity. *Journal of Biological Chemistry*. 1994; **269**: 20548–53.

84. Wang JB, Imai Y, Eppler CM *et al.* mu opiate receptor: cDNA cloning and expression. *Proceedings of the National Academy of Sciences of the United States of America*. 1993; **90**: 10230–4.

85. Pil J, Tytgat J. The role of the hydrophilic Asn230 residue of the mu-opioid receptor in the potency of various opioid agonists. *British Journal of Pharmacology*. 2001; **134**: 496–506.

86. Bond C, LaForge KS, Tian M *et al.* Single-nucleotide polymorphism in the human mu opioid receptor gene alters beta-endorphin binding and activity: possible implications for opiate addiction. *Proceedings of the National Academy of Sciences of the United States of America*. 1998; **95**: 9608–13.

87. Town T, Abdullah L, Crawford F *et al.* Association of a functional mu-opioid receptor allele (+118A) with alcohol dependency. *American Journal of Medical Genetics*. 1999; **88**: 458–61.

88. Bergen AW, Kokoszka J, Peterson R *et al.* Mu opioid receptor gene variants: lack of association with alcohol dependence. *Molecular Psychiatry*. 1997; **2**: 490–4.

89. Sander T, Gscheidel N, Wendel B *et al.* Human mu opioid receptor variation and alcohol dependence. *Alcoholism: Clinical and Experimental Research*. 1998; **22**: 2108–10.

90. Li T, Liu X, Zhu ZH *et al.* Association analysis of polymorphisms in the m opioid gene and heroin abuse in chinese subjects. *Addiction Biology*. 2000; **5**: 181–6.

91. Lotsch J, Zimmermann M, Darimont J *et al.* Does the A118G polymorphism at the mu-opioid receptor gene protect against morphine-6-glucuronide toxicity? *Anesthesiology*. 2002; **97**: 814–9.

92. Hirota T, Ieiri I, Takane H *et al.* Sequence variability and candidate gene analysis in two cancer patients with complex clinical outcomes during morphine therapy. *Drug Metabolism and Disposition*. 2003; **31**: 677–80.

93. Lotsch J, Skarke C, Grosch S *et al.* The polymorphism A118G of the human mu-opioid receptor gene decreases the pupil constrictory effect of morphine-6-glucuronide but not that of morphine. *Pharmacogenetics*. 2002; **12**: 3–9.

94. Klepstad P, Rakvag TT, Kaasa S *et al.* The 118 A>G polymorphism in the human micro-opioid receptor gene may increase morphine requirements in patients with pain caused by malignant disease. *Acta Anaesthesiologica Scandinavica*. 2004; **48**: 1232–9.

95. Janicki PK, Schuler G, Francis D *et al.* A genetic association study of the functional A118G polymorphism of the human mu-opioid receptor gene in patients with acute and chronic pain. *Anesthesia and Analgesia*. 2006; **103**: 1011–7.

96. McQuay H. Opioids in pain management. *Lancet*. 1999; **353**: 2229–32.

97. Zaki PA, Keith Jr DE, Brine GA *et al*. Ligand-induced changes in surface mu-opioid receptor number: relationship to G protein activation? *Journal of Pharmacology and Experimental Therapeutics*. 2000; **292**: 1127–34.

98. Alvarez VA, Arttamangkul S, Dang V *et al*. mu-Opioid receptors: ligand-dependent activation of potassium conductance, desensitization and internalization. *Journal of Neuroscience*. 2002; **22**: 5769–76.

99. Yu Y, Zhang L, Yin X *et al*. Mu opioid receptor phosphorylation, desensitization, and ligand efficacy. *Journal of Biological Chemistry*. 1997; **272**: 28869–74.

100. El Kouhen R, Burd AL, Erickson-Herbrandson LJ *et al*. Phosphorylation of Ser363, Thr370, and Ser375, residues within the carboxyl tail differentially regulates mu opioid receptor internalization. *Journal of Biological Chemistry*. 2002; **276**: 12774–80.

101. Wolf R, Koch T, Schulz S *et al*. Replacement of threonine 394 by alanine facilitates internalization and resensitization of the rat mu opioid receptor. *Molecular Pharmacology*. 1999; **55**: 263–8.

102. Oakley RH, Laporte SA, Holt JA *et al*. Differential affinities of visual arrestin, beta arrestin1, and beta arrestin2 for G protein-coupled receptors delineate two major classes of receptors. *Journal of Biological Chemistry*. 2000; **275**: 17201–10.

103. Bohn LM, Lefkowitz RJ, Gainetdinov RR *et al*. Enhanced morphine analgesia in mice lacking beta-arrestin 2. *Science*. 1999; **286**: 2495–8.

104. Cen B, Xiong Y, Ma L, Pei G. Direct and differential interaction of beta-arrestins with the intracellular domains of different opioid receptors. *Molecular Pharmacology*. 2001; **59**: 758–64.

105. Krupnick JG, Goodman Jr OB, Keen JH, Benovic JL. Arrestin/clathrin interaction. Localization of the clathrin binding domain of nonvisual arrestins to the carboxy terminus. *Journal of Biological Chemistry*. 1997; **272**: 15011–6.

*106. Peyron R, Laurent B, Garcia-Larrea L. Functional imaging of brain responses to pain. A review and meta-analysis. *Neurophysiologie Clinique*. 2000; **30**: 263–88.

107. Ploghaus A, Tracey I, Gati JS *et al*. Dissociating pain from its anticipation in the human brain. *Science*. 1999; **284**: 1979–81.

108. Longe SE, Wise R, Bantick S, Lloyd D *et al*. Counter-stimulatory effects on pain perception and processing are significantly altered by attention: an fMRI study. *Neuroreport*. 2001; **12**: 2021–5.

109. Tracey I, Ploghaus A, Gati JS *et al*. Imaging attentional modulation of pain in the periaqueductal gray in humans. *Journal of Neuroscience*. 2002; **22**: 2748–52.

110. Zubieta JK, Heitzeg MM, Smith YR *et al*. COMT val158met genotype affects mu-opioid neurotransmitter responses to a pain stressor. *Science*. 2003; **299**: 1240–3.

111. Diatchenko L, Nackley AG, Slade GD *et al*. Catechol-O-methyltransferase gene polymorphisms are associated with multiple pain-evoking stimuli. *Pain*. 2006; **125**: 216–24.

112. Diatchenko L, Slade GD, Nackley AG *et al*. Genetic basis for individual variations in pain perception and the development of a chronic pain condition. *Human Molecular Genetics*. 2005; **14**: 135–43.

14

Clinical pharmacology of opioids: adverse effects of opioids

JUAN MANUEL NÚÑEZ OLARTE

Introduction and definition	179	Myoclonus and seizures	187
Classification of important opioid adverse effects	180	Hyperalgesia	188
General etiology and pathophysiology	180	Constipation	189
General epidemiology	180	Nausea and vomiting	190
Overall management strategies	180	Respiratory depression	191
Sedation	184	Tolerance, physical dependence, and addiction	191
Cognitive failure	185	Dry mouth	192
Organic hallucinosis	185	Other side effects	192
Delirium	185	References	192

KEY LEARNING POINTS

- In most cases, a beneficial balance between pain relief and the adverse effects of opioids can be achieved.
- Careful evaluation is needed in order to distinguish the adverse effects of opioids from comorbidities, dehydration, or drug interactions.
- The initial approach should be dose reduction of the systemic opioid.

- When doses cannot be reduced without loss of analgesia, the addition of a coanalgesic or adjuvant, pain-targeting therapies, and regional anesthesia might be helpful.
- If adverse effects still persist, the clinician can choose between symptomatic management of the side effect, opioid rotation, and switching route of systemic administration.

INTRODUCTION AND DEFINITION

Opioid analgesics are certainly the mainstay of cancer pain therapy. The World Health Organization (WHO)'s analgesic "ladder" has been the internationally recommended approach to the pharmacological management of cancer pain for the last two decades.[1, 2] A skillful use of the WHO method for cancer pain relief can achieve success in roughly 80 percent of patients.[3] Whereas excessive concern about opioid toxicity (for example,

addiction) can become an important barrier to adequate pain therapy,[4] improper management of opioid adverse effects might result in decreased quality of life for the patients, and even failures in pain control.

This chapter will review the management of the most important opioid adverse effects. The chapter will try to make the point that in opioid therapy, these effects cannot be avoided, but can and must be minimized. In most cases, a beneficial balance between pain relief and adverse effects can be achieved.

CLASSIFICATION OF IMPORTANT OPIOID ADVERSE EFFECTS

Certain adverse effects of opioids have traditionally been considered most relevant due to their potential impact (i.e. respiratory depression or addiction) or high prevalence (i.e. constipation). On the other hand, skillful management of cancer pain with opioids in the last decades has helped to dispel several myths regarding the relevance of these adverse effects, while highlighting the importance of new ones previously undetected. Consequently, a new group of adverse effects (i.e. sedation, cognitive failure, organic hallucinosis, delirium, myoclonus, seizures, hyperalgesia), sometimes embraced under the term "opioid neurotoxicity," are given due consideration in this classification (see **Box 14.1**).

GENERAL ETIOLOGY AND PATHOPHYSIOLOGY

The likelihood of opioid toxicity has been associated with several factors, such as patient age, organ dysfunction, pharmacodynamic considerations, concurrent use of medications with overlapping toxicity, and the patient's previous experience with opioids.[5] On the other hand, simple hematological and biochemical parameters predictive of morphine intolerance in cancer pain patients have yet to be found.[6]

Box 14.1 Classification of important opioid adverse effects

In the following list, opioid neurotoxicity (ONT) is noted:

- sedation (ONT);
- cognitive failure (ONT);
- organic hallucinosis (ONT);
- delirium (ONT);
- myoclonus and seizures (ONT);
- hyperalgesia (ONT);
- constipation;
- nausea and vomiting;
- respiratory depression;
- tolerance, physical dependence, and addiction;
- dry mouth;
- other:
  - urinary retention;
  - biliary spasm;
  - pruritus and allergy;
  - noncardiac pulmonary edema;
  - hiccups;
  - hypogonadism;
  - adrenal suppression;
  - immunosuppression.

Among adverse effects, there is a substantial variability in their dose response, and even among those where a dose–response relationship is suggested (central nervous system (CNS) side effects) interindividual variability is found. Genetic variability is known to affect the sensitivity to opioid analgesia of several opioids, and it is therefore reasonable to expect a similar role in the predisposition to adverse effects.[7] For example, 118 A>G polymorphism in the human micro-opioid receptor gene has recently been found to increase morphine requirements in cancer pain.[8]

Traditionally, adverse side effects were considered to be a consequence of the binding of opioids at specific receptors in the encephalon, spinal cord, and periphery to either activate or suppress different nerve populations. Apart from its action on the CNS, opioids are known to have effects on the cardiovascular, pulmonary, gastrointestinal (GI), genitourinary, and immune systems, which account for some of their adverse effects.[9] On the other hand, some authors have recently been advocating the role of several nonopioid receptors in the potential mechanisms of morphine neurotoxicity, either through the binding of the parent drug or its metabolites.[10, 11, 12]

The clinical implications of morphine metabolites (morphine-6-glucuronide, morphine-3-glucuronide, and normorphine) in the development of morphine neurotoxicity have been the subject of a heated debate.[13, 14, 15] There is a growing consensus on the importance of these metabolites and their parent drug in the development of certain opioid adverse effects, but their true clinical revelance warrants further investigation.[16, 17, 18, 19, 20]

GENERAL EPIDEMIOLOGY

It is quite difficult to establish overall frequencies of opioid-induced adverse effects due to the multifactorial etiology of the symptoms recorded in cancer patients, where it might be impossible to attribute any given symptom to an opioid adverse effect. Nevertheless, some authors have attempted to study the association of the prevalence of different symptoms with the use of weak or strong opioids within a larger prospective study[21] or to record prospectively the prevalence of opioid adverse effects.[22, 23] The results of these three studies are summarized in **Table 14.1**.

OVERALL MANAGEMENT STRATEGIES

Several global strategies have been proposed that may reduce the adverse effects sometimes associated with opioid therapy. The clinical challenge of selecting the best option is enhanced by the lack of definitive, evidence-based comparative data. Certainly, this aspect of opioid therapy is still surrounded with controversy.

Table 14.1 Prevalence of opioid side effects.

Side effects (N)	Grond et al.[21] (%)	Schug et al.[22] (%)	Cherny et al.[23] (%)
No. of patients	289	550	124.0
(a) Nil			20.1
(b) Somnolence	26 (b+c+d+e+f)		35.4
(c) Cognitive impairment			33.1
(d) Hallucinations			14.5
(e) Myoclonus			8.8
(f) Seizure			1.6
(g) Constipation	42	11.5	21.7
(h) Nausea and vomiting	33+26	6.5	12.9
(i) Respiratory depression			0.8
(j) Urinary retention		4.7	0.8
(k) Itch	6	3.7	0.8
(l) Dizziness			2.4
(m) Sweating	30	2.0	

A recent systematic review of the literature has failed to produce clinical guidelines to manage opioid adverse effects successfully. The lack of well-designed, randomized controlled trials and the heterogeneity of populations and study designs precluded meta-analysis and firm conclusions.[24]

On the contrary, the European Association for Palliative Care (EAPC) has released two reports, one of them evidence-based, with recommendations and strategies to manage the adverse effects of oral morphine.[7, 25] The EAPC Expert Working Group recommends the following strategies for the treatment of opioid adverse effects:

- careful evaluation to distinguish between opioid adverse effects and comorbidities, dehydration, or drug interactions;
- initial consideration of dose reduction of systemic opioid, but when doses cannot be reduced without loss of analgesia, there are several options available to the clinician:
  - addition of a coanalgesic or adjuvant;
  - application of a therapy targeting the cause of the pain (e.g. radiotherapy);
  - application of a regional anesthetic or neuroablative intervention.
- if adverse effects persist, the clinician should consider options of:
  - symptomatic management of the adverse effects;
  - opioid rotation (or switching);
  - switching route of systemic administration;
  - opioid combination (not included in the original EAPC paper).[7]

Addition of a coanalgesic or coadjuvant

If analgesia is satisfactory, a dose reduction of the opioid by 10–25 percent per day until resolution of the adverse

effects has traditionally been considered enough, without compromising pain control. There is no clear evidence to support this assumption. When doses cannot be decreased without loss of analgesia, the addition of a coanalgesic or adjuvant might be a simple and effective approach.

The role of coanalgesic nonopioid drugs to help diminish the opioid dose has also been a contentious issue. Although nonsteroidal anti-inflammatory drugs (NSAIDs) and other adjuvant drugs are widely considered to be one of the basic tenets of cancer pain relief, some authors warn us against indiscriminate use. Caution in their use by applying our knowledge of their indications, pharmacology, and potential for additive and new side effects has long been advocated.[26]

Some authors have raised concerns about the possibility of a "dangerous side" to nonopioid coanalgesic drugs, a new concept that might undermine our previous reliance on these drugs to allow for a reduction in the opioid dose.[27] The evidence presented to support this thesis is not new and relies heavily on studies of adverse effects in different types of population. As relates to cancer pain, there is only anecdotal evidence of the risk of opioid toxicity precipitated by impaired renal function secondary to NSAIDs in the presence of dehydration.[28, 29]

On the other hand, old controlled trials in cancer pain patients have already demonstrated that the addition of a nonopioid can provide analgesia additive to that of opioids,[30, 31] and had supported the role of NSAIDs in the management of malignant bone pain.[32] Newer well-designed cohort studies and randomized controlled trials have readdressed the impact of NSAIDs and have provided evidence of their analgesic efficacy in cancer pain due not only to somatic but also to visceral mechanisms,[33] and also evidence of the opioid-sparing effect of diclofenac in cancer pain.[34, 35][II] This action is not secondary to a modification of morphine or methadone bioavailability induced by diclofenac.[36, 37] Interestingly, sufficient ketorolac has been found to be safe in high-dose, long-term use even in the setting of a frail patient population, with no evidence of precipitating renal dysfunction. In this same case series, ketorolac was useful in reverting opioid bowel syndrome thanks to its morphine-sparing effect.[38][V] This paper is one of the few instances in which the addition of NSAIDs clearly decreased an opioid adverse effect.

A review of the literature concerning the use of NSAIDs as adjuvant analgesics to opioids found nine studies, all of which reported favorable results for the combination of both drugs.[39][I] In summary, the NSAID broad analgesic effect seems to be useful in optimizing the balance between analgesia and side effects in conditions in which increases in opioid dosage cause adverse effects. Nevertheless, further research is needed to assess the safety of NSAIDs as adjuvants on a long-term basis, specifically addressing the significant ulcerogenic gastrointestinal effects of NSAIDs. Finally, a randomized controlled trial has provided some insight into the opioid-sparing possibilities of paracetamol (acetaminophen) in advanced cancer.[40][II]

As regards the potential role of adjuvants, it is important to underline the fact that there are few good studies in the cancer population. Take for example gabapentin, a drug widely tested in benign neuropathic pain, that has been tested only recently in a controlled study versus placebo in malignant neuropathic pain. In this study, gabapentin was able to reduce the need for rescue opioid doses significantly.[41][II]

Symptomatic management of the adverse effects

The EAPC paper mentioned above under Overall management strategies[7] acknowledges the fact that symptomatic drugs to prevent or control opioid adverse effects are commonly employed, but also that the evidence behind this approach is still very poor and largely anecdotal. Nevertheless, these drugs will be discussed under each specific opioid adverse effect. The reader must have in mind the potential risk for interactions, medication burden, and also increased costs.

Opioid rotation

The last 15 years have witnessed a heated debate in the field regarding the potential usefulness of opioid rotation (also called opioid switching or substitution), and even preventive, approach.[42] With the advantage of hindsight and a more recent systematic review of the literature,[43] some conclusions can be proposed.

Opioid rotation has been defined as the practice of reducing opioid adverse effects by switching from the currently administered opioid to an alternative opioid.[7] It is also commonly referred to as opioid switching or opioid substitution, although these alternative terms have lost some of the original emphasis on routine changing of opioids, coupled with hydration, in order to increase the elimination of water-soluble active metabolites and parent opioids.

Not included in this definition is the recent suggestion to stick to the second step of the WHO analgesic ladder when managing mild to moderate pain, if the clinician's main concern is that of avoiding adverse effects. [II] Opioid rotation has traditionally included substitution of third-step opioids by other similar potent opioids – therefore, a switch from a third-step potent opioid to a second-step mild opioid to avoid adverse effects is generally not embraced under the definition. Nevertheless, this is again another widely discussed issue, but some studies merit further comments. In a nonblinded, non-randomized, large study, constipation, neuropsychological symptoms, and pruritus were more frequently found with low-dose morphine than with high-dose tramadol for cancer pain.[44] In another randomized multicenter study, anorexia and constipation were more frequently found in a two-step versus a traditional three-step analgesic ladder. The authors concluded that a direct move to the third step of the WHO analgesic ladder is feasible and could reduce some pain scores, but also requires careful management of adverse effects.[45]

Opioid rotation has been found by different clinicians to be effective in the management of opioid-induced sedation, cognitive failure, hallucinations, delirium, myoclonus, hyperalgesia, nausea and vomiting, constipation, and dry mouth. Nevertheless, in the systematic review mentioned,[43] the search strategy retrieved no randomized controlled trials, therefore the review examined all case reports, uncontrolled and retrospective studies in an attempt to determine the current level of evidence. Fifty-two reports were identified: 23 case reports, 15 retrospective studies/audits, and 14 prospective uncontrolled studies. All reports, apart from one, concluded that opioid rotation is a useful clinical maneuver for improving pain control and/or reducing opioid-related adverse effects. The author concluded that for patients with inadequate pain relief and intolerable opioid-induced toxicity, a switch to an alternative opioid may be the only option for symptomatic relief, even though the evidence supporting the practice is largely anecdotal or based on observational or uncontrolled studies. [III] Clearly, this is a topic that demands further research with randomized trials.

Several papers have been published since the release of the previous systematic review. Four new uncontrolled prospective studies[46, 47, 48, 49] and one retrospective study[50] could now be added to the series. All the studies, apart from one, are again supportive of opioid rotation.

Whereas previous studies focused mainly on morphine as first-line opioid and methadone as second-line, these new studies explore rotations between transdermal fentanyl and methadone and between morphine and transdermal fentanyl.

Guidelines for switching and rotating opioids have been proposed which emphasize:

- the use of conversion tables related to the management of chronic pain;
- that dose conversion tables are guidelines only (e.g. in some cases even reducing the calculated dose by an additional 30–50 percent in order to be on the safe side);
- the need to monitor closely the patients during the switch, to avoid overtreatment or undertreatment.[7]

Several guidelines for opioid rotation have been proposed based on the relevant literature. The ones currently in use in the Hospital General Universitario Gregorio Marañón, Madrid, are outlined in **Tables 14.2, 14.3, 14.4,** and **14.5.** The limitation of these tables has already been discussed and the literature is filled with papers suggesting that relative potency doses are not the same one way or the other (i.e. the dose ratio is not the same when switching from, for example, morphine to methadone, and from methadone to morphine).[52]

Switching route of systemic administration

There are data to suggest that a switch of opioids from the oral or transdermal route to parenteral might improve the adverse effects.[7] A prospective paper evaluated the efficacy of the start of parenteral opioids in 100 cancer patients who had failed on conventional opioids. Adverse effects were present in 78 percent of patients, and resolved completely in 32 percent of patients.[53][III]

Table 14.3 Dose conversion tables of opioids in the setting of cancer pain, part 2.

Oral morphine (mg/day)	Transdermal fentanyl (µg/hour)
40–88	25
89–148	50
149–208	75
209–268	100
269–328	125
329–388	150
389–448	175
449–508	200

Reprinted with permission from Ref. 51.

Table 14.4 Dose conversion tables of opioids in the setting of cancer pain, part 3.

Oral morphine (mg/day)	Transdermal buprenorphine (µg/hour)
30–60	35
90	52.5
120	70

Reprinted with permission from Ref. 51.

Opioid combinations

Some authors have published their preliminary clinical experience combining two opioids in order to improve opioid response in cancer pain. In the 14 patients described, the addition of a second opioid seemed to be effective in maintaining the stability of the first opioid dose.[54][III] We have used this strategy in our institution to avoid the well-demonstrated cardiac toxicity (arrythmia due to prolonged QT interval) from high doses of methadone in patients with good analgesic response to this opioid.

Table 14.2 Dose conversion tables of opioids in the setting of cancer pain.

Opioid	Relative oral potency	Relative parenteral potency
Morphine	1	2 (s.c.), 3 (i.v.)
Oxycodone	1.5–2	3–4
Codeine	1/12	
Dihydrocodeine	1/10	
Dextropropoxyphene	1/15	
Tramadol	1/4	1/10 (of parenteral morphine)
Methadone	1–20	1–20 (of parenteral morphine)
Pethidine (meperidine)		1/8 (of parenteral morphine)
Buprenorphine	60–80 (SL)	30–40 (of parenteral morphine)
Hydromorphone	5	10
Fentanyl		68 (of parenteral morphine)

Reprinted with permission from Ref. 51. SL, sublingual.

Table 14.5 Several examples of relative equianalgesic doses.

Dose

Morphine 10 mg p.o. = hydromorphone 2 mg
    p.o. = hydromorphone 1 mg s.c./i.v.
Morphine 30 mg p.o. = morphine 15 mg s.c. = morphine 10 mg i.v.
Morphine 10 mg p.o. = tramadol 40 mg p.o.
Morphine 10 mg s.c./i.v. = tramadol 100 mg s.c./i.v.

The dose of methadone depends on the dose and time of use of the previous opioid. Indications suggested by Ripamonti et al.[52] should be followed.

SEDATION

Etiology and pathophysiology

Some preliminary evidence suggests that rapidly increasing morphine concentrations cause more sedation than more gradually increasing concentrations.[55] On the other hand, no relationship has been found between plasma morphine, M6G, M6G/M, and pain and sedation scores in another study.[56]

Epidemiology

Data from prospective studies indicate that sedation or drowsiness is observed in 20–60 percent of cancer patients on oral morphine.[7] It has been suggested that in 7–10 percent of advanced cancer patients on opioids, sedation may remain a major problem in spite of opioid dose titration and opioid switch.[57]

Clinical presentation

Sedation is a common adverse effect either when patients are started on opioid analgesics or after receiving a significant increase in dose. After a few days, tolerance to sedation usually develops. It should be noted that in some cases somnolence actually may reflect an increase in comfort after the patient has been relieved from severe pain, rather than true sedation. On the other hand, rapidly progressive sedation in the setting of a stable opioid dose should trigger a review of concurrent medications, and potential complications (metabolic disturbances, sepsis, CNS metastases, etc.), prior to considering somnolence only as an opioid adverse effect.[58]

Evidence–based evaluation of management

The main availiable options are:

- opioid selection;
- opioid rotation and switch of route;
- symptomatic management with amphetamines, caffeine, and donepezil.

Evidence from well-designed open trials suggests that transdermal fentanyl is less sedating than oral morphine for cancer pain.[59, 60, 61][III] In the first of these three studies, significant improvement in morning vigilance was also associated with significant improvement in sleep quality.[59] In the second and larger study, transdermal fentanyl was associated with significantly less daytime drowsiness, but greater sleep disturbance and shorter sleep duration than morphine.[60] On the other hand, a randomized controlled trial that compared subcutaneous morphine and fentanyl in stable hospice patients has not confirmed the range of benefits with fentanyl suggested in other studies.[62][II] Possible explanations for these different findings might be differences in number of patients, the stigma associated with oral morphine acting as a bias, and differences in routes of administration.

Oral methadone may be less sedating than oral morphine, as found in a randomized prospective study.[63][II] As mentioned above, weak opioids used in the second step of the WHO analgesic ladder, such as dextropropoxyphene[64][II] and tramadol[45][III], seem to be less sedating than low-dose oral morphine. On the other hand, tramadol has failed to show this profile in a randomized controlled trial.[65][II]

Opioid rotation and switch of route have been found to be effective, as mentioned above. Summarizing the available data, there is not as yet enough evidence to favor any strong opioid or route of administration as being less sedating than another.

The role of psychostimulants in the management of opioid-induced sedation has been the subject of extensive reviews.[58, 66] Studies in humans have confirmed the enhancement of opioid analgesia by amphetamines shown in animal studies. In addition, clinical studies have demonstrated that psychostimulant drugs produce a decrease in opioid-induced somnolence and an increase in general cognitive abilities. Moreover, the greater alertness allows for the use of larger opioid doses, which can produce a substantial increase in analgesia.[58, 67][I]

Nevertheless, the randomized controlled clinical trials that have addressed the impact of amphetamines in opioid-induced sedation in cancer patients show conflicting results.[67, 68] However, the cumulative evidence of other open studies and retrospective studies, as well as studies on different patient populations, strongly supports the positive influence of amphetamines.

Methylphenidate and dexamphetamine (dextroamphetamine) are usually initiated at doses of 2.5–5 mg once or twice a day (usually in the morning and at noon, in order not to disturb sleep). The dose can be escalated as required and the therapeutic effect is evident within two days of starting the treatment. Experience is greater with methylphenidate.

Psychostimulants can produce adverse effects, such as paranoid ideation, hallucinations, delirium, anorexia, insomnia, and tremulousness. Tolerance can develop to their positive stimulant effects. Amphetamines are contraindicated relatively or even completely in the setting of a previous history of psychiatric disorders, substance abuse, cardiac ischemia, and arrhythmia. Severe extreme adverse effects might also include intracranial hemorrhage.

Caffeine may be useful in the reversal of sedation from opioid analgesics.[69][V] Recently, donepezil at initial doses of 5 mg once a day has started to be studied with promising results.[70, 71, 72][III]

COGNITIVE FAILURE

Introduction and definition

Research has shown that subtle changes in cognitive function in cancer patients can be detected under opioid exposure, see below under Clinical findings. On the other hand, cognitive failure in the terminal cancer population happens usually in the setting of the broader syndromic category of delirium. This section will focus only on cognitive dysfunction without delirium.

Clinical presentation

In most cases, the cognitive failure resembles more a generalized slow down of cognitive function, rather than an increase in number of errors or major errors in judgment.[73, 74, 75]

Clinical findings

A 30 percent increase in the regular opioid dose used for cancer pain relief produces a significant cognitive impairment, measured by specific cognitive tests, that can be detected 45 minutes after receiving the new increased dose. In some cases, this impairment is still detectable one week after the increase in dose.[76, 77]

Cognitive function has been assessed in cancer patients by means of reaction time and compared to other populations.[78, 79, 80, 81, 82, 83] Cancer patients on stable opioid doses have also been tested for their driving ability by means of computerized psychomotor tests originally designed for professional motor vehicle drivers,[84] and by driving regularly on a driving simulator.[85] Similar to the other studies mentioned above, it was concluded that opioids had a slight and selective effect on psychomotor performance, and that long-term stable opioid doses do not necessarily impair driving ability, but with the caveat that each case demands an individual examination.

Evidence-based evaluation of management

The main available options are

- opioid rotation;
- symptomatic management with amphetamines.

In a randomized controlled trial, methylphenidate significantly improved cognitive function as measured by specific testing in patients receiving high doses of opioids subcutaneously.[86][II] Other noncontrolled studies have shown similar results.[87]

ORGANIC HALLUCINOSIS

Introduction and definition

Hallucinations secondary to opioid exposure are usually part of the wider syndromic category of delirium. On the other hand, the syndrome of "organic hallucinosis," characterized by hallucinations in the setting of clear consciousness and intact intellectual function, is considered a separate entity in the Diagnostic and Statistical Manual of Mental Disorders (DSM)-IV[88] and the International Statistical Classification of Diseases (ISCD)-10.[89]

Clinical presentation and findings

Some clinicians have described patients with opioid-induced organic hallucinosis with no evidence of delirium.[90, 91, 92, 93] Hallucinators are more likely to be taking opioids in a hospice population, and it is not clear why some patients on opioids hallucinate and others do not.[94] It was observed that in some cases a transition took place from organic hallucinosis to delirium in spite of opioid rotation, and that most of the patients did not report the presence of hallucinations spontaneously, but they were detected thanks to a sudden change in mood.[94]

Evidence-based evaluation of management

The limited number of cases described in the literature does not allow for a proper discussion of treatment options, but it seems that haloperidol and opioid rotation might be effective options.[94][V]

DELIRIUM

Definition

The definition of delirium in the DSM-IV is based on clinical characteristics considered to be crucial to the diagnosis:

- disturbance of consciousness/impaired attention;
- change in cognition (such as memory deficit, disorientation, language disturbances) or perception disturbances not due to dementia;
- acute presentation and fluctuation during the course of the day;

- evidence of a general medical condition or drugs or several etiologies judged to be etiologically related to the disturbance.[88]

Certain differences exist in the diagnostic criteria established for delirium when comparing DSM-IV and ISCD-10, although the general concept is similar. The ISCD-10 system of classification includes some additional points such as short-term memory impairment with preservation of long-term memory, disorientation, psychomotor disturbances, and sleep problems.[89]

Etiology and pathophysiology

It is important to emphasize that in the medically ill and in cancer patients, opioids are seldom the only causal factor implicated in the genesis of delirium.[90] Multiple etiologies and concomitant conditions may contribute to development of this syndrome, with polypharmacy (especially benzodiazepines and corticosteroids) and toxic-metabolic abnormalities affecting a large percentage of cancer patients.[95]

Nevertheless, it is possible that in certain cases opioids can become the only factor behind the development of delirium. In a prospective study, the only factor associated with a higher frequency of delirious symptoms in terminal cancer patients was higher daily opioid dosage ($p = 0.08$).[96] Some researchers have suggested that oxycodone might be less delirium/hallucinations inducing than morphine,[97] but these claims have not been supported when both drugs were compared in randomized clinical trials.[98, 99]

Several theoretical models have attempted to explain the pathophysiology of delirium in the setting of advanced cancer:

- reduction in cerebral oxidative metabolism;
- imbalance of neurotransmitters acetylcholine versus dopamine;
- stress-induced hypercortisolism;
- neuroanatomic models, changes in endorphin levels.[100]

Epidemiology

Delirium is very prevalent in the advanced cancer population with several studies suggesting that at least one-third of cancer patients admitted for terminal care may develop delirium before death,[97] although in some studies the figure for terminal delirium in the last week of life might increase to 83–88 percent of the patients.[101]

Clinical presentation

Delirium unfortunately still goes unrecognized or is misdiagnosed as depression or dementia. Delirium can present in three categories: hyperactive or agitated,

hypoactive, and mixed. Whereas agitated delirium is easily recognizable, the hypoactive and mixed forms are less easily detectable. Patients' relatives are usually aware of the subtle changes that precede florid delirium. Delirium is very common in advanced cancer patients and is reversible in 50 percent of cases. The most common delirium subtype is mixed.[102]

Delirious patients with advanced cancer are an important stressing factor for relatives and professionals caring for them. There is a tendency to overestimate the intensity of pain in delirious patients by health professionals.[103] Without a high index of suspicion, delirium might go undetected and confound the clinician who might increase the opioid dose in response to the situation, thereby increasing the delirious symptoms of the patient even more. If this "analgesic spiral" goes undetected, a serious deterioration of the patient's condition, and even death, might occur.[104]

Examination and diagnostic criteria

The diagnosis of delirium is primarily clinical and relies on precise criteria. The Mini-Mental State Examination (MMSE) is perhaps the most utilized cognitive screening tool,[105] and its use has long been advocated in the setting of advanced cancer.[106] Although the MMSE is effective in measuring delirium severity, the determination of impairment in the MMSE is not specific to delirium.

A number of instruments have been developed to help to accurately diagnose delirium, and a proper discussion of them is outside the boundaries of this chapter. Nevertheless, let us briefly introduce two:

1. the Confusion Assessment Method (CAM),[107] which has been frequently selected by clinicians and researchers in the field of advanced cancer due to its simplicity;
2. the Memorial Delirium Assessment Scale (MDAS).[108] Although the scale was developed for assessing severity of delirium it may also be useful to establish a diagnosis of delirium in medically ill patients.

Evidence-based evaluation of management

The management of delirium in advanced/terminal cancer can be summarized in the following points:

- provision of a safe environment;
- treatment of underlying etiology – opioid rotation plus hydration;
- psychological interventions;
- pharmacological interventions:
  - tranquilization;
  - sedation;
  - anesthesia.[109]

Despite advanced malignancy, and the fact that the precise etiology can be discovered in less than 50 percent of the cases,[101] managing treatable causes (e.g. hypercalcemia, infection, dehydration, etc.) is perhaps the most effective and rapid method of dealing with delirium. In this setting, it is quite relevant to remember the strategies described above under Overall management strategies for opioid adverse effects. As mentioned before, opioid rotation plus hydration has long been advocated as a way to improve opioid-induced delirium. Morphine, hydromorphone, methadone, oxycodone, and fentanyl have been successfully used for opioid rotation in this setting.

No published studies have formally evaluated psychological approaches to the delirious patient, such as clocks, calendars, reassuring interjections, etc.[110]

Regarding pharmacological interventions, haloperidol is widely considered to be the drug of choice for tranquilization in delirium. Haloperidol is a high-potency, relatively low-toxic neuroleptic, with a wide safety margin and great administration versatility (p.o., p.r., s.c., i.m., i.v.). Adverse effects are rare, except for extrapyramidal reactions. Titration of the dosage against the clinical state is feasible, and oral starting doses are around 0.5–1.5 mg (parenteral doses should be between half and two-thirds of the oral dose). Doses are repeated at regular intervals (2–5 mg at 1 mg/min every 30 minutes i.v. maximum, if rapid tranquilization is necessary), and increased as needed with most advanced cancer patients settling down with a 1.5–20 mg oral total daily dose either every 24, 12, or 8 hours.[109, 110] The newer atypical antipsychotics risperidone and olanzapine might be useful in the setting of complicated delirium when extrapyramidal side effects develop with haloperidol.[111][V] Recently, the use of acetylcholinesterase inhibitors, such as physostigmine and donepezil, has been reported.[112][V]

Sedation with benzodiazepines should be used cautiously because of the risk of worsening the delirium, but occasionally it is unavoidable. Lorazepam, because of its short half-life and lack of active metabolites, is usually preferred, although midazolam is becoming very popular due to its very short half-life, hydrosolubility, and ease of administration. Dose range for midazolam is 30–120 mg parenteral (s.c. or i.v.) total daily dose. As a last resort in very advanced cancer patients, and when everything else has failed, phenobarbitone and propofol can be considered.[109, 110]

Prognosis

In prospective studies, delirium in advanced cancer is reversible in 44–50 percent of cases.[96, 102] Retrospective studies have shown sustained cognitive impairment to be a poor prognosticator for discharge in patients with advanced cancer,[113] with some prospective studies even suggesting an expected survival of less than four weeks in the event of delirium not reverting to normal cognition.[114]

MYOCLONUS AND SEIZURES

Definition

Myoclonus is characterized by sudden, brief, shock-like involuntary movements caused by muscular contractions or inhibitions arising from the CNS. There are various patterns. The amplitude of the jerks can range from small contractions that have no effect on a joint to gross contractions that move limbs, head, or trunk.

Single muscles, or group of muscles, can be involved in a myoclonic jerk with a frequency that ranges from rare, isolated events to several contractions a minute. The distribution of myoclonus in the body can be focal (involving a single region), segmental (involving two or more contiguous regions), or generalized (involving multiple regions of the body). Myoclonic jerks can occur bilaterally (symmetrical or asymmetrical) or unilaterally.[115]

Both myoclonus and seizures can be a manifestation of opioid-induced neurotoxicity. The sequence of events is usually that of nocturnal myoclonus preceding diurnal myoclonus, which in turn might precede convulsions if the opioids are not removed.[116] A theoretical potential exists for myoclonus to become a specific early marker of opioid-induced neuroexcitation.[117]

Etiology and pathophysiology

As with delirium, it is possible that in advanced cancer patients multiple etiologies might be interacting to produce the myoclonic activity. Focal CNS damage, dementias, metabolic encephalopathies, and toxic encephalopathies induced by drugs other than opioids can contribute with the offending opioid in the genesis of myoclonus.[115] Nevertheless, the role of hypomagnesemia and hypoglycemia in opioid-induced myoclonus has been rejected based on the results of two studies,[118, 119] and the role of other metabolic abnormalities, such as hypermagnesemia, hypocalcemia, hypercalcemia, hyponatremia, hypernatremia, hypokalemia, and hyperkalemia seems to be irrelevant.[115]

Myoclonus as a side effect of opioid therapy has already been described after administration of morphine, hydromorphone, diamorphine, meperidine, methadone, and fentanyl.[120] High doses of opioids are not strictly a prerequisite for myoclonus,[120] although they seem to be a prerequisite for seizures.[116]

Our understanding of the pathophysiology of opioid-induced myoclonus is greatly limited by the lack of neurophysiological studies. Animal models have provided evidence of the role of NMDA, GABA, opioid, and serotonin receptors in opioid-induced neuroexcitation.[115]

Epidemiology

The incidence of myoclonus as a side effect of treatment with an opioid in advanced cancer varies widely, ranging from 2.7 to 87 percent depending on the study. This wide discrepancy can be explained by the different nature and methodology of the studies, the absence of validated assessment measures for myoclonus, and different perceptions of myoclonus as an alarming symptom in different settings. There is a very real danger of under-diagnosing myoclonus if it is restricted to sleep.[115]

Clinical presentation and findings

Myoclonus associated with systemic opioid therapy is usually described as uncontrollable jerks affecting the arms, legs, or both. The duration of spasms are commonly about one second, asymmetrical, with varying frequency between patients. Jerking can occur either during night or day or both, with nocturnal myoclonus commonly preceding the appearance of diurnal myoclonus for weeks or months. In cases of low intensity of myoclonus, the phenomenon is not noticed by physicians or nurses, but perceived by patients and/or relatives. Some patients associate myoclonus with poor quality of sleep or feelings of clumsiness, but the true impact of myoclonus as one of the possible etiologies of sleep fragmentation in advanced cancer remains to be determined.[115]

Spinal opioid therapy is particularly associated with focal/segmental myoclonus restricted to myoclonic spasms with spinal jerking distal to the segment of the spinal cord where the tip of the catheter is located, although it might also progress to generalized myoclonus. In this setting, the patient usually complains of a severe increase in his previous pain with the involuntary jerking of spine and lower limbs. Systemic opioid therapy can also induce this type of segmental myoclonus when there is coexistence of pathologic changes within the spine. The risk of developing myoclonus with spinal opioid therapy is highly associated with neural dysfunction due to pathologic damage within the spine.[121]

Diagnostic criteria

Assessment is perhaps one of the most neglected areas of research in myoclonus, and failure to produce a validated tool greatly limits the conclusions of several investigations. A preliminary severity scale for opioid-induced myoclonus has been produced,[115] but still has to undergo appropiate testing to assess its validity and is presented in **Table 14.6**.

Evidence-based evaluation of management

Current standard therapeutic approaches to opioid-induced myoclonus include:

- opioid reduction;
- opioid rotation;
- symptomatic management.[120]

Table 14.6 Marañón's Myoclonus Assessment Scale (MMAS).[115]

Grade	Description
0	Myoclonus absent
1	Myoclonus restricted to sleep that goes undetected
2	Myoclonus restricted to sleep that awakes the patient
3	Myoclonus while awake, not appreciable during a short interview
4	Myoclonus while awake, appreciable during a short interview

Unrestricted escalation of the opioid dosage in the setting of significant myoclonus might trigger a convulsive episode,[117] although epileptic seizures have also been reported with intracerebroventricular and intrathecal morphine bolus with no previous myoclonus warning.[122]

Smaller doses may reduce the myoclonus but also may result in poor pain control, whereas opioid rotation (see above under Opioid rotation), should not be associated with this problem. A specific treatment to control myoclonus has the theoretical advantage that it may allow the continuation of opioid escalation when pain is uncontrolled, whereas an alternate opioid therapy may have a period of poor pain control.[120]

Therefore, the role of supplemental drugs is quite promising but very much under discussion. The balance of present evidence, all of it of anecdotal nature, favors the use of either clonazepam or midazolam. Clonazepam appears to be safe in doses ranging from 0.25 to 2 mg in a single dose at bedtime or twice a day, either p.o. or i.v. in a slow push. The role of other drugs, such as lorazepam, diazepam, baclofen, bupivacaine, dantrolene, haloperidol, phenytoin, carbamazepine, valproic acid, phenobarbital, chlormetiazole, naloxone, gabapentin, dextrometorphan, and ketamine, is either conflicting or difficult to assess in view of the different reports in the literature.[120, 123, 124, 125][V]

HYPERALGESIA

Introduction and definition

Hyperalgesia and allodynia has occasionally been reported following high doses of opioids administered systemically and intrathecally in humans.[126, 127]

Etiology and pathophysiology

Hyperalgesia is presumed to be similar to other manifestations of opioid neurotoxicity with active opioid metabolites playing an important role.

Epidemiology and clinical presentation and diagnostic criteria

Although this is a very rare manifestation of opioid neurotoxicity, it is of clinical relevance because of the real risk of physicians misinterpreting this phenomenon. If not recognized as an opioid adverse effect, the clinician may respond by further increasing the opioid dose in an attempt to control pain, thereby aggravating the problem.

A high degree of suspicion should be exerted whenever a patient experiences a sudden aggravation of pain chronologically linked with the administration of an opioid, and specially if associated with cutaneous hyperalgesia and/or allodynia.[127]

Evidence-based evaluation of management

Opioid switching has been successful in some case reports.[128, 129, 130][V]

Opioid discontinuation and ketamine can improve opioid-induced hyperalgesia dramatically in the author's own limited experience of three cases (unpublished results). [V]

CONSTIPATION

Introduction and definition

Constipation is one of the most frequent and most troublesome adverse effects of opioid analgesia, especially with morphine. Constipated patients might become reluctant to accept the morphine doses that they need to control pain.[131]

Constipation is defined as the passage of small hard feces infrequently and with difficulty. Failure to defecate at least three times per week, straining at stool during more than 25 percent of defecations, hard stools at least 25 percent of the time, and incomplete evacuation at least 25 percent of the time are usually taken as objective indicators of constipation.[132]

Etiology and pathophysiology

In general, opioids inhibit gastrointestinal motility. Their widespread effects on the gut include:

- delayed gastric emptying associated with constriction of the pyloric sphincter;
- increased tone in ileocecal and anal sphincters;
- impaired transit through small intestine and colon;
- reduced intestinal secretion (in animals);
- impaired defecation reflex.[132, 133]

Peripheral opioid receptors on gut smooth muscle presumably mediate these actions.[133] Morphine gastrointestinal effects are preferentially mediated by μ_2-receptors. Central mediation of opioid-induced constipation has been found in animal studies, but its clinical significance in humans remains to be determined.[132, 133]

Constipation in advanced cancer is usually multifactorial, but traditionally opioids have been considered to be an important contributory factor. Dose relation, lack of tolerance to the constipating effect, and large interindividual variability are supposedly common characteristics of opioid-induced constipation.[134] Nevertheless, several studies have challenged these long-held beliefs and suggested that morphine-induced constipation is not dose-dependent, that persistent constipation is more closely related to the patients' condition than to morphine, and that a proportion of patients may become tolerant in the long term to the constipating effects of morphine.[135] Age, female sex, and abdominal tumor involvement have been found to be, along with opioid type, clinical predictors of laxative dose in advanced cancer patients in a retrospective study.[136] Opioids seem to account only for about a quarter of the constipation found in terminally ill cancer patients.[134]

The constipation-inducing capacity of different opioids has been the subject of much recent research and will be discussed as a treatment option. Preclinical evidence from an animal model supports the relatively low incidence of intestinal side effects observed clinically with transdermal fentanyl in comparison with orally administered morphine.[137]

Epidemiology

It is quite difficult to discriminate the amount of constipation due to opioids from that due to other reasons in a physically ill population. Nevertheless, figures ranging from 11.5 to 42 percent of all patients on opioids have been reported for opioid-induced constipation (**Table 14.1**).

Clinical presentation and clinical findings

History-taking, abdominal and rectal examination are essential in the evaluation of constipation and unfortunately easily overlooked.

Diagnostic criteria and critical evaluation of investigations

Investigations are rarely needed in the assessment of constipation. Plain abdominal radiographs may distinguish between constipation and obstruction, but are not useful in the systematic assessment of constipation in advanced cancer.[138]

Mean transit time (MMT-S) has been used as a standard to evaluate stool analysis of transit time (SST) and a standardized estimation of stool form as measures of bowel function in advanced cancer.[139] There is presently no widely accepted measurement tool for constipation, and the lack of it may limit the conclusions of the comparative studies.

Evidence-based evaluation of management

The management of opioid-induced constipation is based on a three-step approach:

1. opioid selection;
2. prevention;
3. symptomatic management with:
   a. oral laxatives;
   b. rectal laxatives;
   c. prokinetics.

An abundance of prospective controlled trials demonstrate that transdermal fentanyl is less constipating than oral morphine and even oral oxycodone.[59, 60, 61, 140, 141, 142, 143, 144, 145][II] This conclusion has been challenged in one of the studies because of the short-term nature of the study and the possibility that opioid withdrawal syndrome might be playing a role.[146] Nevertheless, these criticisms have been convincingly rebutted.[147] Fentanyl is also less constipating than morphine when both are administered subcutaneously.[62][II] Therefore, fentanyl has become the opioid of choice in our institution in the setting of spinal cord compression.

Oral oxycodone has been found to be more constipating than oral morphine in one prospective randomized controlled trial.[98] On the other hand, in a similar study no significant differences were found.[99][II] Anecdotal evidence,[148] retrospective,[136] and prospective randomized studies[63][II] all suggest that oral methadone might be less constipating than oral morphine, and perhaps hydromorphone. Finally, tramadol has induced less constipation than morphine in prospective nonrandomized[44] and randomized[65] studies. [II] The author is not currently recommending clinically any one of these last opioids because of their potential advantages regarding constipation.

Prevention of opioid-induced constipation relies upon:[132, 134]

- encouraging activity;
- increasing fiber and fluid intake if patient still ambulatory and at no risk of GI obstruction;
- altering treatment with constipating drugs if achievable or adding laxatives;
- creating a favorable environment for defecation.

Oral laxatives regularly used in opioid-induced constipation can be classified in:[134, 149]

- agents for colonic lavage (polyethylene glycol – starting low dose 13 g/sachet);
- bulk-forming laxatives;

- cathartic drugs:
  - docusates (starting dose 300 mg);
  - castor oil;
  - anthraquinone derivatives (senna – starting dose 1–2 tablets or 1–2 tbsp);
  - diphenylmethane derivatives (bisacodyl – starting dose 1–2 tablets or 1 suppository);
- lubricants (mineral oil – starting dose 1–2 tbsp);
- osmotic (saline) cathartics (lactulose – starting dose 10–30 mL);
- prokinetics (metoclopramide,[150] cisapride).

A full discussion on these agents is outside the scope of this chapter. Some studies have attempted to compare laxatives in opioid-induced constipation: lactulose and senna in advanced cancer patients,[151] an ayurvedic formulation and senna in the same population,[152] and lactulose–senna–codanthrusate in a volunteer model.[153][II] Also polyethylene glycol has been tested against lactulose in chronic constipation,[154][II] and reported in opioid-induced constipation.[155]

There is increasing interest in the therapeutic possibilities of opioid antagonists in opioid-induced constipation. Several studies have already tested naloxone, methylnaltrexone, and alvimopam and found them to be useful,[156, 157, 158][II] but the potential to precipitate opioid withdrawal with the old antagonists, such as naloxone, is real.

NAUSEA AND VOMITING

Etiology and pathophysiology

It has been suggested that high plasma levels of morphine-3-glucuronide[16] and morphine-6-glucuronide[159] might be associated with chronic nausea in the setting of renal insufficiency.

Whereas typical analgesic doses of opioids are often emetogenic (stimulation of D_2-receptors in the area postrema), very high doses may not be (stimulation of opioid receptors in brainstem).[160]

Epidemiology

The incidence of opioid-induced nausea and vomiting in cancer patients ranges between 8.3 and 18.3 percent for nausea and 22.7 and 40 percent for emesis.[161] A similar study in medical patients with acute pain has found 35.4 percent for nausea and 13.6 percent for emesis.[162]

Evidence-based evaluation of management

Current standard therapeutic approaches to opioid-induced nausea and vomiting include:

- opioid rotation;
- switching route of systemic administration;
- symptomatic management.

Opioid-induced nausea and vomiting have been traditionally managed with antiemetics on an as-needed basis. Antiemetics have been selected according to the putative triggering mechanism:

- delayed gastric emptying – metoclopramide;
- stimulation of vestibular apparatus – antihistamine;
- stimulation of the chemoreceptor trigger zone – haloperidol.[5]

Some authors have reported transdermal hyoscine hydrobromate (scopolamine)[163] and ondansetron[164] to be effective in this setting. In a randomized prospective trial, tropisetron, as a single agent or in combination, was more effective than chlorpromazine plus dexamethasone in the management of nausea and vomiting in advanced cancer patients on opioids.[165] Also, haloperidol has been found to be effective in postoperative nausea and vomiting during epidural analgesia in a randomized controlled trial (RCT).[166] On the other hand, another RCT has found no difference in the antiemetic efficacy of ondansentron, metoclopramide, and placebo in opioid-induced nausea and emesis in cancer patients,[167] and there is a suggestion that morphine might reduce the antiemetic efficacy of serotonin antagonists in the setting of chemotherapy-induced nausea.[168] Recently, olanzapine has been advocated for refractory nausea and vomiting.[169]

In the event of refractory nausea, a trial of an alternative opioid or a switch of route has usually been considered.[7] Few studies have so far been able to show significant differences in the emetogenic capacity of different opioids, but nonetheless there are some. Oxycodone has been found to be both less nausea-inducing[98] and similarly nausea-inducing[99] compared to morphine in controlled trials. Transdermal fentanyl has been found to be less emetogenic than oral morphine in one controlled study,[59] but not in another that compared fentanyl and morphine by the same subcutaneous route.[62] Finally, both oral tramadol[65] and dextropropoxyphene[64] seem to be less emetogenic than oral morphine. [II]

RESPIRATORY DEPRESSION

Opioid-induced respiratory depression in patients treated for cancer pain is a very uncommon circumstance due to the protective nature of pain itself. Morphine does not commonly cause chronic ventilatory impairment when given orally in advanced cancer, even in the setting of preexisting or concurrent respiratory disease.[170][III] Experimental pain has been found to stimulate respiration and attenuate morphine-induced respiratory depression in a controlled study in human volunteers.[171] Furthermore, the mechanisms underlying placebo analgesia and placebo respiratory depression seem to be independent from each other, and might involve different subpopulations of opioid receptors.[172]

In practical terms, caution is advised in patients receiving high doses of opioids in which a change in disease status (e.g. spinal cord compression[173]) or a pain-relieving intervention (e.g. nerve block[174]) may produce rapid pain relief. Also, the clinician has to have in mind those circumstances that might facilitate respiratory depression. For example, extreme heat or fever with trasdermal fentanyl,[175] or difficult opioid rotations to methadone,[176] and certainly renal failure with any opioid.[177] Judicious use of naloxone (trying to revert respiratory depression, but simultaneously avoiding opioid analgesia reversal and withdrawal) might be life-saving in these rare instances.[5] Delayed respiratory depression is a concern with spinal administration of opioids.[9]

TOLERANCE, PHYSICAL DEPENDENCE, AND ADDICTION

Unfortunately, many clinicians, as well as patients, still believe that there is a significant risk of addiction when using opioids for cancer pain. Irrational fears of addiction to opioids are bolstered by professionals with misconceptions about the phenomena of tolerance, physical dependence, and addiction.[4]

Tolerance is defined as a physiological state characterized by a decrease in the effects of a drug (e.g. analgesia) with chronic administration. Tolerance can be induced experimentally in animals, and has been considered to be a bad prognostic factor in the management of cancer pain.[178] Nevertheless, its true clinical relevance seems to be very low. The vast majority of patients that need an increase in their opioid dose do so due to disease progression rather than tolerance.[179] Analgesic tolerance seldom compromises therapy, except perhaps in the setting of previous drug addiction or alcoholism. In those exceptional cases where tolerance is suspected, "burst" ketamine (in isolated "burst" doses) has been reported to be useful.[180][V]

Physical dependence is the physiological adaptation of the body to the presence of an opioid. It is defined by the development of withdrawal symptoms when opioids are discontinued or reduced abruptly, or when an antagonist is administered. It is frequently mistakenly equated with addiction. If the source of pain is successfully treated or removed, physical dependence is easily treated by gradually decreasing the opioid dose (e.g. 75 percent of the previous daily dose).[3, 4]

Addiction is defined by aberrant changes in behavior, with compulsive use of opioids for nonmedical reasons characterized by a craving for mood-altering effects, not pain relief.[4] Addiction is extremely rare in cancer pain and chronic pain patients.[22, 181, 182][II]

DRY MOUTH

Definition

Xerostomia is defined as a the subjective sensation of dryness of mouth.[183]

Etiology and pathophysiology

Xerostomia is usually associated with a low unstimulated whole salivary flow rate, but not the other way round in patients with advanced cancer.[184] There is a positive correlation between low parotid gland salivary flow and severity of symptoms in terminally ill patients.[185]

Epidemiology

Dry mouth is considered to be a very common minor adverse effect of opioids. The prevalence of xerostomia has been variously reported to be anywhere between 30 and 77 percent in advanced cancer patients.[183]

Evidence-based evaluation of management

Dry mouth seems to be less common with methadone[63] and dextropropoxyphene[64] than with morphine. [II] Low-tack chewing gum and pilocarpine hydrochloride have been found to be as effective as artificial saliva in the management of xerostomia in advanced cancer patients in prospective randomized studies.[183, 186, 187][II]

OTHER SIDE EFFECTS

Opioids cause increased bladder and sphincter tone resulting in urgency and retention, most commonly in elderly men. This adverse effect is more likely to occur after spinal administration of opioids.[3, 5, 9]

Biliary spasm is rarely seen, or rather diagnosed, with chronic opioid therapy. Clinically, it mimics gall bladder pain, sometimes associated with an elevation of hepatic and pancreatic enzymes. It is possible with almost every opioid and it has been described with morphine and fentanyl.[9] Both pethidine (meperidine) and tramadol[188] are devoid of this adverse effect. On the other hand, asymptomatic bile duct dilation has been associated with methadone and buprenorphine use.[189] Only a high index of suspicion will help to detect these problems in cancer pain management.

Pruritus is a well known adverse effect of epidural opioids, commonly treated with antihistamines or naloxone.[9] Opioids cause histamine release and this is said to contribute to asthma or urticaria in allergic patients. Some authors consider this to be a rare

phenomenom and not true "allergy".[3] Nevertheless, there have been reports of severe opioid-induced itching refractory to antihistamines responding to transnasal butorphanol.[190] In addition, oral morphine-induced pruritus has been reported to disappear after opioid rotation, in one instance with a previous response to rifampicin.[191, 192][V] Tramadol has been found to induce significantly less pruritus than morphine in a controlled trial.[44]

Noncardiogenic pulmonary edema has been reported in severely debilitated patients treated with high opioid doses.[193] In addition, hiccups have recently been reported with the administration of oral morphine.[194]

Hypogonadotrophic hypogonadism is a common complication of intrathecal opioid therapy in both males and females.[195] Symptomatic hypogonadism is beginning to raise concern in male cancer survivors on chronic opioid therapy.[196, 197, 198] In addition, adrenal suppression from intrathecal morphine has recently been suggested.[199]

Recent studies in animal models suggest that opioids can have an adverse effect on the immune system. Morphine and tramadol have been tested in equianalgesic doses in postoperative pain and found to have different immune effects.[200] The clinical relevance of this observation in cancer pain remains to be found.

REFERENCES

1. World Health Organization. *Cancer pain relief, with a guide to opioid availability*, 2nd edn. Geneva: World Health Organization, 1996.

* 2. Ashby M, Jackson K. When the WHO ladder appears to be failing: approaches to refractory or unstable cancer pain. In: Sykes N, Fallon MT, Patt RB (eds). Cancer pain. In: Rice ASC, Warfield CA, Justins D, Eccleston C (series eds). *Clinical Pain Management*. London: Arnold, 2003: 143–55.

* 3. Hanks GWC, Cherny N. Opioid analgesic therapy. In: Doyle D, Hanks G, Cherny N, Calman K (eds). *Oxford textbook of palliative medicine*, 3rd edn. Oxford: Oxford University Press, 2004: 316–41.

4. Colleau S, Joranson DE. Fear of addiction: confronting a barrier to cancer pain relief. *Cancer Pain Release*. 1998; 11: 1–3.

* 5. Lyss AP, Portenoy RK. Strategies for limiting the side effects of cancer pain therapy. *Seminars in Oncology*. 1997; **24** (Suppl. 16): s28–34.

6. Riley J, Ross JR, Rutter D et al. A retrospective study of the association between haematological and biochemical parameters and morphine intolerance in patients with cancer pain. *Palliative Medicine*. 2004; **18**: 19–24.

* 7. Cherny N, Ripamonti C, Pereira J et al. for the Expert Working Group of the European Association of Palliative Care Network. Strategies to manage the adverse effects of

oral morphine: an evidence-based report. *Journal of Clinical Oncology.* 2001; **19**: 2542–54.

8. Klepstad P, Rakvag TT, Kaasa S *et al.* The 118 A > G polymorphism in the human micro-opioid receptor gene may increase morphine requirements in patients with pain caused by malignant disease. *Acta Anaesthesiologica Scandinavica.* 2004; **48**: 1232–9.

* 9. Lema MJ. Opioid effects and adverse effects. *Regional Anesthesia.* 1996; **21**: 38–42.

10. Centeno C, Bruera E. Uso apropiado de opioides y neurotoxicidad. *Medicina Paliativa.* 1999; **6**: 3–12.

11. Bruera E, Pereira J. Neuropsychiatric toxicity of opioids. In: Jensen TS, Turner JA, Wiesenfeld- Hallin Z (eds). Progress in pain research and management 8. *Proceedings of the VIIIth World Congress on Pain.* Seattle: IASP Press, 1997: 717–38.

12. Thwaites D, McCann S, Broderick P. Hydromorphone neuroexcitation. *Journal of Palliative Medicine.* 2004; **7**: 545–50.

13. Sjogren P. Clinical implications of morphine metabolites. In: Portenoy RK, Bruera E (eds). *Topics in palliative care,* Vol 1. New York: Oxford University Press, 1997: 163–75.

* 14. Portenoy RK, Forbes K, Lussier D, Hanks G. Difficult pain problems: an integrated approach. In: Doyle D, Hanks G, Cherny N, Calman K (eds). *Oxford textbook of palliative medicine,* 3rd edn. Oxford: Oxford University Press, 2004: 438–58.

15. Faura CC, Moore RA, Horga JF *et al.* Morphine and morphine-6-glucuronide plasma concentrations and effect in cancer pain. *Journal of Pain and Symptom Management.* 1996; **11**: 95–102.

16. Wood MM, Ashby MA, Somogyi AA, Fleming BG. Neuropsychological and pharmacokinetic assessment of hospice inpatients receiving morphine. *Journal of Pain and Symptom Management.* 1998; **16**: 112–20.

17. Tiseo PJ, Thaler HT, Lapin J *et al.* Morphine-6-glucuronide concentrations and opioid-related side effects: a survey in cancer patients. *Pain.* 1995; **61**: 47–54.

* 18. Mercadante S. The role of morphine glucuronides in cancer pain. *Palliative Medicine.* 1999; **13**: 95–104.

* 19. Quigley C, Joel S, Patel N *et al.* Plasma concentrations of morphine, morphine-6-glucuronide and morphine-3-glucuronide and their relationship with analgesia and side effects in patients with cancer-related pain. *Palliative Medicine.* 2003; **17**: 185–90.

* 20. Andersen G, Sjogren P, Hansen SH *et al.* Pharmacological consequences of long-term morphine treatment in patients with cancer and chronic non-malignant pain. *European Journal of Pain.* 2004; **8**: 263–71.

* 21. Grond S, Zech D, Diefenbach C, Bischoff A. Prevalence and pattern of symptoms in patients with cancer pain: a prospective evaluation of 1635 cancer patients referred to a pain clinic. *Journal of Pain and Symptom Management.* 1994; **9**: 372–82.

22. Schug SA, Zech D, Grond S *et al.* A long-term survey of morphine in cancer pain patients. *Journal of Pain and Symptom Management.* 1992; **7**: 259–66.

* 23. Cherny NJ, Chang V, Frager G *et al.* Opioid pharmacotherapy in the management of cancer pain. *Cancer.* 1995; **76**: 1288–93.

* 24. McNicol E, Horowicz-Mehler N, Fisk RA *et al.* Management of opioid side effects in cancer-related and chronic noncancer pain: a systematic review. *Journal of Pain.* 2003; **4**: 231–56.

* 25. Hanks GW, de Conno F, Cherny N *et al.* Expert Working Group of the Research Network of the EAPC. Morphine and alternative opioids in cancer pain: the EAPC recommendations. *British Journal of Cancer.* 2001; **84**: 587–93.

26. Portenoy RK, Waldman SA. Preface. Adjuvant analgesics in pain management: part I. *Journal of Pain and Symptom Management.* 1994; **9**: 390–1.

27. Oneschuk D, Bruera E. The "dark side" of adjuvant analgesic drugs. *Progress in Palliative Care.* 1997; **5**: 5–13.

28. Stiefel F, Movant R. Case report: morphine intoxication during acute reversible renal insufficiency. *Journal of Palliative Care.* 1991; **7**: 45–7.

29. Fainsinger RL, Miller MJ, Bruera E. Morphine intoxication during acute reversible renal insufficiency. *Journal of Palliative Care.* 1992; **8**: 52–3.

30. Stambaugh JE, Drew J. The combination of ibuprofen and oxycodone/acetaminophen in the management of chronic cancer pain. *Clinical Pharmacology and Therapeutics.* 1988; **44**: 665–9.

31. Ferrer-Brechner T, Ganz P. Combination therapy with ibuprofen and methadone for chronic cancer pain. *American Journal of Medicine.* 1984; **77**: 78–83.

32. Levick S, Jacobs C, Loukas DF *et al.* Naproxen sodium in treatment of bone pain due to metastatic cancer. *Pain.* 1988; **35**: 253–8.

33. Mercadante S, Cassuccio A, Agnello A *et al.* Analgesic effects of nonsteroidal anti-inflammatory drugs in cancer pain due to somatic or visceral mechanisms. *Journal of Pain and Symptom Management.* 1999; **17**: 351–6.

* 34. Bjorkman R, Ullman A, Hedner J. Morphine-sparing effect of diclofenac in cancer pain. *European Journal of Clinical Pharmacology.* 1993; **44**: 1–5.

* 35. Mercadante S, Sapio M, Caligara M *et al.* Opioid sparing effect of diclofenac in cancer pain. *Journal of Pain and Symptom Management.* 1997; **14**: 15–20.

36. DeConno F, Ripamonti C, Bianchi M *et al.* Diclofenac does not modify morphine bioavailability in cancer patients. *Pain.* 1992; **48**: 401–02.

37. Bianchi M, Clavenna A, Groff L *et al.* Diclofenac does not modify methadone bioavailability in cancer patients. *Journal of Pain and Symptom Management.* 1999; **17**: 227–8.

* 38. Joishy SK, Walsh D. The opioid-sparing effect of intravenous ketorolac as an adjuvant analgesic in cancer pain: application in bone metastases and the opioid bowel syndrome. *Journal of Pain and Symptom Management.* 1998; **16**: 334–9.

* 39. Jenkins CA, Bruera E. Non-steroidal anti-inflammatory
       drugs as adjuvant analgesics in cancer patients. *Palliative
       Medicine.* 1999; **13**: 183–96.
* 40. Stockler M, Vardy J, Pillai A, Warr D. Acetaminophen
       (paracetamol) improves pain and well-being in people
       with advanced cancer already receiving a strong opioid
       regimen: a randomized, double-blind, placebo-controlled
       cross-over trial. *Journal of Clinical Oncology.* 2004; **22**:
       3389–94.
* 41. Caraceni A, Zecca E, Bonezzi C et al. Gabapentin for
       neuropathic cancer pain: a randomized controlled trial
       from the Gabapentin Cancer Pain Study Group. *Journal of
       Clinical Oncology.* 2004; **22**: 2909–17.
* 42. Fallon M. Opioid switching and rotation. In: Sykes N,
       Fallon MT, Patt RB (eds). Cancer pain. In: Rice ASC,
       Warfield CA, Justins D, Eccleston C (series eds). *Clinical
       pain management.* London: Arnold, 2003: 143–55.
* 43. Quigley C. Opioid switching to improve pain relief and
       drug tolerability (review). *Cochrane Database of
       Systematic Reviews.* 2004; **CD004847**.
   44. Grond S, Radbruch L, Meuser T et al. High-dose tramadol
       in comparison to low-dose morphine for cancer pain relief.
       Journal of Pain Symptom Management. 1999; **18**: 174–9.
* 45. Maltoni M, Scarpi E, Modonesi C et al. A validation study
       of the WHO analgesic ladder: a two-step vs three-step
       strategy. *Supportive Care in Cancer.* 2005; **13**: 888–94.
   46. Benitez-Rosario MA, Feria M, Salinas-Martin A et al.
       Opioid switching from transdermal fentanyl to oral
       methadone in patients with cancer pain. *Cancer.* 2004;
       101: 2866–73.
   47. Mercadante S, Ferrera P, Villari P, Cassucio A. Rapid
       switching between transdermal fentanyl and methadone
       in cancer patients. *Journal of Clinical Oncology.* 2005; **23**:
       5229–34.
   48. McNamara P. Opioid switching from morphine to
       transdermal fentanyl for toxicity reduction in palliative
       care. *Palliative Medicine.* 2002; **16**: 425–34.
   49. Morita T, Takigawa C, Onishi H et al. Opioid rotation from
       morphine to fentanyl in delirious cancer patients: an
       open-label trial. *Journal of Pain and Symptom
       Management.* 2005; **30**: 96–103.
   50. Morita T, Tei Y, Inoue S. Agitated terminal delirium and
       association with partial opioid substitution and hydration.
       Journal of Palliative Medicine. 2003; **6**: 557–63.
* 51. Núñez Olarte JM, López Imedio E (eds). *Guía rápida de
       manejo avanzado de síntomas en el paciente terminal.*
       Madrid: Editorial Médica Panamericana, 2007.
* 52. Ripamonti C, Groff L, Brunelli C et al. Switching from oral
       morphine to oral methadone in treating cancer pain: what
       is the equianalgesic dose ratio? *Journal of Clinical
       Oncology.* 1998; **16**: 3216–21.
* 53. Enting RH, Oldenmenger WH, van der Rijt CC et al. A
       prospective study evaluating the response of patients with
       unrelieved cancer pain to parenteral opioids. *Cancer.*
       2002; **94**: 3049–56.
* 54. Mercadante S, Villari P, Ferrera P, Casuccio A. Addition of a
       second opioid may improve opioid response in cancer

       pain: preliminary data. *Supportive Care in Cancer.* 2004;
       12: 762–6.
   55. Christrup LL, Sjogren P, Jensen NH et al. Steady-state
       kinetics and dynamics of morphine in cancer patients: is
       sedation related to the absorption rate of morphine?
       Journal of Pain and Symptom Management. 1999; **18**:
       164–73.
   56. Andersen G, Jensen NH, Christrup L et al. Pain, sedation
       and morphine metabolism in cancer patients during
       long-term treatment with sustained-release morphine.
       Palliative Medicine. 2002; **16**: 107–14.
   57. Bruera E, Brenneis C, Paterson AHG et al. Use of
       methylphenidate as an adjuvant to narcotic analgesics in
       patients with advanced cancer. *Journal of Pain and
       Symptom Management.* 1989; **4**: 3–6.
* 58. Ripamonti C, Bruera E. CNS adverse effects of opioids in
       cancer patients: guidelines for treatment. *CNS Drugs.*
       1997; **81**: 21–37.
   59. The TTS Fentanyl Multicentre Study Group. Transdermal
       fentanyl in cancer pain. *Journal of Drug Development.*
       1994; **6**: 93–7.
   60. Ahmedzai S, Brooks D. on behalf of the TTS-Fentanyl
       Comparative Trial Group. Transdermal fentanyl versus
       sustained-release oral morphine in cancer pain:
       preference, efficacy and quality of life. *Journal of Pain and
       Symptom Management.* 1997; **13**: 254–61.
   61. Payne R, Mathias SD, Pasta DJ et al. Quality of life and
       cancer pain: satisfaction and side effects with transdermal
       fentanyl versus oral morphine. *Journal of Clinical
       Oncology.* 1998; **16**: 1588–93.
   62. Hunt R, Fazekas B, Thorne D, Brooksbank M. A comparison
       of subcutaneous morphine and fentanyl in hospice cancer
       patients. *Journal of Pain and Symptom Management.*
       1999; **18**: 111–19.
   63. Mercadante S, Cassuccio A, Agnello A et al. Morphine
       versus methadone in the pain treatment of advanced
       cancer patients followed up at home. *Journal of Clinical
       Oncology.* 1998; **16**: 3656–61.
   64. Mercadante S, Salvaggio L, Dardanoni G et al.
       Dextropropoxyphene versus morphine in opioid-naive
       cancer patients with pain. *Journal of Pain and Symptom
       Management.* 1998; **15**: 76–81.
   65. Wilder-Smith CH, Schimke J, Osterwalder B, Senn HJ.
       Tramadol oral, un agonista mu opioide, bloqueante de la
       recaptación de monoaminas, y morfina para el dolor fuerte
       relacionado con el cancer. *Annals of Oncology.* 1994; **4**:
       336–41.
   66. Dalal S, Melzack R. Potentiation of opioid analgesia by
       psychostimulant drugs: a review. *Journal of Pain and
       Symptom Management.* 1998; **16**: 245–53.
   67. Bruera E, Chadwick S, Brenneis C et al. Methylphenidate
       associated with narcotics for the treatment of cancer pain.
       Cancer Treatment Reports. 1987; **71**: 67–70.
   68. Wilderding MB, Loprinzi CL, Maillard JA et al. A
       randomized crossover evaluation of methylphenidate in
       cancer patients receiving strong narcotics. *Supportive
       Care in Cancer.* 1995; **3**: 135–8.

69. Sawynok J, Yaksh TL. Caffeine as an analgesic adjuvant: a review of pharmacology and mechanisms of action. *Pharmacological Reviews.* 1993; **45**: 43–85.

70. Slatkin NE, Rhiner M, Bolton TM. Donezepil in the treatment of opioid-induced sedation: report of six cases. *Journal of Pain and Symptom Management.* 2001; **21**: 425–38.

71. Slatkin NE, Rhiner M. Treatment of opiate-related sedation: utility of the cholinesterase inhibitors. *Journal of Supportive Oncology.* 2003; **1**: 53–63.

* 72. Bruera E, Strasser F, Shen L *et al.* The effect of donezepil on sedation and other symptoms in patients receiving opioids for cancer pain: a pilot study. *Journal of Pain and Symptom Management.* 2003; **26**: 1049–54.

73. Zacny JP, Lichtor JL, Flemming D *et al.* A dose-response analysis of the subjective, psychomotor and physiological effects of intravenous morphine in healthy volunteers. *Journal of Pharmacology and Experimental Therapeutics.* 1994; **268**: 1–9.

74. Zacny JP, Lichtor JL, Thapar P *et al.* Comparing the subjective, psychomotor and physiological effects of intravenous butorphanol and morphine in healthy volunteers. *Journal of Pharmacology and Experimental Therapeutics.* 1994; **270**: 579–89.

* 75. Lawlor PG. The panorama of opioid-related cognitive dysfunction in patients with cancer: a critical literature appraisal. *Cancer.* 2002; **94**: 1836–53.

76. Bruera E, MacMillan K, Hanson J, MacDonald RN. The cognitive effects of the administration of narcotic analgesics in patients with cancer pain. *Pain.* 1989; **39**: 13–16.

77. Lepzig RM, Goodman H, Gray G *et al.* Reversible, narcotic-associated mental status impairment in patients with metastatic cancer. *Pharmacology.* 1987; **35**: 47–54.

78. Sjogren P, Banning A. Pain, sedation and reaction time during long-term treatment of cancer patients with oral and epidural opioids. *Pain.* 1989; **39**: 5–11.

79. Banning A, Sjogren P. Cerebral effects of long-term oral opioids in cancer patients measured by continuous reaction time. *Clinical Journal of Pain.* 1990; **6**: 91–5.

80. Banning A, Sjogren P, Kaiser F. Reaction time in cancer patients receiving peripherally acting analgesics alone or in combination with opioids. *Acta Anaesthesiologica Scandinavica.* 1992; **36**: 480–2.

81. Sjogren P, Olsen AK, Thomsen AB, Dalberg J. Neuropsychological performance in cancer patients: the role of oral opioids, pain and performance status. *Pain.* 2000; **86**: 237–45.

82. Larsen B, Otto H, Dorscheid E, Larsen R. Effects of long-term opioid therapy on psychomotor function in patients with cancer pain or non-malignant pain. *Anaesthesist.* 1999; **48**: 613–24.

83. Clemons M, Regnard C, Appleton T. Alertness, cognition and morphine in patients with advanced cancer. *Cancer Treatment Reviews.* 1996; **22**: 451–68.

84. Vainio A, Ollila J, Matikainene E *et al.* Driving ability in cancer patients receiving long-term morphine analgesia. *Lancet.* 1995; **346**: 667–70.

85. Dertwinkel R, Zenz M, Strumpf M *et al.* Drugs and driving. Abstracts of the IVth Congress of the EAPC, 6–9 December 1995, Barcelona (Spain). *European Journal of Palliative Care.* 15.

* 86. Bruera E, Miller MJ, MacMillan K, Kuehn N. Neuropsychological effects of methylphenidate in patients receiving a continuous infusion of narcotics for cancer pain. *Pain.* 1992; **48**: 163–6.

87. Bruera E, Fainsinger R, MacEachern T, Hanson J. The use of methylphenidate in patients with incident cancer pain receiving regular opioids. A preliminary report. *Pain.* 1992; **50**: 75–7.

88. American Psychiatric Association. *Diagnostic and statistical manual of mental disorders*, 4th edn. Washington DC: American Psychiatric Association, 1994.

89. World Health Organization. *International statistical classification of diseases and related health problems,* 10th revision. Geneva: World Health Organization, 1992.

90. Caraceni A, Martini C, DeConno F, Ventafridda V. Organic brain syndromes and opioid administration for cancer pain. *Journal of Pain and Symptom Management.* 1994; **9**: 527–33.

91. Galer BS, Coyle N, Pasternak GW, Portenoy RK. Individual variability in the response to different opioids: report of five cases. *Pain.* 1992; **49**: 87–91.

92. Paix A, Coleman A, Lees J *et al.* Subcutaneous fentanyl and sufentanil infusion for substitution for morphine intolerance in cancer pain management. *Pain.* 1995; **63**: 263–9.

93. Bruera E, Schoeller T, Montejo G. Organic hallucinosis in patients receiving high doses of opiates for cancer pain. *Pain.* 1992; **48**: 397–9.

94. Fountain A. Visual hallucinations: a prevalence study among hospice inpatients. *Palliative Medicine.* 2001; **15**: 19–25.

95. Gaudreau JD, Gagnon P, Harel F *et al.* Psychoactive medications and risk of delirium in hospitalized cancer patients. *Journal of Clinical Oncology.* 2005; **23**: 6712–18.

96. Gagnon PR, Allard P, Masse B. Delirium in terminal cancer: a prospective study on incidence, prevalence and clinical course. Abstract 12th International Congress on Care of the Terminally Ill, Montreal, September 13–17, 1998. *Journal of Palliative Care.* 1998; **14**: 106.

97. Poyhia R, Vainio A, Kalso E. A review of oxycodone's clinical pharmacokinetics and pharmacodynamics. *Journal of Pain and Symptom Management.* 1993; **8**: 63–7.

98. Heiskanen T, Kalso E. Controlled-release oxycodone and morphine in cancer related pain. *Pain.* 1997; **73**: 37–45.

99. Bruera E, Belzile M, Pituskin E *et al.* Randomized, double-blind, cross-over trial comparing safety and efficacy of oral controlled-release oxycodone with controlled-release morphine in patients with cancer pain. *Journal of Clinical Oncology.* 1998; **16**: 3222–9.

100. Stiefel F, Fainsinger R, Bruera E. Acute confusional states in patients with advanced cancer. *Journal of Pain and Symptom Management.* 1992; **7**: 94–8.

101. Bruera E, Miller L, McCallion J et al. Cognitive failure in patients with terminal cancer: a prospective study. Journal of Pain and Symptom Management. 1992; 7: 192–5.

102. Lawlor P, Gagnon B, Mancini I et al. Phenomenology of delirium and its subtypes in advanced cancer patients: a prospective study. Abstract, 12th International Congress on Care of the Terminally Ill, Montreal, September 13–17, 1998. Journal of Palliative Care. 1998; 14: 106.

103. Bruera E, Fainsinger R, Miller MJ, Juehn N. The assessment of pain intensity in patients with cognitive failure: a preliminary report. Journal of Pain and Symptom Management. 1992; 7: 267–70.

104. Coyle N, Breitbart W, Weaber S, Portenoy R. Delirium as a contributing factor to "crescendo" pain: three case reports. Journal of Pain and Symptom Management. 1994; 9: 44–7.

105. Folstein MF, Folstein SE, McHugh PR. "Mini Mental State": a practical method of grading the cognitive state of patients for the clinician. Journal of Psychiatric Research. 1975; 12: 189–98.

106. Núñez Olarte JM. Control de la confusión en pacientes con cáncer en situación terminal. Revista de la Sociedad Española DOLOR. 1995; 2 (Suppl. II): 40–5.

107. Inouye SK, van Dyck CH, Alessi CA et al. Clarifying confusion: the confusion assessment method. Annals of Internal Medicine. 1990; 113: 941–8.

108. Breitbart W, Rosenfeld B, Roth A et al. The Memorial Delirium Assessment Scale. Journal of Pain and Symptom Management. 1997; 13: 128–37.

*109. MacLeod AD. The management of delirium in hospice practice. European Journal of Palliative Care. 1997; 4: 16–120.

110. Núñez JM. Síndromes neuropsicológicos: ansiedad, depresión y confusión. In: Gómez-Batiste X, Planas Domingo J, Roca Casas J, Viladiu Quemada P (eds). Cuidados paliativos en oncología. Barcelona: Editorial Jims, 1996: 229–36.

111. Passik SD, Cooper M. Complicated delirium in a cancer patient successfully treated with olanzapine. Journal of Pain and Symptom Management. 1999; 17: 219–23.

112. Slatkin N, Rhiner M. Treatment of opioid-induced delirium with acetylcholinesterase inhibitors: a case report. Journal of Pain and Symptom Management. 2004; 27: 268–73.

113. Pereira J, Hanson J, Bruera E. The frequency and clinical course of cognitive impairment in patients with terminal cancer. Cancer. 1997; 79: 835–42.

114. Bruera E, Miller MJ, Kuehn N et al. Estimate of survival of patients admitted to a palliative care unit: a prospective study. Journal of Pain and Symptom Management. 1992; 7: 82–6.

*115. Núñez Olarte JM. Opioid-induced myoclonus. European Journal of Palliative Care. 1995; 2: 146–50.

116. Hagen N, Swanson R. Strychnine-like multifocal myoclonus and seizures in extremely high-dose opioid administration: treatment strategies. Journal of Pain and Symptom Management. 1997; 14: 51–8.

117. Núñez Olarte JM. Treatment of opioid-induced myoclonus. Abstract book. 4th Congress of the European Association for Palliative Care, Barcelona, December 1995. European Journal of Palliative Care. 1995; 2: 146–50.

118. Potter JM, Reid DB, Shaw RJ et al. Myoclonus associated with treatment with high doses of morphine: the role of supplemental drugs. British Medical Journal. 1989; 299: 150–3.

119. Taboada R, Juez I, Conti M, Núñez Olarte JM. Papel de la hipomagnesemia en el mioclonus asociado a altas dosis de morfina. Abstract book. 1st International Congress for Palliative Care. Madrid. 1994; February: 78.

*120. Mercadante S. Pathophysiology and treatment of opioid-related myoclonus in cancer patients. Pain. 1998; 74: 5–9.

121. Kloke M, Bingel U, Seeber S. Complications of spinal opioid therapy: myoclonus, spastic muscle tone and spinal jerking. Supportive Care in Cancer. 1994; 2: 249–52.

122. Kronenberg MF, Laimer I, Rifici C et al. Epileptic seizure associated with intracerebroventricular and intrathecal morphine bolus. Pain. 1998; 75: 383–7.

123. Núñez Olarte JM. Opioid-induced myoclonus. Abstract Book. 6th Congress of the European Association for Palliative Care, Geneva. 1999; September: 29.

124. Mercadante S, Villari P, Fulfaro F. Gabapentin for opioid-related myoclonus in cancer patients. Supportive Care in Cancer. 2001; 9: 205–6.

125. Bertran F, Denise P, Letellier P. Nonconvulsive status epilepticus: the role of morphine and its antagonist. Neurophysiologie Clinique. 2000; 30: 109–12.

126. Wilson GR, Reisfield GM. Morphine hyperalgesia: a case report. American Journal of Hospital and Palliative Care. 2003; 20: 459–61.

127. Mercadante S, Ferrera P, Villari P, Arcuri E. Hyperalgesia: an emerging iatrogenic syndrome. Journal of Pain and Symptom Management. 2003; 26: 769–75.

128. Sjogren P, Jonsson T, Jensen NH et al. Hyperalgesia and myoclonus in terminal cancer patients treated with continuous intravenous morphine. Pain. 1993; 55: 93–7.

129. Sjogren P, Jensen NH, Jensen TS. Disappearance of morphine-induced hyperalgesia after discontinuing or substituting morphine with other opioid agonists. Pain. 1994; 59: 313–16.

130. Mercadante S, Arcuri E. Hyperalgesia and opioid switching. American Journal of Hospice and Palliative Care. 2005; 22: 291–4.

131. Sykes N. The treatment of morphine-induced constipation. European Journal of Palliative Care. 1998; 5: 12–15.

*132. Sykes NP. Constipation and diarrhoea. In: Doyle D, Hanks G, Cherny N, Calman K (eds). Oxford textbook of paliative medicine, 3rd edn. Oxford: Oxford University Press, 2004: 483–96.

133. Sykes NP. The relationship between opioid use and laxative use in terminally ill cancer patients. Palliative Medicine. 1998; 12: 375–82.

*134. Derby S, Portenoy RK. Assessment and management of opioid-induced constipation. In: Portenoy RK, Bruera E (eds). *Topics in palliative care*, vol 1. New York: Oxford University Press, 1997: 95–112.

135. Fallon MT, Hanks GW. Morphine, constipation and performance status in advanced cancer patients. *Palliative Medicine*. 1999; **13**: 159–60.

136. Mancini I, Hanson J, Bruera E. Opioid type and other clinical predictors of laxative dose in advanced cancer patients: a retrospective study. *Journal of Pain and Symptom Management*. 1998; **15**: S16.

137. Megens AAHP, Artois K, Vermeire J *et al*. Comparison of the analgesic and intestinal effects of fentanyl and morphine in rats. *Journal of Pain and Symptom Management*. 1998; **15**: 253–8.

138. Bruera E, Suárez-Almazor M, Velasco A *et al*. The assessment of constipation in terminal cancer patients admitted to a palliative care unit: a retrospective review. *Journal of Pain and Symptom Management*. 1994; **9**: 515–19.

139. Sykes NP. Methods of assessment of bowel function in patients with advanced cancer. *Palliative Medicine*. 1990; **4**: 287–92.

140. Donner B, Zenz M, Tryba M, Strumpf M. Direct conversion from oral morphine to transdermal fentanyl: a multicenter study in patients with cancer pain. *Pain*. 1996; **64**: 527–34.

141. Donner B, Zenz M, Strumpf M, Raber M. Long-term treatment of cancer pain with transdermal fentanyl. *Journal of Pain and Symptom Management*. 1998; **15**: 168–75.

142. Zech DFJ, Grond SUA, Lynch J *et al*. Transdermal fentanyl and initial dose-finding with patient-controlled analgesia in cancer pain. A pilot study with 20 terminally ill cancer patients. *Pain*. 1992; **50**: 293–301.

143. Allan L, Hayes H, Jensen NH *et al*. Evidence for better analgesia with transdermal fentanyl in chronic pain treatment: comparison with sustained release morphine in a cross-over efficacy, safety and quality of life trial. Abstract Book. 17th Annual Scientific Meeting, American Pain Society, San Diego. 1998; November: 132.

144. Staats PS, Markowitz J, Schein J. Incidence of constipation associated with long-acting opioid therapy: a comparative study. *Southern Medical Journal*. 2004; **97**: 129–34.

145. Radbruch L, Sabatowski R, Loick G *et al*. Constipation and the use of laxatives: a comparison between transdermal fentanyl and oral morphine. *Palliative Medicine*. 2000; **14**: 111–19.

146. Davis A, Prentice W. Fentanyl, morphine and constipation (letter). *Journal of Pain and Symptom Management*. 1998; **16**: 141–2.

147. Ahmedzai SH. Authors' response (letter). *Journal of Pain and Symptom Management*. 1998; **16**: 142–4.

148. Daeninck PJ, Bruera E. Reduction in constipation and laxative requirements following opioid rotation to methadone: a report of four cases. *Journal of Pain and Symptom Management*. 1999; **18**: 303–09.

149. Klaschik E, Nauck F, Ostgathe C. Constipation – modern laxative therapy. *Supportive Care in Cancer*. 2003; **11**: 679–85.

150. Bruera E, Brenneis C, Michaud M, MacDonald N. Continuous subcutaneous infusion of metoclopramide for treatment of narcotic bowel syndrome. *Cancer Treatment Reports*. 1987; **71**: 1121–2.

151. Agra Y, Sacristan A, Gonzalez M *et al*. Efficacy of senna versus lactulose in terminal cancer patients treated with opioids. *Journal of Pain and Symptom Management*. 1998; **15**: 1–7.

152. Ramesh PR, Kumar KS, Rajagopal MR *et al*. Managing morphine-induced constipation: a controlled comparison of an ayurvedic formulation and senna. *Journal of Pain and Symptom Management*. 1998; **16**: 240–4.

153. Sykes NP. A volunteer model for the comparison of laxatives in opioid-related constipation. *Journal of Pain and Symptom Management*. 1996; **11**: 363–9.

154. Attar A, Lemann M, Ferguson A *et al*. Comparison of a low dose polyethilene glycol electrolyte solution with lactulose for treatment of chronic constipation. *Gut*. 1999; **44**: 226–30.

155. Wirz S, Klaschik E. Management of constipation in palliative care patients undergoing opioid therapy: is polyethylene glycol an option. *American Journal of Hospice and Palliative Care*. 2005; **22**: 375–81.

156. Yuan CS, Foss FJ, O'Connor M *et al*. Methylnaltrexone prevents morphine-induced delay in oral–cecal transit time without affecting analgesia: a double-blind randomized placebo-controlled trial. *Clinical Pharmacology and Therapeutics*. 1996; **59**: 469–75.

157. Holzer P. Treatment of opioid-induced gut dysfunction. *Expert Opinion on Investigational Drugs*. 2007; **16**: 181–94.

158. Liu M, Wittbrodt E. Low-dose oral naloxone reverses opioid-induced constipation and analgesia. *Journal of Pain and Symptom Management*. 2002; **23**: 48–53.

159. Hagen NA, Foley KM, Cerbone DJ *et al*. Chronic nausea and morphine-6-glucuronide. *Journal of Pain and Symptom Management*. 1991; **6**: 125–8.

160. Twycross R, Back I. Nausea and vomiting in advanced cancer. *European Journal of Palliative Care*. 1998; **5**: 39–45.

161. Campora E, Merlini L, Pace M *et al*. The incidence of narcotic-induced emesis. *Journal of Pain and Symptom Management*. 1991; **6**: 428–30.

162. Aparasu R, McCoy RA, Weber C *et al*. Opioid-induced emesis among hospitalized non-surgical patients: effect on pain and quality of life. *Journal of Pain and Symptom Management*. 1999; **18**: 280–8.

163. Ferris FD, Kerr IG, Sone M, Marcuzzi M. Transdermal scopolamine use in the control of narcotic-induced nausea. *Journal of Pain and Symptom Management*. 1991; **6**: 389–93.

164. Mercadante S, Sapio M, Serretta R. Ondansentron in nausea and vomiting induced by spinal morphine. *Journal of Pain and Symptom Management*. 1998; **16**: 259–62.

165. Mystakidou K, Befon S, Liossi C, Vlachos L. Comparison of tropisetron and chlorpromazine combinations in the control of nausea and vomiting in patients with advanced

cancer. *Journal of Pain and Symptom Management*. 1998; **15**: 176–84.

166. Nakata K, Mammoto T, Kita T *et al.* Continuous epidural, not intravenous, droperidol inhibits pruritus, nausea, and vomiting during epidural morphine analgesia. *Journal of Clinical Anesthesia*. 2002; **14**: 121–5.

167. Hardy J, Daly S, McQuade B *et al.* A double-blind, randomised, parallel group, multinational, multicentre study comparing a single dose of ondansentron 24 mg p.o. with placebo and metoclopramide 10 mg t.d.s. p.o. in the treatment of opioid-induced nausea and emesis in cancer patients. *Supportive Care in Cancer*. 2002; **10**: 231–6.

168. Shoji A, Toda M, Suzuki K *et al.* Insufficient effectiveness of 5-hydroxitryptamine-3 receptor antagonists due to oral morphine administration in patients with cisplatin-induced emesis. *Journal of Clinical Oncology*. 1999; **17**: 1926–30.

169. Passik SD, Lundbergh J, Kirsh KL *et al.* A pilot exploration of the antiemetic activity of olanzapine for the relief of nausea in patients with advanced cancer and pain. *Journal of Pain and Symptom Management*. 2002; **23**: 526–32.

*170. Walsh TD, Rivera NI, Kaiko R. Oral morphine and respiratory function amongst hospice inpatients with advanced cancer. *Supportive Care in Cancer*. 2003; **11**: 780–4.

171. Borgbjerg FM, Nielsen K, Franks J. Experimental pain stimulates respiration and attenuates morphine-induced respiratory depression: a controlled study in human volunteers. *Pain*. 1996; **64**: 123–8.

172. Benedetti F, Amanzio M, Baldi S *et al.* The specific effects of prior opioid exposure on placebo analgesia and placebo respiratory depression. *Pain*. 1998; **75**: 313–19.

173. Quevedo F, Walsh D. Morphine-induced ventilatory failure after spinal cord compression. *Journal of Pain and Symptom Management*. 1999; **18**: 140–2.

174. Hanks GC, Twycross RG, Lloyd JM. Unexpected complication of successful nerve block (morphine-induced respiratory depression precipitated by removal of severe pain). *Anaesthesia*. 1981; **36**: 37–9.

*175. Regnard C, Pelham A. Severe respiratory depression and sedation with transdermal fentanyl: four case studies. *Palliative Medicine*. 2003; **17**: 714–16.

*176. Oneschuk D, Bruera E. Respiratory depression during methadone rotation in a patient with advanced cancer. *Journal of Palliative Care*. 2000; **16**: 50–4.

*177. Barnung SK, Treschow M, Borgbjerg FM. Respiratory depression following oral tramadol in a patient with impaired renal function. *Pain*. 1997; **71**: 111–12.

178. Bruera E, Schoeller T, Wenk R *et al.* A prospective multi-center asssessment of the Edmonton staging system for cancer pain. *Journal of Pain and Symptom Management*. 1995; **10**: 348–55.

179. Collin E, Poulain P, Gauvain-Piquard A *et al.* Is disease progression the major factor in morphine "tolerance" in cancer pain treatment? *Pain*. 1993; **55**: 319–26.

180. Mercadante S, Villari P, Ferrera P. Burst ketamine to reverse opioid tolerance in cancer pain. *Journal of Pain and Symptom Management*. 2003; **25**: 302–05.

181. Kanner RM, Foley K. Patterns of narcotic drug use in a cancer pain clinic. *Annals of the New York Academy of Sciences*. 1981; **362**: 161–72.

*182. Cowan DT, Wilson-Barnett J, Griffiths P *et al.* A randomized, double-blind, placebo-controlled, cross-over pilot study to assess the effects of long-term opioid drug consumption and subsequent abstinence in chronic noncancer pain patients receiving controlled-release morphine. *Pain Medicine*. 2005; **6**: 113–21.

183. Davies AN, Daniels C, Pugh R, Sharma K. A comparison of artificial saliva and pilocarpine in the management of xerostomia in patients with advanced cancer. *Palliative Medicine*. 1998; **12**: 105–11.

184. Davies A, Gibbs L, Broadley K. An investigation into the relationship between xerostomia and hyposalivation in patients with advanced cancer. Abstract Book. 6th Congress of the European Association for Palliative Care, Geneva. 1999; September: 21.

185. Waller A, Bercovitch M, Dori S, et al. Sialometry and its relationship to oral symptoms and quality of life parameters in in terminally ill patients. Abstract Book. 6th Congress of the European Association for Palliative Care, Geneva, September, 1999. 1999: 44.

186. Davies AN. A comparison of chewing gum and artificial saliva in the management of xerostomia in patients with advanced cancer. Abstract Book. 6th Congress of the European Association for Palliative Care, Geneva. 1999; September: 20.

187. Mercadante S, Calderone L, Villari P *et al.* The use of pilocarpine in opioid-induced xerostomia. *Palliative Medicine*. 2000; **14**: 529–31.

188. Bamigbade TA, Langford RM. The clinical use of tramadol hydrochloride. *Pain Reviews*. 1998; **5**: 155–82.

189. Zylberberg H, Fontaine H, Correas JM *et al.* Dilated bile duct in patients receiving narcotic substitution: an early report. *Journal of Clinical Gastroenterology*. 2000; **31**: 159–61.

190. Dunteman E, Karanikolas M, Filos KS. Transnasal butorphanol for the treatment of opioid-induced pruritus unresponsive to antihistamines. *Journal of Pain and Symptom Management*. 1996; **12**: 255–60.

191. Katcher J, Walsh D. Opioid-induced itching: morphine sulfate and hydromorphone hydrochloride. *Journal of Pain and Symptom Management*. 1999; **17**: 70–2.

192. Mercadante S, Villari P, Fulfaro F. Rifampicin in opioid-induced itching. *Supportive Care in Cancer*. 2001; **9**: 467–8.

193. Bruera E, Miller MJ. Non-cardiogenic pulmonary edema after narcotic treatment for cancer pain. *Pain*. 1989; **39**: 297–300.

194. Wilcox SK. Persistent hiccups after slow-release morphine. *Palliative Medicine*. 2005; **19**: 568–9.

195. Finch PM, Roberts LJ, Price L *et al.* Hypogonadism in patients treated with intrathecal morphine. *Clinical Journal of Pain*. 2000; **16**: 251–4.

196. Rajagopal A, Bruera E. Improvement in sexual function after reduction of chronic high-dose opioid medication in a cancer survivor. *Pain Medicine*. 2003; **4**: 379–83.

197. Rajagopal A, Vassilopoulou-Sellin R, Palmer JL *et al.* Hypogonadism and sexual dysfunction in male cancer survivors receiving chronic opioid therapy. *Journal of Pain and Symptom Management.* 2003; **26**: 1055–61.

198. Rajagopal A, Vassilopoulou-Sellin R, Palmer JL *et al.* Symptomatic hypogonadism in male survivors of cancer with chronic exposure to opioids. *Cancer.* 2004; **100**: 851–8.

199. Rajagopal A, Kala S, Bruera E. Possible exacerbation of adrenal suppression from intrathecal morphine in a patient receiving pulsed dexamethasone for multiple myeloma. *Journal of Pain and Symptom Management.* 2003; **26**: 786–8.

200. Sacerdote P, Bianchi M, Gaspani L *et al.* The effects of tramadol and morphine on immune responses and pain after surgery in cancer patients. *Anesthesia and Analgesia.* 2000; **90**: 1411–14.

15

Clinical pharmacology and therapeutics: drugs for neuropathic pain in cancer

CARINA SAXBY AND MICHAEL BENNETT

Introduction	200	NMDA receptor antagonists	207
Opioids	202	Local anesthetics and other approaches	208
Antidepressants	205	Drug synergy and sequencing	209
Antiepileptics	206	References	209

KEY LEARNING POINTS

- Neuropathic pain is more common in patients with cancer than in patients with other types of chronic pain and its etiology may be different.
- Because patients with cancer tend to have a lower performance status and may be more susceptible to adverse effects from medication, prescribing should be on an individual patient basis, balancing efficacy with side-effect profile.
- Most evidence for the effectiveness of drugs in neuropathic pain comes from a noncancer setting.

- Evidence supports the use of:
  - opioids;
  - antiepileptics, e.g. gabapentin, pregabalin;
  - antidepressants, e.g. amitriptyline.
- Evidence for the use of NMDA (*N*-methyl-D-aspartate) antagonists and newer antidepressants in cancer patients is less robust.
- Drug synergy may afford improved analgesia for patients with reduced side effects, but evidence for this is only emerging.

INTRODUCTION

According to the International Association for the Study of Pain (IASP), neuropathic pain is initiated or caused by a primary lesion or dysfunction of the nervous system.[1] It has been divided in the past into "physiological" and "pathological" neuropathic pain. The first term defines pain that is generated by ongoing tissue damage around the nerve, e.g. by inflammation, tumor, or trauma. The latter term refers to nerve damage or persistent dysfunction.

Neuropathic pain is best thought of as an abnormal activation of pain pathways that can occur as a result of injury or dysfunction to peripheral nerves and posterior roots (peripheral neuropathic pain) and spinal cord and brain (central pain).

Prevalence

In the general population, a recent UK study showed the prevalence of chronic pain of predominantly neuropathic origin was 8.2 percent in adults.[2] Percentages are higher for specific subgroups of the population, e.g. between 11 and 23 percent of patients with diabetes mellitus. The prevalence of cancer pain inferred to have neuropathic mechanisms was 39.7 percent in an international survey conducted on behalf of the IASP.[3]

Etiology

Patients with cancer may experience neuropathic pain as a direct consequence of the tumor itself, by diagnostic interventions or by treatments such as surgery, chemotherapy, and radiotherapy (see Chapter 3, Cancer pain syndromes and Chapter 29, Pain in cancer survivors). Tumors may infiltrate or cause compression of adjacent nerves, e.g. cranial neuralgias as a result of base of skull metastases. Post-thoracotomy neuropathic pain can occur following surgery for lung tumors. Chemotherapeutic agents, e.g. oxaliplatin, can cause nerve damage, as can radiotherapy. Cancer patients also suffer from neuropathic pains secondary to conditions not directly related to their cancer, such as postherpetic neuralgia.

Patient characteristics

The aim of any pharmacological intervention is to effectively treat the pain without causing any further deterioration in quality of life for the patient. The cancer population is different to the general population in a number of ways and this has implications for approaches to treatments.

In general, the cancer population is older and is therefore likely to have significantly more comorbidities, including cognitive impairment.[4] Performance status may be poor[5] and often there can be a rapidly changing clinical picture which can make drug use and titration more difficult than in the general population. Difficulty in administration of medicines because of the cancer or its treatment, e.g. head and neck cancers, can also impact on drug choice and acceptability. On the other hand, when a patient is entering the more palliative stages of their illness, concerns about the long-term adverse effects of drugs such as opioids are fewer. If the neuropathic pain is caused by local effects of a tumor then oncological options for its treatment may provide an alternative to drug therapy.

In summary, pharmacological treatment of neuropathic pain in cancer patients is different from that in the general population because of the patient characteristics and the changing clinical picture compounded by the fact that research in this area and patient group is lacking.

Table 15.1 gives guidance on the dosing schedule for the drugs used in neuropathic pain in cancer.

Table 15.1 Dosing schedule for medications in cancer neuropathic pain.

Medication	Starting dose	Titration	Maximum dose	Duration of adequate trial
Antiepileptic, e.g. gabapentin				
	100–300 mg nightly or 100–300 mg three times daily	Increase by 100–300 mg/day every 1–7 days as needed and tolerated	3600 mg/day. Reduce dose in renal impairment	1–2 weeks at maximum tolerated dose. May take 3–6 weeks to titrate to maximum dose
Tricyclic antidepressant, e.g. amitriptyline				
	10–25 mg at night	Increase by 10–25 mg every 3–7 days as tolerated	75–150 mg/day	6–8 weeks with 1–2 weeks at maximum tolerated dose
Opioid analgesics, e.g. morphine sulfate				
	2.5–5 mg of immediate release preparation every 4 hours or 5–10 mg twice/day of modified release preparation	Increase regular daily dose by 30–50% every 7 days as tolerated	No maximum with careful titration. Seek specialist advice from pain specialist at doses exceeding 120–180 mg/day	4–6 weeks
NMDA receptor antagonist, e.g. ketamine				
	10 mg orally four times/day or 50–150 mg/day via subcutaneous route	Increase by 5–10 mg per dose orally every 3 days or by 50–100 mg/day subcutaneously	10–100 mg four times/day orally or 50–600 mg/day subcutaneously	1 week

OPIOIDS

Introduction

Opioids would not usually be considered part of the first-line approach to neuropathic pain in noncancer patients. However, cancer patients may already be treated with opioids for existing non-neuropathic pain, and this class of drugs is generally more acceptable as a form of analgesia than in noncancer contexts. In practice, opioids are more commonly used as first-line therapy in this setting. Details of the evidence to support this approach is summarized below.

The term opioid includes naturally occurring, semi-synthetic, and synthetic drugs which combine with opioid receptors to produce their effects. An opiate is a drug derived from the opium poppy, e.g. morphine and codeine.

Three types of opioid receptor are well recognized as mediating analgesia: μ (mu), κ (kappa), δ (delta). The majority of drugs used clinically act at the μ-receptor, e.g. morphine, fentanyl, methadone, etc., and their effects are antagonized by naloxone (**Table 15.2**).

Opioid receptors are found throughout the spinal cord and in many areas of the brain. Within the dorsal horn of the spinal cord, they are located presynaptically on primary afferent neurons. Their mechanism of action here is to reduce transmitter release from nociceptive C-fibers, so that spinal neurons are less excited by incoming painful messages. Additionally, activated opioid receptors may boost the descending inhibitory pathway by blocking GABA release within the midbrain. This results in increased antinociceptive outflow from the midbrain to the spinal cord.

Controversies in neuropathic pain

Opinions on the effectiveness of opioids in neuropathic pain have until recently been divided. Studies in the past have led some investigators to consider that neuropathic pain was inherently resistant to opioids.[6] More recently, evidence has emerged that this is not the case,[7][II], [8][II], [9][III], [10][V], [11][II], [12][II], [13][II] although neuropathic pain

may be less responsive to opioids than nociceptive pain.[8, 9] Neuropathic pain may be relieved by opioids provided that individual titration achieves an optimal balance between maximal analgesia and unmanageable side effects.[14] This is supported by the fact that in a review of cancer patients with neuropathic pain (either pure neuropathic pain or mixed neuropathic/nociceptive pain), the majority gained significant pain relief by following the World Health Organization's (WHO) analgesic ladder. Of the group with pure neuropathic pain, 47 percent required no adjuvants and the authors concluded that opioids and nonopioids produced adequate analgesia.[15][III]

Questions have also been raised as to whether improvements in patient's pain are secondary to the sensory effects of morphine or to the affective effects. Kupers et al.[16] concluded from a small, double-blind, placebo-controlled crossover study that morphine reduced the affective, but not the sensory, dimension of pain sensation in patients with neurogenic pain. Because opioids can modulate the patient's emotional experience of pain, Dellermijn and Vanneste used an active placebo (diazepam) in a trial looking at the analgesic effects of intravenous fentanyl.[17][II] Although fentanyl and diazepam had a similar sedative effect, fentanyl was more effective in decreasing both pain intensity and pain unpleasantness. They concluded that the pain relief achieved by fentanyl was as a result of its intrinsic analgesic effect. Jadad et al.[8] also found no evidence that analgesic responses to morphine in patients with neuropathic pain were due to a change in mood.

A number of reasons exist as to why neuropathic pain may be less sensitive to opioids than nociceptive pain.[18] Genetic variation in receptor sensitivity, and in particular genetic polymorphisms, may influence the effect of opioids between individuals with apparently similar pains. Nerve damage can cause a loss of spinal opioid receptors which results in a reduction in opioid sensitivity. Increases in the levels of cholecystokinin (CCK) which antagonizes opioid actions can be seen following nerve damage. Changes that occur following nerve damage can result in hyperexcitability of spinal neurons, a phenomenon known as "wind up." Increasing doses of opioid may be required to control this. The N-methyl-D-aspartic acid (NMDA) receptor channel complex is felt to

Table 15.2 Opioid activity at receptor sites.

	Mu	Kappa	Delta	NOP	NMDA	Serotonergic	Noradenergic
Morphine	+						
Oxycodone	+	+					
Fentanyl	++						
Tramadol	+					+	+
Methadone	+				−		
Buprenorphine	(+)	−	−				
Diamorphine	+						

+, full agonist; (+), partial agonist; −, antagonist; NOP, nociceptin orphain FQ peptide; NMDA, N-methyl-D-aspartic acid.

play a significant role in the maintenance of these pain states (see below under NMDA receptor antagonists). Trials have shown that the administration of ketamine, an NMDA receptor antagonist, appears to restore opioid sensitivity in patients where wind up is established. Indeed in such patients, opioids (in particular pure μ-agonists) may themselves play a role in inducing excitation when used in large doses.[19] Other opioids that have antagonist activity at certain receptors, for example buprenorphine and methadone, may inhibit the process that leads to excitation.

The classification of neuropathic pain within trial settings is also felt to have added to the controversy about the role of opioids in treating neuropathic pain patients.[14, 20] As several types of neuropathic pain possess distinct mechanisms, each requiring specific treatments, the degree of opioid responsiveness of different neuropathic syndromes may vary. Failure to differentiate types of neuropathic pain may account for disparate responses to opioid medication. Peripheral neuropathic pain may respond better to opioids than central pain[11] and Attal et al.[21][II] showed that opioids appear to selectively reduce spontaneous and touch-evoked allodynia in trials using quantitative methods for sensory testing. Dellermijn and Vanneste,[17] however, found that the type of neuropathic pain did not predict the responsiveness of patients to i.v. fentanyl. Accurate clinical distinction of neuropathic pain can be impossible in some cases and indeed may change because of the inherent plasticity of the neurological system. It remains unclear whether categorizing painful neurological injuries in cancer patients on the basis of inferred pathophysiology is useful when deciding about different treatment options.

Individual drugs

Evidence now supports an important role for opioids in the treatment of neuropathic pain – listed below are the individual opioids and the evidence for their use. Much of the evidence is from trials on patients with noncancer neuropathic pain. Switching between different opioid drugs is advocated in an effort to maximize analgesia and minimize adverse effects, which patients may experience as a result of variations in opioid receptor affinity and side effect profile of each opioid.[22]

MORPHINE

Pharmacology

Morphine is the main pharmacologically active constituent of opium and is the prototypical μ-receptor agonist. Morphine is available orally as an immediate-release elixir or tablets and as sustained-release preparations, as well as in injection form. It is almost completely absorbed after oral administration in the upper small bowel and is metabolized in the liver and other sites to morphine-3-glucuronide (M3G) and morphine-6-glucuronide (M6G). The latter is an active metabolite and is a more potent analgesic than morphine. It is renally excreted and in renal failure the plasma half-life of M6G increases significantly which may lead to toxicity.

Clinical studies

As discussed above, initial studies queried whether the effectiveness of morphine in neuropathic pain was because of its ability to modulate mood, but this has been shown not to be the case. The effectiveness of morphine in treating postherpetic neuralgia and diabetic neuropathy has been established in a number of single-dose and longer-term studies.[7, 8, 12, 23][II] In these studies, morphine was equally effective as standard adjuvant treatments, such as gabapentin and tricyclic antidepressants (TCA). The frequency of adverse effects was similar and in the study comparing morphine with TCAs, patients preferred treatment with opioids.[12] When compared alone and in combination against placebo in a recent trial, the combination of morphine with gabapentin achieved significantly better analgesia at lower doses of each drug than either as a single agent.[23] This may imply synergism between the drugs, but further trials need to be done to establish this finding.

In central neuropathic pain, Attal et al.[21] have demonstrated that intravenous morphine induces analgesic effects on some components, e.g. brush-induced allodynia compared to placebo, but that these effects were less successful in the long term, at one year.

FENTANYL

Pharmacology

Transdermal fentanyl is a self-adhesive patch with a rate-limiting membrane which allows a standard amount of fentanyl to cross each hour from the patch into the skin and the patch is usually changed every 72 hours. It is a potent synthetic μ-receptor antagonist and is approximately 100 times as potent as morphine. Fentanyl is metabolized in the liver to the inactive metabolite nor-fentanyl which undergoes renal excretion. It is safe to use in patients with renal impairment and is less constipating than morphine. Fentanyl is also available as oral transmucosal fentanyl citrate lozenges for absorption on to the buccal mucosa – these are often used to control cancer breakthrough pain.

Clinical studies

A double-blind crossover study involving 53 patients with a variety of neuropathic pains found that an intravenous infusion of fentanyl (5 μg/kg/hour) relieved pain more effectively over eight hours than placebo or diazepam infusion.[17] A follow-up study investigating whether there was a sustained analgesic effect in continued fentanyl therapy (in transdermal form) in the same group of patients was disappointing.[24][III] Only a third of the original patients felt some relief in their pain; the other two-thirds experienced no pain improvement or adverse effects leading to withdrawal.

METHADONE

Pharmacology

Methadone is a synthetic opioid with mixed properties. It is a μ-receptor agonist, an NMDA receptor-channel blocker and a presynaptic blocker of serotonin reuptake. It is well absorbed after oral administration and has a high volume of distribution. Methadone accumulates in the tissues when given repeatedly, creating an extensive reservoir. It has a long and variable half-life (range, 8–80 hours) which is not predicted by age, and is metabolized in the liver to inactive substances. The potency ratio of methadone to morphine has been difficult to establish. Best estimates are that it is five to ten times more potent than morphine with chronic administration.

Clinical studies

There is evidence to suggest that methadone is an analgesic of similar efficacy to morphine in cancer pain.[25] [I] Although there are anecdotal reports of the successful use of methadone in patients with severe cancer neuropathic pain previously treated with morphine, a Cochrane review revealed a lack of evidence to support the superiority of methadone over morphine in this context.[26][I]

OXYCODONE

Pharmacology

Oxycodone is a semi-synthetic opioid which acts on both the μ- and κ-opioid receptors. It is its action at the κ-receptor that has been used to explain its effectiveness in neuropathic pain and a reduction in adverse effects in comparison to morphine. It has a high oral bioavailability and is twice as potent as oral morphine. Oxycodone and its metabolites are excreted renally and renal impairment does cause an increase in its half-life. Available formulations include sustained- and immediate-release preparations, as well as injections.

Clinical studies

Good evidence exists to support the role of oxycodone in neuropathic pain. Two small randomized controlled trials were conducted in postherpetic neuralgia and diabetic neuropathy.[13, 27][II] Both showed significant improvements in the group treated with oxycodone in comparison to the placebo arm. A more recent trial over a six-week period in patients with diabetic neuropathy showed that oxycodone was effective in the treatment of moderate to severe neuropathic pain.[28][II]

BUPRENORPHINE

Pharmacology

Buprenorphine is a potent partial agonist at the μ-receptor. It is also a weak δ- and κ-receptor antagonist. It is available as sublingual tablets and also as transdermal patches which act similarly to fentanyl patches. Buprenorphine is metabolized to inactive substances and is safe to use in renal failure. Animal and volunteer studies suggest that buprenorphine has the highest antihyperalgesic effect of all opioids, i.e. most able to inhibit excitation.[29, 30]

Clinical studies

Case series exist that support the use of buprenorphine in small numbers of patients with mixed and pure neuropathic pain, as well as one that describes the effective use of buprenorphine in postthoractomy neuropathic pain.[31] Another study examined 237 patients with various neuropathic symptoms and pain syndromes and found a clear decrease in the percentage of patients reporting moderate to severe pain after treatment with buprenorphine.[30]

TRAMADOL

Pharmacology

Tramadol is a synthetic opioid which is active at μ-opioid receptors, as well as enhancing central serotonergic and noradrenergic inhibition of pain. The latter sites of activity, while enhancing its analgesic effects, are thought to be responsible for additional antimuscarinic side effects. It is often considered to be a weaker opioid and is five to eight times less potent than morphine. Tramadol is available in normal and sustained release tablets, as well as injections.

Clinical studies

Evidence to support the effectiveness of tramadol in neuropathic pain exists in a number of trials conducted in patients with polyneuropathy, postherpetic neuralgia, and diabetic neuropathy.[32][II], [33][II] A Cochrane review concluded that tramadol was an effective treatment for neuropathic pain with a number needed to treat (NNT) of 3.5, i.e. two patients in every seven will get approximately a 50 percent reduction in their pain with tramadol.[34][I]

DIAMORPHINE

No specific evidence exists for the use of diamorphine in neuropathic pain, although anecdotally some patients do experience greater analgesia with diamorphine via injection or subcutaneous infusion.

ANTIDEPRESSANTS

Clinical pharmacology

TCAs have been widely used for the treatment of neuropathic pain in a variety of noncancer contexts for almost 30 years. Their principal mechanism of action involves inhibiting the presynaptic reuptake of serotonin and noradrenaline in spinal pain pathways, which enhances endogenous pain inhibitory pathways. Secondary amines (nortriptyline and desipramine) are relatively more active on noradrenergic pathways than tertiary amines (amitriptyline and imipramine) which are more balanced, but the latter have additional activity at histamine and muscarinic receptors. As a consequence, tertiary amines are associated with more antimuscarinic and sedating adverse effects than secondary amines. TCAs have been shown to bind to open and inactive sodium channels[35] (the molecular structure of TCAs is very similar to carbamazepine) and may also block voltage-dependent calcium channels.[36]

Selective serotonergic reuptake inhibitors (SSRIs), such as paroxetine and fluoxetine, do not have any activity at noradrenergic or postsynaptic receptors. More recently, a newer class of antidepressants have been developed called serotonin and noradrenergic reuptake inhibitors (SNRIs). These drugs, such as venlafaxine and duloxetine, also do not block postsynaptic receptors. Both SSRIs and SNRIs are better tolerated than TCAs and have minimal adverse effects, the most notable being nausea.

Berger et al.[37] examined a large US health insurance database and identified 956 patients with a diagnosis of cancer and painful neuropathy (the majority of these were probably treatment-related neuropathic pain). A comparison with antiepileptic and antidepressant use revealed that only 14 percent received TCAs, the majority of these were for amitriptyline, suggesting that use of TCAs is relatively low among cancer patients with painful neuropathies.

Tricyclic antidepressants

In controlled clinical trials, TCAs relieve a range of painful peripheral neuropathies (including diabetic neuropathy), postherpetic neuralgia, and central poststroke pain.[38][I], [39] Studies involving patients with phantom limb pain, spinal cord injury pain, or HIV-related neuropathy suggest that TCAs are less effective in these contexts. TCAs relieve neuropathic pain independently of mood and at doses generally lower than those used to treat depression.[40][II]

Systematic reviews have estimated the NNT which is an overall measure of drug efficacy in a particular disease or condition.[38, 39, 41] The NNT usually refers to the number of patients with a condition (e.g. painful diabetic neuropathy) that need to be treated with the drug before one patient experiences 50 percent pain relief. For painful peripheral neuropathy, the NNT for secondary TCAs is 2.5, and for tertiary TCAs it is 2.1. There is a similar pattern in postherpetic neuralgia where NNT values are 3.1 and 2.5 for secondary and tertiary TCAs, respectively. This consistent evidence has led to the view that analgesic efficacy of TCAs is greater with more balanced serotonergic and noradrenergic receptor activity.

Amitriptyline has been studied in cancer neuropathic pain in a randomized, placebo-controlled double blind trial.[42][II] Sixteen patients who were already treated with morphine were randomized to one week of amitriptyline (25 mg for four days, then 50 mg for three days, or half these doses if aged over 65 years) then placebo, or vice versa. At assessment, no difference in global pain intensity or opioid doses were found between treatment arms, although "worst pain" was improved on amitriptyline. Adverse effects were significantly more intense on amitriptyline, but patients did not express a preference for either treatment arm.

Selective serotonin reuptake inhibitors

This group of antidepressants has been examined in painful peripheral neuropathy and, in general, appear to be less effective than TCAs. Paroxetine has shown a small but significant analgesic effect in a trial of painful diabetic neuropathy (n = 20), but fluoxetine is no more effective than placebo in this context.[43][II] The calculated NNT for SSRIs is 6.7. There are no studies of SSRIs in patients with cancer, or cancer treatment-related, neuropathic pain.

Serotonin and noradrenergic reuptake inhibitors

The newer SNRI antidepressants have shown evidence of analgesic effectiveness in peripheral neuropathic pain syndromes. The strongest evidence relates to treatment of painful diabetic neuropathy and both venlafaxine and duloxetine have shown superiority over placebo in double-blind, randomized controlled trials in this condition.[44][II], [45][II] The calculated NNT for the SNRI group is around four, and the number needed to harm (NNH) is not significantly different from that for placebo (i.e. as many patients withdrew on placebo as on active drug in clinical trials).

In cancer neuropathic pain, there is limited direct evidence of the effectiveness of SNRIs. In particular, the small number of studies that exist have examined the effects of venlafaxine on neuropathic pain caused by cancer treatment, rather than caused by the effects of cancer. Studies have shown that perioperative venlafaxine (given one day before, and for two weeks after, mastectomy) significantly reduced the incidence of postmastectomy pain syndrome (PMPS), including chest wall, axilla, and arm pain, at six months follow up.[46] Venlafaxine also appears to be effective in established PMPS in another study of 13 patients who were enrolled into a randomized, placebo-controlled crossover ten-week trial. Although average daily pain intensity was not different between the two groups, average pain relief was.[47][II] Interestingly, the authors describe a potential dose–response relationship in that two poor responders had low serum drug levels, whereas the two patients that were slow drug hydrolyzers had high serum levels and excellent pain relief. This finding is in keeping with larger trials in painful diabetic neuropathy where both venlafaxine and duloxetine have shown increased analgesic efficacy at higher doses.[44, 45]

Summary of evidence

In noncancer neuropathic pain, antidepressants with the most balanced receptor activity (tertiary TCAs and SNRIs) generally have better analgesic efficacy to those that have more selective activity (secondary TCAs and SSRIs). The superior NNT of TCAs over SNRIs, despite similar receptor activity, suggests that other mechanisms may be important and sodium channel blockade is likely to be the most relevant in neuropathic pain.

Systematic reviews in noncancer conditions suggest that a tertiary TCA is likely to be the first choice of antidepressant for cancer neuropathic pain, although trial evidence in support of this is limited.[42] The newer SNRIs may be better tolerated in cancer patients and despite a lower NNT, may prove to be more effective overall. Indeed, a small head to head, crossover trial of venlafaxine versus imipramine in painful diabetic neuropathy demonstrated similar analgesic efficacy and adverse effects.[48][II]

ANTIEPILEPTICS

Clinical pharmacology

Some of the earliest descriptions of neuropathic pain mention "epileptiform neuralgia" referring to the paroxysmal stabbing pains that some patients experience.[49] Based on this concept, phenytoin was one of the first coanalgesic drugs to be used for neuropathic pain over 40 years ago.[50] Since then, antiepileptic drugs have become widely used to treat neuropathic pain.

The principal mechanism of action of some of the older drugs, such as phenytoin and carbamazepine, occurs via blockade of voltage-dependent sodium channels, whereas sodium valproate enhances GABA activity. Given the molecular similarity between carbamazepine and TCAs, some of the analgesic activity of carbamazepine may also occur via serotonergic pathways. More recently developed antiepileptics, such as gabapentin,

pregabalin, lamotrigine, and levetiracetum, have actions on various ion channels, as well as modulation of GABA synthesis, release, and metabolism.[51]

The most important actions of gabapentin and pregabalin appear to be binding to the $\alpha_2\delta$ subunit of voltage-dependent calcium channels.[52] These binding sites are located in the spinal cord, with particularly high density in the superficial laminae of the dorsal horn. The action of both drugs at these sites may inhibit the release of excitatory neurotransmitters and reduce glutamate availability at NMDA and non-NMDA receptors.[53]

The most common adverse effects of antiepileptics are drowsiness, fatigue, and dizziness (ataxia). In longer-term use, weight gain associated with gabapentin is reported. In general, doses of antiepileptics used to treat neuropathic pain are similar to those used in epilepsy. Berger et al.[37] found that only 17 percent of patients with a diagnosis of cancer and painful neuropathy were treated with antiepileptic drugs highlighting the relatively low use of coanalgesic drugs in this context (see Clinical pharmacology under Antidepressants above).

Older antiepileptics

Conventional antiepileptics have been studied in noncancer neuropathic pain and a recently updated Cochrane review calculates a NNT of 2.5 for carbamazepine in trigeminal neuralgia and a NNT of 2.3 in diabetic neuropathy.[54][I] Good quality studies of phenytoin in any neuropathic pain context are more limited, but the estimated NNT in diabetic neuropathy is 2.1.

There is one randomized, double-blind controlled study that examined phenytoin with buprenorphine in patients with difficult to manage cancer pain.[55] The study included, but was not confined to, patients with neuropathic pain features. Phenytoin 100 mg twice daily for one month provided more that 50 percent pain relief to 22 of 25 patients, and buprenorphine provided marginally better analgesia, but at the expense of more adverse effects. Combined therapy provided the most effective analgesia, and doses were lower than when either drug was used alone.

A case report described the successful use of intravenous phenytoin to manage cancer neuropathic pain that was rapidly increasing in intensity.[56] A later randomized controlled study in a noncancer population confirmed the efficacy of this approach (phenytoin given at 15 mg/kg as a two-hour infusion).[57][II]

In cancer neuropathic pain, sodium valproate was evaluated in an observational study that recruited 25 patients with advanced disease and assessed analgesic response over a two-week period.[58] Nineteen patients completed the study and 56 percent experienced a reduction in their pain by one category, e.g. moderate to mild. Around 30 percent of patients experienced a 50 percent reduction in absolute pain score.

Newer antiepileptics

The demands of regulatory bodies have resulted in better quality evidence to support the newer antiepileptic drugs. Gabapentin is undoubtedly the most widely used antiepileptic to treat neuropathic pain and this practice is based on several large, randomized, controlled trials in post-herpetic neuralgia and diabetic neuropathy.[59][II], [60, 61][II] Systematic reviews have calculated a NNT between 3.2 and 3.8 for gabapentin in these conditions.[54]

Gabapentin has been added to opioids for the management of neuropathic pain in a ten-day randomized, double-blind, placebo-controlled trial.[62][II] Pain scores fell by around 30 percent in both placebo and treatment groups (90 percent of latter group were treated with 1200–1800 mg gabapentin daily). However, the study showed that average daily pain scores were significantly better for the treatment group. Further analysis showed that this difference was achieved in the first five days of treatment; thereafter, pain scores were no different between the groups. Overall, the study demonstrated limited additional benefits for combining gabapentin with preexisting opioid treatment.[63] Ross et al.[64][III] later published an open label, non-controlled study in patients with neuropathic pain from either tumor or cancer treatment. In this study, 45 percent of patients experienced a 30 percent reduction in pain score after 15 days of treatment with gabapentin. Taken together, these two studies highlight the need for placebo-controlled trials in palliative care populations in order to quantify treatment and placebo responses.

There are no good quality clinical trials of other newer antiepileptics in cancer neuropathic pain. Case reports exist describing lamotrigine[65] or levetiracetum[66] in the successful management of cancer neuropathic pain and this may stimulate further research.

Summary of evidence

Both older and newer antiepileptics have demonstrated efficacy in neuropathic pain, and in some cases evidence supports their use in cancer neuropathic pain. Newer antiepileptics are generally better tolerated and have more predictable pharmacokinetics than older drugs, making them potentially easier and safer to use in patients with cancer. In clinical practice, gabapentin and pregabalin are likely to remain the first choice of adjuvant analgesic drugs for treating cancer neuropathic pain, but the evidence base for other new antiepileptics will grow. Evidence to date suggests that patients can expect only modest improvements in pain using these drugs.

NMDA RECEPTOR ANTAGONISTS

Background

Glutamate is the main excitatory neurotransmitter in the central nervous system (CNS).[67, 68] Activation of one of the receptors for glutamate, the NMDA receptor, found in the spinal cord seems to be a critical step in the generation of a number of pain states, including prolonged pain states.[68] After initial activation of the alpha-amino-3-hydroxy-5-methylisoxazole-4-proprionic acid (AMPA) receptors in the dorsal horn, repeated stimulation may allow activation of the NMDA receptors with the consequent conversion of a small to large amplitude response and a corresponding increase in pain intensity.[67] The C fiber-induced activity of the dorsal horn nociceptive neurons is enhanced and prolonged – the "wind up" phenomenon. This phenomenon converts simple touch into painful sensation – allodynia. It means that a pain response to any given painful stimulus is magnified – hyperalgesia – and prolonged.

There is substantial animal experimental evidence to show that NMDA antagonists attenuate as well as reverse morphine tolerance.[67, 68] Synergism between NMDA antagonists and morphine have been observed with a reversal of the rightward shift of the opioid dose–analgesic response curve and a reappearance of opioid sensitivity.[69]

Ketamine is the most potent NMDA receptor antagonist available for clinical use. It is a dissociative anesthetic which has analgesic properties in subanesthetic doses. Other NMDA receptor antagonists include dextromethorphan, amantadine, and methadone.

Pharmacodynamics

Ketamine binds to the phencyclidine site when the channels are in an open activated state. At rest, they are blocked by magnesium. It appears that ketamine is most effective in pain states where hyperexcitability is established.[70] Other modes of action which may contribute to ketamine's analgesic properties include interactions with other calcium and sodium channels, cholinergic transmission, noradrenergic and serotoninergic reuptake inhibition, and μ, δ, and κ opioid-like sparing effects.[71] This activity across multiple receptors may explain the variety of unpleasant side effects that ketamine may cause, including confusion, dysphoria, hallucinations, and vivid dreams. It can also cause hypertension and tachycardia. Side effects occur in 40 percent of patients when given ketamine subcutaneously, but less when given by mouth.[72] The incidence of adverse side effects is dose related.[73]

Pharmacokinetics

Commercially available racemic preparations contain equal concentrations of two enantiomers, s(+) ketamine and r(−) ketamine. The S-enantiomer has greater affinity and selectivity for the NMDA receptor; it is three to four times more potent an analgesic and less likely to cause undesirable effects.[71]

Bioavailability following parenteral administration is high (93 percent), but oral bioavailability is only 16 percent. This is because ketamine is poorly absorbed following oral administration and is subject to extensive first-pass hepatic metabolism, the principal metabolite being norketamine.[71, 74] Norketamine is equipotent to ketamine as an analgesic and the maximum blood concentration of norketamine is greater after oral administration than after injection, possibly explaining why an equianalgesic oral dose is approximately 25–50 percent of the previous parenteral dose.[75]

Evidence for use in cancer pain

Ketamine has been used to treat a number of different pains in both cancer and noncancer settings with some success.[76, 77, 78] It is most often used in addition to an opioid when further opioid increments have been ineffective or precluded by unacceptable side effects. The evidence for its use, however, is limited and is mainly from case reports, retrospective studies, and uncontrolled trials. A systematic review examined the use of ketamine as an adjuvant to opioids in the treatment of cancer pain.[79][I] Only four randomized controlled trials (RCT) were identified and two of these were excluded because of poor quality. Of the remaining two, only one specified that the use was for neuropathic pain (the other was for "terminal cancer pain") and the total number of patients between the two trials was 30. Although the trials were positive with regard to the effect of ketamine and noted that it did not cause serious adverse effects, the authors concluded that there was insufficient evidence that ketamine improves the effectiveness of opioid treatment in cancer pain.

Thirty-two case reports, open label audits, or open label, uncontrolled trials were identified during the Cochrane search.[80] The majority demonstrated improved opioid analgesia with ketamine, although the routes of ketamine administration were very varied. The doses also varied greatly and a number of protocols have been suggested for ketamine use.[71, 74, 81] The usual starting doses are 10–25 mg p.o. three or four times a day, or when necessary and 1–2.5 mg/kg/24 hours by the subcutaneous route. The incidence of psychomimetic side effects appears to be reduced by prescription of an antipsychotic, e.g. haloperidol or benzodiazepine, although there is debate as to whether this should be started prophylactically or just given on an as-needed basis.[71, 76]

Intravenous "burst" ketamine is less frequently used, but may have long-term benefits. An open label audit described 39 patients with refractory cancer pain who received a short duration (three to five days) ketamine infusion commencing at 100 mg/24 hours, escalating to 300 mg/24 hours and then to 500 mg/24 hours according to response.[73] In this sample, 67 percent of patients experienced a significant reduction in pain (defined as a 50 percent or greater decrease in mean verbal rating scale (VRS)), but 30 percent experienced psychomimetic side effects. Improvements in pain control lasted up to eight weeks postinfusion in some cases.

Ketamine appears to have a role in the pharmacological management of refractory cancer pain which frequently has a neuropathic element to it. The evidence base is not strong enough to recommend its use before other adjuvants analgesics have been tried. However, it has been shown to be a useful part of the palliative care physicians' formulary.

LOCAL ANESTHETICS AND OTHER APPROACHES

Clinical pharmacology

A range of other pharmacological agents has been used to relieve neuropathic pain because not all such pains are successfully treated with antidepressants, antiepileptics, or opioids. Probably the most commonly used of these other approaches are local anesthetic agents administered systemically, often referred to as antiarrhythmics. These drugs competitively block sodium channels following oral (e.g. mexiletine, flecainide) or parenteral administration (e.g. lidocaine or fosphenytoin). Early studies in animal models of neuropathic pain showed that local anesthetics were capable of blocking ectopic neuroma discharge without affecting nerve conduction and this evidence underpinned clinical application of these drugs.[82]

Other agents, such as lidocaine and capsaicin cream, are used topically. A further group of oral drugs classed as skeletal muscle relaxants include baclofen ($GABA_B$ agonist) and tizanidine (α_2-adrenoreceptor agonist).

Systemic local anesthetics

Intravenous lidocaine relieves noncancer neuropathic pain during and immediately after infusion in placebo-controlled trials.[83][I] Lidocaine was usually administered at doses of 5 mg/kg as an infusion over 30–60 minutes. Adverse effects were generally minor and consisted of light-headedness, nausea, perioral numbness, and drowsiness. The duration of effect, however, appears to be relatively short lived, although there are uncontrolled studies reporting effects lasting several weeks. In contrast, two small randomized controlled trials in cancer patients with neuropathic pain did not show a benefit over placebo.[84, 85][II] Each trial consisted of only ten patients and so may have been underpowered to exclude a treatment effect. However, all patients were being treated with high doses of opioids and any additional analgesic effect of lidocaine may not have been apparent.

Oral agents have also been used to treat neuropathic pain, though only one report describes flecainide in cancer pain.[86] Earlier evidence of the effectiveness of mexiletine in all types of neuropathic pain is weak[83] and its narrow therapeutic index means that its use is frequently complicated by adverse effects. However, a recent systematic review suggests that it has a similar efficacy and adverse effect profile to other analgesics, such as opioids, amitriptyline, and gabapentin.[87][I]

Topical agents and skeletal muscle relaxants

Topical lidocaine patches and capsaicin cream have analgesic efficacy in neuropathic pain and are particularly helpful in pain accompanied by allodynia. Topical approaches have the advantage of low systemic absorption resulting in few adverse effects. Skeletal muscle relaxants, such as baclofen and tizanidine, are also used to treat neuropathic pain, especially in situations complicated by muscle spasm. Further studies are needed in cancer neuropathic pain before these approaches can be recommended for routine use.

DRUG SYNERGY AND SEQUENCING

Therapy for cancer patients with neuropathic pain often involves the use of a number of different drugs either concurrently or sequentially employed to achieve adequate pain relief. There has been a recent drive to develop evidence-based algorithms to guide clinician choices.[39, 88] A number of issues complicate this process as retrospective reviews have to deal with varying study designs, outcome measures, etc. Endeavouring to produce some guidance, while recognizing the limitations of such comparisons, authors[39, 88] have used the concept of NNT and NNH as a means of comparing medications in a practical, clinically relevant manner. NNT and NNH refer, respectively, to the number of patients that need to be treated for one to experience significant pain relief, or significant harm, in comparison with a placebo arm. Where relevant these have been reported in this chapter.

Drug synergy is produced when the effects of a drug combination are greater than when the individual drug effects are simply added together. Based on the nature of the interaction, the mechanism of synergy can be either pharmacodynamic or pharmacokinetic. The former is where two different drugs with unique modes of action target a similar process. Pharmacokinetic synergy is when drug A influences the absorption, distribution, biotransformation, or elimination of drug B.

Given the large number of processes that take place for the development and maintenance of neuropathic pain, it appears logical that targeting separate mechanisms may improve symptoms, but evidence is lacking. Preclinical studies suggest a synergy between opioids and gabapentin and this appears to be supported by more recent clinical studies.[23, 89] Combinations of opioids and other coanalgesics in clinical trials have also suggested possible synergy with tricyclic antidepressants, NMDA receptor antagonists, cholecystokinin antagonists, and in the case of intrathecal administration with clonidine and local anesthetics.[90]

Sequencing of agents and the development of treatment algorithms for neuropathic pain are based largely on NNT and NNH and the limitations of this approach are discussed in a number of texts.[39, 88, 90] Further debate is given to the sequential versus concurrent titration of medications. The former is the approach familiar to most clinicians – the trial of single agents commenced individually and titrated to a clinically effective dose. Concurrent titration is the prescribing of two drugs with the aim of reducing the time to reach a significant clinical improvement, possibly improving compliance by reducing the doses needed to produce such an improvement and the adverse effects of such drugs. This approach may, however, be more harmful in terms of drug interactions.

Using the information from the reviews published to date, a possible treatment algorithm for neuropathic pain in cancer patients can be suggested. It differs from that which may be suggested for neuropathic pain where malignancy is not part of the etiology because of the differences between the patient groups highlighted under Introduction.

Grond et al.[15] showed that by following the WHO guidelines, neuropathic pain in cancer patients can be successfully managed using a stepwise approach incorporating standard nonopioid, "weak" opioid, and "strong" opioid analgesia. A systematic review by Finnerup et al.,[39] has estimated morphine to have a NNT of 2.5 (CI 1.9–3.4), oxycodone of 2.6 (1.9–4.1), and tramadol 3.9 (2.7–6.7). If this approach results in inadequate analgesia, with or without intolerable adverse effects, then adjuvant analgesic drugs can be introduced alongside or to replace standard analgesics. First-line adjuvants would include a tricyclic antidepressant or an antiepileptic, such as gabapentin or pregabalin. The NNT for these drugs are similar and the choice is likely to be based on the side-effect profile of the agents available and the individual patient. Failure on one class of drug after achieving a clinically effective dose for a one to two-week period would indicate that a trial of the alternative class of drug is needed. Further maneuvers in clinical practice are supported by a weaker evidence base, but commonly include opioid switching, a trial of ketamine, or other adjuvants described.

REFERENCES

1. Merskey H, Bogduk N. *Classification of chronic pain.* Seattle: IASP Press, 1994.
2. Torrance N, Smith BH, Bennett M, Lee AJ. The epidemiology of chronic pain of predominantly

neuropathic origin. Results from a general population study. *Journal of Pain.* 2006; **7**: 281–9.

3. Caraceni A, Portenoy RK. An international survey of cancer pain characteristics and syndromes. *Pain.* 1999; **82**: 263–74.

4. Erschler WB. Cancer: a disease of the elderly. *Journal of Supportive Oncology.* 2003; **1** (Suppl. 2): 5–10.

5. Murray S, Kendall M, Boyd K. Illness trajectories and palliative care. *BMJ.* 2005; **330**: 1007–11.

6. Arner S, Meyerson BA. Lack of analgesic effect of opioids on neuropathic and idiopathic forms of pain. *Pain.* 1988; **33**: 11–23.

7. Rowbotham MC, Reisner-Keller LA, Fields HL. Both intravenous lidocaine and morphine reduce the pain of postherpetic neuralgia. *Neurology.* 1991; **41**: 1024–8.

8. Jadad AR, Carroll D, Glynn CJ et al. Morphine responsiveness of chronic pain: double-blind randomised crossover study with patient-controlled analgesia. *Lancet.* 1992; **339**: 1367–71.

9. Cherny NI, Thaler HT, Friedlander-Klar H et al. Opioid responsiveness of cancer pain syndromes caused by neuropathic or nociceptive mechanisms: a combined analysis of controlled, single-dose studies. *Neurology.* 1994; **44**: 857–61.

10. Portenoy RK, Foley KM, Intrurrisi CE. The nature of opioid responsiveness and its implications for neuropathic pain: new hypotheses derived from studies of opioid infusions. *Pain.* 1990; **43**: 273–86.

11. Rowbotham MC, Twilling L, Davies PS et al. Oral opioid therapy for chronic peripheral and central neuropathic pain. *New England Journal of Medicine.* 2003; **348**: 1223–32.

* 12. Raja SN, Haythornthwaite JA, Pappagallo M et al. Opioids versus antidepressants in postherpetic neuralgia A randomized, placebo-controlled trial. *Neurology.* 2002; **59**: 1015–21.

13. Watson CPN, Babul N. Efficacy of oxycodone in neuropathic pain a randomized trial in post herpetic neuralgia. *Neurology.* 1998; **50**: 1837–41.

14. Dellemijn P. Are opioids effective in relieving neuropathic pain? *Pain.* 1999; **80**: 453–62.

* 15. Grond S, Radbruch L, Meuser T et al. Assessment and treatment of neuropathic cancer patients following WHO guidelines. *Pain.* 1999; **79**: 15–20.

16. Kupers RC, Konings H, Adriaensen H, Gybels JM. Morphine differentially affects the sensory and affective pain ratings in neurogenic and idiopathic forms of pain. *Pain.* 1991; **47**: 5–12.

17. Dellemijn P, Vanneste JA. Randomised double-blind active-placebo-controlled crossover trial of intravenous fentanyl in neuropathic pain. *Lancet.* 1997; **349**: 753–8.

18. Dickenson A. The role of receptors in pain and analgesia. *Palliative Care Today.* 2001; **ix**: 46–7.

19. Ballantyne JC, Mao J. Opioid therapy for chronic pain. *New England Journal of Medicine.* 2003; **349**: 1943–53.

* 20. Martin LA, Hagen NA. Neuropathic pain in cancer patients: mechanisms, syndromes, and clinical controversies.

Journal of Pain and Symptom Management. 1997; **14**: 99–117.

21. Attal N, Guirimand F, Brasseur L et al. Effects of IV morphine in central pain: a randomized placebo-controlled study. *Neurology.* 2002; **58**: 554–63.

22. Foley KM. Opioids and chronic neuropathic pain. *New England Journal of Medicine.* 2003; **348**: 1279–81.

* 23. Gilron I, Bailey JM, Dongsheng T et al. Morphine, gabapentin, or their combination for neuropathic pain. *New England Journal of Medicine.* 2005; **352**: 1324–34.

24. Dellemijn PL, van Duijn H, Vanneste JA. Prolonged treatment with transdermal fentanyl in neuropathic pain. *Journal of Pain and Symptom Management.* 1998; **16**: 220–9.

* 25. Bruera E, Palmer JL, Bosnzak S et al. Methadone versus morphine as a first-line strong opioid for cancer pain: a randomised double-blind study. *Journal of Clinical Oncology.* 2004; **22**: 185–92.

26. Nicholson AB. Methadone for cancer pain. *Cochrane Database for Systematic Reviews.* 2006; **CD003971**.

27. Watson CPN, Moulin D, Watt-Watson J et al. Controlled-release oxycodone relieves neuropathic pain; a randomized controlled trial in painful diabetic neuropathy. *Pain.* 2003; **105**: 71–8.

28. Gimbel JS, Richards P, Portenoy RK. Controlled-release oxycodone for pain in diabetic neuropathy: A randomized controlled trial. *Neurology.* 2003; **60**: 927–34.

29. Koppert W, Ihmsen H, Korber N et al. Different profiles of buprenorphine-induced analgesia and hyperalgesia in a human pain model. *Pain.* 2005; **118**: 15–22.

30. Sittl R. Transdermal buprenorphine in cancer pain and palliative care. *Palliative Medicine.* 2006; **20**: s25–30.

31. Benedetti F, Vighetti S, Amanzio M et al. Dose–response relationship of opioids in nociceptive and neuropathic postoperative pain. *Pain.* 1998; **74**: 2005–211.

32. Sindrup SH, Andersen G, Madsen C et al. Tramadol relieves pain and allodynia in polyneuropathy: a randomised, double-blind, controlled trial. *Pain.* 1999; **83**: 85–90.

33. Boureau F, Legallicier P, Kabir-Ahmadi M. Tramadol in post-herpetic neuralgia: a randomized, double-blind, placebo-controlled trial. *Pain.* 2003; **104**: 323–31.

34. Duhmke RM, Cornblath DD, Hollingshead JR. Tramadol for neuropathic pain. *Cochrane Database of Systematic Reviews.* 2004; **CD003726**.

35. Wang GK, Russell C, Wang SY. State-dependent block of voltage-gated Na+ channels by amitriptyline via the local anesthetic receptor and its implication for neuropathic pain. *Pain.* 2004; **110**: 166–74.

36. Shimizu M, Nishida A, Yamawaki S. Antidepressants inhibit spontaneous oscillations of intracellular Ca^{2+} concentration in rat cortical cultured neurons. *Neuroscience Letters.* 1992; **146**: 101–04.

* 37. Berger A, Mercadante S, Oster G. Use of antiepileptics and tricyclic antidepressants in cancer patients with neuropathic pain. *European Journal of Cancer Care.* 2005; **15**: 138–45.

* 38. Saarto T, Wiffen PJ. Antidepressants for neuropathic pain. *Cochrane Database of Systematic Reviews.* 2005; **CD005454.**

* 39. Finnerup NB, Otto M, McQauy HJ *et al.* Algorithm for neuropathic pain treatment: an evidence-based proposal. *Pain.* 2005; **118**: 289–305.

40. Max MB, Culnane M, Schafer SC *et al.* Amitriptyline relieves diabetic neuropathy pain in patients with normal or depressed mood. *Neurology.* 1987; **37**: 589–96.

41. Sindrup SH, Otto M, Finnerup NB, Jensen TS. Antidepressants in the treatment of neuropathic pain. *Basic and Clinical Pharmacology and Toxicology.* 2005; **96**: 399–409.

42. Mercadante S, Arcuri E, Tirelli W *et al.* Amitriptyline in neuropathic cancer pain in patients on morphine therapy: a randomised placebo-controlled, double-blind crossover study. *Tumori.* 2002; **88**: 239–42.

43. Sindrup SH, Gram LF, Brosen K *et al.* The selective serotonin reuptake inhibitor paroxetine is effective in the treatment of diabetic neuropathy symptoms. *Pain.* 1990; **42**: 135–44.

44. Rowbotham MC, Goli V, Kunz NR, Lei D. Venlafaxine extended release in the treatment of painful diabetic polyneuropathy: a double-blind, placebo controlled study. *Pain.* 2004; **110**: 697–706.

45. Goldstein DJ, Lu Y, Detke MJ *et al.* Duloxetine versus placebo in patients with painful diabetic neuropathy. *Pain.* 2005; **116**: 109–18.

46. Reuben SS, Makari-Judson G, Lurie SD. Evaluation of efficacy of the perioperative administration of venlafaxine XR in the prevention of postmastectomy pain syndrome. *Journal of Pain and Symptom Management.* 2004; **27**: 133–9.

47. Tasmuth T, Hartel B, Kalso E. Venlafaxine in neuropathic pain following treatment of breast cancer. *European Journal of Pain.* 2002; **6**: 17–24.

48. Sindrup SH, Bach FW, Madsen CW *et al.* Venlafaxine versus imipramine in painful polyneuropathy: a randomized, controlled trial. *Neurology.* 2003; **60**: 1284–9.

49. Swerdlow M. Anticonvulsant drugs and chronic pain. *Clinical Neuropharmacology.* 1984; **7**: 51–82.

50. Blom S. Trigeminal neuralgia: its treatment with a new anticonvulsant drug. *Lancet.* 1962; **i**: 839–40.

51. Bennett MI, Simpson KH. Gabapentin in the treatment of neuropathic pain. *Palliative Medicine.* 2004; **18**: 5–11.

52. Gee NS, Brown JP, Dissanayake VU *et al.* The novel anticonvulsant drug gabapentin binds to the $\alpha_2\delta$ subunit of a calcium channel. *Journal of Biological Chemistry.* 1996; **271**: 5768–76.

53. Shimoyama M, Shimoyama N, Hori Y. Gabapentin affects glutamatergic excitatory neurotransmission in the rat dorsal horn. *Pain.* 2000; **85**: 405–14.

54. Wiffen P, Collins S, McQuay H *et al.* Anticonvulsant drugs for acute and chronic pain. *Cochrane Database of Systematic Reviews.* 2005; **CD001133.**

55. Yajnik S, Singh GP, Singh G, Kumar M. Phenytoin as a coanalgesic in cancer pain. *Journal of Pain and Symptom Management.* 1992; **7**: 209–13.

56. Chang VT. Intavenous phenytoin in the management of crescendo pelvic cancer-related pain. *Journal of Pain and Symptom Management.* 1997; **13**: 238–40.

57. McCleane GJ. Intravenous infusion of phenytoin relieves neuropathic pain: a randomized, double-blinded, placebo-controlled, crossover study. *Anesthesia and Analgesia.* 1999; **89**: 985–8.

58. Hardy JR, Rees EA, Gwilliam B *et al.* A phase II study to establish the efficacy and toxicity of sodium valproate in patients with cancer-related neuropathic pain. *Journal of Pain and Symptom Management.* 2001; **21**: 204–09.

59. Rice AS, Maton S. Postherpetic Neuralgia Study Group. Gabapentin in postherpetic neuralgia: a randomised, double blind, placebo controlled study. *Pain.* 2001; **94**: 215–24.

60. Backonja A, Beydoun A, Edwards KR *et al.* Gabapentin for the symptomatic treatment of painful neuropathy in patients with diabetes mellitus. *Journal of the American Medical Association.* 1998; **280**: 1831–6.

61. Serpell M. Neuropathic Pain Study Group. Gabapentin in neuropathic pain syndromes: a randomised, double blind, placebo controlled trial. *Pain.* 2002; **99**: 557–66.

* 62. Caraceni A, Zecca E, Bonezzi C *et al.* Gabapentin for neuropathic cancer pain: a randomized controlled trial from the gabapentin cancer pain study group. *Journal of Clinical Oncology.* 2004; **14**: 2909–17.

* 63. Bennett MI. Gabapentin significantly improves analgesia in people receiving opioids for neuropathic cancer pain. *Cancer Treatment Reviews.* 2005; **31**: 58–62.

64. Ross JR, Goller K, Hardy J *et al.* Gabapentin is effective in the treatment of cancer-related neuropathic pain: a prospective, open-label study. *Journal of Palliative Medicine.* 2005; **8**: 1118–26.

65. Devulder JE. Lamotrigine in refractory cancer pain. *a case report. Journal of Clinical Anesthesia.* 2000; **12**: 574–5.

66. Dunteman ED. Levetiracetam as an adjunctive analgesic in neoplastic plexopathies: case series and commentary. *Journal of Pain and Palliative Care Pharmacotherapy.* 2005; **19**: 35–43.

67. Fallon M, Welsh J. The role of ketamine in pain control. *European Journal of Palliative Care.* 1996; **3**: 143–6.

68. Luczak J, Dickenson A, Kotlinska-Lemieszek A. The role of ketamine, an NMDA receptor antagonist, in the management of pain. *Progress in Palliative Care.* 1995; **3**: 127–34.

69. Finlay I. Ketamine and its role in cancer pain. *Pain Reviews.* 1999; **6**: 303–13.

70. Fallon M, Fergus C. Ketamine and other NMDA receptor antagonists. In: Bennett M (ed.). *Neuropathic pain.* Oxford: Oxford Pain Management Library, University Oxford Press, 2006: 97–104.

71. Twycross R, Wilcock A, Charlesworth S, Dickman A. *Palliative care formulary,* 2nd edn. Oxford: Radcliffe Publishing, 2002: 289–93.

* 72. Kannan T, Saxena A, Bhatnagar S, Barry A. Oral ketamine as an adjuvant to oral morphine for neuropathic pain in cancer patients. *Journal of Pain and Symptom Management.* 2002; **23**: 60–3.

73. Jackson K, Ashby M, Martin P *et al.* "Burst" ketamine for refractory cancer pain: an open-label audit of 39 patients. *Journal of Pain and Symptom Management.* 2001; **22**: 834–42.

74. Mercadante S. Ketamine in cancer pain: an update. *Palliative Medicine.* 1996; **10**: 225–30.

75. Fitzgibbon E, Hall P, Schroder C. Low dose ketamine as an analgesic adjuvant in difficult pain syndromes: a strategy for conversion from parenteral to oral ketamine. *Journal of Pain and Symptom Management.* 2002; **23**: 165–70.

76. Fischer K, Hagen N. Analgesic effect of oral ketamine in chronic neuropathic pain of spinal origin: a case report. *Journal of Pain Symptom and Management.* 1999; **18**: 61–6.

77. Mannion S, O'Brien T. Ketamine in the management of chronic pancreatic pain. *Journal of Pain and Symptom Management.* 2003; **26**: 1071–2.

78. Enarson M, Hays H, Woodroffe MA. Clinical experience with oral ketamine. *Journal of Pain and Symptom Management.* 1999; **17**: 384–6.

* 79. Bell R, Eccleston C, Kalso E. Ketamine as an adjuvant to opioids for cancer pain. *Cochrane Database of Systematic Reviews.* 2003; **CD003351**.

80. Bell R, Eccleston C, Kalso E. Ketamine as adjuvant to opioids for cancer pain. *A qualitative systematic review. Journal of Pain and Symptom Management.* 2003; **26**: 867–75.

81. Kotlinska-Lemieszaek A, Luczak J. Subanesthetic ketamine: an essential adjuvant for intractable cancer pain (letter). *Journal of Pain and Symptom Management.* 2004; **28**: 100–02.

82. Devor M, Wall PD, Catalan N. Systemic lidocaine silences ectopic neuroma and DRG discharge without blocking nerve conduction. *Pain.* 1992; **48**: 261–8.

83. Kalso E, Tranmer MR, McQuay HJ, Moore RA. Systemic local anaesthetic type drugs in chronic pain: a systematic review. *European Journal of Pain.* 1998; **2**: 3–14.

84. Ellemann K, Sjogren P, Banning AM *et al.* Trial of intravenous lidocaine on painful neuropathy in cancer patients. *Clinical Journal of Pain.* 1989; **5**: 291–4.

85. Bruera E, Ripamonti C, Brenneis C *et al.* A randomized double-blind crossover trial of intravenous lidocaine in the treatment of neuropathic cancer pain. *Journal of Pain and Symptom Management.* 1992; **7**: 138–40.

86. Dunlop R, Davies RJ, Hockley J, Turner P. Analgesic effects of oral flecainide. *Lancet.* 1988; **20**: 420–1.

87. Challapalli V, Tremont-Lukats IW, McNicol ED *et al.* Systemic administration of local anesthetic agents to relieve neuropathic pain. *Cochrane Database of Systematic Reviews.* 2005; **CD003345**.

* 88. Raja S, Haythornthwaite J. Combination therapy for neuropathic pain – which drugs, which combination, which patients? *New England Journal of Medicine.* 2005; **352**: 1373.

89. Berger A, Dukes E, McCarberg B *et al.* Change in opioid use after the initiation of gabapentin therapy in patients with post herpetic neuralgia. *Clinical Therapeutics.* 2003; **25**: 2809–21.

90. Bennett M. Drug synergy and sequencing. In: Bennett M (ed.). *Neuropathic pain.* Oxford: Oxford Pain Management Library, Oxford University Press, 2006: 145–53.

16

Control of procedure-related pain

IAIN LAWRIE AND COLIN CAMPBELL

Introduction   213
Background   213
Approaching procedure-related pain   214
Nonpharmacological interventions   215
Local and topical techniques   216
Strong opioids   217
Nonsteroidal anti-inflammatory drugs   218
Sedating drugs   218
Conclusions and future directions   219
References   220

KEY LEARNING POINTS

- Diagnostic and therapeutic procedures can cause pain and anxiety, leading to patient distress.
- Distress during procedures is the result of many factors.
- Clinicians should evaluate their practice to identify potential causes of pain and anxiety for their patients.

- Knowledge of a range of pharmacological and nonpharmacological techniques of pain management can result in better tolerated and more successful procedures.
- More widespread adoption of nationally agreed guidelines for managing specific procedures would afford patients a more comfortable and safe experience.

INTRODUCTION

Medical procedures have become increasingly common in the investigation and management of malignant disease. Pain and discomfort experienced by patients undergoing such procedures (procedure-related pain) can add to the physical and emotional burden of their illness. This chapter explores the concept of procedure-related pain, suggests an approach to its management, and examines the evidence for specific strategies.

BACKGROUND

Incidence

In patients with cancer, procedure-related pain can contribute to their global psychological distress and is often poorly managed.[1][IV], [2][IV], [3][IV], [4][III] The incidence of procedure-related pain has not been thoroughly investigated. However, moderate to severe pain has been reported during:

- colonoscopy and double-contrast barium enema (85 and 46 percent, respectively);[5][III]
- bone marrow aspiration (36 percent);[6][II]
- percutaneous liver biopsy (61 percent).[7][III]

Common procedures in pediatric oncology which can cause moderate to severe pain have received more scrutiny:

- venepuncture (49 percent);[3][IV]
- lumbar puncture (62 percent);[3][IV]
- bone marrow aspiration (73 percent).[3][IV]

Provision of analgesia

Procedure-related pain may be compounded by a lack of appropriate analgesia or sedation and inattention to the patient's "total pain." The concept of total pain recognizes that pain is a multidimensional phenomenon and is influenced by physical, social, psychological, and spiritual factors.[8][V]

In one American study, 65 percent of 144 pediatric hematologist/oncologists did not routinely use premedication for bone marrow aspiration or biopsy.[1][IV] Another large pediatric oncology study found premedication drugs used before only 12 percent of bone marrow aspirations and 7 percent of lumbar punctures.[9] [IV] In contrast, intravenous sedation (e.g. benzodiazepine) is routinely used in the UK in upper gastrointestinal endoscopies (more than 90 percent); radiological procedures such as nephrostomy insertion (76 percent);[10] and biliary drainage (66 percent).[10][IV]

In a French study, sedation or premedication was given in only 46 percent of 2084 percutaneous liver biopsies,[11] [IV] known to be among the most painful procedures.[12] [III]

APPROACHING PROCEDURE-RELATED PAIN

Table 16.1 outlines the common medical procedures which can be painful and suggested interventions to manage that pain. **Figures 16.1** and **16.2** show some of these procedures in practice. The delivery of interventional procedures requires forethought and planning. A structured approach, giving due consideration to all relevant factors, will result in better management of procedure-related pain and distress. It is useful to consider such factors in terms of the patient, the physician, and the system (see **Box 16.1**).

Patient factors influence the experience of any procedure. The needs of the individual patient should be considered, and recognition given to the influence of:

- previous experience of medical procedures;[13][III]
- the age of the patient;[14][III]
- gender-specific differences in experience of pain and anxiety;
- personal coping styles;[15][II]
- ethnicity (although evidence for this is not clear);
- patient expectations of a negative outcome;[16][III]
- perception of control;[17][III]
- current and past analgesic use;
- preexisting medical conditions (e.g. arthritis, asthma);
- patient understanding of the procedure and its potential to cause discomfort and anxiety.[18][IV]

However, no single approach will be appropriate, as procedure-related pain varies considerably between individuals. Important aspects of patient assessment are outlined in **Table 16.2**.

Physician factors are important and should be recognized. The clinician's experience of the procedure will determine its success and knowledge of pain management

Table 16.1 Common medical procedures causing pain in cancer patients.

Procedure	Suggested intervention
Mild to moderate pain	
Venepuncture	Topical anesthesia with EMLA or amethocaine
Intravenous cannula insertion	Topical anesthesia with EMLA or amethocaine
Arterial blood sampling	Intradermal infiltration with 1% lidocaine
Fine-needle aspiration	Local anesthetic infiltration with 1% lidocaine
Abdominal paracentesis	Local anesthetic infiltration with 1% lidocaine
Pleural aspiration	Local anesthetic infiltration with 1% lidocaine
Urinary catheterization	Local anesthetic instillation ± midazolam
Moderate to severe pain	
Lumbar puncture	Local anesthetic infiltration ± nonpharmacological intervention; in children ± conscious sedation with: midazolam+pethidine, or OTFC, or midazolam+fentanyl
Bone marrow aspiration	Local anesthetic infiltration ± nonpharmacological intervention; in children ± conscious sedation with: midazolam+pethidine, or OTFC, or midazolam+fentanyl
Gastrointestinal endoscopy	Conscious sedation with midazolam or propofol+pethidine, fentanyl, or alfentanil. Titrate with additional boluses if required
Radiological interventions (urological/biliary)	Conscious sedation with midazolam or propofol+pethidine, fentanyl, or alfentanil. Titrate with additional boluses if required
Painful dressing changes (malignant wounds, pressure sores, debridement)	Conscious sedation with midazolam+pethidine ± topical opioid or OTFC

Note that interventions using sedative or opioid drugs may cause conscious or deep sedation necessitating additional precautions (see **Box 16.6**).
EMLA, eutectic mixture of local anesthetics; OTFC, oral transmucosal fentanyl citrate.

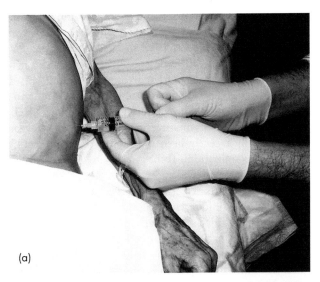

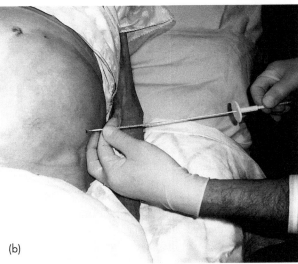

Figure 16.1 (a) Local analgesia for paracentesis. (b) Insertion of a Bonanno catheter for paracentesis.

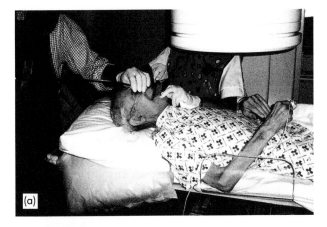

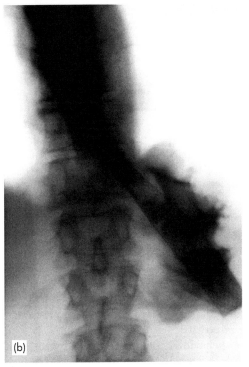

Figure 16.2 (a) Insertion of esophageal stent; (b) esophageal stent *in situ*.

techniques can improve patient care and satisfaction.[20] [III] Physicians may place emphasis on the technical aspects of a procedure rather than assess patient concerns[18] [V] and may display a lack of awareness of the patient's pain and distress,[21] [III] which may result in inadequate analgesia being prescribed.[22] [V]

System factors influence whether pain is a problem during procedures and include:

- the number of procedures on a list;
- the hospital or clinic environment (e.g. noise, temperature, light, privacy) can affect the patient experience;
- procedure duration influences the level of pain experienced,[23] [II] and can be kept to a minimum by an organized approach to care;
- lack of staff can lead to ineffective pain management due to delays in administration of analgesia or insufficient monitoring of pain;[24] [I]

- institutional problems may result in clinicians being reluctant to use adequate analgesia or sedatives, as their use may delay discharge and lead to patients requiring admission.[22] [V]

NONPHARMACOLOGICAL INTERVENTIONS

The use of nondrug interventions, alongside pharmacological agents, can be useful in the management of both pain and anxiety associated with medical procedures. Such interventions are effective in reducing analgesic and sedative requirements.[25] [IV], [26] [III], [27] [II] Clinicians may express skepticism regarding such techniques, but patients may welcome alternative methods to manage discomfort and anxiety. Techniques employed include relaxation,

Box 16.1 Key points to address in preparation for a procedure

- Assess the potential for the procedure to cause pain and anxiety.
- Assess the needs of the individual patient.
- Prepare the patient (and parents if appropriate):
  - give information; answer questions; check understanding.
- Explain clearly what will happen during the procedure.
- Consider and discuss nonpharmacological interventions.
- Consider and discuss pharmacological interventions.

hypnosis, cognitive and behavioral therapy (CBT), acupuncture, and TENS (transcutaneous electrical nerve stimulation).

Hypnosis involves "induction of a state of mind in which a person's normal critical or skeptical [*sic*] nature is bypassed, allowing for acceptance of suggestions"[28][I] and is a state of highly focused attention and intense imaginative involvement. It can be operator- or self-induced and has demonstrated efficacy in reducing pain and anxiety associated with medical procedures.[29][II] More supporting evidence exists for hypnosis for procedural pain in children than for adults. However, a recent systematic review concluded that evidence for the benefits of hypnosis is not yet sufficiently robust for it to be included in best practice guidelines for management of procedure-related pain in pediatric oncology.[30][I]

Cognitive behavioral therapy is a form of psychotherapy which regards internal thoughts as behavior that can be substituted with other, realistic ideas. It has

been proposed that CBT may be used to influence the perception of pain[31][V] and may achieve a 50 percent reduction in procedure-related distress in children.[32][V] However, no significant difference in self-reported fear or fearful anticipation of bone marrow transplantation was found when CBT was compared to general anesthesia in a random-crossover trial of children with leukemia.[14][III]

Acupuncture, originating in China over 3000 years ago, has only recently been the subject of more detailed scientific examination. It has been used with benefit during gastroscopy[33][II] and colonoscopy.[34]

Transcutaneous electrical nerve stimulation is a noninvasive technique, utilizing the "gate control theory" of pain,[35][V] which has been shown to be effective in relieving pain in a variety of conditions.[36][I] TENS has been shown to be beneficial in reducing procedure-related pain in both adults[37][II] and children.[38][II]

LOCAL AND TOPICAL TECHNIQUES

Minor procedures, and those confined to a localized area, can be made less distressing by employing local and topical techniques using either anesthetic or analgesic preparations.

Topical anesthesia can be useful in minimizing the pain of venepuncture and intravenous cannulation and should be considered in patients who have needle phobia, in children, and in those who may require repeated cannulation. EMLA (eutectic mixture of local anesthetics) is an equal mix of lidocaine and prilocaine and is effective in providing dermal anesthesia.[39][I] Due to the risk of methemoglobinemia, its use should be avoided in infants.[40][I]

Other topical anesthetics are available. Tetracaine[39][I] and amethocaine (4 percent) are comparable to EMLA,[41][III] but amethocaine is more expensive and less readily available.

Table 16.2 Assessment of the individual patient.

Patient factors	Clinical relevance
Age (children)	Ability to understand the procedure varies according to the child's developmental stage
	Dose and type of drug may vary according to age/weight
	Parental/guardian anxiety, and their role in supporting the child[19][V]
Age (elderly)	Often have coexisting medical conditions
	Multiple medications
	Declining renal function, with potential for opioid accumulation
Repeated procedures have been distressing	Tendency for increasing anxiety, especially if previous procedure(s)
	Potential for drug accumulation if short intervals between procedures
	Interference with feeding if fasting required before sedation
Psychological	Anticipation of pain heightens anxiety
	Fear associated with life-threatening illness
	Issues around sense of/loss of control

Topical anesthetics tend to cause vasodilation, facilitating systemic absorption, and therefore should be avoided in wounds and mucous membranes. Practical aspects of using topical anesthetic preparations are outlined in **Box 16.2**.

Topical analgesia, in the form of topically applied opioids, has been used in the management of malignant wounds.[42][IV] The opioid is added to a ready-mixed hydrogel wound dressing and applied daily. It is proposed that peripheral opioid receptors are activated in response to tissue inflammation.[43][V]

Local anesthesia, by means of infiltration of a local anesthetic preparation, will provide effective analgesia for many minor procedures. All local anesthetic agents exert their effect by causing a reversible block to conduction of nerve impulses along nerve fibers. Local anesthetics include:

- lidocaine (lignocaine) (the most commonly used local anesthetic currently in use[44][V] and available in different concentrations);
- bupivacaine (slower onset of action, but longer duration of effect);[40][I]
- prilocaine (not for use in infants under six months);[40][I]
- ropivacaine.[40][I]

Practical aspects of using local anesthetic preparations are outlined in **Box 16.3**.

STRONG OPIOIDS

The ideal analgesic for procedure-related pain would have a rapid onset but short duration of action, and many opioids match this description. Strong opioids are used in procedures with potential to cause moderate to severe pain, but are probably underutilized. There is, however, the necessity to monitor the patient for side effects, especially respiratory depression, which can be potentiated by concurrent use of benzodiazepines.[45][I]

Pethidine (meperidine) is still used by some clinicians for painful procedures due to its rapid onset and short duration of action. It is often ineffective in patients taking regular strong opioids, such as those with cancer pain, as the maximum recommended dose of pethidine may be inadequate in these patients. If pethidine is used, clinicians should be aware of its potential to cause hyperexcitability, twitching, and convulsions in patients who accumulate pethidine metabolites as a result of repeated administration. There is a growing tendency to use the fentanyl group of opioids instead of pethidine.

Fentanyl, sufentanil, and alfentanil are synthetic opioids more potent and selective than pethidine for the mu-opioid receptor. They are rapidly absorbed, have a short duration of action and can be given intravenously or by the oral transmucosal route for procedure-related

Box 16.2 Practical aspects of using topical anesthetic preparations

- Apply to the skin as a 2-mm thick layer.
- Cover using an occlusive dressing.
- EMLA requires at least one hour of application to effect local anesthesia.
- Amethocaine requires 35–60 minutes of application for clinical effect.
- Erythema, edema, and pruritus have been reported in association with the use of topical anesthetic agents.
- Other interventions for relieving pain should be remembered, as pain can still be experienced when using topical anesthetic preparations.

Box 16.3 Practical aspects of local anesthesia use

- Allow the liquid to reach room temperature before use.
- Wait 5–10 minutes after infiltration for optimum numbness.
- Administration should be as trauma-free as possible:
  - position the patient adequately;
  - plan the area of infiltration;
  - use small needles.

Note:

- Toxicity, while rare, can occur when recommended doses are exceeded or in procedures which require repeated administration.
- Convulsions and cardiovascular collapse have been reported in cases of inadvertent intravenous injection.

pain. If the intravenous route is used, a bolus or loading dose is given, followed by either a continuous infusion or top-up doses titrated to the patient's response. Oral transmucosal fentanyl citrate (OTFC) in the form of a sweetened matrix lozenge is available in various strengths and is sucked for 30–60 minutes before the procedure. OTFC has shown to be effective for pain relief during lumbar puncture and bone marrow aspiration.[46][III] However, many patients (30–45 percent) experience nausea, although this may be avoided by antiemetic administration.

NONSTEROIDAL ANTI–INFLAMMATORY DRUGS

Nonsteroidal anti-inflammatory drugs (NSAIDs) may play a useful role in amelioration of procedure-related pain. They should be considered before interventions, such as pleural aspiration and dressing of malignant wounds, especially if sedation is not desirable.

SEDATING DRUGS

Midazolam is a benzodiazepine that reduces anxiety and, in therapeutic doses, provides amnesia. It is widely used, either on its own or in conjunction with an opioid, to produce sedation for a variety of painful procedures, notably upper gastrointestinal endoscopy and colonoscopy. Coadministration with an opioid substantially increases the risk of respiratory depression compared with either drug alone.[19][V]

Nitrous oxide mixture (Entonox®) has been used during wound debridement and dressing changes[47][V] and percutaneous liver biopsy[48][II] with beneficial effect on pain. Advantages and disadvantages are outlined in **Box 16.4**.

Ketamine is a rapidly acting, N-methyl-D-aspartic acid (NMDA) receptor antagonist, anesthetic/analgesic agent shown to have analgesic efficacy in subanesthetic doses for minor surgical procedures.[50][I] It has a favorable safety record for use in children and adults[51][V] when used appropriately, and has been used for painful procedures in pediatric cancer units.[52][II] Advantages and disadvantages are outlined in **Box 16.5**.

Propofol is a short-acting hypnotic anesthetic agent which provides amnesia, but minimal analgesia.[53][V] Approximately one-quarter of gastrointestinal endoscopies in the USA are now performed using propofol as an alternative to the use of an opioid and benzodiazepine.[54][IV] It has also been successfully used during endoscopic retrograde cholangiopancreatography (ERCP) due to its short half-life, where propofol is administered as an infusion using a computer-targeted blood concentration, which the patient can then top up with controlled boosts.[55][III] There is, however, awareness that propofol is associated with risks of respiratory depression, and that the drug may increase the likelihood of deep sedation, with all the attendant risks of general anesthesia.[56][V]

Professional organizations have cautioned that the safety profile of both ketamine and propofol is such that their use requires the expertise of a suitably trained professional.[57][I] This is consistent with the need for constant vigilance for signs of hypoxemia and hypotension, and the ability to intubate and ventilate with supplemental oxygen if required.

Conscious sedation

Conscious sedation has been defined as a "… technique in which the use of a drug or drugs produces a state of

---

Box 16.4 Selected advantages and disadvantages to the use of nitrous oxide mixture

Advantages include:

- rapid onset of action and recovery;
- analgesia effective approximately 20 seconds after onset of inhalation, peaking at 40 seconds to 2 minutes;[49][V]
- minimal cardiovascular effects;
- self-administered – mask will drop away if the patient becomes drowsy.[19][V]

Disadvantages include:

- causes excitability and drowsiness at higher concentrations;
- contraindicated in some pulmonary diseases/disorders;
- potential to induce bone marrow suppression, especially with chronic use.[49][V]

Box 16.5 Selected advantages and disadvantages to the use of ketamine

Advantages include:

- rapid onset of action;
- produces conscious sedation, where patients respond to verbal commands, but also experience analgesia;[19][V]
- no need to avoid eating/drinking for long periods before or after the procedure;
- respiratory depression is uncommon, but can happen.[51][V]

Disadvantages include:

- tolerance to repeated doses develops rapidly;
- psychomimetic emergence reactions on recovery occur in 0–30%;[52][II]
- transient laryngospasm can occur;[51][V]
- risks of respiratory depression require facility for full resuscitation and availability of oxygen supplementation.

---

depression of the central nervous system enabling treatment to be carried out, but during which verbal contact with the patient is maintained … [and] … should carry a margin of safety wide enough to render loss of consciousness unlikely."[56][V] Such a state aims to relieve anxiety, enable cooperation, and produce some degree of amnesia.[58][V] Procedures that have the potential to cause pain will require concomitant use of analgesics.

Coexisting medical problems that may make conscious sedation hazardous include:

- diabetes;
- morbid obesity;
- heart disease;
- old age;
- hepatic and renal disease;
- concurrent drug administration;
- sedation within two hours of eating.

Serious complications of sedation are uncommon, but this should not lead to complacency. An American study found that, of 21,000 procedures, the rates of serious cardiorespiratory complications and death with midazolam or diazepam were, respectively, 5.4 and 0.3 per thousand procedures.[59][IV]

The intravenous route is employed for conscious sedation and has several advantages:

- rapid onset of action;
- ease of access;
- both initial bolus and further top-up doses of medication are easily administered;
- continuous background infusion and titration is possible.

The main disadvantage is the narrow safety margin between adequate sedation and analgesia, and toxic side effects, necessitating close patient supervision.[60][V]

Precautions for monitoring conscious sedation are summarized in **Box 16.6**. Guidelines on safe conscious sedation and deep sedation practice have been produced by several professional organizations.[45][I], [57][I], [61][I]

Deep sedation

The term deep sedation has been used by some clinicians and, indeed, sedation is a continuum from anxiolysis through to general anesthesia. However, it should be remembered that deep sedation, effected by use of higher doses of benzodiazepines and opioids or with anesthetic agents, may result in reduction of airway control and spontaneous ventilation[57][I] and thus is akin to general anesthesia. Such sedation should only be initiated by clinicians with the ability to secure a patient's airway and provide positive pressure ventilation, and personnel with advanced life support training should be readily available.[57][I]

CONCLUSIONS AND FUTURE DIRECTIONS

Issues still exist regarding the incidence of pain and distress experienced by patients during procedures. Use of

---

Box 16.6 Guidelines for conscious sedation practice

Before the procedure:

- Sedation used should be adjusted to individual patient requirements.
- Where the intravenous route is used, secure venous access is mandatory. Specific antagonist drugs to reverse potential respiratory depression must be to hand.
- Combinations of drugs, especially sedatives and opioids, should be employed with caution.

During the procedure:

- A suitably trained individual, present throughout the procedure, must have defined responsibility for monitoring patient safety.
- All patient recordings and drugs administered should be documented.
- Continuous monitoring of oxygen saturation and heart rate, and intermittent recording of respiratory rate and blood pressure are essential.
- Oxygen and appropriate delivery devices must be available.
- Appropriate resuscitation facilities must be available.

After the procedure:

- The patient should be observed with the following equipment available:
  - functioning apparatus for endotracheal suction;
  - a means of delivering >90% oxygen and positive pressure ventilation (e.g. bag and mask);
  - laryngoscope and equipment for laryngeal intubation.
- Before being discharged, the patient should be easily rouseable, with protective reflexes intact, and advice on monitoring the patient should be given to the accompanying person.

---

the newer sedative drugs and short-acting opioids has still not gained universal acceptance, with controversy over managing safety concerns. Professional audit of procedures and assessment of patient experience, both locally and at a national level, may lead to improvements in efficacy and safety of pain-relieving measures. Such activities should be used to improve practice and inform regular review of guidelines. The experience of patients undergoing specific procedures may be considerably enhanced by heightened awareness and adoption of guidelines produced by national professional bodies.

REFERENCES

1. Bernstein B, Schechter NL, Hickman T, Beck A. Premedication for painful procedures in children: a national survey. *Journal of Pain and Symptom Management*. 1991; **6**: 190.

2. Klein ER. Premedicating children for painful invasive procedures. *Journal of Pediatric Oncology Nursing*. 1992; **9**: 170–9.

3. McGrath PJ, Hsu E, Cappelli M *et al*. Pain from pediatric cancer: a survey of an outpatient oncology clinic. *Journal of Psychosocial Oncology*. 1990; **8**: 109–24.

4. Weisman SJ, Bernstein B, Schechter NL. Consequences of inadequate analgesia during painful procedures in children. *Archives of Pediatrics and Adolescent Medicine*. 1998; **152**: 147–9.

5. Steine S. Which hurts the most? A comparison of pain rating during double-contrast barium enema examination and colonoscopy. *Radiology*. 1994; **191**: 99–101.

6. Vanhelleputte P, Nijs K, Delforge M *et al*. Pain during bone marrow aspiration: prevalence and prevention. *Journal of Pain and Symptom Management*. 2003; **26**: 860–6.

7. Eisenberg E, Konopniki M, Veitsman E *et al*. Prevalence and characteristics of pain induced by percutaneous liver biopsy. *Anesthesia and Analgesia*. 2003; **96**: 1392–6.

8. Twycross R. *Introducing palliative care*, 3rd edn. Oxford: Radcliffe Medical Press, 1997: 66.

9. Hockenberry MJ, Bologna-Vaughan S. Preparation for intrusive procedures using noninvasive techniques in children with cancer: state of the art vs. new trends. *Cancer Nursing*. 1985; **8**: 97–102.

10. McDermott VG, Chapman ME, Gillespie I. Sedation and patient monitoring in vascular and interventional radiology. *British Journal of Radiology*. 1993; **66**: 667–71.

11. Cadranel J, Rufat P, Degos F. Practices of liver biopsy in France: results of a prospective nationwide survey. *Hepatology*. 2000; **32**: 477–80.

12. Skehan SJ, Malone DE, Buckley N *et al*. Sedation and analgesia in adult patients: evaluation of a staged-dose system based on body weight for use in abdominal interventional radiology. *Radiology*. 2000; **216**: 653–9.

13. Kaplan RM, Atkins CJ, Lenhard L. Coping with a stressful sigmoidoscopy: evaluation of cognitive and relaxation preparations. *Journal of Behavioral Medicine*. 1982; **5**: 67–82.

14. Jay S, Elliott CH, Fitzgibbons I *et al*. A comparative study of cognitive behavioural therapy versus general anesthesia for painful procedures in children. *Pain*. 1995; **62**: 3–9.

15. Stinshoff VJ, Lang EV, Berbaum KS *et al*. Effect of sex and gender on drug-seeking behavior during invasive medical procedures. *Academic Radiology*. 2004; **11**: 390–7.

16. Bayer TL, Coverdale JH, Chiang E, Bangs M. The role of prior pain experience and expectancy in psychologically and physically induced pain. *Pain*. 1998; **74**: 327–31.

17. Litt MD. Self-efficacy and perceived control: cognitive mediators of pain tolerance. *Journal of Personality and Social Psychology*. 1988; **54**: 149–60.

18. Mueller PR, Biswal S, Halpern EF *et al*. Interventional radiologic procedures: patient anxiety, perception of pain, understanding of procedure, and satisfaction with medication – a prospective study. *Radiology*. 2000; **215**: 684–8.

* 19. Agency for Healthcare Policy and Research (AHPCR). Acute pain management: operative or medical procedures and trauma, part 2. *Clinical Pharmacy*. 1992; **11**: 391–413.

20. Jacobson AF. Intradermal normal saline solution, self-selected music, and insertion difficulty effects on intravenous insertion pain. *Heart and Lung*. 1999; **28**: 114–22.

21. Puntillo KA, White C, Morris AB *et al*. Patients' perceptions and responses to procedural pain: results from Thunder Project II. *American Journal of Critical Care*. 2001; **10**: 238–51.

22. Mitchell M. Pain management in day case surgery. *Nursing Standard*. 2004; **18**: 33–8.

23. Kennedy PT, Kelly IM, Loan WC, Boyd CD. Conscious sedation and analgesia for routine aortofemoral arteriography: a prospective evaluation. *Radiology*. 2000; **216**: 660–4.

24. Audit Commission. *Managing pain after surgery. A booklet for nurses*. London: The Stationery Office, 1998. ISBN: 1862401012.

25. Lang EV, Joyce JS, Spiegel D *et al*. Self-hypnotic relaxation during interventional radiological procedures: effects on pain perception and intravenous drug use. *International Journal of Clinical and Experimental Hypnosis*. 1996; **44**: 106–19.

26. Lang EV, Berbaum KS. Educating interventional radiology personnel in nonpharmacologic analgesia: effect on patients' pain perception. *Academic Radiology*. 1997; **4**: 753–7.

27. Schupp CJ, Berbaum K, Berbaum M, Lang EV. Pain and anxiety during interventional radiologic procedures: effect of patients' state anxiety at baseline and modulation by nonpharmacologic analgesia adjuncts. *Journal of Vascular and Interventional Radiology*. 2005; **16**: 1585–92.

28. Stewart JH. Hypnosis in contemporary medicine. *Mayo Clinic Proceedings*. 2005; **80**: 511–24.

29. Liossi C, Hatira P. Clinical hypnosis in the alleviation of procedure-related pain in pediatric oncology patients. *International Journal of Clinical and Experimental Hypnosis*. 2003; **51**: 4–28.

30. Wild MR, Espie CA. The efficacy of hypnosis in the reduction of procedural pain and distress in pediatric oncology: a systematic review. *Journal of Developmental and Behavioral Pediatrics*. 2004; **25**: 207–13.

31. Horn S, Munafo M. Interventions. In: Payne S, Horn S (eds). *Pain: theory, research and intervention.* Buckingham: Open University Press, 1997: 113–29. ISBN: 0335196888.

32. McCarthy AM, Cool VA, Hanrahan K. Cognitive behavioral interventions for children during painful procedures: research challenges and program development. *Journal of Pediatric Nursing.* 1998; **13**: 55–63.

33. Cahn AM, Carayon P, Hill C, Flamant R. Acupuncture in gastroscopy. *Lancet.* 1978; **311**: 182–3.

34. Wang HH, Chang YH, Liu DM. A study of the effectiveness of acupuncture analgesia for colonoscopic examination compared with conventional premedication. *American Journal of Acupuncture.* 1992; **20**: 217–21.

35. Melzack R, Wall PD. Pain mechanisms: a new theory. *Science.* 1965; **150**: 971–9.

36. Sluka KA, Walsh D. Transcutaneous electrical nerve stimulation: basic science mechanisms and clinical effectiveness. *Journal of Pain.* 2003; **4**: 109–21.

37. Hargreaves A, Lander J. Use of transcutaneous electrical nerve stimulation for postoperative pain. *Nursing Research.* 1989; **38**: 159–61.

38. Lander J, Fowler-Kerry S. TENS for children's procedural pain. *Pain.* 1993; **52**: 209–16.

39. Eidelman A, Weiss JM, Lau J, Carr DB. Topical anesthetics for dermal instrumentation: a systematic review of randomized, controlled trials. *Annals of Emergency Medicine.* 2005; **46**: 343–51.

40. British National Formulary. *BNF 51.* London: BMJ Publishing and RPS Publishing, 2006: 648–9. ISBN: 0853696683.

41. Choy L, Collier J, Watson AR. Comparison of lignocaine-prilocaine cream and amethocaine gel for local analgesia before venepuncture in children. *Acta Paediatrica.* 1999; **88**: 961–4.

42. Krajnik M, Zylicz Z, Finlay I *et al.* Potential uses of topical opioids in palliative care – report of 6 cases. *Pain.* 1999; **80**: 121–5.

43. Stein C. Opioid receptors on peripheral sensory neurons. In: Machelska H, Stein C (eds). *Immune mechanisms of pain and analgesia.* Georgetown: Eurekah.com/Landes Bioscience, 2001: 69–76. ISBN: 0306476924.

44. Hatsiopoulou O, Cohen RI, Lang EV. Postprocedure pain management of interventional radiology patients. *Journal of Vascular and Interventional Radiology.* 2003; **14**: 1373–85.

45. Waring JP, Baron TH, Hirota WK *et al.* Standards of Practice Committee, American Society for Gastrointestinal Endoscopy. Guidelines for conscious sedation and monitoring during gastrointestinal endoscopy. *Gastrointestinal Endoscopy.* 2003; **58**: 317–22.

46. Schechter NL, Weisman SJ, Rosenblum M *et al.* The use of oral transmucosal fentanyl citrate for painful procedures in children. *Pediatrics.* 1995; **95**: 335–9.

47. Evans A. Use of Entonox® in the community for control of procedural pain. *British Journal of Community Nursing.* 2003; **8**: 488–94.

* 48. Castèra L, Nègre I, Samii K, Buffet C. Patient-administered nitrous oxide/oxygen inhalation provides safe and effective analgesia for percutaneous liver biopsy: a randomized placebo-controlled trial. *American Journal of Gastroenterology.* 2001; **96**: 1553–7.

49. Pal SK, Cortiella J, Herndon D. Adjunctive methods of pain control in burns. *Burns.* 1997; **23**: 404–12.

* 50. Subramaniam K, Subramaniam B, Steinbrook RA. Ketamine as adjuvant analgesic to opioids: a quantitative and qualitative systematic review. *Anesthesia and Analgesia.* 2004; **99**: 482–95.

* 51. Brown TB, Lovato LM, Parker D. Procedural sedation in the acute care setting. *American Family Physician.* 2005; **71**: 85–90.

52. Marx CM, Stein J, Tyler MK *et al.* Ketamine-midazolam versus meperidine-midazolam for painful procedures in pediatric oncology patients. *Journal of Clinical Oncology.* 1997; **15**: 94–102.

* 53. Nelson DB, Barkun AN, Block KP *et al.* Propofol use during gastrointestinal endoscopy. *Gastrointestinal Endoscopy.* 2001; **53**: 876–9.

54. Cohen LB, Wecsler JS, Gaetano JN *et al.* Endoscopic sedation in the United States: results from a nationwide survey. *American Journal of Gastroenterology.* 2006; **101**: 967–74.

55. Gilham MJ, Hutchinson RC, Carter R, Kenny GNC. Patient-maintained sedation for ERCP with a target-controlled infusion of propofol: a pilot study. *Gastrointestinal Endoscopy.* 2001; **54**: 14–17.

56. Skelly AM. Analgesia and sedation. In: Watkinson AF, Adam A (eds). *Interventional radiology: a practical guide.* Oxford: Radcliffe Medical Press, 1996: 3–11. ISBN: 1857750314.

* 57. American Society of Anesthesiologists Task Force on Sedation and Analgesia by Non-Anesthesiologists. Practice guidelines for sedation and analgesia by non-anesthesiologists. *Anesthesiology.* 2002; **96**: 1004–17.

58. Reid E. Intravenous sedation for short procedures and investigations. *Nursing Standard.* 1997; **12**: 35–8.

59. Arrowsmith JB, Gerstman BB, Fleischer DE, Benjamin SB. Results from the American Society for Gastrointestinal Endoscopy/US Food and Drug Administration collaborative study on complication rates and drug use during gastrointestinal endoscopy. *Gastrointestinal Endoscopy.* 1991; **37**: 421–7.

60. Justins DM, Richardson PH. Clinical management of acute pain. *British Medical Bulletin.* 1991; **47**: 561–83.

* 61. UK Academy of Medical Royal Colleges and their Faculties. *Implementing and ensuring safe sedation practice for healthcare procedures in adults. Report of the Intercollegiate Working Party of the UK Academy of Medical Royal Colleges and their Faculties.* London: Academy of Medical Royal Colleges, 2001.

PART III

NON-DRUG THERAPIES FOR CANCER PAIN

17 Nerve blocks: chemical and physical neurolytic agents   225
    John E Williams

18 Stimulation–induced analgesia   235
    Mark I Johnson, Stephen G Oxberry, and Karen Robb

19 Radiotherapy   251
    Peter J Hoskin

20 Management of bone pain   256
    Peter J Hoskin

21 Complementary therapies   270
    Jacqueline Filshie and Adrian White

22 Management of breakthrough pain   286
    Giovambattista Zeppetella and Russell K Portenoy

23 Psychological interventions in cancer pain management   296
    T Manoj Kumar, C Venkateswaran, and P Thekkumpurath

24 Control of symptoms other than pain   310
    Emma Hall, Nigel Sykes, and Victor Pace

Nerve blocks: chemical and physical neurolytic agents

JOHN E WILLIAMS

Introduction   225
Pathophysiology of neurolysis   226
Chemical neurolytic agents   227
Clinical applications of chemical neurolysis   228

Physical neurolytic agents   231
Summary   233
References   233

KEY LEARNING POINTS

- Chemical and physical neurolysis still has a place in modern pain management practice in conjunction with other therapeutic regimes including pharmacotherapy, physical, and psychological therapies.
- Alcohol and phenol can both be used to block nociceptive transmission.
- The neurolytic celiac plexus block has been widely used and is supported by randomized comparator trials.
- Adverse effects of chemical neurolysis such as motor and sensory loss may be problematical and must be measured against the possible benefits.
- Cryoablation can be used to produce prolonged analgesia without neuritis or neuroma formation.
- Radiofrequency lesioning (RF) can be used to produce a discreet neural lesion.
- Use of modern radiological techniques improves efficacy and safety.
- Use of chemical and physical agents is poorly supported by evidence-based guidelines, long-term outcome studies, and clear guidelines for indications.

INTRODUCTION

Numerous different chemical substances and physical techniques have been applied to elements of the central and peripheral nervous systems in efforts to disrupt pain transmission in a durable yet safe fashion.

Destructive chemical substances include alcohol, phenol, glycerol, and hypertonic saline. Physical methods range from heating nerves with radiofrequency lesions and lasers to cooling the nerves with topical sprays or locally induced ice balls (**Table 17.1**).

Neurolytic procedures with chemical and physical agents have been successfully applied to treat pain since the early part of the twentieth century. **Table 17.2** outlines some of the major early historical developments in the use of neurolytic agents. Over the last two decades, dramatic improvements in the pharmacologic management of pain, such as the development of long-acting opioid preparations and alternative strong opioids, an improved understanding of the role of adjuvant analgesics, and better access to analgesics and acceptance of their role, as well as improvements in anticancer therapies, argue for a more circumscribed role for neurolytic agents in contemporary practice.

Additionally, developments in our understanding of the interactions between nociceptive input and the plasticity of the nervous system suggest that pain is not dependent on hard-wired line-labeled linkages, but is capable of change and modification at all levels throughout the nervous system. This new understanding implies that neurolytic interruption of discrete pathways is unlikely to provide complete pain relief for prolonged intervals. Nevertheless, the varied and complex patterns of pain present in patients with progressive cancer, and the compelling mandate for achieving pain relief in such settings, ensure an essential, although limited, role for neurolysis when pain is intractable. Developments in interventional radiological techniques applied to neurolytic blocks have improved the ease and accuracy of performing the blocks and the risk–benefit ratio.

Although the recent emphasis on the importance of evidence-based medicine has outstripped the availability of controlled trials that accurately depict the relative effect of alternative interventions, potentially useful therapies cannot ethically be withheld while awaiting such data.

The aim of this chapter is to describe the different chemical and physical agents and to outline their role in modern pain management.

Table 17.1 Chemical and physical agents used in current clinical practice.

Chemical agents	Physical agents
50–100% alcohol – intrathecal, sympathetic neurolysis (e.g. celiac), peripheral neurolysis (e.g. intercostal)	Cryoneurolysis – facet joint, selected peripheral nerves
5–15% phenol – intrathecal, epidural, selected peripheral nerves (e.g. intercostal)	Radiofrequency lesioning – facet joint, selected peripheral nerves, percutaneous cordotomy
Glycerol – trigeminal ganglion neurolysis	Laser – endoscopic epidural lysis

Table 17.2 History of chemical neurolysis.

Date	Researcher	Development
1903	Schloesser	Use of alcohol for trigeminal neuralgia
1919	Kappis	Percutaneous celiac plexus block
1926	Swetlow	Neurolytic sympathetic block with alcohol to relieve angina
1929	De Beule	Alcohol celiac plexus block
1931	Dogliotti	Absolute alcohol used intrathecally
1947	Mandl	Phenol for lumbar sympathetic block

PATHOPHYSIOLOGY OF NEUROLYSIS

Chemical and physical neurolytic agents and techniques have a final common pathway in their action on the nerve cells. They are employed with the aim of producing nerve injury sufficient to result in degeneration of the nerve fiber distal to the lesion along with its myelin sheath. This process is called wallerian degeneration[1] and results in a temporary interference in nerve cell transmission resulting in nociceptive block. Wallerian degeneration does not completely disrupt the nerve cell; persistence of the basal lamina of the Schwann cells potentially allows for axonal regrowth with reconnection to the proximal end of the nerve fiber.

If, however, the nerve is surgically cut, there is complete disruption of the neuron and basal lamina which is more likely to result in disorganized regrowth without reconnection of the cut nerve endings, possibly resulting in production of painful neuromata and dysesthetic pain.[2] This difference (**Table 17.3**) justifies reliance on the use of neurolytic agents over surgical interruption of peripheral nerve fibers for the treatment of chronic pain.

Selective neurolysis

It was originally postulated that neurolytic chemicals and physical methods of nerve interruption would produce a differential effect on small nociceptive fibers without interfering with sensory, motor, or autonomic function. Unfortunately, a reliable differential effect has not been shown for any of these methods. Neural tissue appears to be affected nonselectively, with consequent risk of injury to motor and sensory nerves and surrounding tissue. With most modalities, however, there is a concentration effect such that lower concentrations tend to produce a more reversible, less profound degeneration than higher concentrations (**Table 17.4**).

Another difficulty relates to ensuring accurate placement of the chemicals or physical agents at the target area.

Table 17.3 Chemical or physical neurolysis versus surgical sectioning of nerve cell.

		Result
Neurolysis with chemical or physical agent	Surgical cutting of nerve	
Pathological process	Wallerian degeneration	Complete nerve cell disruption
Preservation of basal lamina	Axonal regrowth	
Possible clinical effect	Temporary (1–3 months) block of nociception Dysesthetic pain	Painful neuromata

In the case of alcohol and phenol, image intensification and computed tomography (CT) are used to ensure accurate localization of the needle tip before injection. Physical lesioning using instruments such as the cryoprobe or radiofrequency generator requires accurate localization of the probe tip and should take account of measurement of temperature and duration of application.

CHEMICAL NEUROLYTIC AGENTS

Alcohol, phenol, and glycerol are the only neurolytic agents employed in current clinical practice. Their optimal use depends on producing sufficient damage to result in wallerian degeneration, but not excessive nerve cell disorganization, resulting in adverse effects such as motor and sensory impairment.

Alcohol

Alcohol is the classic neurolytic agent, although today phenol is more commonly used for peripheral neurolysis as it is potentially less toxic. Alcohol is used in concentrations from 3 to 100 percent. It damages sensory,

Table 17.4 Pathophysiological effects of physical and chemical neurolysis.

Chemical or physical agent	Pathophysiological effect
Minimal heat applied to peripheral nerve	Enhanced nerve conduction
Local anesthetic drug applied to peripheral nerve	Totally reversible reduction in nerve conduction
2% lidocaine (lignocaine)	
0.5% bupivacaine	
5–7.5% phenol	Reduction in nerve conduction – usually reversible after weeks or months
50% alcohol	
50% glycerol	
10–15% phenol	Depression of nerve conduction – may be reversible
100% alcohol	
Radiofrequency lesions <44°C	
Cryoprobe causing ice ball	
Radiofrequency lesion temperature >44°C	Potentially irreversible nerve block – permanent lesion
Cryoprobe causing intraneural ice crystals	
Surgical nerve sectioning	Permanent neural lesion, non-wallerian nerve degeneration, possible neuroma formation
Any physical neurolytic measure taken to extreme limits of time and/or temperature	

motor, and autonomic nerves in a nonselective way and is injurious to surrounding soft tissue. It is readily soluble in body fluids, and is hypobaric with respect to cerebrospinal fluid (CSF) and thus will rise, diffusing rapidly from the injection site.[3] Careful positioning of the patient is required to allow the alcohol to act predominantly on the posterior, sensory nerve roots for the treatment of pain (patient in supine position) or anterior motor nerve roots for treatment of spasticity (patient in prone position).

Alcohol works by extracting fatty substances from the myelin sheath and precipitating proteins.[4] This results in degeneration of the nerve fiber and myelin sheath distal to the lesion (wallerian degeneration). Providing the nerve cell is not completely destroyed (i.e. the basal lamina of the Schwann cell is preserved), regeneration usually begins within three to four months. If the entire nerve cell is completely disrupted, regeneration does not occur and effects are prolonged. Despite this, there is a risk of the development of dysesthetic pain as a result of central nervous system (CNS) plasticity or neuroma formation.

Damage to the nerve cells is proportional to the concentration and volume of alcohol used, as well as the rate of instillation, but there is no evidence for selective destruction of nociceptive, motor or sensory fibers (**Table 17.5**).

Phenol

Phenol is commonly used in concentrations of 5–15 percent for neurolysis. Five percent phenol is roughly equivalent to 40 percent alcohol in neurolytic potency. When dissolved in glycerine, it is hyperbaric compared with CSF and therefore patients need to be positioned contrary to that described above under Alcohol (patient needs to be placed in the prone position for the neurolysis to affect the posterior pain fibers). It is also less water soluble than alcohol and therefore may spread less liberally from the injection site.[5]

Table 17.5 Effect of different alcohol concentrations on nerve cell destruction.

Alcohol concentration (%)	Effect
3	Mild local anesthetic effect, usually self-limited
33	Sensory nerve damage, little effect on motor neurons
50	Motor damage, concentration used for celiac plexus blocks
100	Persistent motor paralysis; risk of damage to skin and surrounding tissues

For neuraxial use phenol is formulated in glycerine, which acts as a base from which the glycerine is slowly released, potentially resulting in higher local concentrations. Used peripherally or near the sympathetic axis, phenol is typically compounded with water or saline.

Originally believed to preferentially destroy sensory neurons, destruction is now thought to be nonspecific, although when lower concentrations of phenol are used (e.g. <3 percent) destruction is mild, temporary, and similar to the type of block achieved with a local anesthetic agent. Because of a lower likelihood of producing neuritis, phenol is more widely used than alcohol (**Table 17.6**) and the duration and intensity of block are thought to be less than with alcohol and, therefore, there is a wider margin of safety and complications are more frequently reversible. An exception is that alcohol is traditionally used for neurolytic celiac plexus blockade. This may be because alcohol has theoretically less affinity for vascular structures that are present in the vicinity of the celiac plexus. Phenol may cause ulceration of soft tissues if injected subcutaneously.

Glycerol

Glycerol is used only for peripheral nerve blockade. It is used in the treatment of trigeminal neuralgia when it is injected on to branches of the trigeminal nerve. It may produce less sensory deficit than alcohol, though repeat blocks may be required after a few months.

Ammonium compounds

Ammonium chloride and ammonium hydroxide have been used in 6 percent solutions to produce neurolytic block for pain control. Initially it was thought that a selective, sensory block was achieved, but results are unreliable and unpredictable, and microscopically it was shown that the neurolysis affected all types of nerve fiber.

Hypertonic and hypotonic solutions

Intrathecal injections of these solutions have been used to treat pain. They cause a localized osmotic swelling of the nerve bundle, which reduces nerve conduction. Prolonged exposure may produce more permanent impairment of neurological function, systemic toxicity, and death.

CLINICAL APPLICATIONS OF CHEMICAL NEUROLYSIS

Use of neurolytic chemicals in clinical practice is a balance between yielding potentially beneficial effects and the risk of adverse effects. This balance is dependent on clinical factors such as:

- life expectancy;
- the degree to which reasonable systemic analgesic treatments have been unsuccessful;
- preexisting levels of autonomic, motor, and sensory impairment.

These blocks should be used as adjuncts to systemic treatments as part of a multidisciplinary and multimodal approach to pain management.[6]

Neurolytic celiac plexus block

The celiac plexus block using local anesthetic was first used in 1914 as an adjunct to surgical anesthesia. The neurolytic block using alcohol was first used in 1919 to treat the pain of upper abdominal malignancy

Table 17.6 Neurolytic chemicals in current clinical use.

	Alcohol	Phenol	Glycerol
Concentration	50–100%	4–15%	50–100%
Diluent	Nil	Glycerine Saline Water	Nil
Baricity in CSF	Hypobaric	Hyperbaric	Not used in CSF
Onset	Immediate	15–20 min slow release from glycerine	15–20 min
Position for nociceptive block	Painful side up	Painful side down	–
Complications	Neuritis (common)	Neuritis (uncommon) Toxicity is volume dependent	
Use	Celiac plexus block (50% concentration) Intrathecal Peripheral	Intrathecal Peripheral	Trigeminal neuralgia, facial pain

CSF, cerebrospinal fluid.

(**Table 17.2**). Since then there have been numerous case reports[7] and randomized controlled trials (RCTs) (**Table 17.7**) attesting to its efficacy in the treatment of cancer-related pancreatic pain.

Any pain originating from visceral structures innervated by the celiac plexus can be alleviated by blockade of the plexus. This includes malignant disease of the pancreas, liver, gallbladder, and alimentary tract from the distal esophagus to the transverse colon, including the adrenal glands, although efficacy is poor with ascites and carcinomatosis.

This block may also relieve pain from other upper abdominal malignancies (such as liver and gall bladder) and has been used to treat pain from pancreatitis, but efficacy and durability are reported as being much lower.[12, 13]

There may be additional beneficial effects apart from pain relief, including decreased constipation, decreased nausea, increased appetite, and less sedation as a result of a reduced systemic opioid requirement.

INDICATIONS

Neurolytic celiac plexus block (NCPB) is indicated for patients with visceral pain due to malignancy in one of the sites listed above. Many abdominal malignancies present with mixed visceral and somatic pains as a result of retroperitoneal extension or metastatic spread. NCPB may unmask pains of somatic origin. It is preferable to determine the etiologies of the pain prior to blockade. This can be performed with a diagnostic, temporary block using local anesthetic.

PROCEDURE

Traditionally, the posterior route is taken, using two 7-inch needles to approach the celiac plexus posterolateral

Table 17.7 Evidence for the efficacy of the neurolytic celiac plexus block.

Study	Details of study
Mercadante[8]	Randomized controlled trial ($n = 20$)
	No difference in pain scores between celiac block group and oral morphine group, but fewer side effects with NCPB
Sharfmann and Walsh[9]	Review article
	Efficacy 87% in 418 patients in 15 published series
	Case series studies criticized for methodology
Eisenberg et al.[10]	Meta-analysis; efficacy in 70–90% of patients
Wong et al.[11]	Randomized controlled trial of NCPB versus opioids: improved pain control with NCPB, no difference in quality of life or survival

NCPB, neurolytic celiac plexus block.

to the vertebral bodies under radiographic image intensification. However this approach has now been superseded by use of CT imaging, percutaneous ultrasound, endoscopic ultrasound, or by use of a surgical technique – laparoscopic splanchnectomy.[14, 15, 16]

COMPLICATIONS

Complications have been divided into major and minor. Major complications include paralysis and autonomic dysfunction due to damage to a feeder artery of the spinal cord. The incidence of this may be as high as 1 in 700.[17] Minor complications include hypotension and diarrhea, and are usually transient.

EFFICACY

Case reports of NCPB give an efficacy of 57–95 percent.[7, 18, 19, 20] However, most were retrospective in nature and have been criticized for poor methodology[9] (**Table 17.7**). A meta-analysis of 21 retrospective studies in 1145 patients receiving NCPB reported benefit in 90 percent of patients evaluated after three months.[10]

Data from one RCT comparing the efficacy of the NCPB with oral morphine in 20 patients showed equal visual analog scores in the two groups, but significantly fewer opioid-induced side effects such as sedation and constipation in patients treated with NCPB.[8] A randomized controlled comparison of NCPB versus optimized analgesic therapy plus sham injection showed significantly less pain in the NCPB group but no differences in quality of life or survival.[11] Surgical division of the splanchnic nerves (videothoracoscopic splanchnicectomy) was compared with NCPB and was shown to be effective for controlling pancreatic cancer pain.[21]

There is some controversy over the timing of the block, with some authors advocating early use of the block and others using it only if systemic opioids are ineffective or are associated with toxicity (**Table 17.8**). One study reported less pain, reduced opioid consumption, and better quality of life in patients receiving a NCPB at an early stage in their cancer pain management.[22]

A full assessment of the potential risks versus benefit of the block needs to be discussed with each patient. Duration of block has been variously reported. It is possible that regeneration of new pain pathways or development of deafferentation syndromes may result in pain returning after six to twelve months.[23, 24]

Other neurolytic sympathetic blocks

The sympathetic chain can be blocked with a neurolytic substance at any point along its course. In the treatment of complex regional pain syndromes and other painful neuropathic syndromes of the upper limb, the

Table 17.8 Controversies in neurolytic celiac block.

Factor	Details
Timing	The block has been performed relatively early in the course of malignant disease; others reserve its use for pain unrelieved by systemic opioids
Efficacy	Case series report high efficacy (60–95%)
	Comparative trials have shown efficacy is similar to that of oral opioids
Balance of risk versus benefit	Significant risks of paraplegia in a small proportion of patients
Duration of blockade	Block has been reported to last 6–12 months, which is often adequate
	Longer-term follow up is lacking

sympathetic nerve supply can be blocked by injection of phenol or alcohol into the stellate ganglion. There are risks associated with this procedure, however, with the potential to produce a prolonged Horner syndrome and damage to the brachial plexus and recurrent laryngeal nerve. Traditionally the block is performed using dilute (3–5 percent) phenol.

Neurolytic blockade of the sympathetic supply to the abdomen and pelvis (inferior mesenteric plexus, superior hypogastric plexus block, and ganglion impar block) have been described for the treatment of intractable, cancer-related pelvic pain.[25] One study described the benefits of early superior hypogastric plexus blockade compared with conventional treatment.[22] All of these techniques are associated with infrequent complications and may be suitable for patients with intractable pain and limited life expectancy because sympathetic denervation should not interfere with sensory or motor function.[26]

Intrathecal neurolysis

CLINICAL CONSIDERATIONS

The use of intrathecal neurolysis has declined over the past two decades. This may be because of the increased use of reversible techniques such as neuraxial and opioid delivery systems and because of fears over the side effects of neurolysis, in particular motor, autonomic, and sensory effects. However, in carefully selected patients this type of block may play an important role, particularly when other treatments have not been successful. Intrathecal neurolysis should be performed as part of a multidisciplinary pain strategy. Efficacy and safety may be enhanced when used in conjunction with an image intensifier or in collaboration with an interventional radiologist.

Phenol "saddle" blocks of the lumbo-sacral nerve roots have been described as being effective in reducing pain and opioid requirements for intractable pelvisacral pain.[27]

TECHNIQUE

The effectiveness of intrathecal neurolysis depends on bathing the posterior, sensory, nerve root with neurolytic solution. Either alcohol or phenol can be used. If alcohol is used, the patient is placed on his or her side with the painful side uppermost to allow the hypobaric solution to spread on to the posterior nerve roots. The reverse position, painful side down, is used for phenol, and is often too demanding of patients.

OUTCOME

No controlled data exist comparing the effectiveness of this treatment with other analgesic interventions. Case reports indicate a success rate of between 50 and 75 percent.[28] Success is improved by careful patient selection and meticulous technique and is inversely proportional to the number of dermatomes that need to be blocked. Some patients with a partially effective block may require supplemental oral analgesics.

COMPLICATIONS

Complications following neurolysis include motor paralysis, sensory disturbance, autonomic disturbance, and minor problems such as pain on injection (**Table 17.9**). No controlled data exist regarding the use of intrathecal neurolysis, so it is difficult to estimate the exact incidence of these complications. However, complications are likely to be reduced by accurate needle placement using image intensification where appropriate. The higher concentrations of alcohol, 50 percent and above, are more likely to cause motor paralysis. Dysesthetic pains such as neuralgias are infrequent after injection. After intrathecal neurolysis, an area of numbness may replace the painful area. Some patients may find this distressing.

Alcohol is irritant and painful on injection. After injection it is important to flush the alcohol through the needle with saline to prevent fistula formation.

Epidural neurolytic blockade

Phenol has been injected via the epidural route to achieve a neurolytic sensory block. Theoretical advantages include a lower incidence of autonomic impairment and potentially a less dramatic, more easily titratable, effect.

Single bolus injections of phenol (2 mL of 7 percent) have been used, with some reports of pain relief for as long as nine months.

Racz et al.[29] have developed an epidural catheter that is resistant to the corrosive effects of the neurolytic solution, thus allowing repeated epidural dosing. They reported good pain relief in over 50 percent of patients persisting for three to six months. Repeated dosing was possible if the block receded. Unlike intrathecal administration there

Table 17.9 Complications of intrathecal neurolysis.

Complication	Details
Dysesthetic pain	Painful neuralgias, burning pain, and dysesthetic pain can last for weeks or months, but are rare
	May be related to damage to somatic nerves
Motor paresis	More common with higher volumes
Anesthesia or hypoesthesia	Areas of numbness can occur, which can be distressing
Sphincter disturbance	Bowel and bladder disturbance can occur after intrathecal neurolysis in the sacral area
	Accurate placement of solution is important
Irritation of surrounding tissue	Alcohol is injurious to surrounding tissue; accurate needle placement and injection important
Alcohol toxicity	Alcohol is rapidly absorbed systemically; however, it is unlikely to cause a major problem with the small doses that are used clinically
Pain on injection	Transient

is greater latency to effect, and topographic spread is more variable.

Neurolytic block of peripheral nerves

The use of peripheral nerve neurolysis in cancer pain patients with intractable pain and limited life expectancy has been described.[7] However, these neurolytic blocks may result in neuralgia as the nerves regenerate after neurolysis or in a deafferentation pain syndrome. An exception to this is that neurolytic blockade of the branches of the trigeminal nerve does not usually produce neuralgia during regeneration.

Other neurolytic nerve blocks include paravertebral injections, block of individual branches of the lumbar plexus, ilioinguinal and iliohypogastric blocks, and block of the intercostal nerves.

PHYSICAL NEUROLYTIC AGENTS

Nerves can be cooled or heated in an attempt to interrupt pain transmission. Modern methods of application of these physical techniques include the cryoprobe (cooling), RF (heating), and lasers.

Hypothermia

The application of cold to peripheral nerves results in a reversible block of nerve conduction. This phenomenon has been used to treat pain for many years. Hippocrates described the use of ice and snow packs to relieve pain, and painful limbs were frozen prior to amputation during the Napoleonic wars. Ethyl chloride spray has been used to produce local anesthesia since 1890. Today, cooling is achieved with the use of a cryoprobe.

Cryoanalgesia

In 1976, Lloyd et al.[30] described the use of a probe to apply extreme cold locally to nerves to achieve pain relief by a long-term reversible nerve block called cryoanalgesia. This technique uses the rapid expansion of nitrous oxide or carbon dioxide to produce a temperature of $-20°C$ at the probe tip, which is applied to the nerve. This produces an ice ball, which interferes with nerve cell conduction, and if the probe is placed on the nerve for long enough, the interior of the cell turns into ice crystals, causing a more permanent wallerian degeneration of the nerve cell. The analgesic effect may last for weeks or months. Providing the basal lamina of the neuron has not been damaged, axonal regeneration of the nerve takes place within three months and normal neural function returns. It is possible that the analgesic effect will be more prolonged, and this may be because there has been a more permanent disruption of the nerve cell interior.

One of the disadvantages of the cryoprobe is the size of the probe tip itself, usually more than 3 mm; this can make accurate placement on a nerve difficult (**Table 17.10**).

Cryoneurolysis of the intercostal nerves during surgery is the best-known application of cryotherapy for the treatment of acute post-thoracotomy pain.[31] A number of reports have described effective pain management in this situation, especially when combined with other analgesic treatments.[32, 33] However, the occurrence of chronic dysesthetic pain has led a number of surgeons to abandon its routine use.

Cryolesions have been described for a number of facial nerves,[34] including supraorbital, infraorbital, mandibular, and mental nerves, and in the treatment of groin pain via the iliohypogastric and ilioinguinal nerves.

Hyperthermia

Heating of peripheral nerves initially causes nerve conduction enhancement; if the heat application is continued, a reversible depression is produced (the neuron can regrow following wallerian degeneration) followed by an irreversible depression if the entire nerve is disrupted. Induction heating is a process whereby heated pellets can be inserted into brain tissue and then destroy surrounding tissue. This method has been used in neurosurgery to destroy brain tissue. Because of its relatively

Table 17.10 Advantages and disadvantages of cryoneurolysis.

Advantages	Disadvantages
Potential role in acute and chronic pain	Reports of neuritis and dysesthetic pain
Reversible nerve destruction; duration of analgesia 1–5 months	Lack of comparative studies on efficacy (case reports only)
Relatively easy to use	Large probe tip may make accurate application difficult
Precise placement of probe is necessary, usually under direct vision	

Table 17.11 Advantages and disadvantages of radiofrequency lesioning.

Advantages	Disadvantages
More consistent production of lesions than some other physical methods such as lasers	Potential damage to surrounding tissue, including sensory or motor nerves
Possible to specifically target peripheral nerves, such as trigeminal nerve	Paucity of controlled data describing efficacy
Quantifiable and measurable effects	Paucity of recent descriptions of efficacy
Potentially can selectively destroy pain fibers rather than Aβ-fibers	Requires purchase of expensive equipment and training in its use
Small tip allows discrete placement, and avoids uncertainties of the spread of injected solutions	Pain after lesioning
	Lesion is produced within seconds; accurate placement is required

nonspecific effects, it is not a technique that has been used for pain control.

Lasers

Lasers can be used to heat and cut nerve tissue in the brain and spinal cord. The laser disrupts the interior of the nerve cell, which subsequently undergoes Wallerian degeneration. The perineurium may not be damaged, and regeneration of the nerve cell can take place. Direct visualization of the nerve is required for effective laser treatment. Dorsal root entry zone (DREZ) lesions have been made using a laser. Potential problems include difficulties in quantifying the extent and rapidity of nerve cell destruction and thus variable clinical defects may be produced.[35]

Radiofrequency lesioning

Radiofrequency lesioning (RF) is the use of electricity to generate heat, which can then be used to create a lesion in the nervous system. The radiofrequency probe provides a discrete controllable heat source, which creates a neural lesion when placed directly into the brain or on to peripheral nerves. The size of the lesion is dependent on the temperature of the probe and duration of application. There is some suggestion that the smaller Aδ- and C pain fibers may be preferentially affected by the lesioning. One of the advantages of RF is a precise and measurable application of heat, thus avoiding unwanted and uncontrolled side effects, such as sticking, charring, and formation of explosive gas (**Table 17.11**).

The radiofrequency probe can be applied to the brain (temperatures up to 42°C), or directly on to peripheral nerves (up to 60–70°C). Fluoroscopic guidance may facilitate accurate needle placement.

Clinical application of RF

The best-known indication for RF is lumbar pain emanating from the lumbar facet joints. There are also an increasing number of publications concerning the application of these procedures in thoracic, cervical, and sacroiliac pain syndromes.[36, 37, 38]

FACET JOINT PAIN

The aim of RF is to destroy the nerve supply to the facet joints at multiple vertebral levels. The radiofrequency probe is placed on the nerve to the facet joints; lesions are generated after approximately one minute at 80°C. A recent Cochrane systematic review found seven relevant RCTs assessing RF denervation for neck and back pain which revealed only limited evidence for short-term effectiveness.[39] A review of four prospective trials of the use of RF lesions in treatment of low back pain failed to find more than "sparse evidence" of efficacy.[40] However, a review by Manchikanti et al.[41] found two RCTs and four prospective evaluations and concluded that there was strong evidence of short-term relief and moderate evidence of long-term relief of chronic spinal pain of facet joint origin.[41]

LUMBAR DISCOGENIC PAIN

Radiofrequency lesions have been used to treat lumbar disk pain. Either the gray ramus communicans or the nerves within the disk itself are the targets for RF. The same Cochrane review above[39] showed only limited evidence for efficacy.

TRIGEMINAL NEURALGIA

Radiofrequency lesions have been used to treat facial pain by targeting the trigeminal (Gasserian) ganglion.

SYMPATHETIC CHAIN

Percutaneous RF of the thoracic or lumbar sympathetic chain has been used to treat pain due to sympathetically maintained pain syndromes. Under image intensification, the sympathetic chain is visualized and the radiofrequency lesion generator applied directly to it.

COMPLICATIONS OF RF

The most common complication is post-lesioning neuritis or neuralgia which may occur in up to 10 percent of patients. Other complications include numbness and motor paralysis.

SUMMARY

A variety of different chemical (phenol and alcohol) and physical (heat and cold) neurolytic agents have been used to destroy nerves and reduce afferent nociceptive impulse transmission in the treatment of chronic pain. However, these nerves can regenerate, and the pain can return or a new pain can develop due to deafferentation. Thus, careful consideration of the risk–benefit ratio of the procedure and appropriate patient selection is important. The use of chemical intrathecal neurolysis has diminished over the past 10–20 years with the advent of improved analgesic drugs and the use of reversible infusion pumps and techniques. However, there may still be a role for this technique in intractable pain, especially in cancer pain patients with limited prognosis and functional ability. The neurolytic celiac plexus block is comprehensively described in numerous research studies and may have an important role in the management of intractable upper abdominal pain due to malignancy. Interventional radiology has improved safety and efficacy of the procedure. Physical techniques, such as cryotherapy and RF, are well recognized as treatments for chronic pain problems and have a role within a multidisciplinary therapeutic context. Additional good-quality controlled evidence will help clarify the precise role of these procedures in modern pain practice.

REFERENCES

1. Waller A. Experiments on the section of the glossopharyngeal and hypoglossal nerves of the frog and observations of the alterations produced thereby in the structure of their primitive fibres. *Philosophical Transactions of the Royal Society of London.* 1850; **40**: 423.

2. Sunderland S. The anatomical basis of nerve repair. In: Jewett DL, McCaroll Jr HR (eds). *Nerve repair and regeneration.* St Louis, MO: Mosby, 1980: 14.

3. Swerdlow M. Current views on intrathecal neurolysis. *Anesthesia.* 1978; **33**: 733–40.

4. Rumbsy MG, Finean JB. The action of organic solvents on the myelin sheath of peripheral nerve tissue. *Journal of Neurochemistry.* 1966; **13**: 1509–11.

5. Politis MJ, Schaumburg HH, Spencer PS. Neurotoxicity of selected chemicals. In: Spencer PS, Schaumburg (eds). *Experimental and chemical neurotoxicity.* Baltimore, MD: William and Wilkins, 1980: 613.

* 6. Patt RB. The current status of anesthetic approaches to cancer pain management. In: Payne R, Patt RB, Stratton Hill C (eds). *Assessment and treatment of cancer pain.* Seattle, WA: IASP Press, 1998: 195–213.

7. Bonica JJ, Buckley FP, Moricca G, Murphy TM. Neurolytic blockade and hypophysectomy. In: Bonica JJ, Loeser JD, Chapman CR, Fordyce WE (eds). *The management of pain.* Philadelphia, PA: Lea and Febiger, 1990: 1980–2040.

* 8. Mercadante S. Celiac plexus block versus analgesics in pancreatic cancer pain. *Pain.* 1993; **52**: 187–92.

* 9. Sharfman WH, Walsh TD. Has the analgesic efficacy of neurolytic celiac plexus block been demonstrated in pancreatic cancer pain? *Pain.* 1990; **41**: 267–71.

* 10. Eisenberg E, Carr DB, Chalmers TC. Neurolytic celiac plexus block for treatment of cancer pain. A meta-analysis. *Anesthesia and Analgesia.* 1995; **80**: 290–7.

11. Wong GY, Shroeder DR, Carns PE *et al.* Effect of neurolytic block on pain relief, quality of life, and survival in patients with unresectable pancreatic cancer: a randomised controlled trial. *Journal of the American Medical Association.* 2004; **291**: 1092–9.

12. Bell SN, Cole R, Roberts-Thompson IC. Celiac plexus block for control of pain in chronic pancreatitis. *British Medical Journal.* 1980; **281**: 1604.

13. Waldmann SD. Celiac plexus block. In: Weiner RS (ed.). *Innovations in pain management.* Orlando, FL: PMD Press, 1990: 10–15.

14. Matamala AM, Lopez FV, Martinez LI. The percutaneous anterior approach to the celiac plexus using CT guidance. *Pain.* 1988; **34**: 285–8.

15. Leiberman RP, Nance PN, Cuka DJ. Anterior approach to the celiac plexus during interventional biliary procedures. *Radiology.* 1988; **167**: 562–4.

16. Noble M, Gress FG. Techniques and results of neurolysis for chronic pancreatitis and pancreatic cancer pain. *Current Gastroenterology Reports.* 2006; **8**: 99–103.

17. Davies DD. Incidence of major complications of neurolytic celiac plexus block. *Journal of the Royal Society of Medicine.* 1993; **86**: 264–6.

18. Brown DL, Bulley CK, Quiel EL. Neurolytic celiac plexus block for pancreatic cancer pain. *Anesthesia and Analgesia.* 1987; **66**: 869–73.

19. Orwitz S, Sundararao K. Celiac plexus block: an overview. *Mount Sinai Journal of Medicine*. 1983; **50**: 486–90.

20. Bridenbaugh LD, Moore DC, Campbell DO. Management of upper abdominal cancer pain. *Journal of the American Medical Association*. 1964; **190**: 877–80.

21. Stefaniak T, Basinski A, Vingehoets A *et al*. A comparison of two invasive techniques in the management of intractable pain due to inoperable pancreatic cancer: neurolytic celiac plexus block and videothoracoscopic splanchnicectomy. *European Journal of Surgical Oncology*. 2005; **31**: 768–73.

22. de Oliveira R, dos Reis MP, Prado WA. The effects of early or late neurolytic sympathetic plexus block on the management of abdominal or pelvic cancer pain. *Pain*. 2004; **110**: 400–08.

23. Gorbitz C, Laevens ME. Alcohol block of the celiac plexus for control of upper abdominal pain caused by cancer and pancreatitis. *Journal of Neurosurgery*. 1971; **34**: 575–9.

24. Hegedus V. Relief of pancreatic pain by radiography-guided block. *American Journal of Roentgenology*. 1979; **133**: 1101–03.

25. Kitoh T, Tanaka S, Ono K *et al*. Combined neurolytic block of celiac, inferior mesenteric, and superior hypogastric plexuses for incapacitating abdominal and/or pelvic cancer pain. *Journal of Anesthesia*. 2005; **19**: 328–32.

* 26. de Leon-Casaola OA. Critical evaluation of chemical neurolysis of the sympathetic axis for cancer pain. *Cancer Control*. 2000; **7**: 142–8.

27. Slatkin NE, Rhiner M. Phenol saddle blocks for intractable pain at end of life: report of four cases and literature review. *American Journal of Hospice and Palliative Care*. 2003; **20**: 62–6.

28. Candido K, Stevens RA. Intrathecal neurolytic blocks for the relief of cancer pain. *Best Practice and Research. Clinical Anaesthesiology*. 2003; **17**: 407–28.

29. Racz GB, Heavner J, Haynsworth P. Repeat epidural phenol injections in chronic pain and spasticity. In: Lipton S (ed.). *Persistent pain: modern methods of treatment*. New York: Grune and Stratton, 1985.

30. Lloyd JW, Barnard JDW, Glynn CJ. Cryoanalgesia: a new approach to pain relief. *Lancet*. 1976; **2**: 932–4.

31. Glynn CJ, Lloyd JW, Barnard JD. Cryoanalgesia in the management of pain after thoracotomy. *Thorax*. 1980; **35**: 325–7.

32. Saberski LR. Cryoneurolysis in clinical practice. In: Waldman SD, Winnie AP (eds). *Interventional pain management*. Philadelphia, PA: WB Saunders, 1996.

33. Evans PJD. Cryoanalgesia. *Anaesthesia*. 1981; **36**: 1003–13.

34. Pradel W, Hlawitschka M, Eckelt U *et al*. Cryosurgical treatment of genuine trigeminal neuralgia. *British Journal of Oral and Maxillofacial Surgery*. 2002; **40**: 244–7.

35. Kline MT. Radiofrequency techniques in clinical practice. In: Waldman SD, Winnie AP (eds). *Interventional pain management*. Philadelphia, PA: WB Saunders, 1996.

36. Van Suijlekom JA, Weber WEJ, van Kleef M. Treatment of spinal pain by means of radiofrequency procedures – Part 2; Thoracic and cervical area. *Pain Reviews*. 1999; **6**: 175–91.

37. Gallagher J, Vadi PLP, Wedley JR *et al*. Radiofrequency facet joint denervation in the treatment of low back pain: a prospective controlled double-blind study to assess its efficacy. *Pain Clin*. 1994; **7**: 193–8.

38. Boswell MV, Shah RV, Everett CR *et al*. Interventional techniques in the management of chronic spinal pain: evidence-based practice guidelines. *Pain Physician*. 2005; **8**: 1–47.

* 39. Niemisto L, Kalso E, Malmivaara A *et al*. Radiofrequency denervation for neck and back pain. A systematic review of randomised controlled trials. *Cochrane Database of Systematic Reviews*. 2003; **CD004058**.

* 40. Slipman CW, Bhat AL, Gilchrist DO *et al*. A critical review of the evidence for the use of zygapophysical injections and radiofrequency denervation in the treatment of low back pain. *Spine Journal*. 2003; **3**: 310–16.

* 41. Manchikanti L, Staats PS, Singh V *et al*. Evidence-based practice guidelines for interventional techniques in the management of spinal pain. *Pain Physician*. 2003; **6**: 3–81.

18

Stimulation-induced analgesia

MARK I JOHNSON, STEPHEN G OXBERRY, AND KAREN ROBB

Introduction	235	Summary	246
TENS	236	Acknowledgments	246
SCS	243	References	246
DBS	246		

KEY LEARNING POINTS

- A variety of stimulation techniques are used to alter nervous system activity and may be beneficial for cancer pain or in dying patients.
- Transcutaneous electrical nerve stimulation (TENS) is a noninvasive, inexpensive, safe, and easy to use technique that has a potential role alongside pharmacological management for pain directly or indirectly related to cancer and its treatment.
- There is a lack of available evidence to determine the effectiveness of TENS for cancer pain and evidence

  remains equivocal for other types of pain because of difficulties in trial design.
- Electrical stimulating devices can be implanted into the spinal cord and brain and may prove useful for intractable pain in carefully selected patients who are not responding to other treatments.
- Electrical stimulating devices such as spinal cord stimulation (SCS) and deep brain stimulation (DBS) can be utilized in the management of cancer-related pain but they are expensive and there is currently a lack of evidence surrounding their use in this situation.

INTRODUCTION

Stimulation-induced (produced) analgesia is a term which describes stimulation of the body or the nervous system for pain relief.[1] Stimulation techniques used in physical medicine and rehabilitation and complementary medicine include heat, cold, laser, manipulation, mobilization, massage, traction, ultrasound, vibration, acupuncture, craniosacral therapy, osteopathy, and reflexology (see Chapter 21, Complementary therapies). A role for stimulation-induced analgesia in cancer pain or in dying patients has been recognized.[2] This chapter will focus on the use of electricity to alter nervous system activity for pain relief.

Cave drawings suggest that the Egyptians used electric fish to relieve pain in 2500BC.[3] Publication of the gate control theory of pain revitalized interest in electrical stimulation for pain relief, supported by findings that percutaneous electrical nerve stimulation relieved neuropathic pain[4] and SCS relieved chronic pain.[5] Electrical stimulation of the intact surface of the skin, termed transcutaneous electrical nerve stimulation (TENS), was initially used to predict response prior to implantation of spinal cord stimulators until it was realized that TENS was useful in its own right.[6, 7]

Nowadays, TENS and TENS-like devices are used throughout the world for pain relief.[8] More expensive technologies are used for patients with intractable pain who are resistant to treatment. These include spinal cord stimulation (SCS), deep brain stimulation (DBS), motor cortex stimulation (MCS), and transcranial magnetic stimulation (TMS). The effectiveness of electrical nerve stimulation for nonmalignant pain has been a matter of much debate although evidence tends to support their use. Evidence for the effectiveness for cancer pain remains equivocal.

TENS

TENS is indicated for symptomatic management of acute and chronic pain and may be useful for any type of pain experienced by a patient with cancer (**Table 18.1**).[9, 10, 11, 12, 13] TENS is safe and easy to use and effects are rapid in onset so benefit can be achieved immediately.[9, 10] Ideally, TENS should be prescribed by a healthcare practitioner following a comprehensive assessment to check that the patient does not require additional medical intervention. Patients trying TENS for the first time should be supervised by a practitioner experienced in TENS who can check that the patient is competent in its use. Most patients can administer TENS for themselves. During TENS, pulsed electrical currents are generated by a portable battery powered device which is connected via leads to hydrogel electrodes which are attached to the intact surface of the skin (**Figure 18.1**). Healthcare professionals use the term TENS to describe electrical currents delivered using a "standard" TENS device (**Table 18.2**).[8] TENS devices retail at £20–150 and variations in design between manufacturers are often minor. A variety of shapes, sizes, and colors of electrodes are readily available to suit all needs.

TENS devices enable the user to adjust pulse amplitude, pulse frequency (rate), pulse pattern, and pulse duration (width) of currents, although the search for optimal TENS settings has been futile (**Figure 18.2**, **Table 18.2**). The main determinant for success is to generate an electrical paraesthesia close to the site of pain by titrating TENS intensity (pulse amplitude).[14, 15] It is not possible to predict which patients will respond to TENS.[16] TENS may exacerbate pain, especially if mechanical allodynia is present.

At present, TENS appears to be used only on selected cancer pain patients.[17] A survey of 593 cancer patients treated by a pain service found that TENS was given to support systemic analgesia in only 1 percent of patients with nociceptive pain, 6 percent of patients with neuropathic pain, and 6 percent of patients with mixed nociceptive and neuropathic pain.[18] A ten-year prospective assessment of treatments used to manage cancer pain for 2118 patients by an anesthesiology-based palliative care program revealed that TENS was used in only 3 percent of patients.[19] Reasons may include drug medication adequately managing pain, a lack of knowledge about TENS, weak evidence for TENS effectiveness, and a fear of adverse effects.

Table 18.1 Some examples of painful conditions commonly treated with TENS.

Acute pain	Chronic pain	Cancer-related pain	Non-pain related effects
Postoperative pain	Neuropathic pain (e.g. postamputation, postherpetic, trigeminal neuralgia, poststroke pain)	Pain directly from cancer (e.g. metastatic carcinomas, metastatic bone disease and direct infiltration of nerves)	Reducing symptoms of Alzheimer's dementia
Labor pain	Muscle pain (e.g. myofascial pain/muscle tension/postexercise soreness)	Pain indirectly from cancer (e.g. nerve compression by a neoplasm or enlarged organs, nerve root compression in vertebral collapse)	Neuromuscular stimulating effects (e.g. fecal and urinary incontinence)
Dysmenorrhea	Nociceptive pain (e.g. inflammatory pains, chronic wound pain)	Pain from cancer treatment (e.g. neuropathy from chemotherapy, postsurgical pain, postamputation pain)	Antiemetic effects (e.g. pregnancy, travel sickness, chemotherapy, postoperative opioid medication)
Angina pectoris	Osteoarthritis and rheumatoid arthritis	Pain unrelated to cancer and its treatment	Improving blood flow (Raynaud's disease, wound healing, ischemia due to reconstructive surgery)
Orofacial pain	Low back pain		
Physical trauma (e.g. fractured ribs and minor medical procedures)	Complex regional pain syndrome		

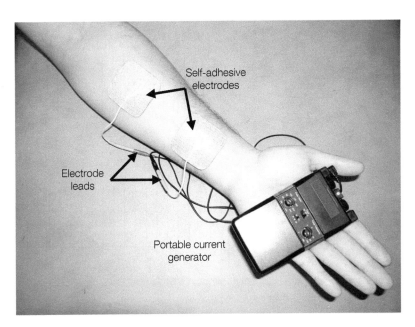

Figure 18.1 TENS.

Table 18.2 Features of a "standard" TENS device (adapted from Refs 8, 11).

Features of a typical TENS device	
Dimensions	$6 \times 5 \times 2$ cm (small device)
	$12 \times 9 \times 4$ cm (large device)
Weight	50–250 g
Cost	£30–150
Channel (electrodes)	1(2) or 2(4)
Batteries	Usually 9 volt or rechargeable
Pulse amplitude (adjustable)	1–50 mA into a 1 kΩ load usually constant current output
Pulse waveform (usually preset)	Monophasic
	Biphasic (symmetrical or asymmetrical)
Pulse duration (usually adjustable)	50–500 µs
Pulse frequency (usually adjustable)	1–200 pulses per second
Pulse pattern (selection of preset options)	Continuous (burst, random frequency, modulated amplitude, modulated frequency, modulated pulse duration)
Additional features	Timer

Concerns have been raised that electrical stimulation of skin overlying a tumor site may cause increased tumor growth through increased blood flow and/or cell proliferation.[20] Possible associations between electromagnetic fields and the risk of malignant diseases[21] and the use of low level direct current therapy to stimulate osteogenesis[22, 23] have fueled the concern. Interestingly, experimental evidence suggests that low level direct current

therapy and ultrasound reduce the cloning efficiency of malignant cells leading to their use as antitumor treatments.[24, 25] To our knowledge, there are no studies that have directly assessed the impact of TENS on tumor growth. Nevertheless, it is generally accepted that in an acute oncology setting electrodes should not be positioned over an active tumor for a patient whose tumor is treatable. In the palliative setting, where the disease is no longer curable, and where pain is a major problem, electrodes can be positioned on areas where there is known disease.

Rationale

The goal of TENS is to selectively activate different populations of peripheral nerves using different TENS techniques (Table 18.3).[9, 10, 11, 12, 26] Conventional TENS is the most common TENS technique used in practice and should be the first treatment option in most situations. The goal of conventional TENS is to activate large diameter non-noxious afferents (i.e. A-beta fibers) without activating small diameter noxious afferents (i.e. A-delta and C fibers) or muscle efferents (i.e. A-alpha, Figure 18.3). This approach inhibits ongoing transmission of nociceptive information in the spinal cord and reduces central sensitization with a rapid onset and offset of action.[27, 28, 29, 30] Conventional TENS is superior to sham TENS in healthy humans experiencing experimentally induced pain,[14, 15] but randomized controlled trials (RCTs) on pain patients are inconclusive due to shortcomings in study designs[31, 32] (see below under Clinical effectiveness).

Other TENS techniques include AL-TENS and intense TENS. AL-TENS is defined as low frequency (e.g. <10 pulses per second (pps)), high intensity stimulation, although many opinion leaders believe that the induction of strong but comfortable muscle contractions is a

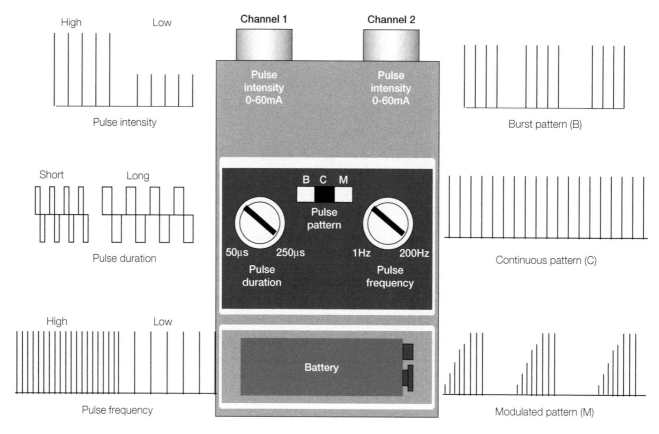

Figure 18.2   Schematic view of TENS controls.

prerequisite for success.[9, 10, 26, 33, 34] This effect is achieved using low frequency bursts of pulses (~2–5 bursts per second of 100 pps) delivered at nonpainful intensities over muscles or motor nerves.[26] The muscle contraction generates small diameter muscle afferent activity which triggers extrasegmental antinociceptive mechanisms and the release of endogenous opioid peptides in the central nervous system (CNS) (**Figure 18.4**).[33, 34, 35, 36] Up to one-third of patients may be resistant to conventional TENS and may benefit from AL-TENS.[26, 37] AL-TENS can be used when electrodes cannot be placed at the site of pain due to altered skin sensations (see Refs 26, 34 for review).

Intense TENS delivers currents that are just tolerable to the patient. Intense TENS activates large (A-beta) and small (A-delta) fibers which block the peripheral transmission of nociceptive information and activate segmental and extrasegmental antinociceptive mechanisms (**Figure 18.5**).[29, 38, 39] It is used to counter intense pains during procedures such as wound dressing and suture removal but can only be administered for short periods of time.[40, 41] The remainder of this chapter will focus on conventional TENS unless otherwise stated.

TENS effects are mediated by opioids at spinal cord and brainstem sites.[42] Antihyperalgesia produced by low frequency TENS may operate via mu opioid receptors[43] and $5-HT_2$ and $5-HT_3$ receptors[44] whereas delta opioid receptors[43] and gamma-aminobutyric acid (GABA) may be involved in high frequency TENS.[45, 46] High frequency,

but not low frequency, TENS reduces aspartate and glutamate release in the spinal cord dorsal horn[47] and low and high frequency TENS activate spinal muscarinic receptors[48] and peripheral alpha-2A adrenergic receptors.[49] Glutamate may have a role in long-term antinociception mediated by intense TENS.[29, 50]

Clinical effectiveness

Clinical experience suggests that TENS is effective for a wide variety of acute and chronic pain conditions of nociceptive and neuropathic origin, irrespective of the presence of a sympathetic component. There is a vast quantity of clinical trials on TENS but evidence from systematic reviews is conflicting and equivocal (for review see Ref. 11), due in the main to difficulties in trial design[51] and underdosing of TENS.[32]

To our knowledge, only one RCT has evaluated the effectiveness of TENS for cancer pain. Robb *et al.*[52] conducted a placebo-controlled evaluation of the effectiveness of TENS and transcutaneous spinal electroanalgesia (TSE) on 41 women with chronic pain associated with breast cancer treatment. TSE is a TENS-like device which uses surface electrodes over the spine and pulse frequencies far greater than a standard TENS device.[8, 53] TENS and TSE reduced pain when compared to baseline but the effect was no greater than that observed with placebo (sham TSE).

Table 18.3 Common TENS techniques (adapted from Refs 8, 11).

	Intention	Patient experience	Electrode location	TENS characteristics	Analgesic profile	Duration of treatment	Analgesic action
Conventional TENS	Selective activation of large diameter non-noxious afferents	Strong comfortable electrical paresthesia with minimal muscle activity	Dermatomal Site of pain	High frequency – 10–200 pulses per second Low amplitude – non-noxious intensity Pulse duration – 100–200 µs Pulse pattern – continuous	Rapid onset and offset within 30 minutes	Continuously when in pain	Segmental
AL-TENS	Indirect activation of small diameter motor afferents through muscle contraction (twitching)	Strong comfortable muscle contractions (twitches)	Myotomal over muscles or motor nerves and/or trigger points and/or acupuncture points	Low frequency bursts of pulses – 1–5 bursts of 100 pulses per second "High" amplitude – non-noxious intensity to generate muscle contractions Pulse duration – 100–200 µs Pulse pattern – burst	Rapid onset but delayed offset of over 1 hour	~30 minutes per session	Extrasegmental Segmental
Intense TENS	Activation of small diameter noxious afferents	Electrical paresthesia that is uncomfortable but tolerable with poststimulation hypoesthesia	Main nerve bundle from origin of pain	High frequency – 50–200 pulses per second High amplitude – noxious intensity Pulse duration > 500 µs Pulse pattern – continuous	Rapid onset and delayed offset over 1 hour	~15 minutes per session	Peripheral Extrasegmental Segmental

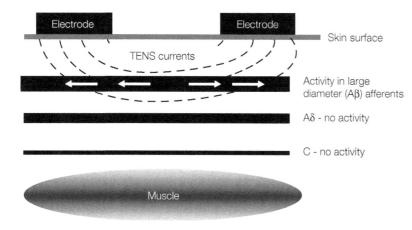

Figure 18.3 Conventional TENS. Current amplitude is titrated to cause selective activation of large diameter (Aβ) afferents. Arrows indicate direction of nerve impulses.

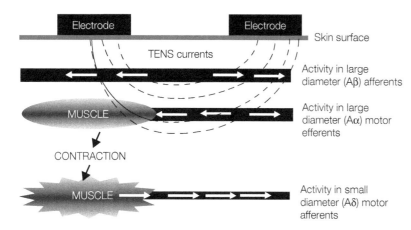

Figure 18.4 AL-TENS. Current amplitude is titrated to cause activation of large diameter (Aα) motor neurons. Trains (bursts) of electrical pulses are used and the resultant phasic muscle contraction produces activity in small diameter (Aδ) motor afferents. Arrows indicate direction of nerve impulses.

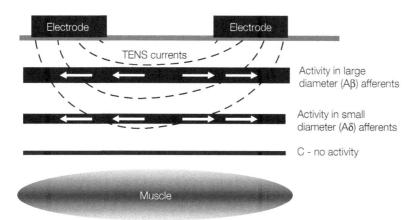

Figure 18.5 Intense-TENS. Current amplitude is titrated to cause activation of small diameter (Aδ) afferents. Arrows indicate direction of nerve impulses.

Most published research is anecdotal but suggests that TENS may provide immediate benefits for pain directly or indirectly due to cancer (**Table 18.4**).[6, 54, 55, 56, 57, 58, 59, 60, 61, 62, 63][III] This includes pains from metastatic carcinomas, metastatic bone disease, direct infiltration of nerves, nerve compression by a neoplasm or vertebral collapse, or enlarged organs. TENS may provide benefit for pain from chemotherapy, postsurgery (e.g. post-thorocotomy, post-mastectomy pain) and postamputation (e.g. phantom breast or limb pain). Responses appear to decline over time which may be due to worsening pain condition, habituation to TENS, or an initial placebo response to TENS. Cancer-related pains in extremities and trunk have been reported to respond better than perineum and pelvic pain.[61]

Avellanosa and West[54] evaluated TENS on 60 patients with a variety of intractable cancer pains from metastatic carcinomas, surgery, irradiation, and amputation. Excellent or fair pain relief was experienced by 39 patients at two weeks but this declined to 20 patients at three months. Patients reported awkwardness with using TENS

Table 18.4 TENS effectiveness for cancer-related pain: available evidence.

Reference	Type	Patients (n)	TENS treatment (n)	Results for pain	Comment
Robb et al.[52]	Double blind, randomized sham controlled crossover trial on TENS versus TSE versus sham TSE n = 41	Breast cancer with chronic pain of at least 6 months duration and secondary to treatment for breast cancer	TENS: strong but comfortable paresthesia over site of pain TSE: Full intensity, without a noticeable sensation, either paravertebrally at C3–C4 for pains in arm head and neck, or on the spinous processes of T1 and T10 for pains below the neck	Reductions in pain for all groups when compared to baseline. No significant differences between any groups for pain measures although more patients continued to use TENS on completion of the trial (15) when compared to TSE (5) and sham TSE (6)	Patients encountered difficulties with reporting pain relief with inconsistencies between pain diary pain relief scores and the Brief Pain Inventory
Avellanosa and West[54]	Pre-post TENS evaluation n = 60	Intractable cancer pain metastatic carcinoma (24), lumbosacral plexitis (8), brachial plexitis (6), postherpetic neuralgia (7), postsurgical pain (4), chemo-drug infiltration (4), tumor infiltration (2) others (5)	Away from pain followed by nerve trunk close to pain followed by over painful site. Tolerance of the patient-strong non-noxious TENS paresthesia	2 weeks of TENS 17/60 excellent relief 22/60 fair relief 21/60 no relief 3 months of TENS 9/60 excellent relief 11/60 fair relief 40/60 no relief	TENS effect rapidly declined after 2 weeks of treatment and depended on location and source of pain with extremity/trunk > perineal/pelvic pain
Ostrowski[55]	Pre-post TENS evaluation n = 9	Advanced carcinomas of breast (3), uterine body, mouth, prostate, bronchus, sarcoma of radius and Hodgkin disease-metastases in spine (7), pulmonary (1), jaw (1)	Strong non-noxious TENS paresthesia at trigger zones, peripheral nerves and/or acupuncture points	Immediate effect of TENS 7/9 good relief 1/9 partial relief 1/9 no relief 3/9 used TENS for more than 6 months	8/9 used TENS until condition worsened or patient died. Effect of TENS declined as condition worsened
Long[6]	Pre-post TENS evaluation n = 5	Chronic pain mixed population (197) including 5 malignancies	Strong non-noxious TENS paresthesia at site of pain	3/5 good relief 2/5 no relief	
Hardy[56]	Pre-post TENS evaluation n = 4	Chronic pain mixed population (53) including 4 malignancies	Strong non-noxious TENS paresthesia at site of pain	2/4 good relief 2/4 no relief	

(Continued over)

Table 18.4 TENS effectiveness for cancer-related pain: available evidence (continued).

Reference	Type	Patients (n)	TENS treatment (n)	Results for pain	Comment
Loeser et al.[57]	Pre–post TENS evaluation n = 7	Mixed population pain patients (198) including 7 malignancies	Strong non-noxious TENS paresthesia at site of pain	3/7 partial relief 4/7 no relief	TENS reduced analgesic intake
Ventafridda et al.[58]	Pre–post TENS evaluation n = 37	Cancer pain or pain in which cancer was the primary cause	Strong non-noxious TENS paresthesia	1–10 days 36/37 good relief 28/37 improved activity 30 days 4/37 good relief 7/37 improved activity	Authors concluded long-term effects poor but worthy of a trial for head pain, neck pain, phantom limb pain and postherpetic neuralgia
Bates and Nathan[59]	Pre–post TENS evaluation over 7 year period n = 5	Mixed population treatment-resistant pain patients (161) including 5 with cancer	Strong non-noxious TENS paresthesia at site of pain	Overall 4/5 good relief 1/5 = no relief	In this mixed pain population there was no relationship between TENS outcome and disease or pain and 50% of patients returned TENS at 1 month and 25% still using TENS at 2 years
Rafter[60] cited in Librach[61]	Pre–post TENS evaluation n = 49	Variety of malignancies including myeloma and bony metastases, head and neck cancer, and pain of musculoskeletal origin	High frequency TENS 80–200 pulses per second. Location and intensity not stated	Overall 36/49 good sustained relief 1/49 good temporary relief 4/49 no relief	Average duration of TENS treatment = 5.2 month (range 1–23 months). Myeloma and bony metastases responded better than head and neck cancer – due to difficulty of electrode location
Dil'din et al.[62] Abstract only	Pre–post TENS evaluation n = 84	Tumor-induced pain (84) including advanced tumor pain (11), intraoperative anesthesia (29), postoperative pain (54)	Soviet-made transcutaneous electrostimulation device– unknown whether this was a typical TENS device	Overall 55/84 good 29/84 partial	
Grond et al.[63]	Survey	593 cancer patients treated by a pain service		TENS given as adjunct to drug medication in 1% patients with nociceptive pain and 6% neuropathic pain and 6% mixed	Analgesic treatment resulted in a significant pain relief in all groups of patients

and difficulty in achieving paresthesia over large areas of pain (e.g. cutaneous carcinomas, postradiotherapy skin, and subcutaneous fibrosis). The authors concluded that TENS may be an effective part of the overall pain control programme.

Ventafridda et al.[58] reported that TENS reduced pain in 35 of 37 patients with cancer-related pain within the first ten days of treatment. This effect rapidly declined to four patients by 30 days, although drug intake was reduced in 20 patients at this follow up. The authors concluded that short-term effects of TENS may be useful for pain arising from compression by large masses over the cervical nerve trunks or neoplastic involvement on maxillofacial tissues. Ostrowski[55] reported that TENS outcome was good in seven of nine patients with various carcinomas and metastases in the spine, lung, and jaw. TENS effect declined over time although reductions in drug intake were observed. A congress presentation by Rafter[60] cited in Librach[61] described benefit from TENS in 36 of 49 patients with a variety of malignancies. Myeloma and bony metastases responded better than head and neck cancer, although this appeared to be due to difficulties in applying electrodes to the scalp. The effect of TENS on small numbers of patients within larger case series provides similar findings (**Table 18.4**).[6, 56, 57, 59, 63] No serious complications from TENS were reported in any of these published trials.

It is claimed that TENS can reduce chemotherapy-induced nausea when applied to the P6 acupuncture point.[64, 65, 66] However, a Cochrane review concluded that noninvasive electrostimulation (TENS) was unlikely to have a clinically meaningful outcome for chemotherapy-induced nausea and vomiting although electro-acupuncture and self-administered acupressure appeared to be of benefit.[67] TENS has also been reported to be successful for the management of lymphedema.[68]

Clinical technique

Any patient with cancer who is in pain may respond to TENS. Outcomes will depend on appropriate technique. Activation of large diameter afferents is recognized by a "strong but comfortable" paresthesia beneath the electrodes and patients titrate pulse amplitude to achieve this effect. Hypothetically, high frequency pulses (~10–200 pps) with pulse durations between 50 and 500 µs are optimal for differential recruitment of large diameter afferents[69] although in practice patients are encouraged to experiment with settings according to what is comfortable for them at that moment in time.[16, 70] TENS effects are maximal when TENS paresthesia is present, so patients may need to use TENS throughout the day. TENS users have been shown to stimulate for over eight hours per day although this is punctuated by periods where TENS is switched off.[16] Individual treatments often last no more than 40 minutes at a time.

Electrodes must be positioned on healthy innervated skin where sensation is intact, so skin sensation should be checked prior to using TENS. For most pains, TENS electrodes are placed on healthy skin around the painful site so that paresthesia can be directed into the painful area (**Figure 18.6**). Exceptions include:

- pain directly over an active tumor in the acute oncology setting;
- skin that is allodynic, hypolgesic, hypoesthesic, or dysesthesic;
- a pain made worse by TENS;
- skin that is frail or damaged, such as irradiated skin in the immediate four to six weeks after radiotherapy.

In these situations electrodes are positioned along the main nerves proximal to the site of pain, on a contralateral dermatome or paravertebrally at the appropriate spinal segment. Four electrodes (dual channel TENS) should be used for large areas of pain. Examples include patients with postmastectomy pain and associated shoulder pain and stiffness or patients with widespread metastatic disease in the spine and mixed nociceptive/neuropathic pain at different spinal levels. Patients can leave electrodes in situ and deliver TENS intermittently throughout the day. Skin underneath the electrodes should be monitored regularly to prevent skin irritation.

Contraindications and precautions to TENS are few (**Table 18.5**). Manufacturers list cardiac pacemakers, pregnancy, and epilepsy as absolute contraindications because it may be difficult to exclude TENS as a potential cause of a problem in a medicolegal case. TENS could be used in these patients providing it is not applied locally and the patient's progress is carefully monitored. TENS can be used at bedtime providing the device has a timer so that it automatically switches off. TENS can be used on children providing they understand what to expect.

SCS

SCS was first used in the 1960s using radiofrequency stimulation of plate electrodes placed directly over the dorsal columns.[5] Nowadays electrodes are implanted in the epidural space and powered by a small pulse generator which is usually implanted (similar to a cardiac pacemaker).[71] SCS appears to be more effective for ischemic pain and neuropathic pain than nociceptive pain (**Table 18.6**).[72, 73] At present, SCS is seldom used for cancer-related pain.

Rationale

The goal of SCS is to generate electrical paresthesia over a region of pain. Originally, it was thought that SCS

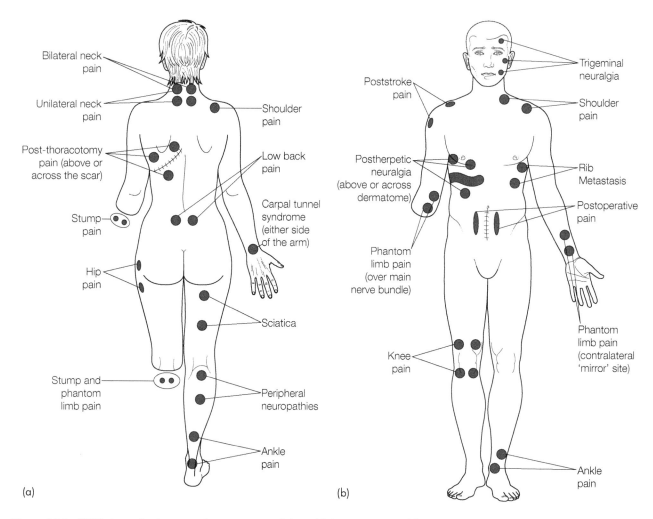

Figure 18.6 TENS electrode placement for common conditions. (a) Anterior aspect. (b) Posterior aspect. Adapted from Refs 11, 12.

inhibited ongoing transmission of nociceptive information at the first synapse in the posterior horn by stimulating A-beta fibers in the spinal cord. The mechanism is more complex and involves spinal and supraspinal structures, including descending pain inhibitory pathways, the autonomic nervous system, and visceral pathways in the posterior columns.[74]

Clinical effectiveness

Systematic reviews conclude that SCS confers significant benefit over comparative therapy for refractory neuropathic back and leg pain from failed back surgery syndrome (FBSS),[75, 76] for chronic low back pain,[77] complex regional pain syndrome (CRPS) (type 1),[75, 76, 78, 79, 80] and chronic critical limb ischemia.[81, 82][I] Good quality RCTs suggest that SCS is effective for refractory angina pectoris[83, 84, 85, 86] and diabetic neuropathy.[87] Careful patient selection is critical for success and careful consideration should be given to risk–benefit, especially where patients have advanced malignancy. Decision-analytic models find that two-year cost-effectiveness for patients with FBSS

ranged from 30,370 to 63,511 euros.[88, 89] Over the lifetime of patients with FBSS, SCS was more effective and less costly than conventional medical management and potentially cost-effective in the short term. For this reason, SCS should not be discounted as a possible treatment option for patients with cancer.

There is a lack of evidence to judge the effectiveness of SCS in cancer pain, with no known RCTs. SCS outcome has been variable in published case studies for cancer pain. Meglio *et al.*[90] found no clinical usefulness in 11 patients with cancer pain whereas Shimoji *et al.*[91] reported over 50 percent pain reduction in patients with carcinoma/sarcoma. Eisenberg and Brecker[92] reported success in one patient with lower extremity neuropathic pain due to removal of a C1 meningioma.

Clinical technique

"Wire" or "catheter" electrodes are often used and inserted percutaneously into the posterior epidural space under local anesthetic so that patients can report the exact location of paresthesia. These systems may dislodge and

Table 18.5   Contraindications and precautions.

Contraindication/Precaution	Advice
Contraindication	
Cardiac pacemakers	Seek approval from cardiologist – monitor progress frequently
Pregnancy	Seek approval from obstetrician and midwife – do not apply over abdomen/pelvic region
Epilepsy	Seek approval from neurologist – do not apply on neck or head
Cardiovascular conditions	Seek approval from cardiologist – and monitor progress frequently. TENS is frequently used for angina
Nonadherent patients	Assess patient's competency
Precaution	
Active malignancy	Electrodes should not be positioned over an active tumor for a patient whose tumor is treatable. Position electrodes along the main nerves proximal to the tumor/site of pain or on a contralateral dermatome or paraverterbrally at the appropriate spinal segment. Monitor progress frequently
Dermatological conditions/frail skin (e.g. irradiated skin within 6 weeks of radiotherapy)	Apply electrodes to healthy skin at appropriate dermatomes. Consider AL-TENS
Inappropriate electrode sites	Do not apply on anterior neck, around the eyes, over testes, through the chest (i.e. anterior and posterior electrode positions) or over damaged skin or open wounds
Presence of dysethesia/hypoesthesia/allodynia/ hyperalgesia	Test skin sensation prior and apply TENS to skin with normal sensation. Position electrodes along main nerves proximal to pain or on a contralateral dermatome or paraverterbrally at the appropriate spinal segment. Ensure TENS does not exacerbate the pain
Contact dermatitis	Change type of electrodes (e.g. use hypoalergenic electrodes)
Autonomic reactions to TENS	Supervise first TENS treatment
Operating hazardous equipment	Advise not to use TENS when driving or when using hazardous equipment

Table 18.6   Indications for spinal cord stimulation (adapted from Refs 72, 73).

Likely to respond	May respond	Unlikely to respond
Neuropathic pain	Neuropathic pain	Central pain
Limb pain following lumbar or cervical spine surgery (FBSS/FNSS)	Stump pain	Spinal cord injury
Secondary to peripheral nerve damage	Axial pain following spinal surgery	Perineal anorectal pain
Postirradiation brachial plexopathy	Postherpetic neuralgias	Complete cord transaction
Peripheral vascular disease	Spinal cord damage	Nonischemic nociceptive pain
Angina	Peripheral neuropathic pain syndromes	Nerve root avulsion

FBSS, failed back surgery syndrome; FNSS, failed neck surgery syndrome.

are less electrically efficient. Alternatively, plate or surgical electrodes can be used which are more secure and potentially more effective but require laminectomy or partial laminectomy. SCS may exacerbate the patient's pain so some practitioners undertake a trial stimulation with an external pulse generator prior to implantation. Reports that the trial period has a predictive value for SCS success have been challenged when long-term data are assessed. Patients can adjust pulse frequency, pulse duration, and pulse amplitude and can alter the polarity and montage of electrodes.[71, 72, 73]

Contraindications are similar to those for TENS and include demand-type cardiac pacemakers and implanted cardiac defibrillators, diathermy, uncontrolled bleeding disorders, ongoing anticoagulant therapy, sepsis, and noncompliant patients. Some magnetic resonance imaging (MRI) scanners interfere with SCS function so individual SCS–MRI compatibility must be established with an experienced neuroradiologist. SCS may activate security systems (e.g. at airports). Patients should not drive with the stimulator switched on as, from a legal perspective, it may be difficult to exclude SCS as a contributing factor in a motor accident. Major complications are rare. Neurological damage may occur for percutaneous and plate electrodes as a result of electrode migration or breakage. Infection can be a potentially serious problem and electrode infection mandates the removal of the system.

DBS

Electrical stimulation of the gray matter deep brain structures, termed DBS, has been used for decades. In 1954, Heath[93] described alleviation of cancer pain in one patient by stimulating the septal area which was replicated on several cancer patients.[94] Nowadays, periventricular and periaqueductal gray matter (PVG/PAG) are stimulated for nociceptive pain, and sensory thalamus (ventroposterior lateral (VPL) and ventroposterior medial (VPM) nuclei) and internal capsule for neuropathic pain. Success rates vary and depend on the appropriate selection of patients.[95, 96]

Rationale

In 1969, Reynolds observed that stimulation of the PVG of rats produced antinociception during surgery[97] and the finding was replicated in chronic pain patients in 1977.[98, 99] The PVG/PAG lie on descending pain inhibitory pathways and elevations in endogenous opioids and naloxone reversibility have been demonstrated.[100] Pathways ascending from the PVG/PAG may also be involved, including the internal capsule system in a similar manner to SCS.[101]

Clinical effectiveness

A meta-analysis of six studies on nonmalignant pain found that DBS provided better long-term success for nociceptive pains than neuropathic pain.[102] Over 80 percent of patients with intractable low back pain (FBSS) achieved long-term success, with best results when PVG/PAG or the PVG/PAG plus sensory thalamus/internal capsule were stimulated. These results are impressive and suggest that DBS is of benefit in well-selected patients. To our knowledge, no RCTs exist on DBS for cancer pain.

Observations of 17 patients with treatment-resistant pain due to progressive malignancies concluded that DBS was safe and effective with 13 patients reporting total pain relief and only four of 17 patients requiring analgesics at hospital discharge.[103] Kumar and colleagues[104, 105] evaluated a small number of cancer patients within a larger population of pain patients and found that they only responded to DBS in the short term.

Clinical technique

DBS electrodes are implanted stereotactically via a burr hole under local anesthesia and localization achieved with MRI. Electrodes are externalized during trial stimulation and a stimulator implanted if the trial is successful. Electrode insertion has the potential for hemorrhage, infection, or seizures and such complication rates are unknown although often reported to be few.[103] Serious morbidity or mortality is always a possibility.

Recent techniques and developments

Motor cortex stimulation has been used for over a decade[106] and may have a role for intractable neuropathic pain[107] and for patients who no longer respond to DBS.[108] Intraoperative neuronavigation and cortical mapping is used for site targeting on the contralateral primary motor cortex. There are reports of superiority over SCS and DBS and success may depend on the type of pain.[109] Transcranial magnetic stimulation allows noninvasive stimulation of discrete brain cortical areas and it is claimed that it can induce plastic changes in the cortex at the site of stimulation and at connected sites, including the spinal cord.[110] Lefaucheur et al.[111] reported that TMS over the motor cortex produced greater reductions in pain than sham TMS in 18 patients with intractable neurogenic pain. TMS may be useful to select patients for the surgical implantation of a cortical stimulator or as a analgesic treatment on its own in the future.

SUMMARY

TENS is an inexpensive, safe, and easy to use technique with the potential to relieve cancer pain and/or allow dose reduction of drugs. When used in cancer pain management, it is important that disease status and treatment is regularly reviewed by the pain therapist and the cancer care team. More expensive stimulation techniques such as SCS and DBS may have a role for very carefully selected cancer patients who are resistant to other forms of treatment.

ACKNOWLEDGMENTS

This chapter is adapted and expanded from Stannard C. Stimulation-induced analgesia in cancer pain management. In: Sykes N, Fallon MT and Patt RB (eds). *Clinical Pain Management: Cancer Pain*, 1st edn. London: Hodder Arnold, 245–252. The authors wish to thank Dr Karen Simpson for her advice during manuscript preparation.

REFERENCES

1. Charlton J. Stimulation-produced analgesia. In: Charlton J (ed.). *Task force on professional education*. Seattle: IASP Press, 2005: 93–6.

2. Pan CX, Morrison RS, Ness J et al. Complementary and alternative medicine in the management of pain, dyspnea, and nausea and vomiting near the end of life. A systematic review. *Journal of Pain and Symptom Management*. 2000; **20**: 374–87.

3. Gildenberg PL. History of electrical neuromodulation for chronic pain. *Pain Medicine*. 2006; **7** (Suppl 1): S7–S13.

4. Wall PD, Sweet WH. Temporary abolition of pain in man. *Science*. 1967; **155**: 108–09.

5. Shealy CN, Mortimer JT, Reswick JB. Electrical inhibition of pain by stimulation of the dorsal columns: preliminary clinical report. *Anesthesia and Analgesia*. 1967; **46**: 489–91.

6. Long DM. External electrical stimulation as a treatment of chronic pain. *Minnesota Medicine*. 1974; **57**: 195–8.

7. Shealy CN. Transcutaneous electrical stimulation for control of pain. *Clinical Neurosurgery*. 1974; **21**: 269–77.

8. Johnson M. Transcutaneous electrical nerve stimulation (TENS) and TENS-like devices. Do they provide pain relief? *Pain Reviews*. 2003; **8**: 121–8.

9. Walsh D. *TENS. Clinical applications and related theory*, 1st edn. New York: Churchill Livingstone, 1997.

10. Barlas P, Lundeberg T. Transcutaneous electrical nerve stimulation and acupuncture. In: McMahon S, Koltzenburg M (eds). *Melzack and Wall's textbook of pain*. Philadelphia: Elsevier Churchill Livingstone, 2006: 583–90.

* 11. Johnson MI. Transcutaneous electrical nerve stimulation. In: Watson T (ed.). *Electrotherapy: evidence-based practice*. Edinburgh: Churchill Livingstone, 2008.

* 12. Thompson J, Filshie J. Transcutaneous electrical nerve stimulation (TENS) and acupuncture. In: Doyle D, Hanks G, MacDonald N (eds). *Oxford textbook of palliative medicine*, 2nd edn. Oxford: Oxford University Press, 1998: 421–37.

13. Berkovitch M, Waller A. Treating pain with transcutaneous electrical nerve stimulation (TENS). In: Doyle D, Hanks G, Cherny NI, Calman K (eds). *Oxford textbook of palliative medicine*. Oxford: Oxford University Press, 2005: 405–10.

14. Chesterton LS, Foster NE, Wright CC et al. Effects of TENS frequency, intensity and stimulation site parameter manipulation on pressure pain thresholds in healthy human subjects. *Pain*. 2003; **106**: 73–80.

15. Johnson MI, Tabasam G. An investigation into the analgesic effects of interferential currents and transcutaneous electrical nerve stimulation on experimentally induced ischemic pain in otherwise pain-free volunteers. *Physical Therapy*. 2003; **83**: 208–23.

16. Johnson MI, Ashton CH, Thompson JW. An in-depth study of long-term users of transcutaneous electrical nerve stimulation (TENS). Implications for clinical use of TENS. *Pain*. 1991; **44**: 221–9.

17. Hoskin PJ, Hanks GW. The management of symptoms in advanced cancer: experience in a hospital-based continuing care unit. *Journal of the Royal Society of Medicine*. 1988; **81**: 341–4.

18. Grond S, Radbruch L, Meuser T et al. Assessment and treatment of neuropathic cancer pain following WHO guidelines. *Pain*. 1999; **79**: 15–20.

19. Zech DF, Grond S, Lynch J et al. Validation of World Health Organization Guidelines for cancer pain relief: a 10-year prospective study. *Pain*. 1995; **63**: 65–76.

20. Sicard-Rosenbaum L, Danoff JV, Guthrie JA, Eckhaus MA. Effects of energy-matched pulsed and continuous ultrasound on tumor growth in mice. *Physical Therapy*. 1998; **78**: 271–7.

21. Hardell L, Holmberg B, Malker H, Paulsson LE. Exposure to extremely low frequency electromagnetic fields and the risk of malignant diseases – an evaluation of epidemiological and experimental findings. *European Journal of Cancer Prevention*. 1995; **4**: 3–107.

22. Goh JC, Bose K, Kang YK, Nugroho B. Effects of electrical stimulation on the biomechanical properties of fracture healing in rabbits. *Clinical Orthopaedics and Related Research*. 1988; **233**: 268–73.

23. Wang Q, Zhong S, Ouyang J et al. Osteogenesis of electrically stimulated bone cells mediated in part by calcium ions. *Clinical Orthopaedics and Related Research*. 1998; **348**: 259–68.

24. Lejbkowicz F, Salzberg S. Distinct sensitivity of normal and malignant cells to ultrasound in vitro. *Environmental Health Perspectives*. 1997; **105**: 1575–8.

25. Griffin DT, Dodd NJ, Zhao S et al. Low-level direct electrical current therapy for hepatic metastases. I. Preclinical studies on normal liver. *British Journal of Cancer*. 1995; **72**: 31–4.

26. Sjölund B, Eriksson M, Loeser J. Transcutaneous and implanted electric stimulation of peripheral nerves. In: Bonica J (ed.). *The management of pain*. Philadelphia: Lea and Febiger, 1990: 1852–61.

27. Garrison DW, Foreman RD. Decreased activity of spontaneous and noxiously evoked dorsal horn cells during transcutaneous electrical nerve stimulation (TENS). *Pain*. 1994; **58**: 309–15.

* 28. Sluka KA, Walsh D. Transcutaneous electrical nerve stimulation: basic science mechanisms and clinical effectiveness. *Journal of Pain*. 2003; **4**: 109–21.

29. Sandkühler J, Chen JG, Cheng G, Randic M. Low-frequency stimulation of afferent Adelta-fibers induces long-term depression at primary afferent synapses with substantia gelatinosa neurons in the rat. *Journal of Neuroscience*. 1997; **17**: 6483–91.

30. Ma YT, Sluka KA. Reduction in inflammation-induced sensitization of dorsal horn neurons by transcutaneous electrical nerve stimulation in anesthetized rats. *Experimental Brain Research*. 2001; **137**: 94–102.

31. Carroll D, Moore RA, McQuay HJ et al. Transcutaneous electrical nerve stimulation (TENS) for chronic pain. *Cochrane Database of Systematic Reviews (Online : Update Software)*. 2003; **CD003222**.

* 32. Bjordal JM, Johnson MI, Ljunggreen AE. Transcutaneous electrical nerve stimulation (TENS) can reduce postoperative analgesic consumption. A meta-analysis with assessment of optimal treatment parameters for postoperative pain. *European Journal of Pain*. 2003; **7**: 181–8.

33. Sjölund B, Eriksson M. Electro-acupunture and endogenous morphines. *Lancet.* 1976; **2**: 1085.

* 34. Johnson M. The analgesic effects and clinical use of acupuncture-like TENS (AL-TENS). *Physical Therapy Reviews.* 1998; **3**: 73–93.

35. Sjölund B. Peripheral nerve stimulation suppression of C-fiber-evoked flexion reflex in rats. Part 2: Parameters of low-rate train stimulation of skin and muscle afferent nerves. *Journal of Neurosurgery.* 1988; **68**: 279–83.

36. Sjölund B, Terenius L, Eriksson M. Increased cerebrospinal fluid levels of endorphins after electro-acupuncture. *Acta Physiologica Scandinavica.* 1977; **100**: 382–4.

37. Eriksson MB, Sjölund BH, Nielzen S. Long term results of peripheral conditioning stimulation as an analgesic measure in chronic pain. *Pain.* 1979; **6**: 335–47.

38. Ignelzi RJ, Nyquist JK. Excitability changes in peripheral nerve fibers after repetitive electrical stimulation. Implications in pain modulation. *Journal of Neurosurgery.* 1979; **51**: 824–33.

39. Chung JM. Antinociceptive effects of peripheral nerve stimulation. *Progress in Clinical and Biological Research.* 1985; **176**: 147–61.

40. Jeans M. Relief of chronic pain by brief, intense transcutaneous electrical stimulation-a double blind study. In: Bonica J, Liebeskind J, Albe-Fessard D (eds). *Advances in pain research and therapy.* New York: Raven Press, 1979: 601–06.

41. Melzack R, Vetere P, Finch L. Transcutaneous electrical nerve stimulation for low back pain. A comparison of TENS and massage for pain and range of motion. *Physical Therapy.* 1983; **63**: 489–93.

42. Ainsworth L, Budelier K, Clinesmith M *et al.* Transcutaneous electrical nerve stimulation (TENS) reduces chronic hyperalgesia induced by muscle inflammation. *Pain.* 2006; **120**: 182–7.

43. Kalra A, Urban MO, Sluka KA. Blockade of opioid receptors in rostral ventral medulla prevents antihyperalgesia produced by transcutaneous electrical nerve stimulation (TENS). *Journal of Pharmacology and Experimental Therapeutics.* 2001; **298**: 257–63.

44. Radhakrishnan R, King EW, Dickman JK *et al.* Spinal 5-HT(2) and 5-HT(3) receptors mediate low, but not high, frequency TENS-induced antihyperalgesia in rats. *Pain.* 2003; **105**: 205–13.

45. Duggan AW, Foong FW. Bicuculline and spinal inhibition produced by dorsal column stimulation in the cat. *Pain.* 1985; **22**: 249–59.

46. Sluka KA, Deacon M, Stibal A *et al.* Spinal blockade of opioid receptors prevents the analgesia produced by TENS in arthritic rats. *Journal of Pharmacology and Experimental Therapeutics.* 1999; **289**: 840–6.

47. Sluka KA, Vance CG, Lisi TL. High-frequency, but not low-frequency, transcutaneous electrical nerve stimulation reduces aspartate and glutamate release in the spinal cord dorsal horn. *Journal of Neurochemistry.* 2005; **95**: 1794–801.

48. Radhakrishnan R, Sluka KA. Spinal muscarinic receptors are activated during low or high frequency TENS-induced antihyperalgesia in rats. *Neuropharmacology.* 2003; **45**: 1111–19.

49. King EW, Audette K, Athman GA *et al.* Transcutaneous electrical nerve stimulation activates peripherally located alpha-2A adrenergic receptors. *Pain.* 2005; **115**: 364–73.

50. Sandkühler J. Long-lasting analgesia following TENS and acupuncture: Spinal mechanisms beyond gate control. In: Devor M, Rowbotham MC, Wiesenfeld-Hallin Z (eds). *9th World Congress on Pain: Progress in Pain Research and Management*, Vol. 16. Austria: IASP Press, 2000: 359–69.

51. Bjordal J, Greve G. What may alter the conclusions of systematic reviews? *Physical Therapy Reviews.* 1998; **3**: 121–32.

52. Robb KA, Newham DJ, Williams JE. Transcutaneous electrical nerve stimulation versus transcutaneous spinal electroanalgesia for chronic pain associated with breast cancer. *Journal of Pain and Symptom Management.* 2007; **33**: 410–19.

53. Macdonald ARJ, Coates TW. The discovery of trancutaneous spinal electroanalgesia and its relief of chronic pain. *Physiotherapy.* 1995; **81**: 653–60.

54. Avellanosa AM, West CR. Experience with transcutaneous electrical nerve stimulation for relief of intractable pain in cancer patients. *Journal of Medicine.* 1982; **13**: 203–13.

55. Ostrowski MJ. Pain control in advanced malignant disease using transcutaneous nerve stimulation. *British Journal of Clinical Practice.* 1979; **33**: 157–62.

56. Hardy RW. Current techniques in the management of pain. *Cleveland Clinic Quarterly.* 1974; **41**: 177–83.

57. Loeser J, Black R, Christman A. Relief of pain by transcutaneous electrical nerve stimulation. *Journal of Neurosurgery.* 1975; **42**: 308–14.

58. Ventafridda V, Saganzerla EP, Fochi C *et al.* Transcutaneous nerve stimulation in cancer pain. In: Bonica J, Ventafridda V (eds). *Advances in pain research and therapy.* New York: Raven Press, 1979: 509–15.

59. Bates JA, Nathan PW. Transcutaneous electrical nerve stimulation for chronic pain. *Anaesthesia.* 1980; **35**: 817–22.

60. Rafter J. TENS and cancer pain. In: Canada AFO (ed.) *Congress on Acupuncture Techniques*, Toronto, Canada, 1986.

61. Librach S. The use of transcutaneous electrical nerve stimulation (TENS) for the relief of pain in palliative care. *Palliative Medicine.* 1988; **2**: 15–20.

62. Dil'din AS, Tikhonova GP, Kozlov SV. [Transcutaneous electrostimulation – method leading to a permeation system of electroanalgesia in oncological practice]. *Voprosy Onkologii.* 1985; **31**: 33–6.

63. Grond S, Radbruch L, Meuser T *et al.* Assessment and treatment of neuropathic cancer pain following WHO guidelines. *Pain.* 1999; **79**: 15–20.

64. Dundee JW, Yang J, McMillan C. Non-invasive stimulation of the P6 (Neiguan) antiemetic acupuncture point in

cancer chemotherapy. *Journal of the Royal Society of Medicine.* 1991; **84**: 210–12.

65. McMillan C, Dundee JW, Abram WP. Enhancement of the antiemetic action of ondansetron by transcutaneous electrical stimulation of the P6 antiemetic point, in patients having highly emetic cytotoxic drugs. *British Journal of Cancer.* 1991; **64**: 971–2.

66. Pearl ML, Fischer M, McCauley DL *et al.* Transcutaneous electrical nerve stimulation as an adjunct for controlling chemotherapy-induced nausea and vomiting in gynecologic oncology patients. *Cancer Nursing.* 1999; **22**: 307–11.

67. Ezzo J, Streitberger K, Schneider A. Cochrane systematic reviews examine P6 acupuncture-point stimulation for nausea and vomiting. *Journal of Alternative and Complementary Medicine.* 2006; **12**: 489–95.

68. Waller A, Bercovitch M. Treatment of lymphoedema with TENS. In: Twycross R, Jenns K, Todd J (eds). *Lymphoedema.* Oxford: Radcliffe Medical Press, 2000: 27–184.

69. Howson DC. Peripheral neural excitability. Implications for transcutaneous electrical nerve stimulation. *Physical Therapy.* 1978; **58**: 1467–73.

70. Johnson MI, Ashton CH, Thompson JW. The consistency of pulse frequencies and pulse patterns of transcutaneous electrical nerve stimulation (TENS) used by chronic pain patients. *Pain.* 1991; **44**: 231–4.

71. Bradley K. The technology: the anatomy of a spinal cord and nerve root stimulator: the lead and the power source. *Pain Medicine.* 2006; **7**: S27–34.

∗ 72. Simpson K, Stannard C (eds). *Spinal cord stimulation for the management of pain: recommendations for best clinical practice.* London: British Pain Society, 2005.

73. Simpson B. Spinal cord stimulation. In: Bennett M (ed.). *Neuropathic pain.* Oxford: Oxford University Press, 2006: 125–33.

74. Linderoth B, Foreman RD. Mechanisms of spinal cord stimulation in painful syndromes: role of animal models. *Pain Medicine.* 2006; **7**: S14–26.

75. Taylor RS, Van Buyten JP, Buchser E. Spinal cord stimulation for chronic back and leg pain and failed back surgery syndrome: a systematic review and analysis of prognostic factors. *Spine.* 2005; **30**: 152–60.

76. Turner JA, Loeser JD, Deyo RA, Sanders SB. Spinal cord stimulation for patients with failed back surgery syndrome or complex regional pain syndrome: a systematic review of effectiveness and complications. *Pain.* 2004; **108**: 137–47.

77. Turner JA, Loeser JD, Bell KG. Spinal cord stimulation for chronic low back pain: a systematic literature synthesis. *Neurosurgery.* 1995; **37**: 1088–95; discussion 95–6.

78. Mailis-Gagnon A, Furlan AD, Sandoval JA, Taylor R. Spinal cord stimulation for chronic pain. *Cochrane Database of Systematic Reviews.* 2004; **CD003783**.

79. Grabow TS, Tella PK, Raja SN. Spinal cord stimulation for complex regional pain syndrome: an evidence-based medicine review of the literature. *Clinical Journal of Pain.* 2003; **19**: 371–83.

80. Boswell MV, Shah RV, Everett CR *et al.* Interventional techniques in the management of chronic spinal pain: evidence-based practice guidelines. *Pain Physician.* 2005; **8**: 1–47.

81. Ubbink DT, Vermeulen H. Spinal cord stimulation for non-reconstructable chronic critical leg ischaemia. *Cochrane Database of Systematic Reviews.* 2005; **CD004001**.

82. Ubbink DT, Vermeulen H. Spinal cord stimulation for critical leg ischemia: a review of effectiveness and optimal patient selection. *Journal of Pain and Symptom Management.* 2006; **31**: S30–5.

83. Ekre O, Eliasson T, Norrsell H *et al.* Long-term effects of spinal cord stimulation and coronary artery bypass grafting on quality of life and survival in the ESBY study. *European Heart Journal.* 2002; **23**: 1938–45.

84. Hautvast RW, DeJongste MJ, Staal MJ *et al.* Spinal cord stimulation in chronic intractable angina pectoris: a randomized, controlled efficacy study. *American Heart Journal.* 1998; **136**: 1114–20.

85. Mannheimer C, Eliasson T, Augustinsson LE *et al.* Electrical stimulation versus coronary artery bypass surgery in severe angina pectoris: the ESBY study. *Circulation.* 1998; **97**: 1157–63.

86. de Jongste MJ, Hautvast RW, Hillege HL, Lie KI. Efficacy of spinal cord stimulation as adjuvant therapy for intractable angina pectoris: a prospective, randomized clinical study. Working Group on Neurocardiology. *Journal of the American College of Cardiology.* 1994; **23**: 1592–7.

87. Tesfaye S, Watt J, Benbow SJ *et al.* Electrical spinal-cord stimulation for painful diabetic peripheral neuropathy. *Lancet.* 1996; **348**: 1698–701.

88. Taylor RS, Taylor RJ, Van Buyten JP *et al.* The cost effectiveness of spinal cord stimulation in the treatment of pain: a systematic review of the literature. *Journal of Pain and Symptom Management.* 2004; **27**: 370–8.

89. Taylor RJ, Taylor RS. Spinal cord stimulation for failed back surgery syndrome: a decision-analytic model and cost-effectiveness analysis. *International Journal of Technology Assessment in Health Care.* 2005; **21**: 351–8.

90. Meglio M, Cioni B, Rossi GF. Spinal cord stimulation in management of chronic pain. A 9-year experience. *Journal of Neurosurgery.* 1989; **70**: 519–24.

91. Shimoji K, Hokari T, Kano T *et al.* Management of intractable pain with percutaneous epidural spinal cord stimulation: differences in pain-relieving effects among diseases and sites of pain. *Anesthesia and Analgesia.* 1993; **77**: 110–16.

92. Eisenberg E, Brecker C. Lumbar spinal cord stimulation for cervical-originated central pain: a case report. *Pain.* 2002; **100**: 299–301.

93. Heath RG. Psychiatry. *Annual Review of Medicine.* 1954; **5**: 223–36.

94. Gol A. Relief of pain by electrical stimulation of the septal area. *Journal of the Neurological Sciences.* 1967; **5**: 115–20.

95. Hamani C, Schwalb JM, Rezai AR *et al.* Deep brain stimulation for chronic neuropathic pain: Long-term

outcome and the incidence of insertional effect. *Pain.* 2006; **125**: 188–96.

96. Owen SL, Green AL, Stein JF, Aziz TZ. Deep brain stimulation for the alleviation of post-stroke neuropathic pain. *Pain.* 2006; **120**: 202–06.

97. Reynolds DV. Surgery in the rat during electrical analgesia induced by focal brain stimulation. *Science.* 1969; **164**: 444–5.

98. Richardson DE, Akil H. Pain reduction by electrical brain stimulation in man. Part 1: Acute administration in periaqueductal and periventricular sites. *Journal of Neurosurgery.* 1977; **47**: 178–83.

99. Richardson DE, Akil H. Long term results of periventricular gray self-stimulation. *Neurosurgery.* 1977; **1**: 199–202.

100. Millan M, Czlonkowski A, Herz A. Evidence that mu-opioid receptors mediate midbrain "stimulation-produced analgesia" in the freely moving rat. *Neuroscience.* 1987; **22**: 885–96.

101. Sillery E, Bittar RG, Robson MD *et al.* Connectivity of the human periventricular-periaqueductal gray region. *Journal of Neurosurgery.* 2005; **103**: 1030–4.

*102. Bittar RG, Kar-Purkayastha I, Owen SL *et al.* Deep brain stimulation for pain relief: a meta-analysis. *Journal of the Neurological Sciences.* 2005; **12**: 515–19.

103. Young RF, Brechner T. Electrical stimulation of the brain for relief of intractable pain due to cancer. *Cancer.* 1986; **57**: 1266–72.

104. Kumar K, Wyant GM, Nath R. Deep brain stimulation for control of intractable pain in humans, present and future: a ten-year follow-up. *Neurosurgery.* 1990; **26**: 774–81; discussion 81–2.

105. Kumar K, Toth C, Nath RK. Deep brain stimulation for intractable pain: a 15-year experience. *Neurosurgery.* 1997; **40**: 736–46; discussion 46–7.

106. Tsubokawa T, Katayama Y, Yamamoto T *et al.* Chronic motor cortex stimulation in patients with thalamic pain. *Journal of Neurosurgery.* 1993; **78**: 393–401.

107. Brown JA, Pilitsis JG. Motor cortex stimulation. *Pain Medicine.* 2006; **7**: S140–5.

108. Katayama Y, Tsubokawa T, Yamamoto T. Chronic motor cortex stimulation for central deafferentation pain: experience with bulbar pain secondary to Wallenberg syndrome. *Stereotactic and Functional Neurosurgery.* 1994; **62**: 295–9.

109. Katayama Y, Yamamoto T, Kobayashi K *et al.* Motor cortex stimulation for post-stroke pain: comparison of spinal cord and thalamic stimulation. *Stereotactic and Functional Neurosurgery.* 2001; **77**: 183–6.

110. Pridmore S, Oberoi G, Marcolin M, George M. Transcranial magnetic stimulation and chronic pain: current status. *Australasian Psychiatry.* 2005; **13**: 258–65.

111. Lefaucheur JP, Drouot X, Keravel Y, Nguyen JP. Pain relief induced by repetitive transcranial magnetic stimulation of precentral cortex. *Neuroreport.* 2001; **12**: 2963–5.

19

Radiotherapy

PETER J HOSKIN

Introduction	251	Nerve pain	254
Specific indications for radiotherapy in cancer pain management	251	Special comments	254
		References	255
Soft tissue pain	252		

KEY LEARNING POINTS

- Radiotherapy is valuable in the treatment of malignant pain due to bone, soft tissue, and nervous system tumor infiltration.
- Palliative doses as low as single exposures of 10 Gy in nonsmall cell lung cancer (NSCLC) and 12 Gy in two fractions for cerebral metastases are effective for pain control.

- Fractionated treatments in liver metastases and splenomegaly reduce toxicity and are effective.
- Mesothelioma may be helped by local radiotherapy but is more resistant.
- Pituitary ablation can also be achieved by focused radiotherapy for intractable pain.

INTRODUCTION

Radiotherapy has far ranging application in the management of cancer pain. It should be considered in any situation where localized tumor growth is the underlying cause of pain. This may be due to bone metastasis (see Chapter 20, Management of bone pain), soft tissue infiltration, or neuropathic pain from tumor encroaching upon sensory nerves. A brief overview of the process by which radiotherapy is delivered, potential side effects, and complications will be found in Chapter 20, Management of bone pain.

The mechanism for the analgesic action of radiotherapy remains uncertain. Pain relief can often be achieved by low doses of radiation exemplified by the treatment of bone metastasis where a nontumor effect on humoral mediators of pain has been proposed. Where there is soft tissue infiltration or neuropathic pain, tumor shrinkage reducing local pressure and thereby the physical pain stimulus may be important but again a direct effect upon the release of chemical pain mediators and nerve conduction cannot be excluded. However, the degree of shrinkage required for symptomatic as distinct from radiographic response may be very small and thus the concept of radiosensitivity as applied to the curative situation should not be used to deny patients local radiotherapy for cancer pain. It is important to realize that after radiation doses of only 2 Gy, 50–80 percent of the cell population in common cancers will fail to survive in experimental cultures. In contrast, a radical course of radiotherapy aiming at tumor cure would deliver 30–35 doses of 2 Gy, giving a total dose of 60–70 Gy.

SPECIFIC INDICATIONS FOR RADIOTHERAPY IN CANCER PAIN MANAGEMENT

Bone pain

This is by far the most common indication for radiotherapy in cancer pain management, accounting for up to 20 percent of all radiotherapy treatment given in some departments. This has been discussed in detail in Chapter 20, Management of bone pain.

Soft tissue pain

The main indications for radiotherapy in soft tissue pain are given in **Table 19.1**. By far the most common indications are local chest pain from carcinoma of the bronchus, reflecting its high incidence, and headache from cerebral metastasis.

Nerve pain

The main indications for radiotherapy in nerve pain are given in **Table 19.2**.

Often it is not possible to readily distinguish the three categories of pain described above. For example, bone metastases in the spine are often associated with both local pain in the involved bone and neuropathic pain from nerve root irritation; soft tissue infiltration into the presacral space or pelvic side wall will result in both local pelvic pain and neuropathic pain radiating from the lumbar sacral plexus.

SOFT TISSUE PAIN

Chest pain

Malignant chest pain may arise because of carcinoma of the bronchus where it is seen in 40–70 percent of cases[1, 2, 18][II] or where there is pleural infiltration either from a primary mesothelioma or blood-borne metastasis. In general, pleural infiltration is far more troublesome with regard to pain than a central chest tumor.

In the treatment of carcinoma of the bronchus there is published evidence from randomized trials using specific symptom score cards to show that radiotherapy is effective in controlling chest pain in over 70 percent of patients.[1, 2][II] This can be achieved with simple pragmatic courses of treatment, the randomized trials demonstrating that a dose of 17 Gy in two fractions is as good as 30 Gy in ten fractions,[1] and indeed in poor performance status patients equivalent pain control can be achieved with a single dose of 10 Gy.[2]

There is less evidence to support the use of radiotherapy in pleural disease although it is a relatively common practice when faced with symptomatic mesothelioma or metastatic deposits. One small series of 19 patients with pain from mesothelioma reports pain relief in 13 (68 percent) at one month, but longer-term pain control was poor with only four patients having sustained relief at three months.[19][V] An additional advantage for radiotherapy in this setting is the prevention of tumor growth through drain sites in the chest wall, although the evidence in support is equivocal.[3][I]

Headache

Headache may arise from an expanding mass within the skull and in the context of malignant disease this may be

Table 19.1 Indications for radiotherapy in soft tissue pain.

Site of pain	Cause of pain	Published response rate (%)	Level of evidence
Chest pain	Primary ca bronchus	70–80[1, 2]	[II]
	Mesothelioma	68[3]	[I]
Headache	Primary glioma	Not stated[4]	
	Cerebral metastases	70–80[5, 6, 7]	[II]
Liver pain	Primary hepatocellular ca	Not available	
	Liver metastases	55–74[8, 9]	[II]
Splenic pain	Leukemia/lymphoma	91[10]	[I]
Loin pain	Renal cancer	Not available	
Back pain	Paraaortic nodes	Not available	
Pelvic pain	Ca uterus	83[11]	[I]
	Ca ovary	44[12]	[I]

Table 19.2 Indications for radiotherapy in nerve pain.

Site of pain	Cause of pain	Published response rate (%)	Level of evidence
Pelvic pain	Presacral mass e.g. ca rectum	70[13]	[I]
	Lumbosacral plexus infiltration	100[14]	[I]
Shoulder/upper limb	Apical ca lung (Pancoast's)	30–79[15, 16]	[I]
	Axillary nodes, e.g. ca breast	77[17]	[I]

either a primary or secondary tumor. In the population at large, primary brain tumors are rare and the majority of intracranial neoplasms will be cerebral metastases. Radiotherapy may well have a role in the treatment of a primary brain tumor, but the randomized controlled trials focus principally upon survival rather than symptom control. Performance status and quality of life is undoubtedly improved with local radiotherapy for high grade gliomas in selected patients who are aged under 65, present with fits alone, and who have no major neurological deficits.[4][II] There is now phase III trial evidence that this is improved when radiotherapy is given with adjuvant temozolamide.[5][II] In older patients and those with more advanced disease at presentation, hypofractionated radiotherapy delivering 30 Gy in six fractions improved functional status, as measured by the Barthel index, in 38 percent of patients with a further 39 percent remaining stable; specific data relating to pain are not reported.[6][III]

In contrast, there are prospective randomized data[7, 8, 9] [II] to strongly support the use of radiotherapy in the management of headache due to cerebral metastasis. The two largest series performed by the Radiotherapy Therapy Oncology Group (RTOG) in the United States[7][II] some years ago reported control of headache in 70– 80 percent of patients and, across their series of studies including over 2000 patients, it was shown that this could be achieved with relatively low doses of radiation, down to 20 Gy in five daily fractions over one week, with no difference when compared with longer treatments over four weeks. More recent data from the UK Royal College of Radiologists' randomized trial[9][II] compared 12 Gy in two fractions with 30 Gy in ten fractions and again showed equivalent responses and control of headache in over 90 percent of patients. This has therefore become common treatment in the UK for brain metastasis and elsewhere one- to two-week courses of radiotherapy are generally given with good effect for control of headache. However, it is important to note that further recent studies have cast doubt on the value of radiotherapy in patients with significant neurological deficits, poor performance status, and in particular those with primary lung cancer.[10][IV] Careful patient selection is therefore required to ensure optimal use of radiotherapy in cerebral metastases.

Liver pain

Rapid expansion of the liver with progressive hepatic metastasis results in right-sided abdominal pain due to stretching of the liver capsule. In tumors which are sensitive to chemotherapy or hormone therapy this is usually the most appropriate treatment alongside systemic steroids. In many cases, however, progressive, painful liver metastases will reflect advanced disease either insensitive to systemic anticancer therapy or having relapsed after

earlier exposure. Two randomized trials[11, 12][II] have evaluated the role of hepatic irradiation in these circumstances and have demonstrated control of liver pain in over 50 percent from relatively low doses of radiation delivering 20–30 Gy over two to three weeks to the liver. One of the major difficulties and reservations with regard to hepatic irradiation relates to the associated toxicity with nausea, vomiting, and general malaise recognized problems. The published data,[11, 12][II] however, suggests that the benefits in terms of liver shrinkage and improved well-being as a result of improved liver function outweigh these toxicities which can be minimized by avoiding irradiation to the whole liver if possible and using appropriate anti-emetic cover.

Splenic pain

Pain from the spleen may arise because of progressive enlargement, typically due to hematological malignancies such as chronic granulocytic leukemia or non-Hodgkin's lymphoma. In many circumstances, the treatment of choice will be surgical removal or chemotherapy but, in advanced cases or where the patient is unfit for surgery, splenic irradiation is entirely appropriate. Very low doses of irradiation will cause significant splenic shrinkage and considerable pain relief. A greater effect with doses above 5 Gy has been reported and typical schedules will deliver doses of around 10 Gy in up to ten daily treatments over two weeks. Reduction in splenic size is reported in 60 percent and pain relief occurred in 91 percent maintained for up to six months.[20][IV]

Loin pain

Both primary renal cancer and retroperitoneal sarcoma can present severe loin and back pain. This will reflect infiltration of the retroperitoneal tissues from tumors which are locally advanced and inoperable. In these circumstances local radiotherapy may be of value, although the dose will be limited by the surrounding tissues which are relatively sensitive to radiation, in particular the small bowel, stomach, liver, and normal kidney. Nonetheless, useful pain control may be achieved although published data to support this are scanty.

Para–aortic lymphadenpathy

Enlargement of the para-aortic lymph nodes causes a characteristic persistent back ache. When due to chemotherapy-sensitive tumors such as lymphoma or germ cell tumors, then chemotherapy is the best approach but in chemo-resistant tumors, local radiotherapy delivering doses of 20–30 Gy in two to three weeks is traditionally delivered. Anecdotally good pain control can be achieved although there are few published data to support this impression.

Pelvic pain

Advanced or recurrent tumors within the pelvis frequently present with local pain which may be of a visceral nature or neuropathic (see below under Nerve pain). Visceral pain is typically related to gynecological primary tumors, in particular in the cervix and ovary. Results from palliative radiotherapy to recurrent ovarian cancer delivering a median dose of 35 Gy report pain relief in 83 percent of 47 treatments[13] [IV] and in advanced uterine cancer pain relief was seen in 44 percent after single dose treatment with 10 Gy.[14] [IV]

NERVE PAIN

Bone metastasis may be a cause of nerve root compression and associated neuropathic pain which is successfully treated with local radiotherapy as discussed in Chapter 20, Management of bone pain.

Pelvic pain

Pelvic pain may be associated with pain in the sciatic nerve distribution radiating into the buttocks and down the leg due to infiltration of the lumbosacral plexus. The common situations in which this is encountered are due to presacral recurrence of colorectal tumor and central pelvic recurrence from uterine tumors. In patients who have not received chemotherapy this should be considered, but where there are local symptoms and previous radiotherapy has not been given then pelvic radiotherapy may be of value. One series has evaluated the response of pelvic pain reporting success in 80 percent of patients who received either a single dose of 10 or 35 Gy in 15 fractions with no difference between the two radiation dose schedules.[17] [III] One series of 13 patients with neuropathic pain from lumbosacral plexus involvement with tumor reports pain relief in all patients after doses of either 17 Gy in two fractions or 20 Gy in five fractions.[15] [III]

Upper limb pain

Upper limb pain may arise because of tumor in the apex of the lung, axilla, or lower neck. The typical situation is that of the Pancoast tumor which is an apical primary NSCLC. Another common situation is metastatic lymph nodes which may be axillary from carcinoma of the breast, low deep cervical lymph nodes from carcinoma of the bronchus, or left-sided supraclavicular nodes arising from intra-abdominal malignancy. A wide range of doses

for radiotherapy in this setting have been reported ranging from single doses of 10 to 58 Gy in 31 fractions.[16] [IV] "Significant" pain relief is reported in up to 77 percent of patients with metastatic breast cancer, with similar response rates for Pancoast's tumor also. However, one retrospective series of treatment to apical lung cancer suggests that no more than 30 percent of patients receiving radiotherapy will achieve durable pain control.[21] [IV] A dose response effect has been reported with Pancoast's tumor,[22] [IV] although other studies report no improvement with increasing dose.[21] [IV]

Pituitary ablation

This is rarely performed today but has been reported as a useful technique in intractable pain. Local radiotherapy has been used as a means of achieving this.[23] [IV] Similarly, thalamic ablation using stereotactic irradiation has been described[24] [III] and the proponents of this approach have reported response rates in patients with intractable pain of up to 90 percent.

SPECIAL COMMENTS

Radiotherapy will rarely be used as a sole agent in the management of cancer pain. Within the indications mentioned above, it will be used alongside analgesics and adjuvant analgesics as detailed in Part II and elsewhere in Part III of this volume. The relative merits of each approach will vary from patient to patient. The need for radiotherapy where regular analgesia can control pain is less certain unless there is undue associated toxicity with the drug regimen when local radiotherapy may provide a means of reducing or even withdrawing the need for regular systemic medication. However, there is a strong indication for local radiotherapy where simple drug schedules fail to adequately control pain. Associated symptoms may also be an important consideration in seeking radiotherapy as effective palliation; for example where there is chest pain and associated hemoptysis from NSCLC, radiotherapy is indicated for both symptoms and similarly the presence of motor weakness with headache due to brain metastases presents a situation where local radiotherapy may have a dual indication, even if the headache can be controlled with steroids and analgesics.

Radiotherapy should therefore be considered as one component of a multimodality approach to cancer pain within the specific indications discussed above. The application of the basic principles of careful patient assessment, pain identification, and diagnosis of underlying pathological mechanisms will allow individualized treatment for each patient incorporating radiotherapy where appropriate.

REFERENCES

1. Medical Research Council Lung Cancer Working Party. Prepared on behalf of the working party and all its collaborators by Bleehen NM, Girling DJ, Machin D, Stephens RJ. Inoperable non-small-cell lung cancer (NSCLC): a Medical Research Council randomised trial of palliative radiotherapy with two fractions or ten fractions. *British Journal of Cancer.* 1991; **63**: 265–70.

* 2. Medical Research Council Lung Cancer Working Party. Prepared on behalf of the working party and all its collaborators by Bleehen NM, Girling DJ, Machin D, Stephens RJ. A Medical Research Council (MRC) randomised trial of palliative radiotherapy with two fractions or a single fraction in patients with inoperable non-small-cell lung cancer (NSCLC) and poor performance status. *British Journal of Cancer.* 1992; **65**: 934–41.

* 3. Ung YC, Yu E, Falkson C et al. The role of radiation therapy in malignant pleural mesothelioma: a systematic review. *Radiotherapy and Oncology.* 2006; **80**: 13–18.

4. Bleehen NM, Stenning SP. On behalf of the Medical Research Council Brain Tumour Working Party. A Medical Research Council trial of two radiotherapy doses in the treatment of grades 3 and 4 astrocytoma. *British Journal of Cancer.* 1991; **64**: 769–74.

5. Stupp R, Mason WP, van den Bent MJ et al. Radiotherapy plus concomitant and adjuvant temozolomide for glioblastoma. *New England Journal of Medicine.* 2005; **352**: 987–96.

* 6. Thomas R, James N, Guerro D et al. Hypofractionated radiotherapy as a palliative treatment in poor prognosis patients with high grade glioma. *Radiotherapy and Oncology.* 1994; **33**: 113–16.

* 7. Borgelt B, Gelber R, Kramer S et al. The palliation of brain metastases: final results of the first two studies by the Radiation Therapy Oncology Group. *International Journal Radiation Oncology Biology Physics.* 1980; **6**: 1–9.

8. Harwood AR, Simpson JW. Radiation therapy of cerebral metastases: A randomized prospective clinical trial. *International Journal Radiation Oncology Biology Physics.* 1977; **2**: 1091–4.

9. Priestman TJ, Dunn J, Brada M et al. Final results of the Royal College of Radiologists' trial comparing two different radiotherapy schedules in the treatment of cerebral metastases. *Clinical Oncology.* 1996; **8**: 308–15.

10. Lock M, Chow E, Pond GR et al. Prognostic factors in brain metastases: can we determine patients who do not benefit from whole-brain radiotherapy? *Clinical Oncology.* 2004; **16**: 332–8.

11. Borgelt B, Gelber R, Brady LW et al. The palliation of hepatic metastases: results of the Radiation Therapy Oncology Group pilot study. *International Journal of Radiation Oncology, Biology, Physics.* 1981; **7**: 587–91.

12. Leibel SA, Pajak TF, Massullo V et al. A comparison of Misonidazole sensitized radiation therapy to radiation therapy alone for the palliation of hepatic metastases: results of a Radiation Therapy Oncology Group randomized prospective trial. *International Journal of Radiation Oncology, Biology, Physics.* 1987; **13**: 1057–64.

13. Corn BW, Lanciano RM, Boente M et al. Recurrent ovarian cancer. Effective radiotherapeutic palliation after chemotherapy failure. *Cancer.* 1994; **74**: 2979–83.

14. Halle JS, Rosenman JG, Varia MA et al. 1000cGy single dose palliation for advanced carcinoma of the cervix or endometrium. *International Journal of Radiation Oncology, Biology, Physics.* 1986; **12**: 1947–50.

15. Russi EG, Pergolizzi S, Gaeta M et al. Palliative-radiotherapy in lumbosacral carcinomatous neuropathy. *Radiotherapy and Oncology.* 1993; **26**: 172–3.

16. Ampil FL. Radiotherapy for carcinomatous brachial plexus plexopathy. *Cancer.* 1985; **56**: 2185–8.

17. Allum WH, Mack P, Priestman TJ, Fielding JWL. Radiotherapy for pain relief in locally recurrent colorectal cancer. *Annals of the Royal College of Surgeons of England.* 1987; **69**: 220–1.

18. Collins TM, Ash DV, Close HJ, Thorogood J. An evaluation of the palliative role of radiotherapy in inoperable carcinoma of the bronchus. *Clinical Radiology.* 1988; **39**: 284–6.

19. Bissett D, Macbeth FR, Cram I. The role of palliative radiotherapy in malignant mesothelioma. *Clinical Oncology.* 1991; **3**: 315–17.

20. Paulino AC, Reddy SP. Splenic irradiation in the palliation of patients with lymphoproliferative and myeloproliferative disorders. *American Journal of Hospice and Palliative Care.* 1996; **13**: 32–5.

21. Watson PN, Evans RJ. Intractable pain with lung cancer. *Pain.* 1987; **29**: 163–73.

22. Morris RW, Abadir R. Pancoast tumour: the value of high dose radiation therapy. *Radiology.* 1979; **132**: 717–19.

23. Kuttig H. Radiotherapy of cancer pain. *Recent Results in Cancer Research.* 1984; **89**: 190–4.

24. Leksell L, Meyerson BA, Forster DMC. Radiosurgical thalamotomy for intractable pain. *Confinia Neurologica (Basel).* 1972; **34**: 264.

Management of bone pain

PETER J HOSKIN

Introduction and definition	256	Hormone treatment	265
Etiology and pathophysiology	256	Surgery	266
Clinical presentation	257	Prognosis	267
Diagnostic criteria	257	Special comments	267
Evidence-based evaluation of management	258	References	267
Chemotherapy	264		

KEY LEARNING POINTS

- Bone metastases are a result of osteoclast activation by malignant cells.
- Diagnosis should be confirmed on x-ray, isotope bone scan, computed tomography (CT), or magnetic resonance imaging (MRI).
- Initial treatment is with analgesics according to the World Health Organization (WHO) ladder with nonsteroidal anti-inflammatory drugs (NSAIDs).
- Single dose radiotherapy delivering 8–10 Gy is effective for local bone pain and neuropathic pain but may require retreatment in 25 percent of patients.

- Multiple sites of pain are effectively treated with single-dose wide-field external beam irradiation or radioisotope therapy.
- Chemotherapy has a role in breast and lung cancer and myeloma.
- Surgery is important for actual and impending pathological fracture and spinal instability.
- Bisphosphonates are indicated for prophylaxis in myeloma and high-risk breast cancer; they may also have a role in pain relief.

INTRODUCTION AND DEFINITION

Bone pain secondary to cancer is an extremely common symptom reflecting its prevalence in the common cancers, in particular breast, lung, and prostate cancer. Whilst the vast majority of patients with malignant bone pain have bone metastasis, it is also a feature of primary bone tumors both benign and malignant. The incidence of bone metastasis at post-mortem in various primary sites is shown in **Table 20.1**.[1][III]

It is always important to consider other causes of bone pain in the cancer patient who presents with this symptom, as outlined in **Table 20.2**.

ETIOLOGY AND PATHOPHYSIOLOGY

Bone pain due to tumor infiltration is usually a result of blood-borne metastasis. Rarely, there may be direct infiltration of a bone where a tumor arises adjacent to that site, for example in the paravertebral region from a retroperitoneal sarcoma or in the head and neck region with direct infiltration into the skull base.

The pathophysiology of bone metastasis has been well described.[2][III] The series of events from a tumor cell arriving at the bone surface is coordinated through the release of chemical agents which activate the osteoclasts within the bone. These include prostaglandins, kinins,

Table 20.1 Incidence of bone metastases based on post-mortem data.

Primary site	Percentage of cases having bone mets	Total number bone mets yearly/ 1,00,000[a]
Breast	73	60
Prostate	68	34
Thyroid	42	0.8
Bronchus	36	29
Kidney	35	2.5
Rectum	11	3
Esophagus	6	0.6

[a]Based on UK incidence rates.

Table 20.2 Causes of bone pain in cancer patients.

Cause
Metastases
Fracture
Degenerative bone disease
Bone marrow pain
Nonmetastatic hypertrophic osteoarthropathy
Other bone disease, e.g. Pagets

substance P, and parathyroid hormone-related peptides, collectively termed osteoclast-activating factors (OAFs). Osteoclast activation is mediated through binding of RANK ligand on the surface of the osteoclast and this has been identified as an important biochemical target for agents acting against osteoclast activation. The osteoclast activity results in bone destruction, allowing entry of the malignant cells into the bone. In response to this, possibly mediated by various growth factors of which osteoprotogerin (OPG) is one of the more important, there is an osteoblastic reaction in which the bone attempts to repair the damaged areas by laying down osteoid. The balance between osteoclast and osteoblast activity defines the morphological features of the bone metastasis, those where osteoclastic activity predominates being seen as lytic bone disease and those where osteoblastic activity predominates being seen as osteosclerotic metastasis.

The actual cause of pain as a result of this process is not well understood. Various suggestions have included the effects of direct damage to the bone and the surrounding periosteum where the principal sensory nerve fibers exist and changes in the intra-osseous pressure. The final pain pathway is mediated through large C fibers stimulated by various neurochemicals including many of the OAFs, several of which, in particular the kinins, prostaglandins, and substance P, are recognized as mediators involved in pain and nociception.

CLINICAL PRESENTATION

Malignant bone pain may present in the context of a patient with a known primary tumor or as the initial presentation of either metastatic bone disease or a primary bone tumor.

Typical features of malignant bone pain include its character, which tends to be dull and persistent occurring through the night as well as the daytime, but made worse on weight-bearing. On clinical examination the area is usually locally tender, there may be local swelling and in the case of a particularly vascular tumor an audible bruit over the bone metastasis; this is said to be typical of renal cancer.

DIAGNOSTIC CRITERIA

The presence of malignant tumor within a bone will be detected on either plain x-ray, isotope bone scan, CT scan, or MRI. It is usual to work up this hierarchy. Isotope bone scan has the advantage of demonstrating the overall distribution of bone metastasis, but can be relatively nonspecific and distinction between spinal metastasis and degenerative disease can be difficult. It is, however, far more sensitive than a plain x-ray, except in the case of predominantly lytic disease such as that seen in multiple myeloma where the bone scan may be entirely negative because of the minimal osteoblastic response. CT and MR imaging will give far better definition of the anatomical extent of the bone tumor. MR is superior to CT for imaging the spine and long bones, whereas CT often gives better definition of flat bones such as the pelvis and scapula.[3, 4][III] Bone metastases will also be demonstrated on positron emission tomography (PET) and where this is undertaken as part of staging an early cancer, previously unexpected metastases may be identified.

Whilst supportive evidence may also be obtained from biochemical tests such as the serum alkaline phosphatase and acid phosphatase, these are rarely diagnostic although a very high serum alkaline phosphatase should raise the question of Paget's disease as an alternative or coexisting diagnosis. In the case of prostate cancer then a raised serum prostate specific antigen (PSA), with levels above 20 ng/mL, is associated in over 90 percent of cases with bone metastasis,[5][III] a proportion of which may be occult at the time of initial diagnosis.

In a patient presenting with no known underlying primary tumor, then histological confirmation of metastatic disease in the bone is required if the primary cannot be identified by subsequent investigations. In the light of the known distribution and frequency of bone metastasis (**Table 20.1**), in all patients the neck should be examined and a chest x-ray performed to exclude bronchial and thyroid cancer, in a male patient the prostate should be examined and a serum PSA measured and in a woman the breasts and axillae should be examined with bilateral mammograms. Where lesions are predominantly lytic then serum should be sent for protein electrophoresis and urine for Bence–Jones proteins to exclude multiple myeloma, the other cause of predominantly lytic bone metastasis being renal cancer which may be diagnosed on abdominal ultrasound.

EVIDENCE-BASED EVALUATION OF MANAGEMENT

Pharmacological management of malignant bone pain

Pharmacological management of malignant bone pain using basic pharmacological techniques will not differ from that of other examples of cancer pain following the analgesic ladder principles of stepwise escalation monitoring response to each period of change (see Chapter 10, Clinical pharmacology: principles of analgesic drug management). Incident pain may be a particular problem in bone pain. Opioid drugs can be effective but satisfactory control of incident pain may require doses associated with opioid-related adverse effects.[6][II]

NSAIDs have a major role in the management of musculoskeletal pain in keeping with the recognized role of prostaglandins in the etiology of metastatic bone pain (see Chapter 11, Clinical pharmacology and therapeutics: non-opioids). Whilst this is a well-established principle in reviews and textbooks on the subject,[7][V] objective data on their efficacy for metastatic bone pain are not so readily available. When used alone as the primary means of pain control, pain relief is seen in only 20 percent of patients.[8] [III] This is in keeping with data on the use of the WHO analgesic ladder in which NSAIDs together with simple analgesics are classified as level 1 analgesia, found to be effective alone in only 11 percent of one series of 1229 patients.[9][III] A meta-analysis[10][I] of trials of NSAIDs in cancer pain identified three trials which specifically addressed their use in bone pain, of which only two were included in the analysis. Peak pain intensity was reduced from 55 to 40 percent in the one single dose study and from 33 to 23 percent in the multidose study. There is no data to recommend one NSAID over any other and choice will, in general, be based upon individual preference and tolerance of side effects of which gastrointestinal symptoms, dizziness, and drowsiness predominate. One study[11][III] has suggested a dose-response for naproxen in metastatic bone pain comparing 550 mg eight-hourly with 275 mg eight-hourly but more side effects are seen at the higher dose.

In most patients with metastatic bone pain, NSAIDs will be used as an adjuvant alongside opioid analgesics and the additional measures described below.

Radiotherapy

Whilst the use of analgesics and NSAIDs will form the initial management of the patient presenting with malignant bone pain, for many patients definitive treatment will be required to achieve optimal pain relief. Details of the management of primary bone tumors is outside the scope of this chapter but in general a combination of chemotherapy and local treatment, either surgery or radiotherapy, will be indicated for chemosensitive tumors, such as osteosarcoma and Ewing's tumor, whilst the mainstay of treatment for chondrosarcoma is surgery.

For metastatic bone pain, radiotherapy has a major role. Treatment may be delivered with either external beam radiotherapy or the use of radioactive isotopes which selectively concentrate in bone. Techniques are chosen dependent upon the distribution and sites of pain.

LOCALIZED BONE PAIN

For localized sites of bone pain, simple external beam radiotherapy is the most effective and appropriate. This should not be undertaken without definitive evidence of metastasis at the site of pain and having excluded other causes such as degenerative disease as the primary cause of the pain. It is also important in weight-bearing areas to have excluded pathological fracture for which internal fixation will be indicated. High risk lesions can be identified based on the extent of cortical erosion.[12][II] Having confirmed metastatic bone pain then the radiotherapy technique will be chosen to give a homogeneous radiation dose across the involved bone, while as far as possible avoiding sensitive normal structures, a particular concern when treating ribs where there is underlying lung and the lumbo-sacral spine and pelvis where abdominal contents will encroach. The radiotherapy procedure follows a series of defined steps as follows.

Immobilization

It is important that the treated area is stable within the treatment beam and that there is not significant movement while the treatment is delivered. In general, this will require simple cooperation from the patient and a comfortable position. With this in mind, it is important when patients attend for radiotherapy that adequate analgesia is provided and in particular that they do not miss doses of analgesia whilst attending the Radiotherapy Department.

Localization

Localization refers to the need to accurately define the painful site incorporating both clinical evaluation and radiographic evidence:

- for superficial bones, palpation may be sufficient so that for example a painful rib may be identified and the treatment area defined on the patient's skin;
- for deeper bones, a treatment simulator which produces diagnostic x-ray pictures simulating the therapy x-ray beam may be used to accurately

identify the sites of metastasis and define the beam size and shape required to cover the area.

Increasingly, CT is used for treatment planning to give more accurate definition of bone and soft tissue. Once defined, skin marks will be used to enable relocation of the beam on the treatment machine.

Planning

Planning is rarely complex when treating bone metastasis. Occasionally, in the case of a spinal metastasis with a para-spinal mass, two or three beams may be focused on the treatment area to enable accurate coverage but otherwise for the majority of bone metastasis single or matched opposed beams will be used.

For superficial bones, a beam with limited penetration may be chosen. In modern departments this will be achieved using an electron beam whose depth of penetration is defined by its energy, for example a 10-MeV electron beam will deliver its high dose region to a depth of between 3 and 3.5 cm, which is adequate for most chest wall treatments. An alternative is to use a low energy x-ray beam of 250–300 KV. This does not have such a sharp cut-off in its dose distribution and delivers a higher dose to deeper tissues, a particular disadvantage when treating ribs where there is underlying lung but rarely of clinical significance in a patient with advanced disease.

For other bones such as the spine, long bones, and pelvis, then high energy x-ray beams from a linear accelerator of 4–6 MV, or if not available then a cobalt 60 gamma-ray beam will be used. For the spine, a single beam directed at the appropriate area will be chosen, for other sites two beams opposing each other will be used to give an even distribution of dose across the bone.

Treatment delivery

Treatment delivery is a simple matter of transferring the above processes to the actual treatment machine. Delivery of radiotherapy for the patient is little different to a diagnostic x-ray exposure lasting only a few minutes with no associated immediate side effects.

Radiation side effects and complications

Toxicity from radiotherapy is divided into two main groups based upon their timing in relation to treatment.

Acute side effects occur during treatment, usually as a direct result of epithelial cell damage and are related to the site of treatment. Thus, radiation including the bowel will result in acute bowel toxicity with nausea from the upper bowel and diarrhea from the large bowel; irradiation of the skin causes a typical reaction ranging from skin erythema to dry desquamation to moist desquamation as there is progressive epithelial damage; treatment to the oral cavity causes mucositis and to the mediastinum results in oesophagitis. In principle, acute radiation effects are self-limiting and, provided the patient is supported through the symptomatic period, will heal as basal cells repair the damaged surface epithelium.

Late radiation damage is a distinct entity typically occurring from nine months after treatment and often manifest many years later, in most instances being irreversible and often progressive. Examples include late bowel damage with strictures causing subacute obstruction or fistula formation, progressive pneumonitis and lung fibrosis, skin fibrosis, and telangiectasia.

Whilst acute side effects may be seen with palliative treatment, dose fractionation schedules will be chosen to minimize toxicity and where anticipated for example a large field including bowel, prophylactic antiemetics or antidiarrheal agents will be given. Late toxicity is not expected after palliative treatments except for the rare occasions where successive retreatment may have been given. This is partly due to the relatively short period of risk for most patients whose life expectancy will be only a few months, whereas most late toxicity will be seen some years after treatment but principally because the doses used will not reach the threshold for late damage to be induced. This threshold is sometimes referred to as "radiation tolerance dose" and is the dose beyond which a significant level (usually defined at >5 percent) of late effects may be anticipated. The most sensitive structures for late effects are the bowel which will tolerate no more than around 40 Gy in 20 daily fractions and the spinal cord which may become a dose-limiting structure when treating bone metastases in the spine repeatedly. Cumulative doses greater than 50 Gy in 25 fractions or its equivalent will exceed spinal cord tolerance. It should be noted that there is very little recovery of tolerance in the short term and hence in the palliative setting retreatment may exceed a conventional tolerance dose. This is only considered where there is a reasonable expectation of further clinically useful response and either the patient is aware of the risks of late tissue damage or the prognosis is so poor that it would never be expressed in the patient's lifespan.

RADIATION DOSE AND BONE PAIN

The optimal dose for treatment of metastatic bone pain has been defined from extensive clinical trial data culminating in three meta-analyses,[13, 14, 15][I] each of which comes to the same conclusion that there is no evidence for a dose response effect for pain relief at doses above 8 Gy as a single dose, as shown in **Figure 20.1**. This applies to all parameters of pain, including rate of onset and overall incidence of pain relief. A large bone pain trial from the UK Collaborative Group[16][II] confirms that duration of pain relief up to one year after treatment is equivalent comparing a single dose of 8 Gy with a five or ten fraction treatment, shown in **Figure 20.2**. There is therefore little justification in routine practice for patients to receive more than a single dose of 8–10 Gy to the painful site.

The toxicity from treating sites such as the cervical spine, ribs, and long bones is negligible and the main

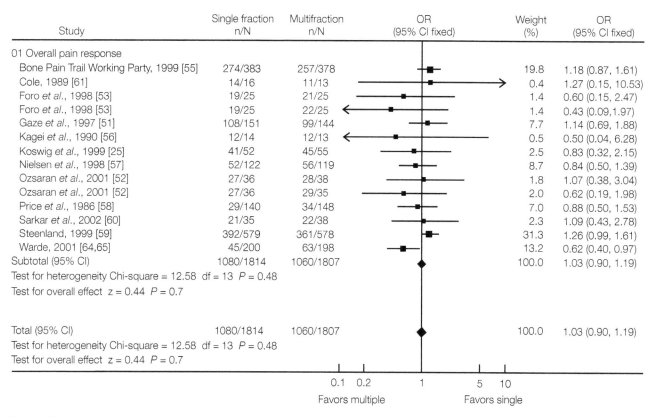

Figure 20.1 Meta-analysis of trials comparing single doses with multifraction treatments for metastatic bone pain. Redrawn with permission from *Clinical Oncology*, 15, Sze WM, Shelley MD, Held I *et al.*, Palliation of metastatic bone pain: single fraction versus multifraction radiotherapy – a systematic review of randomised trial, 345–52, © Elsevier (2003). For full details of the studies listed, see Ref. 14.

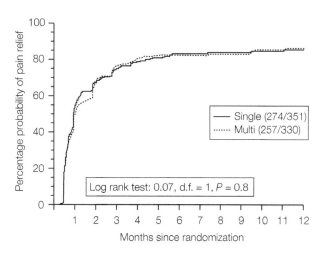

Figure 20.2 Rate of onset of pain relief after localized radiotherapy for metastatic bone pain delivering either 8 Gy as a single dose or 30 Gy in ten daily fractions. Redrawn with permission from *Radiotherapy and Oncology*, 6, Price P, Hoskin PJ, Easton D *et al.*, Prospective randomised trial of single and multifraction radiotherapy schedules in the treatment of painful bony metastases, 247–55, © Elsevier (1986).

issue focuses upon whether treatments to the lumbosacral spine and pelvis are associated with more nausea, vomiting, and diarrhea when delivered with single doses than with multiple doses. The evidence base for treatment-related toxicity is less strong than for treatment effect in the randomized trials included in the meta-analyses. Two trials[16, 17][II] have looked at the incidence of toxicity systematically and in neither of these is there an effect of treatment dose upon the incidence of toxicity.

Neuropathic pain may be related to bone metastasis. This has been the specific subject of a multicenter randomized trial in the UK and Australasia comparing single doses with multi-fraction doses.[18][II] The overall response rates were 53 percent after a single dose of 8 Gy and 61 percent after 20 Gy in five fractions which was not statistically different; complete response rates were 26 and 27 percent respectively and, as shown in **Figure 20.3**, there was no significant difference in response duration.

The one area where single dose treatment may be inferior to multiple higher dose treatment is in the rate of retreatment which in the meta-analysis[14, 15][I] is consistently greater after a single dose, being given in around 25 percent of patients as shown in **Figure 20.4**. There are limited data on the efficacy of retreatment but reanalysis of the largest trial in the literature from the Dutch Bone Pain group shows that when retreatment effect is excluded, there remains no difference between the two dose levels studied.[19][II] Retrospective data also suggest that retreatment once or even twice has the same chance of response as primary treatment and that this is not necessarily related to the initial response, pain relief being seen even in patients who do not respond initially.[20][III] There is a multinational trial under way at present to evaluate this further.

Estimated percentage not failed
100
80
60
40
20
0
8/1
20/5
P = 0.056
0 3 6 9 12 15 18 21 24 27 30
Months following randomization
Number at risk
8/1 137 33 19 11 5 3 3 3 3 2 2
20/5 135 58 24 19 10 5 5 2 2 2 1

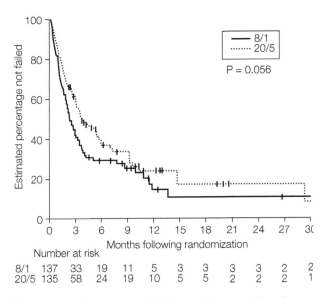

Figure 20.3 Response to radiotherapy of neuropathic pain, comparing a single dose of 8 Gy with 20 Gy in five fractions. Redrawn with permission from *Radiotherapy and Oncology*, 75, Roos DE, Turner SL, O'Brien PC *et al.*, Randomized trial of 8 Gy in 1 versus 20 Gy in 5 fractions of radiotherapy for neuropathic pain due to bone metastases (TROG 96.05), 54–63, © Elsevier (2005).

BONE PAIN IN MULTIPLE SITES

Because the nature of bone metastasis is to develop by blood-borne spread, it is usual for there to be multiple sites of metastasis. Despite this, pain may occur from only a limited area when local radiotherapy is appropriate. However, there are patients who will develop pain in multiple sites which cannot be encompassed in a single localized radiation beam covering one bone area. These patients can still be offered radiation therapy which, if possible, will remain the most effective treatment for their pain. In selected cases, which will be discussed below under Chemotherapy and Hormone treatment, chemotherapy or hormone therapy are also entirely appropriate.

WIDE FIELD IRRADIATION

Wide field irradiation or hemibody radiotherapy covers a wide anatomical area where there is scattered pain. The techniques are similar to those described above but the radiation field is considerably larger and focused on a region of the body where pain may predominate. However, there are limits to the extent which can be safely treated to avoid the risk of bone marrow failure if too great a marrow volume is included. It is possible to cover the upper, lower, or mid half-bodies, selected according to the predominant sites of pain as illustrated in **Figure 20.5**. One further limitation is the size of x-ray beam which can be delivered from a linear accelerator typically no bigger than 40 cm^2 on the patient's skin. This can, however, be overcome by extending the treating distance so that the patient is further away from the beam, the size of the beam then increasing by simple geometry.

Typical doses are 8 Gy to the lower half body but only 6 Gy to the upper half-body, greater doses than this resulting in significant lung damage. These doses are prescribed to the center of the body, i.e. midway between two

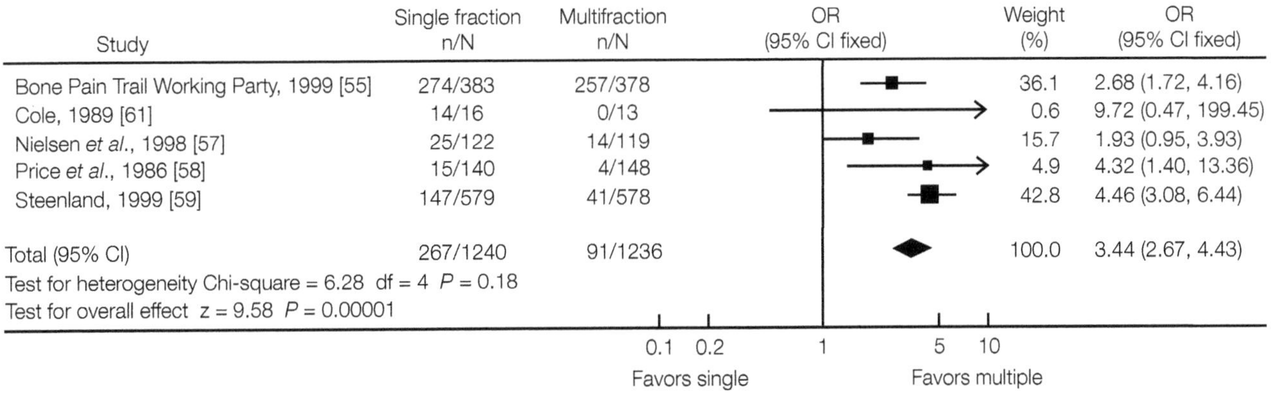

Study
Single fraction n/N
Multifraction n/N
OR (95% CI fixed)
Weight (%)
OR (95% CI fixed)
Bone Pain Trail Working Party, 1999 [55] 274/383 257/378 36.1 2.68 (1.72, 4.16)
Cole, 1989 [61] 14/16 0/13 0.6 9.72 (0.47, 199.45)
Nielsen et al., 1998 [57] 25/122 14/119 15.7 1.93 (0.95, 3.93)
Price et al., 1986 [58] 15/140 4/148 4.9 4.32 (1.40, 13.36)
Steenland, 1999 [59] 147/579 41/578 42.8 4.46 (3.08, 6.44)
Total (95% CI) 267/1240 91/1236 100.0 3.44 (2.67, 4.43)
Test for heterogeneity Chi-square = 6.28 df = 4 P = 0.18
Test for overall effect z = 9.58 P = 0.00001
0.1 0.2 1 5 10
Favors single
Favors multiple

Figure 20.4 Probability of retreatment after a single dose or multiple dose radiotherapy for metastatic bone pain from meta-analysis. Redrawn with permission from *Clinical Oncology*, 15, Sze WM, Shelley MD, Held I *et al.*, Palliation of metastatic bone pain: single fraction versus multifraction radiotherapy – a systematic review of randomised trial, 345–52, © Elsevier (2003). For full details of the studies listed, see Ref. 14.

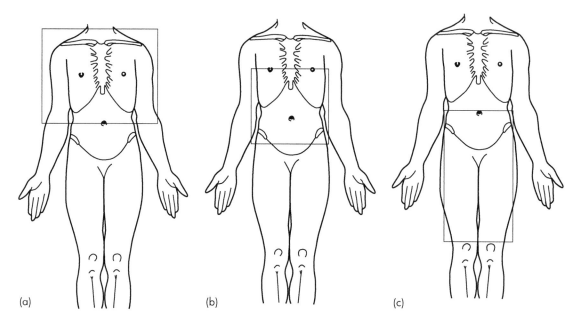

(a)   (b)   (c)

Figure 20.5 Examples of hemibody radiation fields (a) to upper hemibody, (b) to mid-hemibody, (c) to lower hemibody.

beams, front and back, opposing each other to give equal dose distribution across the treated area. They may also be corrected for the increased transmission through lungs, ideally using a CT scan to determine the lung depth.

There has been no randomized comparison of this technique against "best supportive care." Efficacy has been defined in single arm studies[21, 22, 23, 24, 25][III] and the results are similar to those achieved with external beam radiotherapy. More rapid responses than with localized irradiation, often within 24 hours, may be seen with up to 80 percent of patients reporting improved pain at one month. One randomized dose trial has compared 8 Gy in two fractions with 15 Gy in five fractions and 12 Gy in four fractions, showing no advantage for the higher dose schedules.[26][II] There is, however, undoubtedly an increased incidence of acute toxicity as a result of which wide field irradiation is perhaps relatively underused. The principal toxicities are outlined in **Table 20.3**.

RADIOISOTOPE THERAPY

Radioisotope therapy is an alternative to wide field irradiation. It involves the intravenous administration of a radioisotope which will be selectively taken up at sites of bone metastases. Isotopes in common use are shown in **Table 20.4**. The ideal isotope will deliver radiation through decay to predominantly beta particle irradiation of limited range, 2–4 mm, to deposit its energy within the bone metastasis in which it is localized. A small component of low energy gamma irradiation is also of value as it can be detected by a gamma camera to give pictures analogous to a diagnostic bone scan showing the distribution of the isotope uptake.

Table 20.3 Toxicity of wide field (hemibody) radiotherapy.

Site		
All sites	Bone marrow	Transfusion requirements
		Measured falls in WBC and platelets
Upper body	Lungs	Interstitial pneumonitis
	Stomach	Nausea
	Liver	Nausea
		Subclinical hepatitis
Lower body	Small and large bowel	Diarrhea

Table 20.4 Radioisotopes for metastatic bone pain.

Element	Isotope	Chemical form for clinical use
Isotopes with intrinsic bone seeking activity		
Phosphorus	^{32}P	PO_4
Strontium	^{89}Sr	$SrCl_2$
Radium	^{223}Ra	RaCl
Isotopes targeting by conjugation with bisphosphonate		
Samarium	^{153}Sm	Sm EDTMP
Rhenium	^{186}Re	Re EDTP
	^{188}Re	Re EDTP
Tin	^{117}Sn	Sn DTPA

Strontium

Strontium (^{89}Sr) is the most commonly used radioisotope for the treatment of metastatic bone pain. This decays entirely by beta emission and has a radioactive half-life of 50.5 days. Its beta particles have an energy of 1.46 MeV, which means they will penetrate up to 8 mm in tissue. Chemically, strontium is similar to calcium and therefore taken up into bone and incorporated into hydroxyapatite. Areas of active mineralization will therefore concentrate strontium and this will include all sites of osteoblastic response to bone metastasis.

One of the major advantages of strontium is its ease of administration, requiring a simple intravenous injection which can be given as an outpatient. Because it produces short-range beta irradiation, there are few if any major radiation hazards associated with its use and no acute toxicity. The only significant contraindications to strontium use are where there is extensive bone marrow depression, since its widespread uptake into bone will result in a radiation dose being delivered to the bone marrow with suppression of hemopoeisis. Urinary incontinence is also a relative contraindication since strontium is excreted in the urine and if there is spillage on to the patient's skin, clothing, or bed, then contamination will occur. This may be overcome by urethral catheterization for incontinent patients. Renal failure will impair excretion of strontium, prolonging its half-life, and is also a relative contraindication.

The pattern of pain relief with radioactive strontium is different to that with external beam treatment and in general follows a longer time course with many patients taking up to 12 weeks to achieve their maximum response.[27][IV] For this reason, patients who have a life expectancy of less than this may benefit more from external beam treatment or appropriate pharmacological manipulations.

Strontium has been evaluated in both formal phase II dose escalation studies[28][III] and a randomized double-blind placebo controlled trial[29][II] in which it was found to be superior to placebo in its effective dose of 150 MBq. It has also been compared in a randomized trial with external beam radiotherapy[30][II] in which it was found to be equivalent. A case control comparison with wide field irradiation[31][III] has shown equivalence for pain control but less associated toxicity and in particular fewer blood and platelet transfusion requirements after treatment.

Current licensed indications in the UK for strontium are restricted to prostate cancer where the initial evaluation has been focused due to the osteoblastic nature of its metastases, but activity in other primary tumor types has also been demonstrated.[32][III]

Whilst most patients will receive a single dose of strontium in their management, there is limited experience of repeated doses[32][III] which appear to be equally effective to the initial exposure and may be considered at three- to six-monthly intervals.

Samarium

Samarium (^{153}Sm) is available as an alternative to strontium. This is conjugated with a phosphonate compound ethylene diamine tetraline tetramethyline phosphonic acid (EDTMP) and thereby preferentially taken up after intravenous administration into sites of bone remineralization. It is a beta particle emitter with an average energy of 233 KeV and a range of 3 mm in soft tissue. In addition, samarium produces low energy gamma rays at 103 KeV which gives the advantage that it can be imaged using a gamma camera, as shown in **Figure 20.6**. Administration is by single intravenous injection and formal phase I and II dose escalation studies[33][III] have shown optimal effect at a dose of 1 mCi/kg. It has been evaluated in randomized placebo-controlled double-blind trials[34][II] and found to have a demonstrable analgesic effect in hormone-resistant prostate cancer and breast cancer. Transient myelosuppression is seen from radiation dose to the bone marrow, which is rarely of clinical consequence and multiple doses of samarium at eight-week intervals have been described.

Iodine

Radioactive iodine has a specific indication in bone metastasis from metastatic differentiated thyroid cancer. Up to 80 percent of such tumors retain the characteristics of thyroid tissue and avidly concentrate radio-iodine. The

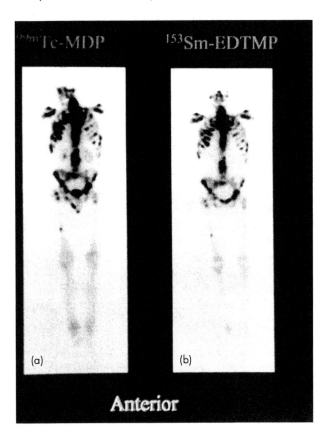

Figure 20.6 Gamma camera pictures of (a) technetium uptake in diagnostic bone scan and (b) samarium uptake after therapeutic administration.

[131]I isotope is used therapeutically.[35][III] Again, this isotope produces both beta and gamma emissions and can therefore be imaged on gamma camera scanning, in addition to delivering a localized radiation dose through its beta emission. Whilst the use of radio-iodine is well established in the management of thyroid cancer, it has in fact not been subject to randomized controlled trial evaluation. Single arm studies confirm lengthy survival in patients with metastatic thyroid cancer treated in this way and indeed radiographic remission of isotope concentrating metastases can be shown. Paradoxically, the effect on bone pain may be less striking and one paper[36][III] has suggested external beam radiotherapy may be more effective than radioisotope therapy in this situation.

Phosphorous

The isotope ^{32}P has in the past been evaluated for the treatment of metastatic bone pain. It is also used in the treatment of polycythemia since it is widely taken up in bone and will suppress bone marrow function. This is a major disadvantage when used for metastatic bone pain and with the development of more selective isotopes, including strontium and samarium, it is rarely used.

Rhenium

Rhenium has also been developed conjugated with a phosphonate compound [1-1-hydroethylidene diphosphate] analogous to the samarium compound. Two isotopes of rhenium are available, ^{186}Re and ^{188}Re. Most data are available for ^{186}Re-HEMP which appears very similar to samarium in its efficacy and pattern of response.[37][III] ^{188}Re has a potential advantage in being supplied in a rhenium generator which can be used to provide multiple doses of isotope relatively inexpensively.

CHEMOTHERAPY

When metastatic bone pain is due to widespread disease and particularly where, as may be the case, there is associated soft tissue metastasis as well, then systemic chemotherapy should be considered. The major limitations relate to the chemosensitivity of the primary sites commonly presenting with bone metastasis, as shown in **Table 20.5**. From this it will be apparent that there are perhaps four major indications for chemotherapy in metastatic bone pain.

1. Breast cancer has a greater than 50 percent response rate to most first-line chemotherapy.[38] [II] Many patients who present with bone metastasis will, however, have previously been exposed to adjuvant chemotherapy and this will be an increasing problem as more adjuvant chemotherapy is used. In the majority of cases the patient will be offered systemic chemotherapy, the drug combinations varying according to their

Table 20.5 Chemosensitivity of primary tumors commonly metastasizing to bone.

Primary site	Sensitivity[a]
Myeloma	High
Breast	High
Prostate	Low
Thyroid	Low
Bronchus	High
Kidney	Low
Rectum	Mid
Esophagus	Mid/low

[a]High >50% response rate; mid 25–50% response rate; low <25% response rate.

previous exposure. There are few published data on the efficacy of systemic chemotherapy in metastatic breast cancer specifically relating to bone pain relief. One review[39][III] has suggested that response in bone metastasis lags behind that in soft tissue with a median time to maximal response of 32 weeks.

2. Small cell lung cancer (SCLC) is a highly chemoresponsive disease. Patients presenting with metastatic disease will usually be offered some form of chemotherapy, specific drug combinations varying from time to time. A randomized trial reported by the United Kingdom Medical Research Council[40][II] has suggested that combination drug therapy may be better than single drug therapy using etoposide, although the actual gains are relatively modest. The role of chemotherapy at relapse is a little more controversial, but one published randomized trial[41][II] does support the use of second-line combination chemotherapy, with better symptom control than patients treated with "best supportive care."

3. Nonsmall cell lung cancer (NSCLC) is less sensitive to chemotherapy than SCLC but the results of randomized trials[42, 43][II] support the use of chemotherapy in NSCLC with improved quality of life and approximately two months survival advantage when compared to best supportive care. The common drugs used are combinations of cisplation or carboplatin with gemcitabine, paclitaxel, docetaxel, or vinorelbine in symptomatic patients. There has been no randomized comparison with radiotherapy and many patients have both chemotherapy and radiotherapy at different times in their disease.

4. Multiple myeloma is routinely treated with chemotherapy. First-line treatment will involve the use of either oral melphalan in combination with prednisolone and thalidomide[44][II] or combination chemotherapy containing high doses

of dexamethasone in combination with vincristine and adriamycin or idarubicin.[45][III] There are high response rates to this treatment both in terms of pain relief and suppression of the paraprotein, which is a useful marker of disease activity. However, few patients are cured, although younger patients achieving a good initial response will be selected to proceed to even more intensive treatment with high-dose chemotherapy resulting in prolonged periods of remission. At relapse, the role of chemotherapy is less certain but most patients will be re-exposed either to oral melphalan or cyclophosphamide or to high-dose dexamethasone-containing schedules[46][III] which can result in further remission in over 40 percent percent of patients. There is no randomized comparison of second-line chemotherapy against "best supportive care" in multiple myeloma.

Other primary sites may metastasize to bone and in some of these chemotherapy may be entirely appropriate. In general, hematological malignancies including lymphomas will be highly chemosensitive. Ovarian cancer and colorectal cancer are other less common sources of bone metastasis which may benefit.

HORMONE TREATMENT

Among the common sites that metastasize to bone, breast and prostate are hormone-sensitive and this may result in dramatic improvements in pain control for responsive patients.

Prostate cancer

Prostate cancer in virtually all cases is androgen-dependent at the time of presentation. Hormone therapy therefore aims to block androgen activity either pharmacologically using oral anti-androgens such as bicalutamide or flutamide, gonadotrophin-releasing hormone analogs such as goserelin or leuprolide, or surgical castration by orchidectomy. These individual methods of androgen ablation have been compared in multicenter randomized trials[47, 48] [II] and no advantage for one against the other has emerged. Similarly, whilst there have been advocates for "maximal androgen blockade," incorporating a central androgen blockade, such as goserelin, with peripheral androgen blockade using an oral anti-androgen drug meta-analysis[49][II] suggests there is no significant advantage for maximal androgen blockade in patients with metastatic disease. Single agent anti-androgen therapy is therefore indicated with response rates of 80 to 90 percent for pain relief which may occur dramatically within 24 hours of starting treatment. The duration of response to androgen therapy is limited with an average duration of two to three years, during which time androgen-independent cells emerge; further short-lived responses may be obtained by switching to second-line hormone therapy or adding a second anti-androgen to achieve maximal androgen blockade. Chemotherapy using single agent taxotere has been shown to improve quality of life and extend survival by two months in this group of patients.[50][II] It is in this group of "hormone-resistant" patients that wide field irradiation and systemic isotope therapy has been widely evaluated and has a major role.

Breast cancer

In many cases, breast cancer will also be hormone-sensitive. This is particularly the case in the postmenopausal woman when around 60 percent of patients will have demonstrable estrogen receptors on the surface of their malignant cells; this compares to approximately half that rate in premenopausal women.[51][III] The standard treatment for hormone-responsive breast cancer has been tamoxifen but newer aromatase inhibitor drugs such as anastrazole are replacing this. Many women now receive adjuvant hormone therapy at the time of their primary presentation as adjuvant treatment. Women who have not been previously exposed to tamoxifen or anastrazole should have this at the time of relapse with bone metastasis; those who have had previous adjuvant hormone therapy will be considered for second-line hormone therapy, such as a progestogen such as medroxyprogesterone or megestrol, and up to 50 percent of women may achieve a second response with objective tumor shrinkage. The impact of this on pain control is less well documented and radiotherapy is often also required in this setting.

Endometrium

Carcinoma of the endometrium is responsive to progestogens. Bone metastases are relatively unusual in this tumor but when encountered, progestogens in the form of megestrol or medroxyprogesterone acetate may be of value for multiple sites of bone pain.

Bisphosphonates

Bisphosphonates are a class of drug originally developed for use in metabolic bone disease, such as osteoporosis and Paget's disease. The first generation drugs such as etidronate have subsequently been replaced with the development of more potent drugs. The most commonly used currently are clodronate, pamidronate, and zolendronate, which have an increasing role in the management of metastatic bone disease. Their mode of action is through inhibiting the function of osteoclasts. Since the initial response in the process of a bone metastasis being established is osteoclast activation, they have been investigated as a potential means of inhibiting the development of bone metastasis in patients who are at high risk. There are now phase III randomized placebo-controlled trial data supporting this effect in myeloma[52] [II] and breast cancer.[53, 54][II] Although the magnitude of effect is relatively modest, bisphosphonates are standard adjuvant treatment in myeloma and breast cancer patients at high risk of bone metastases.

A second role for bisphosphonates in the management of bone metastasis is in the treatment of established disease. Single arm studies in patients with metastases, predominantly from breast cancer and thyroid cancer, have demonstrated radiological and biochemical responses with x-ray bone healing of lytic lesions and a reduction in markers of osteoclast activity[55][III] such as urinary deoxypyridinoline, urinary calcium, and serum IL6. It is also clear that a number of patients with metastatic bone pain have good pain relief with the use of bisphosphonate drugs. This has now been shown in both single arm studies and double-blind placebo-controlled trials[56][II] using clodronate or pamidronate. Whilst the greatest body of data is in patients with breast cancer, several other sites have been included in these studies with no apparent difference in their response, albeit within small subgroups.

The relative role of bisphosphonates alongside the other measures for pain relief remains uncertain. A Cochrane review has identified four randomized controlled trials addressing this issue, all of which confirm efficacy for pain relief, but concluded that they could not be considered standard treatment and should be reserved for those patients failing to respond to analgesics, NSAIDs, and radiotherapy.[57][I]

SURGERY

Surgery has an important role in the management of impending or actual pathological fracture associated with bone metastasis. Occasionally, this may be the first presentation of the malignancy when diagnostic information from the bone biopsy at the time of fixation is also of vital importance.

Patients with advanced lytic disease are at high risk of fracture. Specific criteria for internal fixation to prevent fracture have been defined:[58][V]

- lytic lesions > 2.5 cm in diameter;
- > 50 percent cortical destruction;
- diffuse lytic disease in a weight-bearing area.

In established pathological fracture of a long bone, then internal fixation, where possible and appropriate, is undoubtedly the best management for early pain relief and mobility. The other indication for surgery is vertebral collapse where there is associated compression of the spinal canal and spinal instability. In this setting, radiotherapy alone is not adequate and anterior spinal stabilization and fusion is indicated.[59, 60][II]

Following surgery for pathological fracture, postoperative radiotherapy is generally recommended. Whilst this is standard practice, there is limited evidence supporting its value.[61][IV] It is based on the hypothesis that surgery does not eradicate or even suppress residual tumor within the bone and anecdotally areas of internal fixation left alone have subsequent complications with further bone destruction. In practice, postoperative

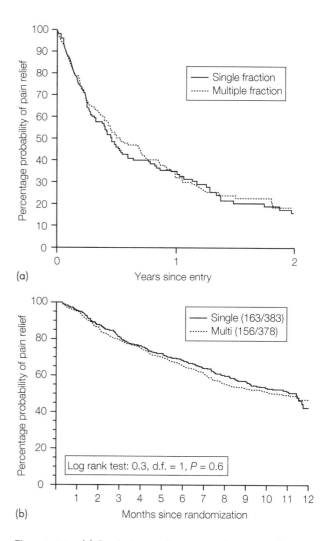

Figure 20.7 (a) Survival curve for patients from time of localized radiotherapy for metastatic bone pain (redrawn with permission from *Radiotherapy and Oncology*, 6, Price P, Hoskin PJ, Easton D *et al.*, Prospective randomised trial of single and multifraction radiotherapy schedules in the treatment of painful bony metastases, 247–55, © Elsevier (1986); (b) Survival curve for patients from time of localized radiotherapy for metastatic bone pain in a population selected for a projected survival of at least one year from the time of treatment (redrawn with permission from *Radiotherapy and Oncology*, 52, Bone Pain Trial Working Party, 8 Gy single fraction radiotherapy for the treatment of metastatic skeletal pain: randomised comparison with a multifraction schedule over 12 months of patient follow-up, 111–21, © Elsevier (1999).

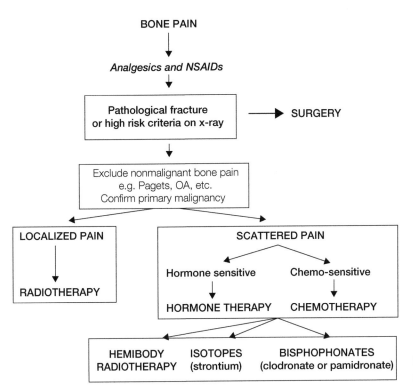

Figure 20.8 Overview of the management of metastatic bone pain.

radiotherapy is selected for patients with a life expectancy of more than three months following fixation.

PROGNOSIS

The prognosis for metastatic bone pain is relatively good with over 80 percent of patients having pain relief and up to one-third achieving complete control of pain. The onset of pain relief with radiotherapy will be seen within four to six weeks and in patients who survive, prolonged relief for many weeks and months can be expected. There is also evidence that if pain returns, retreatment with radiotherapy is of equal value to initial treatment.[20][III]

The efficacy of radiotherapy in metastatic bone pain has been subject to a meta-analyses,[13, 14, 15][I] which included all trials in which there was objective measurement of pain and recorded response rates. One of these[13] [I] has reported results in terms of the number of patients needed to treat (NNT) for an effect. For any pain response, the NNT was 3.6 and for complete pain response the NNT was 3.9.

In contrast, the prognosis for survival in patients with bone metastasis is poor, as shown in a representative survival curve of patients treated for bone metastasis in **Figure 20.7a**. Since these will also represent a selected sample of patients fit enough to attend for radiotherapy, it is likely the actual survival of the entire population of patients with bone metastasis is even worse, reflecting the presence of widespread disseminated cancer often accompanied by soft tissue disease and poor performance status, which in the absence of an effective systemic anticancer therapy results in death within a few months.

The small number of patients surviving for a year or more are typically those with breast or prostate cancer who have not previously received hormone therapy. Even when patients are selected for longer survival, the actual survival is poor, as demonstrated in **Figure 20.7b** from a trial in which the entry criteria was an expected survival of more than one year. It can be seen that even in this group the actual survival is poor.

SPECIAL COMMENTS

Bone metastases result in considerable morbidity. A range of treatments are available which are largely complementary and should be considered as a comprehensive strategy to enable pain control and retain the performance status of the patient. This is illustrated in **Figure 20.8**.

Finally, metastatic bone pain should not be considered in isolation. Few patients with advanced cancer have a single site or cause of pain and this applies as much, if not more so, to bone metastasis as any other scenario. In particular, associated musculoskeletal pain, neuropathic pain, nerve compression with the associated problems of motor weakness, and degenerative bone disease must all be considered in the overall management of the patient.

REFERENCES

1. Abrams HL, Spiro R, Goldstein N. Metastases in carcinoma. Analysis of 1000 autopsied cases. *Cancer.* 1950; 3: 74–85.
2. Ross Garrett I. Bone destruction in cancer. *Seminars in Oncology.* 1993; 20 (Suppl. 2): 4–9.

3. Cranston PE, Patel RB, Harrison RB. Computed tomography for metastatic lesions of the osseous pelvis. *Journal of Computer Assisted Tomography.* 1984; **8**: 582.

4. Rimmer WD, Berquist TH, McLeod RA *et al.* Bone tumours: magnetic resonance imaging versus computed tomography. *Radiology.* 1985; **155**: 709–15.

5. Spencer JA, Chng WJ, Hudson E *et al.* Prostate specific antigen level and Gleason score in predicting the stage of newly diagnosed prostate cancer. *British Journal of Radiology.* 1998; **71**: 1130–5.

6. Mercadante S, Fulfaro F, Casuccio A. A randomised controlled study on the use of anti-inflammatory drugs in patients with cancer pain on morphine therapy: effects on dose escalation and a pharmacoeconomic analysis. *European Journal of Cancer.* 2002; **38**: 1358–63.

7. McQuay HJ, Moore A. Non-opioid analgesics. In: Doyle D, Hanks GW, Cherny N, Calman K (eds). *Oxford textbook of palliative medicine*, 3rd edn. Oxford: Oxford University Press, 2004: 342–8.

8. Coombes RC, Munro Neville A, Gazet J-C *et al.* Agents affecting osteolysis in patients with breast cancer. *Cancer Chemotherapy and Pharmacology.* 1979; **3**: 41–4.

9. McQuay H, Moore A. *An evidence-based resource for pain relief.* Oxford: Oxford University Press, 1998: 196.

＊ 10. Eisenberg E, Berkey CS, Carr DB *et al.* Efficacy and safety of nonsteroidal anti-inflammatory drugs for cancer pain: a meta-analysis. *Journal of Clinical Oncology.* 1994; **12**: 2756–65.

11. Levick S, Jacobs C, Loukas D *et al.* Naproxen sodium in the treatment of bone pain due to metastatic cancer. *Pain.* 1988; **35**: 253–8.

12. van der Linden YM, Kroon HM, Dijkstra PD *et al.* Simple radiographic parameter predicts fracturing in metastatic femoral bone lesions: results from a randomized trial. *Radiotherapy and Oncology.* 2003; **69**: 21–31.

＊ 13. McQuay HJ, Carroll D, Moore RA. Radiotherapy for painful bone metastases: a systematic review. *Clinical Oncology.* 1997; **9**: 150–4.

＊ 14. Sze WM, Shelley MD, Held I *et al.* Palliation of metastatic bone pain: single fraction versus multifraction radiotherapy – a systematic review of randomised trial. *Clinical Oncology.* 2003; **15**: 345–52.

＊ 15. Wu JS, Wong R, Johnston M *et al.* Meta-analysis of dose-fractionation radiotherapy trials for the palliation of painful bone metastases. *International Journal of Radiation Oncology, Biology, Physics.* 2003; **55**: 594–605.

16. Bone Pain Trial Working Party. 8Gy single fraction radiotherapy for the treatment of metastatic skeletal pain: randomised comparison with a multifraction schedule over 12 months of patient follow-up. *Radiotherapy and Oncology.* 1999; **52**: 111–21.

17. Price P, Hoskin PJ, Easton D *et al.* Prospective randomised trial of single and multifraction radiotherapy schedules in the treatment of painful bony metastases. *Radiotherapy and Oncology.* 1986; **6**: 247–55.

18. Roos DE, Turner SL, O'Brien PC *et al.* Randomized trial of 8Gy in 1 versus 20Gy in 5 fractions of radiotherapy for neuropathic pain due to bone metastases (TROG 96.05). *Radiotherapy and Oncology.* 2005; **75**: 54–63.

19. van der Linden YM, Lok JJ, Steenland E *et al.* Single fraction radiotherapy is efficacious: a further analysis of the Dutch Bone Metastasis Study controlling for the influence of retreatment. *Radiotherapy and Oncology.* 2004; **59**: 528–37.

20. Mithal NP, Needham PR, Hoskin PJ. Retreatment with radiotherapy for painful bone metastases. *International Journal of Radiation Oncology, Biology, Physics.* 1994; **29**: 1011–14.

21. Salazar OM, Rubin P, Hendricksen F *et al.* Single-dose half body irradiation for palliation of multiple bone metastases from solid tumours. *Cancer.* 1986; **58**: 29–36.

22. Hoskin PJ, Ford HT, Harmer CL. Hemibody irradiation (HBI) for metastatic bone pain in two histological distinct groups of patients. *Clinical Oncology.* 1989; **1**: 67–9.

23. Fitzpatrick PJ. Wide-field irradiation of bone metastases. In: Weiss L, Gilbert HA (eds). *Bone metastasis.* Boston: GK Hall, 1981: 83–113.

24. Qasim MM. Half body irradiation (HBI) in metastatic carcinomas. *Clinical Radiology.* 1981; **32**: 215–19.

25. Douglas P, Rossier Ph, Mirimanoff R-O, Coucke PA. Third-body irradiation as an effective palliative treatment for painful multiple bone metastases resistant to chemo- or hormonal treatment. *Radiotherapy and Oncology.* 1993; **28**: 76–8.

＊ 26. Salazar OM, Sandhu T, DaMotta NW *et al.* Fractionated half body irradiation (HBI) for the rapid palliation of widespread symptomatic metastatic bone disease: a randomised phase III trial of the International Atomic Energy Agency (IAEA). *International Journal of Radiation Oncology, Biology, Physics.* 2001; **50**: 765–75.

27. Hoskin PJ. Strontium. In: Dollery C (ed.). *Drug therapy supplement 2.* Edinburgh: Churchill Livingstone, 1994.

28. Laing AH, Ackery DM, Bayly RJ *et al.* Strontium-89 chloride for pain palliation in prostatic skeletal malignancy. *British Journal of Radiology.* 1991; **64**: 816–22.

29. Lewington VJ, McEwan AJ, Ackery DM *et al.* A prospective randomized double-blind crossover study to examine the efficacy of strontium-89 in pain palliation in patients with advanced prostate cancer metastatic to bone. *European Journal of Cancer.* 1991; **27**: 954–8.

＊ 30. Quilty PM, Kirk D, Bolger JJ *et al.* A comparison of the palliative effects of strontium-89 and external beam radiotherapy in metastatic prostate cancer. *Radiotherapy and Oncology.* 1994; **31**: 33–40.

31. Dearnaley DP, Bayley RJ, A'Hern RP *et al.* Palliation of bone metastases in prostate cancer: Hemibody irradiation or strontium-89. *Clinical Oncology.* 1992; **4**: 101–07.

32. Kasalicky J, Krajska V. The effect of repeated strontium therapy on bone pain palliation in patients with skeletal cancer metastases. *European Journal of Nuclear Medicine.* 1998; **25**: 1362–7.

33. Resche I, Chatal J-F, Pecking A *et al.* A dose-controlled study of [153] Sm-Ethylenediaminetetramethylenephosphonate

(EDTMP) in the treatment of patients with painful bone metastases. *European Journal of Cancer.* 1997; **33**: 1583–91.

* 34. Sartor O, Reid RH, Hoskin PJ *et al.* Samarium-153-Lexidronam complex for treatment of painful bone metastases in hormone-refractory prostate cancer. *Urology.* 2004; **63**: 940–5.

35. Tubiana M, Lacour J, Monnier MD *et al.* External radiotherapy and radioiodine in the treatment of 359 thyroid cancers. *British Journal of Radiology.* 1975; **48**: 894–907.

36. Brown AP, Greening WP, McCready VR *et al.* Radioiodine treatment of metastatic thyroid carcinoma: The Royal Marsden Hospital experience. *British Journal of Radiology.* 1984; **57**: 232–7.

37. Maxon III HR, Schroder LE, Hertzberg VS *et al.* Rhenium-186(Sn)HEDP for treatment of painful osseous metastases: Results of a double-blind crossover comparison with placebo. *Journal of Nuclear Medicine.* 1991; **32**: 1877–81.

38. Honig SF. Hormonal therapy and chemotherapy. In: Harris JR, Lippman M, Morrow M, Hellman S (eds). *Diseases of the breast.* Philadelphia: Lippincott Raven, 1996: 669–734.

39. Smith IE, Macaulay V. Comparison of different endocrine therapies in management of bone metastases from breast carcinoma. *Journal of the Royal Society of Medicine.* 1985; **78** (Suppl. 9): 15–21.

40. Medical Research Council Lung Cancer Working Party. Comparison of oral etoposide and standard intravenous multidrug chemotherapy for small-cell lung cancer: a stopped multicentre randomised trial. *Lancet.* 1996; **348**: 563–6.

41. Spiro SG, Souhami RL, Geddes DM *et al.* Duration of chemotherapy in small cell lung cancer: A Cancer Research Campaign trial. *British Journal of Cancer.* 1989; **59**: 578–83.

42. Ellis PA, Smith IE, Hardy JR. Symptom relief with MVP (mitomycin C, vinblastine and cisplatin) chemotherapy in advanced non-small-cell lung cancer. *British Journal of Cancer.* 1995; **71**: 366–70.

* 43. Schiller JH, Harrington D, Belani C *et al.* Comparison of four chemotherapy regimens for advanced non-small-cell lung cancer. *New England Journal of Medicine.* 2002; **346**: 92–8.

* 44. Palumbo A, Bringen S, Caravita T *et al.* Oral melphalan and prednisone chemotherapy plus thalidomide compared with melphalan and prednisone alone in elderly patients with multiple myeloma: randomised controlled trial. *Lancet.* 2006; **367**: 825–31.

45. Cook G, Clark RE, Morris TC *et al.* A randomized study (WOS MM1) comparing the oral regime Z-Dex (idarubicin and dexamethasone) with vincristine, adriamycin and dexamethasone as induction therapy for newly diagnosed patients with multiple myeloma. *British Journal of Haematology.* 2004; **126**: 792–8.

46. Alexanian R, Dimopoulos MA, Delasalle K, Barlogie B. Primary dexamethasone treatment of multiple myeloma. *Blood.* 1992; **80**: 887–90.

47. Newling DW. Anti-androgens in the treatment of prostate cancer. *British Journal of Urology.* 1996; **77**: 776–84.

48. Galbraith SM, Duchesne GM. Androgens and prostate cancer: biology, pathology and hormonal therapy. *European Journal of Cancer.* 1997; **33**: 545–54.

* 49. Prostate Cancer Trialists Collaborative Group. Maximum androgren blockade in advanced prostate cancer: an overview of 33 randomised trials with 3283 deaths in 5710 patients. *Lancet.* 1995; **346**: 265–9.

50. Tannock IF, de Wit R, Berry WR *et al.* Docetaxel plus prednisone or mitoxantrone plus prednisone for advanced prostate cancer. *New England Journal of Medicine.* 2004; **351**: 1502–12.

51. Honig SF. Hormonal therapy and chemotherapy. In: Harris JR, Lippman ME, Morrow M, Hellmann S (eds). *Diseases of the breast.* Philadelphia: Lippincott-Raven Publishers, 1996: 669–734.

* 52. McCloskey EV, MacLennan ICM, Drayson MT *et al.* A randomized trial of the effect of clodronate on skeletal morbidity in multiple myeloma. MRC Working Party on Leukaemia in Adults. *British Journal of Haematology.* 1998; **100**: 317–25.

53. Paterson AH, Powles TJ, Kanis JA *et al.* Double-blind controlled trial in patients with bone metastases from breast cancer. *Journal of Clinical Oncology.* 1993; **11**: 59–65.

54. Diel IJ, Solomayer E-F, Costa SD *et al.* Reduction in new metastases in breast cancer with adjuvant clodronate treatment. *New England Journal of Medicine.* 1998; **339**: 357–63.

55. Coleman RE, Houston S, Purohit OP *et al.* A randomised phase II study of oral pamidronate for the treatment of bone metastases from breast cancer. *European Journal of Cancer.* 1998; **34**: 820–4.

56. Bloomfield DJ. Should bisphosphonates be part of the standard therapy of patients with multiple myeloma or bone metastases from other cancers? An evidence-based review. *Journal of Clinical Oncology.* 1998; **16**: 1218–25.

* 57. Wong R, Wiffen PJ. Bisphosphonates for the relief of pain secondary to bone metastases. *Cochrane Database of Systematic Reviews.* 2002; **CD002068**.

58. Harrington KD. Impending pathological fractures from metastatic malignancy: Evolution and management. *Instructional Course Lectures.* 1986; **35**: 357–81.

59. Siegal T, Siegal T. Surgical decompression of anterior and posterior malignant epidural tumours compressing the spinal cord: A prospective study. *Neurosurgery.* 1985; **17**: 424–32.

60. Patchell R, Tibbs PA, Regine WF *et al.* Direct decompressive surgical resection in the treatment of spinal cord compression caused by metastatic cancer: a randomised trial. *Lancet.* 2005; **366**: 643–8.

61. Hardman PDJ, Robb JE, Kerr GR *et al.* The value of internal fixation and radiotherapy in the management of upper and lower limb bone metastases. *Clinical Oncology.* 1992; **4**: 244–8.

21

Complementary therapies

JACQUELINE FILSHIE AND ADRIAN WHITE

Introduction	270	Massage and aromatherapy	277
Acupuncture	271	Healing (UK and elsewhere) equivalent to therapeutic	
Herbal medicine (phytotherapy)	274	touch (US)	278
Homeopathy	275	Music therapy	278
Hypnosis	275	Conclusions	279
Relaxation, distraction, and visualization	277	References	279

KEY LEARNING POINTS

- Complementary therapies are used by to 84 percent of cancer patients, mainly for symptom control and psychological support. This could imply a significant need that is not met in conventional health care.
- Acupuncture is a needling therapy that modulates endogenous analgesic systems and other substances for pain and symptom control.
- Herbal preparations may alter the bioavailability of conventional medications including chemotherapeutic agents and hormones. Patients should be routinely asked about their use of complementary therapies.

- Hypnosis and self-hypnosis can reduce pain and other symptoms, such as anticipatory nausea and vomiting.
- Massage therapy, music therapy, and healing and homeopathy are widely used but more evidence is required on their effectiveness.
- Patients need to be aware that, along with the potential benefits of complementary therapies, there are possible dangers including exploitation by unscrupulous practitioners and claims that are unfounded in evidence.

INTRODUCTION

Complementary therapies are methods of treatment which provide a range of physical and emotional support, but are usually regarded as falling outside mainstream medicine. Some are not far removed from it, having something of a scientific basis: this includes therapies such as acupuncture, hypnosis, and massage therapy. Other therapies, such as crystal healing and iridology, use concepts that are very different from conventional treatment and are often considered to be implausible. This range of therapies is reflected in the labels that are commonly used, from "integrative" through "complementary" to "alternative"

medicine. Complementary therapists often stress their "holistic" attitude, but of course healthcare staff in mainstream medicine are also aware of the importance of the therapeutic relationship and attention to every aspect of a person's physical and emotional needs, particularly at critical times in life such as after a diagnosis of cancer has been made.

Complementary medicine (CM) is increasingly popular among the general public, and cancer patients are no exception. A review of 26 surveys of use of CM by cancer patients in 13 different countries found that the rate varied from 7 to 64 percent, with an average of about 31–34 percent.[1] Molassiotis et al.[2] showed a range of use of 15–73 percent (average 36 percent) in European countries, often involving more than one therapy.[2] Among children, rates of use were up to 84 percent.[3] Patients who used CM tended to be younger, were more likely to be female, and to come from a higher socioeconomic group than those who made no use of CM.[4] The most common therapies used by oncology patients in the UK were healing, relaxation, visualization, diet, homeopathy, vitamins, and herbal therapy. In children, factors associated with CM use include poor prognosis, higher parental education, faith, and previous use of CM.[5]

In one survey of CM usage (using a highly inclusive definition) among breast cancer patients in the USA, the most popular therapy was prayer (76 percent), followed by exercise (38 percent), spiritual healing (29 percent), and megavitamins (25 percent).[6] A survey of healthcare professionals identified five therapies of greatest interest, namely: acupuncture, massage therapy, hypnosis or self-hypnosis, therapeutic touch, and biofeedback.[7]

The reasons why patients with cancer turn to CM have been explored.[8, 9] Fundamental, unsurprisingly, is the fact that orthodox medicine has not delivered a cure. The fact that interest in CM is increasing can be seen as part of the rise in consumerism, particularly the wish for self-empowerment and the desire to cope, both physically and psychologically. Patients are looking for therapies that are natural and gentle and which emphasize caring – partly as a reaction to the perceived deficiencies of conventional medicine, which has become increasingly objective and technical. Further, CM is more widely available and accessible, and the public are more aware of it because of increased exposure in the media. Not least, patients may have an underlying but unstated wish for a magical cure. This may leave them open to exploitation, particularly via the internet. Complementary therapies are accessed at any point in the cancer journey, from diagnosis, through therapy, at tumor recurrence, and in late stage cancer. In a systematic review on patients' reasons for accessing CM, Verhoef and colleagues[10] found these included the need for a therapeutic response, wanting control, a strong belief in CM, CM as a last resort, and finding hope.

The attitude of medical, nursing, and allied professions towards CM is changing from antagonism towards productive coexistence.[11, 12] Many people working in the caring professions feel more comfortable with the role of touch, time, support, and care, in a wider, holistic approach to medicine for palliation of symptoms. Far from continuing to reject all unconventional approaches, medical staff are increasingly willing to integrate therapies that seem to have something valuable to offer.[13] These include:

- therapies directed at control of symptoms: mainly pain, but also anxiety, nausea, and vomiting;
- mind-body therapies that help patients come to terms with their disease and adopt a positive approach;

- sensible nutritional advice plus exercise or relaxation therapies that improve general health;
- psychosocial support.

On the other hand, medical staff continue to be appropriately suspicious of other aspects of alternative therapies which have no supporting evidence and may be potentially harmful, including:

- severe dietary regimens, particularly damaging to debilitated patients;
- herbs, megavitamins, and food supplements: promotion of bogus cures is a "scam" with a long history;[8] such cures may even sometimes be promoted by state authorities on anecdotal evidence, as in the "di Bella" episode;[14]
- spiritual or psychological interventions which emphasize the individual's emotions or behavior as the cause of cancer, and therefore create guilt and misery in patients;
- therapists who have little experience of dealing with cancer and who raise false hopes, believing they can correct "fundamental imbalances"; this is particularly likely to be misleading when their treatment happens to coincide with a remission due to conventional therapy.

There are, therefore, numerous reasons why patients and their practitioners of all kinds increasingly need access to high quality information about the evidence for or against CM use in cancer.

ACUPUNCTURE

History and introduction

The first known text on acupuncture, The Yellow Emperor's Classic of Internal Medicine (*Huang Ti Nei Ching*), dates from about 200BC,[15] though it has been suggested that acupuncture may have originated in the Eurasian continent 2000 years earlier because of tattoos, corresponding to acupuncture points, that were found on the Alpine hunter Ötzi, whose body was preserved in a glacier.[16]

The traditional Chinese approach, with an elaborate system of diagnosis and therapy involving needling precise locations to "harmonize Yin and Yang",[17] is challenged by western understanding of anatomy and physiology, and there is increasing interest in a western approach to acupuncture, based on neurophysiological and neuropharmacological evidence. Western medical acupuncturists use a combination of traditional, segmental, and trigger points for their effects on the nervous system. This approach is commensurate with conventional medical practice.[18, 19]

The various approaches to treatment with acupuncture include:

- traditional Chinese acupuncture, in which manual stimulation of the needles elicits "De Qi," a strange sensation of heaviness and numbness. Needles are usually retained for about 20 minutes. Moxibustion, a thermal stimulation from burning a special herb, may also be used;[20]
- western medical acupuncture, within conventional medical treatment; the strength and duration of needling are variable;[18, 19]
- continuous treatment with indwelling needles, typically in the shape of tiny drawing-pins, to prolong the effects of acupuncture without the need to attend clinic;[21]
- electroacupuncture at low or high frequency (2 Hz up to 100 Hz) for pain relief, and for acupuncture analgesia;[22]
- laser therapy (using low power, nonthermal laser) used at acupuncture points with the aim of reducing pain and enhancing tissue healing;[23]
- auriculoacupuncture, or ear acupuncture, used for a variety of painful and nonpainful conditions,[24] and other "micro-systems" such as scalp acupuncture,[25] needling areas of rich innervation;
- ryodoraku is a Japanese form of acupuncture in which disease states are assessed from skin impedance and supposedly addressed by electrical stimulation;[26]
- acupressure (Shiatsu) involves pressure on traditional acupuncture points and is often regarded as a weaker form of stimulation than needle acupuncture.

Acupuncture is the first-line treatment for many painful and nonpainful conditions in China and is increasingly available in both primary and secondary care in the west, for example in about 85 percent of chronic pain services in the UK.[27, 28]

A typical course of treatment for noncancer chronic pain would be once weekly for six weeks (or twice weekly for three weeks) with further "top ups" as necessary. For treating cancer pain, a more gentle approach is necessary and the "dose" should be modified depending on the patient's response. If there is no pain relief whatsoever after three treatments, it is probably better to stop when life expectancy is short. However, a small but significant number of patients obtain significant relief after six treatments – this is the minimum number of treatments that has been shown to be necessary for the relief of pain of mixed origin.[29]

Clinical trial evidence

The balance of evidence supports the role of acupuncture in the treatment of some painful conditions including dental pain,[30][II] experimental pain,[31][II] headache,[32][II] knee osteoarthritis,[33][I] and low back pain[34, 35][I] when compared with sham acupuncture or with usual care.

Kotani et al.,[36][II] in a well-designed study on postoperative pain following upper and lower gastrointestinal surgery, showed that semipermanent indwelling needles inserted preoperatively reduced postoperative pain and analgesic requirements, as well as nausea and vomiting, compared with sham semipermanent needles. Considering postoperative or "acute" pain in cancer patients, two studies by Poulain and colleagues[37] on patients undergoing major abdominal surgery are relevant. In an open, randomized controlled trial (RCT), 250 patients who received electroacupuncture before and during surgery needed lower doses of conventional analgesic drugs.[37] In a double-blinded study in 42 patients, electroacupuncture given peroperatively produced superior analgesia to sham acupuncture (Poulain, personal communication, 1993). Both studies also suggested that acupuncture enhanced postoperative recovery. A further RCT showed that acupuncture increased mobility and reduced pain after breast surgery with axillary lymph node removal.[38][II]

Studies of acupuncture for treatment of cancer pain were reviewed by Lee et al.[39] Seven studies (n = 368) were included: three RCTs (n = 214) and four uncontrolled studies (n = 154). One of the three RCTs was of high quality (score five points); the other two were of poor quality, scoring only one point each (for randomization). Major methodological limitations of the included studies were small sample size, the lack of a statistical comparison between treatments, use of unreliable or subjective outcome measures, lack of consistent protocols, and poor reporting.

The one high-quality RCT in 90 patients with chronic central or neuropathic pain recruited at a pain management unit found that ear acupuncture significantly reduced pain intensity, on a visual analog scale (VAS), compared with placebo ear acupuncture at day 30 (p = 0.02) and day 60 (p < 0.001).[40][II] The pain reduction at two months in the acupuncture group was 36 percent compared with 2 percent in the placebo group (p < 0.0001). The remaining poor-quality RCTs (n = 48 and n = 76) found mixed results: one found no significant difference between body acupuncture and control, while the other found body acupuncture improved chest pain. thus the results were "unproved not disproved."

Three of the four uncontrolled studies (n ranged from 10 to 92) found pain relief with acupuncture; the other study found no effect on pain. Three studies reported mild or no adverse effects; the other four studies did not mention adverse effects.

The evidence is therefore somewhat sparse at present. Another review found eight clinical trials, and concluded that, "Although most of these studies were positive and demonstrated the effectiveness of acupuncture in cancer pain control, the findings have limited significance because of methodologic weakness …".[41]

Despite the lack of rigorous controlled trials of acupuncture for cancer pain, a number of observational studies show that acupuncture can produce considerable benefit for patients in pain. As early as 1973, Mann *et al.*[42] described short-lived pain relief in eight patients with intractable cancer pain. In Hong Kong, Wen[43] described using several electroacupuncture sessions daily for terminal cancer patients, gradually reducing the number of sessions once pain control was established. This treatment was successful in treating pain in patients who were resistant to opioids or who had pain and opioid toxicity. Filshie and colleagues[44, 45] summarize two audits of the use of acupuncture for pain control in a heterogeneous cancer population whose pain had not responded to conventional pharmacological approaches. The results from both studies are presented here, representing 339 patients who were given a course of at least three weekly treatments of manual acupuncture. Between 52 and 56 percent of patients had worthwhile long-lasting relief after three weekly sessions, though subsequent top-ups were necessary. The interval between treatments could usually be increased progressively. Pain related to oncological treatment (postsurgical and irradiation) showed more prolonged analgesia than that due to metastatic disease. A further 21–30 percent had short-lived analgesia of up to two days and may have benefited from more frequent treatments per week. Between 18 and 22 percent had no significant pain relief. It was noted that the greater the tumor load, the shorter acting the relief. Patients who developed new metastatic disease often suddenly experienced a shorter duration of pain relief than they had previously enjoyed with acupuncture; once the metastasis was treated, the patients often responded to acupuncture again. Muscle spasm was particularly helped by acupuncture treatment and mobility often increased substantially.

In a further audit of treatment for pain in breast cancer patients associated with surgery, radiotherapy or tumor in the chest, axilla, and arm, psychological profiles were recorded. After one month of acupuncture, statistically significant reductions were seen in average pain, worst pain, interference with lifestyle, distress, pain behavior, and depression.[46] Other studies have shown equally good results, and clearly more comparative trials are urgently needed.

An audit of a palliative care physician's first year of acupuncture practice found that 31 of 50 (62 percent) complaints of pain showed a "good" or "excellent" response, as measured by a verbal rating scale.[47]

The problem of maintaining the pain-relieving effects of acupuncture in late stage disease has been overcome by the use of semi-permanent indwelling acupuncture needles inserted into a tender area in the ear.[48] In a sample of 28 patients in a hospice setting, massaging the studs at times of intense pain resulted in a statistically significant reduction in pain.

Mechanisms of action

The neurophysiology of acupuncture is summarized in numerous articles and reviews.[49, 50, 51, 52, 53] The salient evidence is as follows:

- Many acupuncture points are richly innervated.[54]
- The effects of acupuncture are prevented by prior local anesthetic injection.[55, 56]
- Acupuncture analgesia appears to depend on stimulation of small unmyelinated nerve fibers.[57]
- Acupuncture has considerable influence on the limbic system, which is the probable explanation for its ability to reduce the affective component of pain.[53, 58]
- There is little evidence to support the meridian theories, though they may be explained by the referral patterns from trigger points which are often close to traditional acupuncture points.[59] Another hypothesis involves conduction of electrical signals via liquid crystal formation of collagen fibers.[60]
- Acupuncture releases β endorphins, enkephalins, and dynorphins which act on mu, delta, and kappa receptors, respectively, though not specifically. At least 15 lines of evidence have been advanced to support the opioidergic theory of acupuncture analgesia.[49]
- Cholecystokinin is also released by acupuncture, yet is antagonistic to endogenous opioids. This may in part explain the phenomenon of tolerance to acupuncture.[61]
- Acupuncture may also act by diffuse noxious inhibitory control.[62]
- Serotonin, a neurotransmitter involved in analgesia and mood elevation, is released by acupuncture.[63]
- Oxytocin, which has both analgesic and anxiolytic properties in addition to its other functions, is released by sensory stimulation such as acupuncture.[64]
- Myofascial trigger points often overlap with acupuncture points,[65, 66] and treatment by dry needling is used for many myofascial pain syndromes.[67, 68, 69]
- Acupuncture has been found to release adrenocorticotropic (ACTH)[70] hormone and therefore has the potential to reduce inflammation.
- Acupuncture has widespread autonomic effects on blood flow, blood pressure, and gastric motility.[71, 72]
- There is increasing evidence that changes in expression of pain inhibitory transmitters may contribute to the sustained effects of acupuncture.[73, 74]

Acupuncture for cancer symptoms other than pain

Beneficial side effects, such as coincidental alleviation of other longstanding symptoms, can often be an unexpected bonus of treatment with acupuncture. A Cochrane review of 26 trials showed that acupuncture at the point PC6, near the wrist, reduces postoperative nausea and the need for rescue antiemetics, compared with the sham treatment.[75][I]

In another Cochrane review, acupuncture was also shown to reduce the nausea of chemotherapy.[76][I] Self-administered acupressure appears to have a protective effect for acute nausea and can readily be taught to patients, though these studies did not involve placebo control.

In a pilot study, acupuncture has been shown to be effective for treating dyspnea in 14 out of 20 patients with advanced, cancer-related breathlessness.[77] There was statistically significant subjective benefit as well as reduction in the respiratory rate, measured objectively. A significant reduction of anxiety accompanied the relief. Semi-permanent indwelling studs were inserted to prolong relief.

Several studies have shown that acupuncture increases salivary flow in patients with Sjogren's syndrome or radiation damage to the salivary glands.[51, 78, 79] Acupuncture has helped to heal radionecrotic ulcers, which normally have an extremely poor prognosis.[80] Hot flushes induced by treatment, such as tamoxifen, were reduced by manual acupuncture, with the addition of indwelling acupuncture studs in resistant cases.[21, 81, 82] Recent work has also shown the benefit of acupuncture treatment for vasomotor symptoms induced by therapy of prostate cancer.[83] For further details of the actions of acupuncture on non-pain symptoms, refer to Thompson and Filshie.[84]

Complications and contraindications

Side effects of acupuncture have been classified as follows:

- infective (single use disposable needles should always be used);
- traumatic, for example pneumothorax (good anatomical knowledge is essential; particular care necessary in cachectic patients);
- needle fracture;
- miscellaneous, including syncope, bruising, and sedation.

Severe adverse effects are rare, but there are some 700 reports of serious adverse events in the literature over 30 years.[85] In cancer patients, acupuncture should be avoided in any area of spinal instability, as it may reduce protective muscle spasm and expose the patient to the risk of cord compression or transection.[86] It should also be avoided in any lymphedematous limbs or limbs prone to lymphedema, such as postaxillary dissection.[87] Severely disordered clotting function is a further contraindication. Electroacupuncture should not be used in patients with a demand pacemaker.

HERBAL MEDICINE (PHYTOTHERAPY)

Herbs are part of traditional medicine in most cultures, and a variety of herbal, mineral, and animal products and combinations are frequently promoted for use in cancer. In some studies, over 50 percent of cancer patients use herbs because of the perception that natural products are less toxic than conventional prescribed medicines.[88, 89] Yet the majority did not tell their oncologists about this and a significant proportion of treatments they took were contraindicated. Parents are increasingly using herbs for children with cancer. Some herbs are used with the aim of controlling symptoms, such as nausea (ginger) and depression (St John's wort), but others are used apparently in the hope of possible effects on survival.

Several herbs are currently being intensively investigated for antitumor potential shown *in vitro*, such as induction of apoptosis, immune enhancement, antioxidant activity, and inhibition of angiogenesis.[90] A general review suggested that there is more evidence for prevention than for treatment.[91] One meta-analysis suggests positive benefits of Chinese herbal medicine as an adjunct to chemotherapy for hepatocellular carcinoma.[92] Other reviews are optimistic but ultimately inconclusive.[93, 94]

Mistletoe is widely promoted for cancer, commonly as the preparation Iscador®. It contains several active chemicals, some of which have immunostimulating properties.[95] One problem in designing rigorous clinical trials is that blinding is difficult since mistletoe is given as a series of subcutaneous injections which produce strong local reactions.

Two systematic reviews were published in the same year, giving different interpretations of the literature. In the first, because of methodological problems, the authors concluded that rigorous trials of mistletoe extracts fail to demonstrate efficacy of this therapy.[96] In the second, 23 studies were included of which 12 showed one or more statistically significant, positive results, another seven showed at least one positive trend, three showed no effect and one had a negative trend. These authors concluded that further properly designed trials should be encouraged.[97]

Essaic, a combination of burdock root, Indian rhubarb, sheep sorrel, and the inner bark of slippery elm, is well known in North America and claims to be effective in strengthening the immune system, improving appetite, and relieving pain, as well as reducing tumor size and prolonging life in many types of cancer.[98] However, a review by the Task Force of the Canadian Breast Cancer Research Initiative found no controlled trials and concluded there was "some weak evidence of its effectiveness and [Essaic is] ... unlikely to cause serious side effects when used as directed."[98]

The use of herbs specifically for pain control in cancer patients seems to be rarely documented. There is some evidence of a positive effect on pain due to rheumatological conditions.[99]

Cannabinoids are of considerable current interest, with mixed reports of possible antitumor effects, and for their potential benefit for pain, nausea, and vomiting and for increasing appetite. One systematic review concluded that their analgesic effect was no stronger than codeine and their depressant effects limited their use in practice.[100]

Capsaicin cream, derived from cayenne pepper, reduced "jabbing" pain but not steady pain in an RCT when applied topically in postmastectomy syndrome;[101] blinding is a problem because of side effects.

Chinese herbs are usually prescribed according to a complex traditional diagnosis. Li *et al.*[102] reported a controlled study in which a mixture of Chinese herbs appeared to give relief of acute pain following abdominal surgery for liver cancer. However, the numbers were small and details of the methods are sparse, so no firm conclusions can be drawn.

In view of the number and potency of the chemicals in plants, it is hardly surprising that medicinal herbs commonly have side effects[90] and may interact with orthodox medication.[103] Patients may self-administer Chinese herbs in order to reduce the side effects of conventional hormone therapy for cancer: herbs which block estrogen receptors may reduce the effectiveness of relevant treatments.

Another problem seen with herbs is the quality of their preparation. In one recent example, a major trial of PC-SPES for prostatic cancer in the US was halted because of contamination of the PC-SPES preparation with synthetic estrogens.[104]

Herbal medicines are now subject to regulation, and only those with a long history of indication or trial evidence of effectiveness may be promoted. Medical staff are advised to be alert to the possibility that their patients are using herbs or supplements and to question them routinely. It is currently safest to advise patients not to take anything other than one multivitamin tablet per day while on active chemotherapy, hormone manipulation, or radiotherapy. Also, doctors should avoid uncritical encouragement[88] as it is theoretically possible that prescribers could expose themselves to criticism and even litigation.[105]

HOMEOPATHY

The homeopathic method of treatment was first described in 1790 by the physician Samuel Hahnemann in Germany. The practice of homeopathy (*homeo* = similar, *pathos* = illness) rests on two fundamental principles: the first is "similia similibus curentur" or "let like be cured with like" in which the toxic symptoms of a substance are carefully recorded, and that substance is then used as a remedy for patients who present with those symptoms. The second principle stated by Hahnemann was that repeated dilution of the remedy, with vigorous shaking, increased its power of action, a process called "potentization." Extreme dilutions may be used in which no molecules remain. Claims that diluting the material increases its strength appear biologically implausible.

The evidence on homeopathy for cancer pain is slim. There is anecdotal support of its role in difficult cases,[106] and an observational study showing its use within the National Health Service (NHS) for pain, fatigue, and hot flushes[107] with high satisfaction.[108]

There are some positive clinical trials,[109, 110] but a systematic review of eight controlled trials of homeopathy found insufficient evidence to recommend it.[111][III]

Homeopathy is likely to be a safe intervention but there is insufficient evidence to incorporate it in routine care. Homeopathic consultations are long and detailed, which may contribute to the beneficial effects on patients.

HYPNOSIS

Trance experiences have been described as far back as the time of the ancient Greeks, but hypnosis was first identified as a formal psychotherapeutic interest in the eighteenth century by Anton Mesmer, who used "animal magnetism" for a range of psychosomatic conditions.

Hypnosis is an altered state of consciousness which provides access to unconscious processes and a change in memory or perception. Spiegel and Moore[112] define it as a "a natural state of aroused, attentive local concentration coupled with a relative suspension of peripheral awareness" with three main components, absorption, dissociation, and suggestibility. When subjects are hypnotized they become so absorbed in the experience that there is a distortion of time awareness, thoughts, memories, and perception of activities around them. They experience a curious degree of dissociation from the environment, emotions, and sensations. Some of their critical faculty is bypassed so that suggestions implanted in this state can continue to affect them after the therapy, a phenomenon known as "posthypnotic suggestion." Hypnotizability is a stable and measurable state.[113, 114] Approximately two-thirds of the normal adult population are hypnotizable and up to 10 percent are highly responsive. There are numerous methods of directly inducing the hypnotic state which rely more on the individual subject than the skill of the hypnotist.[115] An indirect method of inducing hypnosis with a gentle, permissive, and less power implicit technique can be successful even in cancer patients with low susceptibility,[116, 117] although Reeves *et al.*[118] found poor results in a controlled trial using the "indirect" method of hypnosis for acute pain of hyperthermia treatment in cancer patients.

There are numerous aims for hypnosis in respect of pain:

- anxiety reduction;
- guided imagery and progressive relaxation;
- displacement of pain or symptoms of nausea and vomiting, using many techniques;

- alteration of the meaning of pain so it is less important and debilitating, for example, "although the pain is there it ceases to bother or disturb you";
- regression to an earlier pain-free time;
- amnesia for previous pain experience.

These techniques can be supplemented by prolonged relaxation, a boosting of self-esteem (so called "ego strengthening"), psychological support, and improvement in body image. Additionally, hypnosis can be used to access and purge unpleasant memories which are inaccessible to the conscious mind but profoundly effect behavior. This technique requires great skill. Self-hypnosis can be taught in the hypnotized state to enhance self-control and to give the patient a degree of mastery over pain.[113]

A distinguished panel of experts who assessed the efficacy of behavioral and relaxation approaches for the treatment of chronic pain and insomnia concluded that there was strong evidence for the use of hypnosis in alleviating pain associated with cancer and for the use of relaxation techniques in reducing chronic pain.[119][V]

One critical review of treatment, however, highlighted confusion over nomenclature and re-emphasized the need for clarity in trial methodology.[120] The term "hypnosis" can have negative connotations as shown when an identical treatment was viewed differently by patients, depending on whether it was labeled as hypnosis, relaxation, or passive relaxation with guided imagery.[121]

Hypnotic interventions have been reviewed by Stam[122] and further details of hypnotic techniques for cancer pain control are outlined.[123, 124, 125] Trijsburg et al.[126] have critically reviewed trial methodology for cancer patients undergoing psychological treatment.

One trial by Spiegel and Bloom[127][II] showed that 34 women with metastatic breast cancer obtained a significant reduction in pain and suffering with hypnosis compared with a control group. Additionally, long-term follow up showed that the treatment group lived on average 36 months, compared with 18 months for the control group.[128][II] However, part of the success was undoubtedly the skilful psychotherapy involved in the "supportive expressive group therapy" given in addition to the hypnosis.[112]

Syrjala et al.[129][II] found that superior pain control for mucositis of bone marrow transplantation was achieved from individualized hypnosis with imagery compared with an untreated control group, a group with usual therapist contact, and a fourth group who were taught cognitive-behavioral coping skills.

Pediatric procedure-related pain

In many parts of the world, sedation is employed instead of general anesthesia, and is used almost routinely for children requiring painful procedures, such as lumbar punctures and bone marrow aspiration, but this can sometimes be inadequate so hypnosis has been used in addition. Many studies have shown that hypnosis is helpful in reducing the pain of such procedures in children with cancer. Zeltzer and colleagues[130, 131][II] have shown that hypnosis can reduce procedure-related pain and chemotherapy-related distress in children. The whole field of hypnosis for children and adolescents with cancer has been reviewed,[132, 133, 134, 135, 136] and many studies included, for example Refs. 137, 138, 139, 140, 141, 142. The use of hypnosis plus local anesthesia was more useful than local anesthesia alone or local anesthesia plus attention in an RCT of procedure-related pain.[143][II] More recently, Richardson et al.,[144] in a systematic review on the use of hypnosis for procedure-related pain and distress in children, showed positive results despite methodological limitations.[144]

Other symptoms

Hypnosis can be helpful for chemotherapy-related nausea and vomiting.[145][II] Reviews have included the treatment of anxiety, stress, and chemotherapy-related nausea and vomiting.[135, 136] Shorter hospital stay after head and neck surgery was found by Rapkin et al.[146][II] when patients were given hypnosis, as compared with standard care. Liossi and White[147][II] showed an improvement in quality of life, anxiety, and depression in an RCT comparing hypnosis with standard care. This was the only RCT cited in a systematic review on the use of hypnosis for symptom control in terminally ill patients.[148] Most of the observational studies showed subjective patient improvements, but the poor quality of the studies and heterogeneity of the population limited conclusions. Hypnosis is also useful in the treatment of dissociative disorders, post-traumatic stress disorders, anxiety, and smoking. However, the use of hypnosis for forensic purposes has aroused controversy.[149, 150]

Side effects

A skilful hypnotherapist should be able to manage a catharsis as this can be very distressing if it occurs during therapy. One retrospective survey of the use of hypnosis for relaxation and coping in 52 palliative care patients found that 61 percent (49) were able to cope better with their illness, whilst 7 percent (three) had negative effects.[151] One of the three patients reported coping was "more difficult," one found the hypnotherapy an "emotionally and physically disturbing experience," and one found it an "adverse experience."

Mechanisms

It is still far from certain how hypnosis works for pain reduction.

- Hypnosis is an altered state of consciousness with electroencephalogram (EEG) patterns of alert wakefulness.[152]

- Spira and Spiegel[123] described the state more akin to intense concentration than to sleep.
- There is some evidence that hypnosis is not reversible by naloxone,[153] but this does not entirely rule out an endogenous opioid mechanism.
- Pederson[154] reviewed early experimental work which provided supporting evidence that the hypnotic state is a largely a right hemisphere-oriented task.
- Gruzelier[155] has shown that hypnosis is much more complex than initially thought, with highly susceptible hypnotic subjects showing prehypnosis asymmetry in favor of the left hemisphere, which is reversed by hypnosis. The opposite effects were seen in subjects who had low susceptibility to hypnosis. The author describes frontal inhibition and accentuation of posterior right-sided hemisphere functions in the hypnotic state.
- When hypnosis alters perception, there is evidence that it alters the event-related potentials to somatosensory stimuli. When highly hypnotized subjects imagine that a visual stimulus is blocked, their visual cortical response to those stimuli is reduced, particularly in the right hemisphere.[156]
- Dissociation of sensory and affective components of pain occurs under hypnosis.[157]
- The specific pain dimension on which hypnotic suggestions act depends on the content of the instructions and is not a characteristic of hypnosis itself.[158]
- Positron emission tomography (PET) has shown changes in the activity of the anterior cingulate cortex associated with hypnotic suggestions designed to alter the unpleasantness, or affective component, of pain.[159]

With the increasing availability of imaging techniques such as PET and functional magnetic resonance imaging (fMRI) scans for research purposes, further scientific evidence for the mechanisms of hypnosis is accumulating.

Hypnotherapy appears to have a positive role in the treatment of pain and treatment-related pain in cancer patients and merits further clinical trials. The success of hypnosis may depend on the skill and interaction of the patient and therapist more than in many other treatments. Any nonhypnotizable subjects should be offered another form of supportive therapy.[123]

RELAXATION, DISTRACTION, AND VISUALIZATION

Relaxation and visualization are other "mind–body" approaches used in cancer patients. They can be considered to be on a continuum with hypnosis, but seem to be viewed by patients with less suspicion.[121] Distraction is used by almost every patient in some form, whether it is work, relationships, television, etc. Music is selected more often than comedy by cancer patients.[160] Children who are encouraged by their families to use their imagination have a greater ability to obtain help by magic and fantasy than those brought up to use intellect and reason, although the latter may respond better to a combination of relaxation and instruction.[161] Kuttner et al.[162][II] compared three forms of treatment on children undergoing bone marrow aspiration. The first group received standard medical management using reassurance and support, the second group were taught a distraction technique, and the third group were encouraged to involve their imagination, becoming totally absorbed as in hypnosis. Imaginative involvement was more helpful for the three to six year olds, whereas both distraction and imaginative involvement were helpful in the seven to ten year olds. In the distraction group, coping skills needed to be learned over one or more sessions.

An RCT comparing relaxation training, by tapes or nurses, compared with no training showed a reduction in pain and a reduced need for breakthrough medication in a cancer hospital.[163][II]

Guided imagery and relaxation were compared with a control group in elderly patients having colorectal surgical resections.[164][II] Whilst well accepted by patients, the interventions failed to positively influence the postoperative course.

Visualization with guided imagery, such as imagining white blood cells killing cancer cells, was popularized by Simonton et al.[165] Claims that this method is effective have not been backed up by any convincing evidence. While seemingly benign, any failure to control the disease might add to a patient's burden of unwarranted guilt.[112]

The role of psychoneuroimmunomodulation is very complex.[166, 167] Further clinical studies which highlight any specific interactions between the immune system and psychology studies are eagerly awaited.

MASSAGE AND AROMATHERAPY

Massage is defined as manipulation of the soft tissues of the body performed by the hands for the purpose of producing effects on the vascular, muscular, and nervous systems of the body. Aromatherapy massage involves the use of essential oils which are combined with a carrier oil or cream to manipulate the soft tissues of the body.[168] These treatments are generally used with the intention of relieving stress and improving well-being, rather than the control of specific symptoms such as pain.

The touch that massage offers may convey psychological messages such as caring, comfort, and support to patients who are stressed and vulnerable. Massage and aromatherapy are widely available in hospices and palliative care units.[169]

There are two main types of massage therapy. Massage (also known as Swedish massage) includes techniques from slow, gentle stroking to more vigorous movements such as friction, kneading/rolling movements (petrissage), and flicking/clapping movements (tapotement). Shiatsu massage is a more forceful form of treatment which aims to "release blocked energy" by strong, sustained pressure at specific points. It is not commonly used for cancer patients.

In addition to any psychological effects, massage may have physical effects including:

- relaxation;
- relief of muscle spasm;
- nociceptive inhibition through Gate Control theory;
- improvement of circulation;
- reduction of swelling associated with lymphedema (this is not discussed here; for a review see Ko et al.[170]).

In one RCT, Weinrich and Weinrich[171] compared the effect on pain of a single ten-minute Swedish massage of the back with a "visitation" control who had no massage, in a relatively small sample of 28 patients. Massage was associated with a significant fall in pain scores in men immediately after treatment but not after one or two hours; there was no significant pain relief in women. The initial pain scores were higher in men than in women. The sample size was too small for these results to be definitive, and the effect of repeated treatment in patients with moderate or severe pain are worth exploring further. The treatment in this study was given by senior nurses who had received only one hour's training in massage therapy which may be insufficient.

Grealish and colleagues[172] gave two ten-minute sessions of massage, compared with quiet time for the control group: only the treatment group showed a significant reduction of pain. Wilkie and colleagues[173] gave 30–50-minute sessions of massage to 20 patients twice a week for two weeks, showing a trend to greater pain reduction in the massage group.

A Cochrane review included eight RCTs, three of which measured pain as an outcome and concluded that massage and aromatherapy massage confer short-term benefits on psychological well-being.[168][III] There is limited evidence of an effect on anxiety. The impact on pain may be apparent in subgroups (men, or more severe pain) rather than the whole patient population. Evidence is mixed as to whether aromatherapy enhances the effects of massage to a clinically significant level.

Another review[174][III] reached a similar conclusion, and commented, "The oncologist should feel comfortable discussing massage therapy with patients and be able to refer patients to a qualified massage therapist as appropriate."

Cassileth and Vickers,[175] in a subsequent large observational study on 1290 patients, showed an improvement of multiple symptoms including pain throughout the 48-hour observation period.

There is a theoretical risk that massage could mobilize dormant cancer cells, although there are no reports of this happening. However, this possibility should be borne in mind when assessing the benefit/risk ratio for an individual patient. Clearly, massage should not be performed close to tumors or venous thrombosis, or in patients with grossly abnormal clotting function. Possible adverse effects of the essential oils, including skin reactions, have been reported and should be monitored.

Massage and other forms of sensory stimulation release oxytocin which is both anxiolytic[64] and analgesic.[176] Perhaps this goes part way to explain the analgesic and sedative qualities of massage.

HEALING (UK AND ELSEWHERE) EQUIVALENT TO THERAPEUTIC TOUCH (US)

Healing usually involves the practitioner passing his or her hands over the patient's clothed body, usually without making physical contact (despite the term "therapeutic touch"). Various explanatory models are offered, including the channeling of energy, or the reestablishment of the patient's own energy flow. Some forms are associated with particular religious beliefs, but usually patients are not required to hold any particular form of faith or belief. Various forms exist including spiritual healing, Reiki, and therapeutic touch. Patients are often aware of tingling or warmth during the session and relief of symptoms afterwards.

It is important that patients do not misinterpret the word "healing" to indicate that the treatment is likely to heal their cancer.

Several studies showed that healing can help with relaxation, pain, and sleep in palliative care patients.[177] For patients who were undergoing radiotherapy for breast or gynecological cancer, an improvement was found for measures of quality of life for vitality, pain, and physical functioning in favor of healing versus mock healing.[178]

Reiki healing, using light physical contact, was compared with rest periods of the same duration in an RCT in patients with advanced cancer receiving opioids for pain.[179] Of 53 patients recruited, data are available on 24. Two sessions of Reiki in four days were each followed by short-term, significantly superior reduction in pain scores than rest alone, as well as a significant improvement in the quality of life. There was no difference in opioid consumption.

It appears that the outcome from a healing intervention may be largely due to expectation, relaxation and other nonspecific effects. No adverse effects have been recorded.

MUSIC THERAPY

Music therapy has been defined as the "creative and professionally informed use of music in a therapeutic relationship for physical, social, and spiritual help."[180]

Music therapists use various techniques such as song writing, improvization, guided imagery and music, lyric analysis, singing, instrument playing, and music-associated relaxation techniques to improve the quality of life. Music therapists are integrated into the care provided by many hospices.

A Cochrane review of RCTs that tested just listening to music as a treatment for acute or chronic pain, or cancer pain, concluded that listening to music reduces pain intensity levels and opioid requirements, but the magnitude of these benefits is small and, therefore, its clinical importance unclear.[181]

In a systematic review of 11 studies of various designs, and sources including masters theses and conference proceedings,[182][IV] two uncontrolled studies of reasonable size ($n = 90$, $n = 80$) showed a significant reduction of pain, as well as anxiety or relaxation, after music therapy. One very small ($n = 8$) crossover study also found a significant reduction of pain in the period during which patients listened to music on headphones, compared with the control period. Other studies provided conflicting results on the effect of music therapy on quality of life in patients in hospice and palliative care.

CONCLUSIONS

Many CM therapies can be described as complex interventions, and it is recognized that the formal evaluation of complex interventions is challenging.[183] Therefore, it would be wrong to dismiss CM therapies completely on the existing evidence, and methods need to be developed to find out which components are effective, and whether they can play an effective role in improving healthcare.

A significant unmet need in conventional health care drives many patients to seek CM therapies and healthcare professionals need to communicate more effectively with the patients and have access to information about CM in order to advise patients about the risks and benefits of treatment.[184] Indeed, significant numbers of patients enrolling on phase I clinical trials of chemotherapy were taking a range of nonpharmacological CM treatments.[185] Asking patients if they use CM is vital in case they need to be advised to stop taking anything which could interact with or adversely affect the efficacy of the trial drug(s).

Complementary therapies are becoming increasingly popular with the general public, including cancer patients. Conventional medical personnel are now less inclined than previously to dismiss the use of such approaches, and should be aware when their patients are using them. Patients should be advised when they are at risk from practitioners who raise false hopes, from therapies that may harm them directly, and from therapies that may interfere with conventional treatments. A recent systematic review of the efficacy of CM treatments for pain[186] concluded that hypnosis, imagery, support groups, acupuncture, and healing confer some benefit,

and that future research should focus on methodologically sound RCTs to determine their efficacy.

To summarize the current evidence for CM treatment of cancer pain presented in this chapter, hypnosis offers a variety of approaches and is probably the therapy that is best supported by expert consensus opinion, as well as the limited experimental evidence that exists. There is also reasonable trial evidence that both hypnosis and the related technique of imagery can be useful for procedure-related pain, particularly in children. Other therapies such as acupuncture, massage, and aromatherapy have shown promise as useful techniques for the palliation of symptoms in cancer patients. More and better quality studies are awaited before they can be considered an integral part of management. There is also some evidence supporting the use of herbal preparations of mistletoe, but it is not conclusive. The value of approaches using healing or homeopathy in the management of cancer pain is still not known.

REFERENCES

1. Ernst E, Cassileth B. The prevalence of complementary/alternative medicine in cancer. *Cancer.* 1998; **83**: 777–82.
2. Molassiotis A, Fernadez-Ortega P, Pud D *et al.* Use of complementary and alternative medicine in cancer patients: a European survey. *Annals of Oncology.* 2005; **16**: 655–63.
3. Kelly KM, Jacobson JS, Kennedy DD *et al.* Use of unconventional therapies by children with cancer at an urban medical center. *Journal of Pediatric Hematology/Oncology.* 2000; **22**: 412–6.
4. Downer SM, Cody MM, McCluskey P *et al.* Pursuit and practice of complementary therapies by cancer patients receiving conventional treatment. *British Medical Journal.* 1994; **309**: 86–9.
5. Fernandez CV, Stutzer CA, MacWilliam L, Fryer C. Alternative and complementary therapy use in pediatric oncology patients in British Columbia: prevalence and reasons for use and nonuse. *Journal of Clinical Oncology.* 1998; **16**: 1279–86.
6. VandeCreek L, Rogers E, Lester J. Use of alternative therapies among breast cancer outpatients compared with the general population. *Alternative Therapies in Health and Medicine.* 1999; **5**: 71–6.
7. Sellick SM, Zara C. Critical review of 5 nonpharmacologic strategies for managing cancer pain. *Cancer Prevention and Control.* 1998; **2**: 7–14.
8. Cassileth BR, Brown H. Unorthodox cancer medicine. *Cancer Journal for Clinicians.* 1988; **38**: 176–86.
* 9. Cassileth BR, Chapman CC. Alternative cancer medicine: a ten-year update. *Cancer Investigation.* 1996; **14**: 396–404.
10. Verhoef MJ, Balneaves LG, Boon HS, Vroegindewey A. Reasons for and characteristics associated with

complementary and alternative medicine use among adult cancer patients: a systematic review. *Integrative Cancer Therapies.* 2005; **4**: 274–86.

11. Baum M. Quack cancer cures or scientific remedies. *Journal of the Royal Society of Medicine.* 1996; **89**: 543–7.

12. Cosh J, Sikora K. Conventional and complementary treatment for cancer. [letter]. *British Medical Journal.* 1989; **298**: 1200–1 (letter).

13. Burke C, Sikora K. Complementary and conventional cancer care: the integration of two cultures. *Clinical Oncology.* 1993; **5**: 220–7.

14. Remuzzi G, Schieppati A. Lessons from the Di Bella affair. *Lancet.* 1999; **353**: 1289–90.

15. Veith I. *The Yellow Emperor's classic of internal medicine*, 3rd printing. Berkley: University of California Press, 1972.

16. Dorfer L, Moser M, Bahr F *et al.* A medical report from the stone age? *Lancet.* 1999; **354**: 1023–5.

17. *Essentials of chinese acupuncture.* Beijing: Foreign Languages Press, 1980.

18. Filshie J, White A (eds). *Medical acupuncture: a western scientific approach.* Edinburgh: Churchill Livingstone, 1998.

19. Ernst E, White A (eds). *Acupuncture: a scientific appraisal.* Oxford: Butterworth-Heinemann, 1999.

20. Birch S, Kaptchuk T. History, nature and current practice of acupuncture: an East Asian perspective. In: Ernst E, White A (eds). *Acupuncture: a scientific appraisal.* Oxford: Butterworth-Heinemann, 1999: 11–30.

21. Filshie J, Bolton T, Browne D, Ashley S. Acupuncture and self acupuncture for long-term treatment of vasomotor symptoms in cancer patients – audit and treatment algorithm. *Acupuncture in Medicine.* 2005; **23**: 171–80.

22. White A. Electroacupuncture and acupuncture analgesia. In: Filshie J, White A (eds). *Medical acupuncture: a western scientific approach.* Edinburgh: Churchill Livingstone, 1998: 153–75.

23. de Bie RA, Verhagen AP, Lenssen AF *et al.* Efficacy of 904 nm laser therapy in the management of musculoskeletal disorders: a systematic review. *Physical Therapy Reviews.* 1998; **3**: 59–72.

24. Nogier PFM. *Treatise of auriculotherapy.* France: Maisonneuve, 1972.

25. Yamamoto T, Yamamoto H. *Yamamoto new scalp acupuncture YNSA.* Axel Springer Japan Publishing Inc, 1998.

26. Yoshino N, Yamashita K. *Ryokaraku acupuncture.* Ryokaraku Research Institute Limited, 1977.

27. Woollam CH, Jackson AO. Acupuncture in the management of chronic pain. *Anaesthesia.* 1998; **53**: 593–5.

28. National Review of Pain Services and Standards for the Clinical Standards Advisory Group (CSAG). Department of Health Publication, 2000.

29. Ezzo J, Berman B, Hadhazy VA *et al.* Is acupuncture effective for the treatment of chronic pain? A systematic review. *Pain.* 2000; **86**: 217–25.

30. Ernst E, Pittler MH. The effectiveness of acupuncture in treating acute dental pain: a systematic review. *British Dental Journal.* 1998; **184**: 443–7.

31. White A. Neurophysiology of acupuncture analgesia. In: Ernst E, White A (eds). *Acupuncture: a scientific appraisal.* Oxford: Butterworth-Heinemann, 1999.

32. Melchart D, Linde K, Fischer P *et al.* Acupuncture for recurrent headaches: a systematic review of randomized controlled trials. *Cephalalgia.* 1999; **19**: 779–86.

33. White A, Foster NE, Cummings M, Barlas P. Acupuncture treatment for chronic knee pain: a systematic review. *Rheumatology (Oxford).* 2007; **46**: 384–90.

34. Manheimer E, White A, Berman B *et al.* Meta-analysis: acupuncture for low back pain. *Annals of Internal Medicine.* 2005; **142**: 651–63.

35. Furlan A, Tulder M, Cherkin D *et al.* Acupuncture and dry-needling for low back pain. *Cochrane Database of Systematic Reviews.* 2005; **CD001351**.

* 36. Kotani N, Hashimoto H, Sato Y *et al.* Preoperative intradermal acupuncture reduces postoperative pain, nausea and vomiting, analgesic requirement, and sympathoadrenal responses. *Anesthesiology.* 2001; **95**: 349–56.

37. Poulain P, Pichard Leandri E *et al.* Electroacupuncture analgesia in major abdominal and pelvic surgery: a randomised study. *Acupuncture in Medicine.* 1997; **XV**: 10–13.

38. He JP, Friedrich M, Ertan AK *et al.* Pain-relief and movement improvement by acupuncture after ablation and axillary lymphadenectomy in patients with mammary cancer. *Clinical and Experimental Obstetrics and Gynecology.* 1999; **26**: 81–4.

39. Lee H, Schmidt K, Ernst E. Acupuncture for the relief of cancer-related pain – a systematic review. *European Journal of Pain.* 2005; **9**: 437–44.

40. Alimi D, Rubino C, Pichard-Leandri E *et al.* Analgesic effect of auricular acupuncture for cancer pain: a randomized, blinded, controlled trial. *Journal of Clinical Oncology.* 2003; **21**: 4120–6.

* 41. National Cancer Institute. Effect of acupuncture on cancer pain. Bethesda, MD, USA: National Cancer Institute. Last updated November 20, 2007; cited April 16, 2007. Available from: www.cancer.gov/cancertopics/pdq/cam/acupuncture/HealthProfessional/page5.

42. Mann F, Bowsher D, Mumford J *et al.* Treatment of intractable pain by acupuncture. *Lancet.* 1973; ii: 57–60.

43. Wen HL. Cancer pain treated with acupuncture and electrical stimulation. *Modern Medicine of Asia.* 1977; **13**: 12–15.

44. Filshie J, Redman D. Acupuncture and malignant pain problems. *European Journal of Surgical Oncology.* 1985; **11**: 389–94.

* 45. Filshie J. Acupuncture and malignant pain problems. *Acupuncture in Medicine.* 1990; **8**: 38–9.

46. Filshie J, Scase A, Ashley S, Hood J. A study of the acupuncture effects on pain, anxiety and depression in

patients with breast cancer. *Pain Society Meeting*, 1997. Abstract.

47. Leng G. A year of acupuncture in palliative care. *Palliative Medicine*. 1999; **13**: 163–4.

48. Dillon M, Lucas CF. Auricular stud acupuncture in palliative care patients: an initial report. *Palliative Medicine*. 1999; **13**: 253–4.

49. Stux G, Pomeranz B. *Basics of acupuncture*, 4th edn. Berlin: Springer-Verlag, 1998.

50. Bowsher D. Mechanisms of acupuncture. In: Filshie J, White A (eds). *Medical acupuncture: a western scientific approach*. Edinburgh: Churchill Livingstone, 1998: 69–82.

51. Lundeberg T. Effects of sensory stimulation (acupuncture) on circulatory and immune systems. In: Ernst E, White A (eds). *Acupuncture: a scientific appraisal*. Oxford: Butterworth-Heinemann, 1999: 93–106.

∗ 52. Han JS. Acupuncture and endorphins. *Neuroscience Letters*. 2004; **361**: 258–61.

∗ 53. Cho ZH, Hwang SC, Wong EK *et al.* Neural substrates, experimental evidences and functional hypothesis of acupuncture mechanisms. *Acta Neurologica Scandinavica*. 2006; **113**: 370–7.

54. Dung HC. Anatomical features contributing to the formation of acupuncture points. *American Journal of Acupuncture*. 1984; **12**: 139–43.

55. Chiang C-Y, Chang C-T, Chu H-L, Yang L-F. Peripheral afferent pathway for acupuncture analgesia. *Scientia Sinica*. 1973; **16**: 210–17.

56. Dundee JW, Ghaly G. Local anesthesia blocks the antiemetic action of P6 acupuncture. *Clinical Pharmacology and Therapeutics*. 1991; **50**: 78–80.

57. Chung JM, Fang ZR, Hori Y *et al.* Prolonged inhibition of primate spinothalamic tract cells by peripheral nerve stimulation. *Pain*. 1984; **19**: 259–75.

∗ 58. Pariente J, White P, Frackowiak RS, Lewith G. Expectancy and belief modulate the neuronal substrates of pain treated by acupuncture. *Neuroimage*. 2005; **25**: 1161–7.

59. Filshie J, Cummings M. Western medical acupuncture. In: Ernst E, White A (eds). *Acupuncture: a scientific appraisal*. Oxford: Butterworth-Heinemann, 1999.

60. Ho MW, Knight DP. The acupuncture system and the liquid crystalline collagen fibers of the connective tissues. *American Journal of Chinese Medicine*. 1998; **26**: 251–63.

61. Han JS, Ding XZ, Fang SG. Cholecystokinin octapeptide (CCK-8): antagonism to electroacupuncture analgesia and a possible role in electroacupuncture tolerance. *Pain*. 1986; **27**: 101–15.

62. Le Bars D, Villanueva L, Willer JC, Bouhassira D. Diffuse noxious inhibitory controls (DNIC) in animals and in man. *Acupuncture in Medicine*. 1991; **IX**: 47–56.

∗ 63. Han J, Terenius L. Neurochemical basis of acupuncture analgesia. *Annual Review of Pharmacology and Toxicology*. 1982; **22**: 192–220.

64. Uvnas-Moberg K. Physiological and endocrine effects of social contact. *Annals of the New York Academy of Sciences*. 1997; **807**: 146–63.

65. Melzack R, Stillwell DM, Fox EJ. Trigger points and acupuncture points for pain, correlations and implications. *Pain*. 1977; **3**: 3–23.

66. Dorsher PT. Poster 196 Myofascial pain: rediscovery of a 2000-year-old tradition. *Archives of Physical Medicine and Rehabilitation*. 2004; **85**: E42.

∗ 67. Travell JG, Simons DG. *Myofascial pain and dysfunction. The trigger point manual*. Baltimore: Williams and Wilkins, 1983.

∗ 68. Baldry PE. *Acupuncture, trigger points and musculo-skeletal pain*, 2nd edn. Edinburgh: Churchill Livingston, 1993.

∗ 69. Hong C-Z, Simons DG. Pathophysiologic and electrophysiologic mechanisms of myofascial trigger points. *Archives of Physical Medicine and Rehabilitation*. 1998; **79**: 863–72.

70. Roth LU, Maret-Maric A, Adler RH, Neuenschwander BE. Acupuncture points have subjective (needing sensation) and objective (serum cortisol increase) specificity. *Acupuncture in Medicine*. 1997; **15**: 2–5.

71. Han JS. *The neurochemical basis of pain relief by acupuncture*. Beijing: Beijing Medical University Press, 1987.

72. Filshie J, White A. The clinical use of, and evidence for, acupuncture in the medical systems. In: Filshie J, White A (eds). *Medical acupuncture: a western scientific approach*. Edinburgh: Churchill Livingstone, 1998: 225–94.

73. Lee JH, Beitz AJ. The distribution of brain-stem and spinal cord nuclei associated with different frequencies of electroacupuncture analgesia. *Pain*. 1993; **52**: 11–28.

74. Guo HF, Tian J, Wang X *et al.* Brain substrates activated by electroacupuncture of different frequencies (1): comparative study on the expression of oncogene c-fos and genes coding for three opioid peptides. *Molecular Brain Research*. 1996; **43**: 157–66.

∗ 75. Lee A, Done M. Stimulation of the wrist acupuncture point P6 for preventing postoperative nausea and vomiting. *Cochrane Database of Systematic Reviews*. 2004; CD003281.

∗ 76. Ezzo JM, Richardson MA, Vickers A *et al.* Acupuncture-point stimulation for chemotherapy-induced nausea or vomiting. *Cochrane Database of Systematic Reviews*. 2006; CD002285.

77. Filshie J, Penn K, Ashley S, Davis CL. Acupuncture for the relief of cancer-related breathlessness. *Palliative Medicine*. 1996; **10**: 145–50.

78. Johnstone PA, Niemtzow RC, Riffenburgh RH. Acupuncture for xerostomia: clinical update. *Cancer*. 2002; **94**: 1151–6.

79. Johnstone PAS, Peng YP, May BC *et al.* Acupuncture for pilocarpine-resistant xerostomia following radiotherapy for head and neck malignancies. *International Journal of Radiation Oncology, Biology, Physics*. 2001; **50**: 353–7.

80. Filshie J. The non-drug treatment of neuralgic and neuropathic pain of malignancy. In: Hanks GW (ed.). *Pain and cancer*. Oxford: Oxford University Press, 1988: 161–93.

81. Towlerton G, Filshie J, O'Brien M, Duncan A. Acupuncture in the control of vasomotor symptoms caused by tamoxifen. *Palliative Medicine*. 1999; **13**: 445.

82. de Valois B. Using acupuncture to manage hot flushes and night sweats in women taking tamoxifen for early breast cancer. PhD thesis, Thames Valley University, 2006.

83. Frisk J, Spetz AC, Hjertberg H *et al.* Two modes of acupuncture as a treatment for hot flushes in men with prostate cancer – a prospective multicenter study with long-term follow-up. *European Urology*. 2008; Feb 14 (Epub ahead of print).

* 84. Thompson JW, Filshie J. Transcutaneous electrical nerve stimulation (TENS) and acupuncture. In: Doyle D, Hanks G, Macdonald N (eds). *Oxford textbook of palliative medicine*, 2nd edn. Oxford: Oxford Medical Publications, 1997: 421–37 (3rd edition in press).

* 85. White A. A cumulative review of the range and incidence of significant adverse events associated with acupuncture. *Acupuncture in Medicine*. 2004; **22**: 122–33.

* 86. Filshie J. Safety aspects of acupuncture in palliative care. *Acupuncture in Medicine*. 2001; **19**: 117–22.

* 87. Filshie J, Hester J. Guidelines for providing acupuncture treatment for cancer patients – a peer-reviewed sample policy document. *Acupuncture in Medicine*. 2006; **24**: 172–82.

88. Werneke U, Earl J, Seydel C *et al.* Potential health risks of complementary alternative medicines in cancer patients. *British Journal of Cancer*. 2004; **90**: 408–13.

89. Citrin DL, Gupta D, Birdsall TC *et al.* Prevalence of use of herbal therapies in adult cancer patients: Potential for herb–drug interactions. *Journal of Clinical Oncology*. 2005; **23**: 549s.

* 90. Spaulding-Albright N. A review of some herbal and related products commonly used in cancer patients. *Journal of the American Dietetic Association*. 1997; **97**: S208–15.

* 91. Boon H, Wong J. Botanical medicine and cancer: a review of the safety and efficacy. *Expert Opin Pharmacother*. 2004; **5**: 2485–501.

92. Lian Z, Niwa K, Onogi K *et al.* Anti-tumor effects of herbal medicines on endometrial carcinomas via estrogen receptor-alpha-related mechanism. *Oncology Reports*. 2006; **15**: 1133–6.

93. McCulloch M, See C, Shu XJ *et al.* Astragalus-based Chinese herbs and platinum-based chemotherapy for advanced non-small-cell lung cancer: meta-analysis of randomized trials. *Journal of Clinical Oncology*. 2006; **24**: 419–30.

94. Block KI, Mead MN. Immune system effects of echinacea, ginseng, and astragalus: a review. *Integrative Cancer Therapies*. 2003; **2**: 247–67.

95. Hajto T, Hostanska K, Frei K *et al.* Increased secretion of tumor necrosis factor alpha, interleukin 1, and interleukin 6 by human mononuclear cells exposed to b-galactoside-specific lectin from clinically applied mistletoe extract. *Cancer Research*. 1990; **50**: 3322–6.

* 96. Ernst E, Schmidt K, Steuer-Vogt MK. Mistletoe for cancer? A systematic review of randomised clinical trials.

International Journal of Cancer. 2003; **107**: 262–7.

* 97. Kienle GS, Berrino F, Bussing A *et al.* Mistletoe in cancer – a systematic review on controlled clinical trials. *European Journal of Medical Research*. 2003; **8**: 109–19.

* 98. Kaegi E. Unconventional therapies for cancer: 1. Essiac. *Canadian Medical Association Journal*. 1998; **158**: 897–902.

99. Ernst E, Chrubasik S. Phyto-antiinflammatories: a systematic review of randomized, placebo-controlled, double-blind trials. In: Woolf AD (ed.). *Bailliere's Best Practice and Research in Clinical Rheumatology*. Philadelphia: WB Saunders, 2000.

*100. Campbell FA, Tramer MR, Carroll D *et al.* Are cannabinoids an effective and safe treatment option in the management of pain? A qualitative systematic review. *British Medical Journal*. 2001; **323**: 13–16.

101. Watson CP, Evans RJ. The postmastectomy pain syndrome and topical capsaicin: a randomized trial. *Pain*. 1992; **51**: 375–9.

102. Li QS, Cao SH, Xie GM *et al.* Relieving effects of Chinese herbs, ear-acupuncture and epidural morphine on postoperative pain in liver cancer. *Chinese Medical Journal*. 1994; **107**: 289–94.

103. Boyle FM. Adverse interaction of herbal medicine with breast cancer treatment. *Medical Journal of Australia*. 1997; **167**: 286.

104. Oh WK, Kantoff PW, Weinberg V *et al.* Prospective, multicenter, randomized phase II trial of the herbal supplement, PC-SPES, and diethylstilbestrol in patients with androgen-independent prostate cancer. *Journal of Clinical Oncology*. 2004; **22**: 3705–12.

105. Cohen MH, Eisenberg DM. Potential physician malpractice liability associated with complementary and integrative medical therapies. *Annals of Internal Medicine*. 2002; **136**: 596–603.

106. Thompson E, Hicks F. Intrathecal baclofen and homeopathy for the treatment of painful muscle spasms associated with malignant spinal cord compression. *Palliative Medicine*. 1998; **12**: 119–21.

107. Thompson EA, Reilly D. The homeopathic approach to symptom control in the cancer patient: a prospective observational study. *Palliative Medicine*. 2002; **16**: 227–33.

108. Clover A, Last P, Fisher P *et al.* Complementary cancer therapy: a pilot study of patients, therapies and quality of life. *Complementary Therapies in Medicine*. 1995; **3**: 129–33.

109. Oberbaum M. Experimental treatment of chemotherapy-induced stomatitis using a homeopathic complex preparation: a preliminary study. *Biologicial Medicine*. 1998; **3**: 104–08.

110. Oberbaum M, Yaniv I, Ben Gal Y *et al.* A randomized, controlled clinical trial of the homeopathic medication TRAUMEEL S in the treatment of chemotherapy-induced stomatitis in children undergoing stem cell transplantation. *Cancer*. 2001; **92**: 684–90.

111. Milazzo S, Russell N, Ernst E. Efficacy of homeopathic therapy in cancer treatment. *European Journal of Cancer.* 2006; **42**: 282–9.

*112. Spiegel D, Moore R. Imagery and hypnosis in the treatment of cancer patients. *Oncology.* 1997; **11**: 1179–95.

*113. Hilgard ER, Hilgard JR. *Hypnosis in the relief of pain.* Los Altos, CA: William Kaufmann, 1975.

114. Spiegel H, Spiegel D. *Trance and treatment; Clinical uses of hypnosis.* New York: Basic Books, 1978.

115. Orne MT. Hypnotic control of pain. Towards a clarification of the different psychological processes involved. In: Bonica JJ (ed.). *Pain,* Vol. 58. New York: Raven Press, 1980: 155–72.

116. Barber J, Gitelson J. Cancer pain: psychological management using hypnosis. *CA: A Cancer Journal for Clinicians.* 1980; **30**: 130–6.

117. Barber J. Incorporating hypnosis in the management of chronic pain. In: Barber J, Adams C (eds). *Psychological approaches to the management of pain.* New York: Brunner/Mazel, 1984: 40–59.

118. Reeves JL, Redd WH, Storm FK, Minagawa RY. Hypnosis in the control of pain during hyperthermia treatment of cancer. In: Bonica JJ *et al.* (eds). *Advances in pain research and therapy,* Vol. 5. New York: Raven Press, 1983: 857–61.

*119. NIH Technology Assessment Panel on integration of Behavioral and Relaxation Approaches into the Treatment of Chronic Pain and Insomnia. Integration of behavioral and relaxation approaches into the treatment of chronic pain and insomnia. *Journal of the American Medical Association.* 1996; **276**: 313–18.

*120. Jay SM, Elliott C, Varni JW. Acute and chronic pain in adults and children with cancer. *Journal of Consulting and Clinical Psychology.* 1986; **54**: 601–07.

121. Hendler CS, Redd WH. Fear of hypnosis: the role of labeling in patients' acceptance of behavioral intervention. *Behavior Therapy.* 1986; **17**: 2–13.

122. Stam HJ. From symptom relief to cure. In: Spanos NP, Chaves JF (eds). *Hypnosis: the cognitive-behavioral perspective.* Buffalo, NY: Prometheus Books, 1989: 313–39.

*123. Spira JL, Spiegel D. Hypnosis and related techniques in pain management. *Hospital Journal.* 1992; **8**: 89–119.

124. Chaves JF. Recent advances in the application of hypnosis to pain management. *American Journal of Clinical Hypnosis.* 1994; **37**: 117–29.

125. Levitan AA. The use of hypnosis with cancer patients. *Psychiatric Medicine.* 1992; **10**: 119–31.

*126. Trijsburg RW, van Knippenberg FCE, Rijpma SE. Effects of psychological treatment on cancer patients: a critical review. *Psychosomatic Medicine.* 1992; **54**: 489–517.

*127. Spiegel D, Bloom JR. Group therapy and hypnosis reduce metastatic breast carcinoma pain. *Psychosomatic Medicine.* 1983; **45**: 333–9.

*128. Spiegel D, Bloom JR, Kraemer HC, Gottheil E. Effect of psychosocial treatment on survival of patients with metastatic breast cancer. *Lancet.* 1989; **2**: 888–91.

129. Syrjala KL, Cummings C, Donaldson GW. Hypnosis or cognitive behavioral training for the reduction of pain and nausea during cancer treatment: a controlled clinical trial. *Pain.* 1992; **48**: 137–46.

*130. Zeltzer L, LeBaron S. The hypnotic treatment of children in pain. In: Wolraich ML, Routh DK (eds). *Advances in developmental and behavioral pediatrics,* Vol. 7. Greenwich, CT: JAI Press, 1986: 197–234.

131. Zeltzer LK, Dolgin MJ, LeBaron S, LeBaron C. A randomized, controlled study of behavioral intervention for chemotherapy distress in children with cancer. *Pediatrics.* 1991; **88**: 34–42.

*132. Steggles S, Fehr R, Aucoin P. Hypnosis for children and adolescents with cancer: an annotated bibliography 1960–1985. *Journal of the Association of Pediatric Oncology Nurses.* 1986; **3**: 23–5.

*133. Sutters KA, Miaskowski C. The problem of pain in children with cancer: a research review. *Oncology Nursing Forum.* 1992; **19**: 465–71.

134. Ellis JA, Spanos NP. Cognitive-behavioral interventions for children's distress during bone marrow aspirations and lumbar punctures: a critical review. *Journal of Pain and Symptom Management.* 1994; **9**: 96–108.

*135. Genuis ML. The use of hypnosis in helping cancer patients control anxiety, pain, and emesis: a review of recent empirical studies. *American Journal of Clinical Hypnosis.* 1995; **37**: 316–25.

136. Steggles S, Damore-Petingola S, Maxwell J, Lightfoot N. Hypnosis for children and adolescents with cancer: an annotated bibliography, 1985–1995. *American Journal of Clinical Hypnosis.* 1997; **39**: 187–200.

137. Olness K. Imagery (self-hypnosis) as adjunct therapy in childhood cancer: clinical experience with 25 patients. *American Journal of Pediatric Hematology/Oncology.* 1981; **3**: 313–21.

138. Hilgard JR, LeBaron S. relief of anxiety and pain in children and adolescents with cancer: quantitative measures and clinical observations. *International Journal of Clinical and Experimental Hypnosis.* 1982; **XXX**: 417–42.

139. Zeltzer L, LeBaron S. Hypnosis and nonhypnotic techniques for reduction of pain and anxiety during painful procedures in children and adolescents with cancer. *Journal of Pediatrics.* 1982; **101**: 1032–5.

140. Kellerman J, Zeltzer L, Ellenberg L, Dash J. Adolescents with cancer. Hypnosis for the reduction of the acute pain and anxiety associated with medical procedures. *Journal of Adolescent Health Care.* 1983; **4**: 85–90.

141. Katz ER, Kellerman J, Ellenberg L. Hypnosis in the reduction of acute pain and distress in children with cancer. *Journal of Pediatric Psychology.* 1987; **12**: 379–94.

142. Wall VJ, Womack W. Hypnotic versus active cognitive strategies for alleviation of procedural distress in pediatric oncology patients. *American Journal of Clinical Hypnosis.* 1989; **31**: 181–91.

143. Liossi C, White P, Hatira P. Randomized clinical trial of local anesthetic versus a combination of local anesthetic with self-hypnosis in the management of pediatric

procedure-related pain. *Health Psychology.* 2006; **25**: 307–15.

144. Richardson J, Smith JE, McCall G, Pilkington K. Hypnosis for procedure-related pain and distress in pediatric cancer patients: a systematic review of effectiveness and methodology related to hypnosis interventions. *Journal of Pain and Symptom Management.* 2006; **31**: 70–84.

145. Jacknow DS, Tschann JM, Link MP, Boyce WT. Hypnosis in the prevention of chemotherapy-related nausea and vomiting in children: a prospective study. *Journal of Developmental and Behavioral Pediatrics.* 1994; **15**: 258–64.

146. Rapkin DA, Straubing M, Holroyd JC. Guided imagery, hypnosis and recovery from head and neck cancer surgery: an exploratory study. *International Journal of Clinical and Experimental Hypnosis.* 1991; **XXXIX**: 215–26.

147. Liossi C, White P. Efficacy of clinical hypnosis in the enhancement of quality of life of terminally ill cancer patients. *Contemporary Hypnosis.* 2001; **18**: 145–60.

148. Rajasekaran M, Edmonds PM, Higginson IL. Systematic review of hypnotherapy for treating symptoms in terminally ill adult cancer patients. *Palliative Medicine.* 2005; **19**: 418–26.

149. Spiegel D. Uses and abuses of hypnosis. *Integrative Psychiatry.* 1989; **6**: 211–18.

150. Spiegel D, Cardena E. New uses of hypnosis in the treatment of posttraumatic stress disorder. *Journal of Clinical Psychiatry.* 1990; **51**: 4–8.

151. Finlay IG, Jones OL. Hypnotherapy in palliative care. *Journal of the Royal Society of Medicine.* 1996; **89**: 493–6.

152. Alman M, Lambrou P. *Self-hypnosis: the complete manual for health and self-change*, 2nd edn. London: Souvenir Press, 1993.

153. Spiegel D, Albert LH. Naloxone fails to reverse hypnotic alleviation of chronic pain. *Psychopharmacology.* 1983; **81**: 140–3.

∗154. Pedersen DL. Hypnosis and the right hemisphere. *Proceedings of the British Society of Medical and Dental Hypnosis.* 1984; **5**: 2–13.

∗155. Gruzelier J. The state of hypnosis: evidence and applications. *QJM.* 1996; **89**: 313–17.

156. Spiegel D, Cutcomb S, Ren C, Pribram K. Hypnotic hallucination alters evoked potentials. *Journal of Abnormal Psychology.* 1985; **94**: 249–55.

157. Meier W, Klucken M, Soyka D, Bromm B. Hypnotic hypo- and hyperalgesia: divergent effects on pain ratings and pain-related cerebral potentials. *Pain.* 1993; **53**: 175–81.

158. Rainville P, Carrier B, Hofbauer RK *et al.* Dissociation of sensory and affective dimensions of pain using hypnotic modulation. *Pain.* 1999; **82**: 159–71.

159. Rainville P, Duncan GH, Price DD *et al.* Pain affect encoded in human anterior cingulate but not somatosensory cortex. *Science.* 1997; **277**: 968–71.

160. Rhiner M, Dean GE, Ducharme S. Nonpharmacologic measures to reduce cancer pain in the home. *Home Health Care Management and Practice.* 1996; **8**: 41–7.

161. LeBaron S, Zeltzer L. Imaginative involvement and hyponotizability in childhood. *International Journal of Clinical and Experimental Hypnosis.* 1988; **36**: 284–95.

162. Kuttner L, Bowman M, Teasdale M. Psychological treatment of distress, pain, and anxiety for young children with cancer. *Journal of Developmental and Behavioral Pediatrics.* 1988; **9**: 374–81.

163. Sloman R, Brown P, Aldana E, Chee E. The use of relaxation for the promotion of comfort and pain relief in persons with advanced cancer. *Contemporary Nurse.* 1994; **3**: 6–12.

164. Haase O, Schwenk W, Hermann C, Muller JM. Guided imagery and relaxation in conventional colorectal resections: a randomized, controlled, partially blinded trial. *Diseases of the Colon and Rectum.* 2005; **48**: 1955–63.

165. Simonton OC, Simonton MS, Creighton S. *Getting well again.* Los Angeles: JP Tarcher, 1978.

166. Besedovsky HO, Rey AD. Physiology of psychoneuroimmunology: a personal view. *Brain, Behavior, and Immunity.* 2007; **21**: 34–44.

167. Walker LG, Eremin O. Psychoneuroimmunology: a new fad or the fifth cancer treatment modality? *American Journal of Surgery.* 1995; **170**: 2–4.

168. Fellowes D, Barnes K, Wilkinson S. Aromatherapy and massage for symptom relief in patients with cancer. *Cochrane Database of Systematic Reviews.* 2004; **CD002287**.

169. Wilkes E. Complementary therapy in hospice and palliative care. Report for Trent Palliative Care Centre, 1992.

170. Ko D, Lerner R, Klose G, Cosini AB. Effective treatment of lymphoedema of the extremities. *Archives of Surgery.* 1998; **133**: 452–8.

171. Weinrich SP, Weinrich MC. The effect of massage on pain in cancer patients. *Applied Nursing Research.* 1990; **3**: 140–5.

172. Grealish L, Lomasney A, Whiteman B. Foot massage. A nursing intervention to modify the distressing symptoms of pain and nausea in patients hospitalized with cancer. *Cancer Nursing.* 2000; **23**: 237–43.

173. Wilkie DJ, Kampbell J, Cutshall S *et al.* Effects of massage on pain intensity, analgesics and quality of life in patients with cancer pain: a pilot study of a randomized clinical trial conducted within hospice care delivery. *Hospice Journal.* 2000; **15**: 31–53.

174. Corbin L. Safety and efficacy of massage therapy for patients with cancer. *Cancer Control.* 2005; **12**: 158–64.

175. Cassileth BR, Vickers AJ. Massage therapy for symptom control: outcome study at a major cancer center. *Journal of Pain and Symptom Management.* 2004; **28**: 244–9.

176. McCarthy MM, Altemus M. Central nervous system actions of oxytocin and modulation of behavior in humans. *Molecular Medicine Today.* 1997; **3**: 269–75.

177. Sayre Adams J, Wright S. *Therapeutic touch.* London: Churchill Livingstone, 2001.

178. Cook CA, Guerrerio JF, Slater VE. Healing touch and quality of life in women receiving radiation treatment for cancer: a randomized controlled trial. *Alternative Therapies in Health and Medicine.* 2004; **10**: 34–41.

179. Olson K, Hanson J, Michaud M. A phase II trial of Reiki for the management of pain in advanced cancer patients. *Journal of Pain and Symptom Management.* 2003; **26**: 990–7.

180. Filshie J, Rubens CN. Complementary and alternative medicine. *Anesthesiology Clinics.* 2006; **24**: 81–111, viii.

181. Cepeda MS, Carr DB, Lau J, Alvarez H. Music for pain relief. *Cochrane Database of Systematic Reviews.* 2006; **CD004843**.

182. Hilliard RE. Music therapy in hospice and palliative care: a review of the empirical data. *Evidence-based Complementary and Alternative Medicine.* 2005; **2**: 173–8.

183. Campbell NC, Murray E, Darbyshire J *et al.* Designing and evaluating complex interventions to improve health care. *British Medical Journal.* 2007; **334**: 455–9.

184. Hart J. Complementary therapies for cancer survivors: communicating with patients about risks and benefits. *Alternative and Complementary Therapies.* 2006; **208**: 13.

185. Dy GK, Bekele L, Hanson LJ *et al.* Complementary and alternative medicine use by patients enrolled onto phase I clinical trials. *Journal of Clinical Oncology.* 2004; **22**: 4810–5.

*186. Bardia A, Barton DL, Prokop LJ *et al.* Efficacy of complementary and alternative medicine therapies in relieving cancer pain: a systematic review. *Journal of Clinical Oncology.* 2006; **24**: 5457–64.

22

Management of breakthrough pain

GIOVAMBATTISTA ZEPPETELLA AND RUSSELL K PORTENOY

Introduction	286	Symptomatic interventions	289
Definition of breakthrough pain	287	Transmucosal formulations	291
Characteristics of breakthrough pain	287	Parenteral formulations	292
Management of breakthrough pain	288	Nonpharmacologic therapies	292
Primary interventions	288	Summary	292
Treatment of the neoplasm or comorbid conditions	289	References	293
Treatment of precipitating factors	289		

KEY LEARNING POINTS

- Breakthrough pain is a transient increase in pain intensity over background pain that occurs commonly in cancer patients; it is a distinct component of cancer pain and requires specific management.
- Breakthrough pain is a heterogeneous phenomenon that is typically of fast onset, short duration, and feels similar to background pain except that it may be more severe.
- Despite the self-limiting nature of breakthrough pain, it can have a profound impact on both patients and carers quality of life.

- Several subtypes of breakthrough pain have been recognized including incident pain, spontaneous pain, and end-of-dose failure.
- Management of breakthrough pain involves a combination of pharmacological and nonpharmacological treatment strategies.
- Pharmacological management is usually in the form of supplemental analgesia (also known as rescue medication) which is best administered before or soon after the onset of breakthrough pain.
- The ideal rescue medication should be potent, absorbed and excreted rapidly, easy to administer, and produce minimal adverse effects.

INTRODUCTION

For the patient with cancer, pain may be a frightening and debilitating symptom, which adds to the burden of illness and undermines quality of life for both patients and their caregivers. Although management strategies have improved over several decades of clinical research, cancer pain remains a clinical challenge and novel therapies that address unmet needs continue to be sought. One such need relates to the observation that patients with cancer pain often report daily fluctuations in the pain, which may include severe exacerbations that compromise function, even if the pain overall is relatively well controlled. Indeed, most cancer patients are able to identify two distinct components of their pain: persistent background pain, which is present most of the time, and transient breakthrough pain, which temporarily increases above the background pain.

As a result of these observations, breakthrough pain began to be studied as a discrete pain state.[1] During the past 15 years, cancer-related breakthrough pain has become recognized as an important clinical problem in its own right and an increasing number of published studies have appeared, which have led to an ongoing discussion about the definition, assessment, and management of this problem.

DEFINITION OF BREAKTHROUGH PAIN

The term breakthrough pain has been used to describe a phenomenon in which pain intensity suddenly increases to "break through" the background pain that is otherwise controlled by a fixed schedule, "around-the-clock" (ATC) opioid regimen (**Figure 22.1**). Although originally described in opioid-treated cancer patients, this phenomenology is neither specific to cancer nor opioid therapy. Accordingly, although many studies apply a definition that requires opioid-treated, adequately controlled background pain,[1] others define breakthrough pain irrespective of analgesic regimen or in patients with uncontrolled background pain who experience exacerbations.[2] This inconsistency in the definition of breakthrough pain was highlighted by an international study, which found that the term "breakthrough pain" is either defined or recognized differently in different countries.[3]

This lack of consensus on a formal definition of breakthrough pain can lead to difficulties when comparing studies and recommending management strategies. Even the term "breakthrough pain" is not one that is universally accepted and some clinicians prefer alternative terms, such as episodic pain, or use a variety of terms – such as end-of-dose failure, incident pain, pain flare, transient pain, and transitory pain – interchangeably.[4]

The need to build consensus about the definition of breakthrough pain has been recognized.[4] All the suggested

definitions begin with the concept that the label applies to a temporal phenomenology characterized by a transitory increase in pain intensity over the background pain. A relatively stringent definition applies the term only to the cancer population, in which it was first defined, and posits that breakthrough pain is a transitory, severe, or excruciating pain, which lasts seconds to hours and is superimposed on a background pain controlled to a moderate or better intensity by an opioid regimen. This definition can be contrasted with one that is very broad: breakthrough pain can refer to any severe, transient pain with intensity exceeding baseline. Given the imprecision in the latter definition, the potential to confuse breakthrough pain with poorly controlled background pain, the more stringent definition will be used in this discussion. Moreover, the term "incident pain," which has been used synonymously with breakthrough pain by some authors, will herein be defined, perhaps more traditionally, as a type of breakthrough pain precipitated by a voluntary action of the patient. Likewise, the term "end-of-dose failure" will refer to another type of breakthrough pain, this one characterized by the temporal occurrence of the pain at the end of the dosing interval when the fixed schedule opioid regimen involves repeated doses.

CHARACTERISTICS OF BREAKTHROUGH PAIN

Studies have evaluated the characteristics of breakthrough pain in patients attending cancer centers and pain clinics, and in patients managed through hospice inpatient units or outpatients services.[5] These studies have varied in their sampling procedures and their inclusion and exclusion criteria; some have specifically addressed breakthrough pain, while others describe breakthrough pain as an incidental finding. In the more detailed reports, breakthrough pain is usually characterized according to its location, severity, temporal characteristics, relationship to the fixed schedule analgesic regimen, precipitating factors, predictability, pathophysiology, etiology, and palliative factors.[6]

The reported prevalence of breakthrough pain has varied from 20 to 95 percent,[5] depending on the population and survey methodology. The daily frequency of the pains vary greatly as well; the modal experience is three to four pains per day. Breakthrough pains may be predictable or unpredictable, and their location is usually related to the location of the background pain. The onset of breakthrough pain is typically fast (reaching a maximum severity within five minutes) and the duration is usually relatively short (most subside within 30 minutes). The quality in most cases is similar to the background pain. Like the background pain, the pathophysiology of breakthrough pain may be visceral, somatic, neuropathic, or mixed, and the etiology may be directly due to cancer, cancer treatment, or it may be unrelated to the cancer.

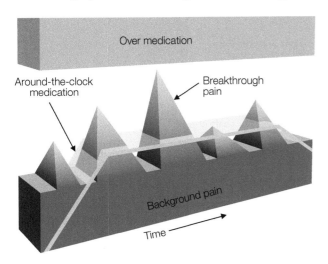

Figure 22.1 Model of breakthrough pain. Figure © Cephalon, Inc.

Despite the self-limiting nature of breakthrough pain, it can pose a significant physical, psychological, or economic burden on patients and their caregivers. Patients with breakthrough pain are often less satisfied with their analgesic therapy, have decreased functioning because of their pain, and may experience social and psychosocial consequences such as increased levels of anxiety and depression.[7] Breakthrough pain can be a poor prognostic indicator,[8, 9] and the site of breakthrough pain may predict response to treatment.[10] Furthermore, inadequately relieved breakthrough pain can place additional burden on the healthcare system, with increases in emergency and medical visits, more hospital admissions, and longer hospital stays.[11]

The epidemiology of the subtypes of breakthrough pain has been described in several studies. Incident pain has been reported in between 32 and 94 percent of patients.[12, 13] Because these pains are precipitated by voluntary action, such as walking, they are usually predictable; their occurrence is associated with a poor response to pharmacological therapy.[9, 14] Spontaneous pain has been reported in between 28 and 45 percent of patients.[1, 13] These pains may occur in the absence of a specific trigger or may be precipitated by nonvoluntary phenomena, such as fullness of the bladder, bowel movement, or cough. These pains may also be predictable or unpredictable. Breakthrough pain that occurs reliably at the end of the dosing interval of an analgesic drug, or end-of-dose failure, has been reported in between 2 and 29 percent of patients.[1, 13] The occurrence of these pains suggests that the prescribed dose is too low or the interval between administrations is too long. As noted, although most authors consider end-of-dose failure a subtype of breakthrough pain, some interpret the occurrence of these pains as evidence of uncontrolled background pain.

MANAGEMENT OF BREAKTHROUGH PAIN

Successful management of breakthrough pain, like the pain syndrome overall, is predicated on a comprehensive assessment, good communication, education, and reassurance of the patient and family, and efforts to encourage the participation of patients and caregivers in the treatment plan. The specific management of the breakthrough pain must be integrated into the overall plan of care, and should be appropriate for the status of the disease and the goals of care (**Table 22.1**).

As a plan of care evolves for the treatment of breakthrough pain, concurrent interventions should be considered to address the impact of these pains on function or quality of life. For example, the simple provision of a walking aid may make mobility easier around the house for patients with incident pain. If appropriate, referral to an occupational therapist for an assessment of functional outcomes should be considered.

PRIMARY INTERVENTIONS

As a general rule, the effective control of a specific pathology is a useful strategy in the management of cancer pain. The pathological processes responsible for breakthrough pain include those directly related to the underlying neoplasm or a comorbid condition, and others that may be specific precipitants for the pain.

Table 22.1 Strategies for the management of breakthrough pain.

Strategies for the management of breakthrough pain		
Foundation for effective treatment	Comprehensive assessment	
	Ongoing communication with the patient and caregivers	
	Education and reassurance of the patient and caregivers	
	Encouragement of patients and caregivers to participate in pain assessment and treatment	
	Integration of breakthrough pain treatment into the overall plan of care	
	Consideration of the status of the disease and the goals of care	
Primary interventions	Treat underlying disease, if possible and appropriate	
	Treat specific precipitating causes of breakthrough pain	
Pharmacological management	Optimize regular analgesics	Nonopioids
		Opioids
		Adjuvant analgesics
	Optimize the rescue analgesics	Nonopioids
		Opioids
		Adjuvant analgesics
Nonpharmacological management (see **Table 22.2**)		

TREATMENT OF THE NEOPLASM OR COMORBID CONDITIONS

Antineoplastic therapies include chemotherapy, biological therapies such as cytokines and monoclonal antibodies, hormonal therapies, radiation therapy, and surgery. Cytotoxic chemotherapy, biological therapies, and hormonal therapy have diverse and characteristic antitumor activities, sites of action, and toxic effects. Drugs may be used either singly or in combination, and may be combined with surgery or radiotherapy. Relief of breakthrough pain is likely to occur only when the response to chemotherapy is substantial, and if the goals of care warrant consideration of primary antineoplastic therapy, consultation with an oncologist may be valuable when developing a plan of care for breakthrough pain.

Radiotherapy is often used primarily for pain control and should be considered when breakthrough pain is associated with a discrete neoplastic lesion, even if the tumor type is known to be relatively radioresistant. Radiation is particularly effective for pain associated with bone metastases, which may cause incident or spontaneous breakthrough pain.[15][I] Pain relief can be achieved with hypofractionated therapy, thereby minimizing inconvenience and cost.[16][I]

Surgery may be used as an antineoplastic approach to achieve local tumor control, or may be appropriate for management of specific comorbidies. For example, tumor excision and fixation of a pathological fracture may be highly effective in relieving severe incident pain, and surgical treatment of intestinal or urinary obstruction, if possible and appropriate, can eliminate breakthrough pains associated with these lesions. Surgery is usually considered when conservative approaches have failed, the patient's performance status is favorable, the disease is not widespread, and the patient is agreeable to this option.

Treatment of infection is another primary intervention that has the potential to yield improvement in breakthrough pain. Although infection is usually obvious, some clinical scenarios are challenging and suggest the value of empirical therapy. For example, worsening breakthrough pain in a previously irradiated region or a region adjacent to a pressure ulcer may be related to concomitant infection, the diagnosis of which may be difficult.

TREATMENT OF PRECIPITATING FACTORS

Breakthrough pains may be precipitated by numerous processes, some of which are amenable to therapy. This therapy may be pharmacologic or nonpharmacologic. Pain related to cough or constipation, for example, may be effectively ameliorated by an anti-tussive or laxative, respectively. Pain related to joint movement may be addressed in some cases by an orthotic that limits the mobility of the joint. The assessment of the patient with breakthrough pain should identify all potential precipitants in the hope that primary interventions against the precipitating process can be implemented and thereby reduce reliance on symptomatic therapy.

SYMPTOMATIC INTERVENTIONS

Pharmacotherapy: optimizing the baseline therapy

Oral pharmacological management is usually the first line in the treatment of pain in patients with cancer. Management often follows the principles of the World Health Organization's (WHO) analgesic ladder, which popularized the notion that analgesics should be selected according to the severity of the pain and not the severity of the disease.[17] This strategy is applied to the management of breakthrough pain by optimizing both the fixed schedule, ATC regimen and a co-administered "as needed" drug for the breakthrough pain.[18][V]

In the absence of treatment-limiting side effects, an increase in the ATC opioid dose is often considered in an effort to reduce the frequency or intensity of breakthrough pains. The evidence for this approach is limited, however. An open-label study of patients with incident pain showed that titrating the dose beyond analgesia to the point of adverse effects prevented or limited breakthrough pain,[19][V] and another reported a 32–70 percent reduction in breakthrough pain within one week of increasing both the ATC analgesic and adjuvant analgesics.[10] However, another study of 137 oncology outpatients with pain from bone metastases appeared to show that patients using opioids only as needed had pain relief similar to patients taking opioids ATC despite using lower daily doses of opioid.[20][IV] Adjusting the fixed schedule opioid regimen is most clearly appropriate in patients with end-of-dose failure, for whom the usual intervention is to increase the dose or decrease the dosing interval. If an adjustment in the ATC dose leads to side effects between episodes of breakthrough pain (**Figure 22.2**), the dose should again be lowered.

Although the mainstay approach to the management of cancer pain is an opioid regimen, nonopioid analgesics and adjuvant analgesics can play important roles. Paracetamol and the nonsteroidal anti-inflammatory drugs (NSAIDs) are widely used in the management of mild cancer pain. The evidence of the analgesic efficacy of paracetamol is primarily in acute postoperative pain,[21][I] and although included in a systematic review of cancer pain treatments,[22] it could not be analyzed separately due to insufficient data. Studies examining a possible additive analgesic effect of paracetamol during concurrent opioid therapy in cancer patients have had conflicting results.[23, 24] The evidence for NSAIDs from systematic reviews suggests they are effective analgesics in cancer pain, both when studied in single doses and with chronic

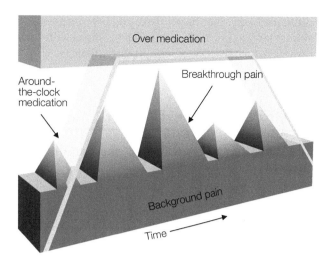

Figure 22.2 Titrating arround-the-clock analgesia: possibility of over-medication. Figure © Cephalon, Inc.

dosing,[23, 25, 26, 27][II] although the heterogeneity of study designs and outcome measures make analysis difficult.

Adjuvant analgesics are drugs that have an indication other than pain, but are capable of producing an analgesic effect.[28] Adjuvant analgesics should be considered at all stages of the patient's illness and at each step of the WHO analgesic ladder. It is important to explain to patients that these drugs have a nonanalgesic primary indication so as to avoid confusion.

The most commonly used adjuvant analgesics in the cancer population are those that may be efficacious for neuropathic pain. Although there are very few studies of drugs for cancer-related neuropathic pain, treatment generally is extrapolated from experience with noncancer pain. The best studied drugs are specific anticonvulsants and antidepressants.[29, 30][I] Other classes, including corticosteroids and membrane-stabilizing drugs,[31][II] are also tried for this indication. Paroxysmal neuropathic pains can be among the most challenging breakthrough pains and the addition of one or more drugs specific for neuropathic pain to the opioid regimen often is a valuable strategy to reduce or prevent them.

Patients with metastatic bone pain are also candidates for several classes of adjuvant analgesics. The most important are the corticosteroids and the bisphosphonates.[32] The bisphosphonates are drugs that inhibit osteoclast-mediated bone resorption and are usually prescribed to reduce the incidence of skeletal complications of metastases.[33][I] If bone pain responds overall to these therapies, movement-related breakthrough pains may be less likely to occur.

Corticosteroids are also used as adjuvant analgesics for a variety of other syndromes. These include pain from raised intracranial pressure, obstruction of hollow viscus, and organ infiltration. Breakthrough pains associated with any of these syndromes should be considered targets for a trial

of a corticosteroid coadministered with the opioid. At low doses, they also increase general well-being.

Pharmacotherapy: rescue dosing

Rescue dosing refers to the "as needed" use of a symptomatic medication for breakthrough pain, either prophylactically for predicable pains, or more commonly, as soon as pain starts. Conventionally, rescue dosing usually involves the coadministration of an immediate-release, short-acting opioid formulation in combination with the ATC opioid regimen. Occasionally, paracetamol or an NSAID is used empirically, and there have been reports of other drugs, including nitrous oxide, ketamine, midazolam, and cannabinoids.[34, 35, 36, 37, 38] The evidence for the latter treatments is mostly in the form of case reports or small controlled studies and is sometimes conflicting. Although one review confirmed that NSAIDs are effective analgesics for cancer pain, and may be comparable to morphine in single doses,[25][I] the maximal analgesic effectiveness of the nonopioid analgesics, their side effects, and the relatively slow onset of action and long duration of effect limit their value overall in the treatment of breakthrough pain.

The ideal rescue medication should be efficacious, have a rapid onset of action, a relatively short duration of effect, and minimal adverse effects (**Figure 22.3**), Oral opioids have been the mainstay approach for patients who are receiving an oral or transdermal baseline opioid regimen. Recently, new formulations that deliver a lipophilic opioid, fentanyl, directly through mucous membranes have been developed in an effort to provide a more rapid onset of effect, and one or two of these formulations are now in use in some countries. Novel delivery systems for other lipophilic drugs are in development. Alternative nonoral routes are also available, including the parenteral and rectal, and these may play a role in selected populations with breakthrough pain.

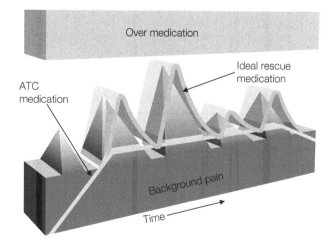

Figure 22.3 Ideal rescue medication. Figure © Cephalon, Inc.

Oral rescue dosing

The most common approach to rescue dosing involves the use of an immediate-release formulation of morphine, hydromorphone, or oxycodone, either as a single entity formulation or as a combination product combined with paracetamol or an NSAID.[39] The latter formulations have a ceiling dose imposed by the toxicity of the nonopioid component and are only used when the ATC dose is relatively low. Other opioids, either in single entity formulations (such as oxymorphone) or in combination products (such as hydrocodone plus paracetamol) are also available in some countries. Occasionally, methadone is used for rescue,[40] typically in patients receiving methadone as the baseline therapy; this approach must be undertaken cautiously because of concerns about accumulation of a long half-life drug with repeated administration.[39]

The dose selected for oral rescue is based largely on anecdotal observations. Various guidelines have been suggested, most of which suggest that the dose of an oral or parenteral rescue medication should be within the parameters of 5–15 percent of the total daily dose.[18][V] This selection of the rescue dose as a percentage of the total daily dose is consistent with the known relationship between plasma drug concentration and effects, which becomes linear when plotted on a log-linear scale. Given this relationship, there is a greater likelihood of a reliable change in effects when transiently increasing the dose if the increment is a percentage of the baseline dose. Paradoxically, recent controlled trials of transmucosal fentanyl formulations did not confirm that the effective dose for breakthrough pain was proportionate to the baseline opioid dose (see below under Transmucosal formulations), and for this reason, the "5–15 percent rule" should be applied only to oral or parenteral rescue doses.

The time–action relationship of an orally administered opioid rescue dose, which may be characterized by an onset of meaningful analgesia up to an hour after administration and a duration that may last four hours or more, may not be ideal for breakthrough pains that peak rapidly and persist for less than an hour[39] (**Figure 22.4**). This mismatch between pharmacokinetics and phenomenology has driven the development of transmucosal opioid formulations that have a more rapid onset of effect.

TRANSMUCOSAL FORMULATIONS

Transmucosal formulations comprise a variety of delivery systems that present the drug to the oral, nasal, bronchial, or rectal mucosa. Rectal administration has been used for many years and a number of short-acting opioids are commercially available in rectal formulations. These drugs may be useful when patients are temporarily unable to tolerate oral medication, or the parenteral route becomes compromised by a bleeding disorder or generalized edema. The use of rectal drugs for breakthrough pain is

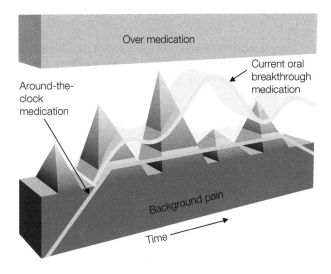

Figure 22.4 Mismatch between breakthrough pain and oral rescue medication. Figure © Cephalon, Inc.

compromised by dose-to-dose variability in absorption and effects, and limited patient acceptance for long-term use.

The sublingual route of administration has also been used historically for patients with advanced disease who become unable to tolerate oral medication. The only drug currently licensed by this route in the United Kingdom is buprenorphine, which has a relatively slow onset and long duration of analgesia, and is therefore not ideally suited to the management of breakthrough pain. Sublingual administration of injectable formulations, including morphine, is sometimes tried in the clinical setting, but the response is variable.[41, 42, 43, 44, 45] Sublingual formulations of fentanyl and other lipophilic opioids are in development for cancer-related breakthrough pain and are likely to provide a reliable alternative for rapid-onset analgesia when they become available.

Other transmucosal formulations of fentanyl are already available in some countries, and others are also in development. These drugs, and other formulations of lipophilic alternatives such as sufentanil, are being studied as treatments for breakthrough pain that may address an unmet need by providing a more rapid onset of effect than oral drugs. Presumably, a proportion of patients with breakthrough pain that peaks rapidly would indeed gain substantial benefit from these rapid-onset rescue dose formulations. Given the lack of trials comparing these formulations with currently available oral rescue drugs, however, the size and characteristics of this subgroup are not known, and oral drugs are generally tried first because of cost.

Oral transmucosal fentanyl citrate (OTFC), a fentanyl-impregnated lozenge, was the first transmucosal fentanyl formulation developed specifically for the management of breakthrough cancer pain. OTFC is rapidly absorbed through the oral mucosa and may produce analgesia in minutes.[46] A number of trials have confirmed the efficacy, safety, and tolerability of OTFC, including two randomized controlled studies[47, 48][I] and a long-term follow-up study.[49]

The second transmucosal fentanyl formulation to become commercially available is the fentanyl buccal tablet. This tablet, which has been approved in the United States for the management of breakthrough pain in opioid-treated patients with cancer, provides rapid penetration of fentanyl through the buccal mucosa by using effervescence to cause pH shifts that enhance the rate and extent of fentanyl absorption. Compared to OTFC, the buccal tablet provides a larger proportion of the dose transmucosally (48 versus 22 percent) and has an earlier T_{max} (47 versus 91 minutes).[50] The efficacy of this formulation has been shown in an open-label trial[51] and a placebo-controlled study of patients with cancer-related breakthrough pain;[52][II] as expected, the latter study demonstrated an onset of effect more rapid than would be expected from oral therapy.

The controlled clinical trials of OTFC and the fentanyl buccal tablet determined that the successful dose of these formulations did not correspond to the ATC dose. Accordingly, it is recommended that treatment with these formulations always start with a low dose, which should then be titrated to identify the effective dose.

The use of inhaled opioids for postoperative pain has been described in several studies,[53, 54, 55][III] but there are few data on patients with breakthrough pain.[56][V] Although traditional nebulizers may not be acceptable to some patients and may be an inefficient method of drug delivery,[57] several newer types of systems to aerosolize opioids are now in trials. The drugs under study include a formulation of free and liposome-encapsulated nebulized fentanyl, which can provide a more precise patient-controlled analgesia system.

Nasal administration is another approach to transmucosal delivery. Reports describing the nasal administration of morphine, fentanyl, alfentanil, or sufentanil suggest that this route provides a rapid onset of action.[43, 58, 59, 60, 61, 62][V] Although the relatively small volume of drug accommodated by the nose can be a disadvantage, the use of highly potent drugs, such as fentanyl, circumvents the problem. Nasal formulations are currently being tested.

Other transmucosal formulations are in development. For example, fentanyl and alfentanil bio-erodible muco-adhesive patches have been developed, which adhere to the buccal mucosa and rapidly release drug through the mucous membrane.[63] Like most other transmucosal formulations, these systems have been designed to yield a rapid onset of effect in the hope that this profile better meets the analgesic needs of patients with breakthrough pain.

PARENTERAL FORMULATIONS

Intravenous morphine has been shown to be effective, well-tolerated, and safe for the inpatient management of breakthrough pain,[64, 65][V] and hydromorphone has been delivered subcutaneously using a "pain pen."[51][V] In these studies, the successful rescue dose was proportionate to the ATC dose. Although the use of a parenteral rescue dose may not be practical in most cases, it is commonly considered when patients are receiving long-term parenteral opioid therapy by means of continuous subcutaneous or intravenous administration, and may be considered for short-term therapy when pain is very severe and rapid titration of doses with quick peak effects would be advantageous.[66]

NONPHARMACOLOGIC THERAPIES

Nonpharmacological approaches should also be considered in the management of breakthrough pain (**Table 22.2**). Although none of these therapeutic strategies have been studied specifically for breakthrough pain, their use in selected patients is supported by clinical observations. All of these approaches may be used in combination with conventional pharmacotherapy.

The nonpharmacological approaches can be divided into interventional strategies, including injection therapy and neural blockade, and other approaches. The latter include a diverse group of rehabilitative, psychological, and complementary therapies. To optimize the treatment of the heterogeneous population of patients with cancer-related breakthrough pain, the clinician should have access to professionals who can assist in the assessment of patients with challenging or refractory pain, and provide these strategies as appropriate.

SUMMARY

The successful management of cancer pain depends on a comprehensive assessment, which must take into account both background and breakthrough pain. Despite the

Table 22.2 Examples of nonpharmacological treatments for breakthrough pain.

Examples of nonpharmacological treatments for breakthrough pain	
Interventional therapies	Injection therapies
	Neural blockade
Physical medicine approaches	Transcutaneous electrical nerve stimulation
	Heat/cold/vibration
	Physiotherapy
Psychological approaches	Distraction, relaxation therapy
Complementary approaches	Massage
	Aromatherapy
	Acupuncture

self-limiting nature of each breakthrough pain, the repeated episodes of severe pain can have a significant impact on both patients' and caregivers' quality of life. Breakthrough pains are heterogeneous and vary in frequency, onset, duration, predictability, precipitants, pathophysiology, and etiology. Given this variation, management must begin with a comprehensive assessment. Treatment should consider whether the underlying disease, comorbidities, or precipitating events are amenable to primary interventions. Symptomatic therapy relies on both efforts to optimize the analgesic regimen for the background pain and coadministration of a rescue dose specifically for the breakthrough pain. In some cases, treatment may require a combination of pharmacological and nonpharmacological treatment strategies. Most of the evidence for the management of breakthrough pain is based on case studies and larger observational studies. Controlled trials have been carried out with rapid onset formulations containing fentanyl, but there have been no comparative trials. Guidelines remain empirical and more studies are needed to evaluate the different treatment options.

REFERENCES

∗ 1. Portenoy RK, Hagen NA. Breakthrough pain: definition, prevalence and characteristics. *Pain*. 1990; **41**: 273–81.

2. Petzke F, Radbruch L, Zech D *et al*. Temporal presentation of chronic cancer pain: Transitory pains on admission to a multidisciplinary pain clinic. *Journal of Pain and Symptom Management*. 1999; **17**: 391–401.

3. Caraceni A, Portenoy RK. An international survey of cancer pain characteristics and syndromes: IASP Task Force on Cancer Pain, International Association for the Study of Pain. *Pain*. 1999; **82**: 263–74.

∗ 4. Mercadante S, Radbruch L, Caraceni A *et al*. Episodic (breakthrough) pain: consensus conference of an expert working group of the European Association for Palliative Care. *Cancer*. 2002; **94**: 832–9.

∗ 5. Zeppetella G, Ribeiro MDC. Pharmacotherapy of cancer-related episodic pain. *Expert Opinion on Pharmacotherapy*. 2003; **4**: 493–502.

6. Portenoy RK. Treatment of temporal variations in chronic cancer pain. *Seminars in Oncology*. 1997; **24**: S16-7-16-12.

7. Portenoy RK, Payne D, Jacobsen P. Breakthrough pain: characteristics and impact in patients with cancer pain. *Pain*. 1999; **81**: 129–34.

8. Bruera E, Fainsinger R, MacEachern T *et al*. The use of methylphenidate in patients with incident cancer pain receiving regular opiates: A preliminary report. *Pain*. 1992; **50**: 75–7.

9. Mercadante S, Maddaloni S, Roccella S, Salvaggio L. Predictive factors in advanced cancer pain treated only by analgesics. *Pain*. 1992; **50**: 151–5.

10. Hwang SS, Chang VT, Kasimis B. Cancer breakthrough pain characteristics and responses to treatment at a VA medical center. *Pain*. 2003; **101**: 55–64.

11. Fortner BV, Okon TA, Portenoy RK. A survey of pain-related hospitalizations, emergency department visits, and physician office visits reported by cancer patients with and without history of breakthrough pain. *Journal of Pain*. 2002; **3**: 38–44.

12. Banning A, Sjøgren P, Henriksen H. Treatment outcome in a multidisciplinary cancer pain clinic. *Pain*. 1991; **47**: 129–34.

13. Swanwick M, Haworth M, Lennard RF. The prevalence of episodic pain in cancer: a survey of hospice patients on admission. *Palliative Medicine*. 2001; **15**: 9–18.

14. Bruera E, Scholler T, Wenk R *et al*. A prospective multicentre assessment of the Edmonton staging system for cancer pain. *Journal of Pain and Symptom Management*. 1995; **10**: 348–55.

∗ 15. McQuay HJ, Collins SL, Carroll D, Moore RA. Radiotherapy for the palliation of painful bone metastases. *Cochrane Database of Systematic Reviews*. 1999; **CD001793**.

∗ 16. Sze WM, Shelley MD, Held I *et al*. Palliation of metastatic bone pain: single fraction versus multifraction radiotherapy – a systematic review of randomised trials. *Clinical Oncology*. 2003; **15**: 345–52.

17. World Health Organization. *Cancer pain relief*, 2nd edn. Geneva: World Health Organization, 1996.

∗ 18. Hanks GW, De Conno F, Cherny N *et al*. Morphine and alternative opioids in cancer pain: the EAPC recommendations. *British Journal of Cancer*. 2001; **84**: 587–93.

19. Mercadante S, Villari P, Ferrera P, Casuccio A. Optimization of opioid therapy for preventing incident pain associated with bone metastases. *Journal of Pain and Symptom Management*. 2004; **28**: 505–10.

20. Miaskowski C, Mack KA, Dodd M *et al*. Oncology patients with pain from bone metastases require more than around-the-clock dosing of analgesia to achieve adequate pain control. *Journal of Pain*. 2002; **3**: 12–20.

∗ 21. Moore A, Collins S, Carroll D *et al*. Single dose paracetamol (acetaminophen), with and without codeine, for postoperative pain. *Cochrane Database of Systematic Reviews*. 1998; **CD001547**.

∗ 22. McNicol E, Strassels S, Goudas L *et al*. Nonsteroidal anti-inflammatory drugs, alone or combine with opioids, for cancer pain: a systematic review. *Journal of Clinical Oncology*. 2004; **22**: 1975–92.

23. Axelsson B, Borup S. Is there an additive analgesic effect of paracetamol at step 3? A double-blind randomized controlled study. *Palliative Medicine*. 2003; **17**: 724–5.

24. Stockler M, Vardy J, Pillai A, Warr D. Acetaminophen (paracetamol) improves pain and well-being in people with advanced cancer already receiving a strong opioid regimen: a randomized, double-blind, placebo-controlled cross-over trial. *Journal of Clinical Oncology*. 2004; **22**: 3389–94.

* 25. Eisenberg E, Berkey CS, Carr DB *et al*. Efficacy and safety of nonsteroidal anti-inflammatory drugs for cancer pain: a meta-analysis. *Journal of Clinical Oncology*. 1994; **12**: 2756–65.

26. Alkhenizan A, Librach L, Beyene J. NSAIDs: are they effective in treating cancer pain? *European Journal of Palliative Care*. 2004; **11**: 5–8.

* 27. Carr DB, Goudas LC, Balk EM *et al*. Evidence report on the treatment of pain in cancer patients. *Journal of the National Cancer Institute. Monographs*. 2004; **32**: 23–31.

28. Lussier D, Huskey AG, Portenoy RK. Adjuvant analgesics in cancer pain management. *Oncologist*. 2004; **9**: 571–91.

* 29. Wiffen P, Collins S, McQuay H *et al*. Anticonvulsant drugs for acute and chronic pain. *Cochrane Database of Systematic Reviews*. 2005; **CD001133**.

* 30. Saarto T, Wiffen PJ. Antidepressants for neuropathic pain. *Cochrane Database of Systematic Reviews*. 2005; **CD005454**.

* 31. Kalso E, Tramer MR, Moore RA, McQuay HJ. Systemic local-anaesthetic-type drugs in chronic pain: a systematic review. *European Journal of Pain*. 1998; **2**: 3–14.

* 32. Wong R, Wiffen PJ. Bisphosphonates for the relief of pain secondary to bone metastases. *Cochrane Database of Systematic Reviews*. 2002; **CD002068**.

* 33. Djulbegovic B, Wheatley K, Ross J *et al*. Bisphosphonates in multiple myeloma. *Cochrane Database of Systematic Reviews*. 2002; **CD003188**.

34. Parlow JL, Milne B, Tod DA *et al*. Self-administered nitrous oxide for the management of incident pain in terminally ill patients: a blinded case series. *Palliative Medicine*. 2005; **19**: 3–8.

35. Enting RH, Oldenmenger WH, van der Rijt CC *et al*. Nitrous oxide is not beneficial for breakthrough cancer pain. *Palliative Medicine*. 2002; **16**: 257–9.

36. Mercadante S, Arcuri E, Tirelli W, Casuccio A. The analgesic effect of intravenous ketamine in cancer patients on morphine therapy: a randomised double-blind cross-over double-dose study. *Journal of Pain and Symptom Management*. 2000; **20**: 246–52.

37. del Rosario MA, Martin AS, Ortega JJ, Feria M. Temporary sedation with midazolam for control of severe incident pain. *Journal of Pain and Symptom Management*. 2001; **21**: 177–8.

38. Campbell FA, Tramer MR, Carroll D *et al*. Are cannabinoids an effective and safe treatment option in the management of pain? A qualitative systematic review. *British Medical Journal*. 2001; **323**: 1–6.

* 39. Bennett D, Burton AW, Fishman S *et al*. Consensus panel recommendations for the assessment and management of breakthrough pain. Part 2 Management. *Pharmacy and Therapeutics*. 2005; **30**: 354–61.

40. Fisher K, Stiles C, Hagen NA. Characterization of the early pharmacodynamic profile of oral methadone for cancer-related breakthrough pain: a pilot study. *Journal of Pain and Symptom Management*. 2004; **28**: 619–25.

* 41. Coluzzi PH. Sublingual morphine: efficacy reviewed. *Journal of Pain and Symptom Management*. 1998; **16**: 184–92.

42. Zeppetella G. Sublingual fentanyl citrate for cancer-related breakthrough pain: a pilot study. *Palliative Medicine*. 2001; **15**: 323–38.

43. Duncan A. The use of fentanyl and alfentanil sprays for episodic pain. *Palliative Medicine*. 2002; **16**: 550.

44. Gardner-Nix J. Oral transmucosal fentanyl and sufentanil for incident pain. *Journal of Pain and Symptom Management*. 2001; **22**: 627–30.

45. McQuay HJ, Moore RA, Bullingham RE. Sublingual morphine, heroin, methadone and buprenorphine: kinetics and efficacy. In: Foley KM, Inturrisi CE (eds). *Opioid analgesics in the management of clinical pain, advances in pain research therapy*, Vol. 8. New York: Raven Press, 1986: 407–12.

46. Hanks G. Oral transmucosal fentanyl citrate for the management of breakthrough pain. *European Journal of Palliative Care*. 2001; **8**: 6–9.

* 47. Farrar JT, Cleary J, Rauch R *et al*. Oral transmucosal fentanyl citrate: randomized, double-blind, placebo-controlled trial for the treatment of breakthrough pain in cancer patients. *Journal of the National Cancer Institute*. 1998; **90**: 611–16.

* 48. Coluzzi PH, Schwartzberg L, Conroy JD *et al*. Breakthrough cancer pain: a randomized trial comparing oral transmucosal fentanyl citrate (OTFC) and morphine sulfate immediate release (MSIR). *Pain*. 2001; **91**: 123–30.

49. Payne R, Coluzzi P, Hart L *et al*. Long-term safety of oral transmucosal fentanyl citrate for breakthrough cancer pain. *Journal of Pain and Symptom Management*. 2001; **22**: 575–83.

50. Darwish M, Kirby M, Robertson P Jr *et al*. Comparative bioavailability of the novel fentanyl effervescent buccal tablet formulation: an open-label crossover study. Poster presented at the American Pain Society annual meeting, May 3–6, 2006, San Antonio, TX.

51. Enting RH, Mucchiano C, Oldenmenger WH *et al*. The 'pain pen' for breakthrough cancer pain: a promising treatment. *Journal of Pain and Symptom Management*. 2005; **29**: 213–17.

* 52. Portenoy R, Taylor D, Messina J, Tremmel L. A randomized, placebo-controlled study of fentanyl buccal tablet for breakthrough pain in opioid-treated patients with cancer. *Clinical Journal of Pain*. 2006; **22**: 805–11.

53. Worsley MH, MacLeod AD, Brodie MJ *et al*. Inhaled fentanyl as a method of analgesia. *Anaesthesia*. 1990; **45**: 449–51.

54. Thipphawong JB, Babul N, Morishige RJ *et al*. Analgesic efficacy of inhaled morphine in patients after bunionectomy surgery. *Anesthesiology*. 2003; **99**: 693–700.

55. Higgins MJ, Asbury AJ, Brodie MJ. Inhaled nebulised fentanyl for postoperative analgesia. *Anaesthesia*. 1991; **46**: 973–6.

56. Zeppetella G. Nebulized and intranasal fentanyl in the management of cancer-related breakthrough pain. *Palliative Medicine*. 2000; **14**: 57–8.

57. Clay MM, Clarke SW. Wastage of drug from nebulisers: a review. *Journal of the Royal Society of Medicine*. 1987; **80**: 38–9.

∗ 58. Dale O, Hjortkjaer R, Kharasch ED. Nasal administration of opioids for pain management in adults. *Acta Anaesthesiologica Scandinavica*. 2002; **46**: 759–70.

59. Pavis H, Wilcock A, Edgecombe J *et al.* Pilot study of nasal morphine-chitosan for the relief of breakthrough pain in patients with cancer. *Journal of Pain and Symptom Management*. 2002; **24**: 598–602.

60. Fitzgibbon D, Morgan D, Dockter D *et al.* Initial pharmacokinetic, safety and efficacy evaluation of nasal morphine gluconate for breakthrough pain in cancer patients. *Pain*. 2003; **106**: 309–15.

61. Zeppetella G. An assessment of the safety, efficacy, and acceptability of intranasal fentanyl citrate in the management of cancer-related breakthrough pain: a pilot study. *Journal of Pain and Symptom Management*. 2000; **20**: 253–8.

62. Jackson K, Ashby M, Keech J. Pilot dose finding study of intranasal sufentanil for breakthrough and incident cancer-associated pain. *Journal of Pain and Symptom Management*. 2002; **23**: 450–2.

63. Sprintz M, Benedetti C, Ferrari M. Applied nanotechnology for the management of breakthrough cancer pain. *Minerva Anestiologica*. 2005; **71**: 419–23.

64. Mercadante S, Villari P, Ferrera P *et al.* Safety and effectiveness of intravenous morphine for episodic (breakthrough) pain using a fixed ratio with the oral daily morphine dose. *Journal of Pain and Symptom Management*. 2004; **27**: 352–9.

65. Mercadante S, Villari P, Ferrera P *et al.* Safety and effectiveness of intravenous morphine for episodic breakthrough pain in patients receiving transdermal buprenorphine. *Journal of Pain and Symptom Management*. 2006; **32**: 175–9.

66. Walker G, Wilcock A, Manderson C *et al.* The acceptability of different routes of administration of analgesia for breakthrough pain. *Palliative Medicine*. 2003; **17**: 219–21.

23

Psychological interventions in cancer pain management

T MANOJ KUMAR, C VENKATESWARAN, AND P THEKKUMPURATH

Introduction	296	Psychological interventions for pain in children with	
Psychology of pain	297	cancer	304
Overview of the chapter	297	Cognitive-behavioral techniques and coping skills	305
Psychological interventions in adult populations	297	Overall conclusions	306
Pain and other symptoms	303	References	306

KEY LEARNING POINTS

- The evidence base for the use of psychosocial interventions in managing cancer pain is increasing.
- Psycho-educational programs are effective and should be integrated with physical pain management.
- Supportive psychotherapy is probably effective but understudied.
- There is evidence for efficacy for a number of techniques grouped together as cognitive-behavioral therapy (CBT).

- The best evidence is for hypnosis and consideration should be given for using it at least as an adjunctive treatment.
- While the evidence-base is better in adults, there is sufficient evidence of efficacy in children to suggest that hypnosis and other cognitive behavioral therapy techniques should be offered to children as well.

INTRODUCTION

Interest in nonpharmacological management of cancer pain has grown in line with the use of increasingly sophisticated pharmacological options. Over the last decade, in parallel with the attention paid to better symptom control in palliative care, there has been increased attention on the psychological aspects of the pain management in patients with advanced cancer too. Many of the principles involved in nonpharmacological management of pain are illustrated in an article by Abrahm in 1999, on a hypothetical patient with terminal illness.[1] However, most of the attention is still on getting the medications right and all that the hypothetical patient appears to require is "psychological support" from the pastor and resumption of attending Sunday church services. To a large extent, this is truly indicative of the current situation with nonpharmacological interventions still at the periphery of physicians' choices.

However, there is increasing interest in interventions other than pharmacological, as reflected by an increasing level of published evidence. These range from case reports to systematic reviews and meta-analyses, covering a range of interventions from psycho-education, massage, guided imagery, relaxation techniques, supportive psychotherapy, and cognitive-behavioral therapy (CBT).

In line with the increase in interest in cognitive-behavioral interventions for almost all psychological conditions, there is an increased interest in the use of cognitive-behavioral techniques in pain management as well. There is also increasing recognition that pain as a symptom coexists and interacts with other symptoms such as fatigue and emotional distress. Fleishman[2] suggests that there may be a "cross over" effect on other symptoms when an established treatment for a particular symptom is used.

PSYCHOLOGY OF PAIN

Bond[3] points out that the psychological mechanisms in chronic pain are different to those in acute pain conditions. Pain in cancer gives rise to unique psychological issues so that the experience of pain may not be proportional to the extent of tissue damage. Whether due to cancer or not, common patterns seen in people with chronic pain include those who fail to cope with pain and those in whom there is a somatoform presentation where there is little or no evidence of physical disease or injury to explain the pain. Distress arising from, and failing to cope with, pain are common in acute pain presentations as well. It is no wonder that psychological interventions have been the focus of interest in cancer-related pain.

Bond[3] describes a biopsychosocial model for pain. The biological and social elements of pain are outside the scope of this chapter but have important management implications. In terms of the psychological aspects, most models focus on the cognitive processes linking physical and emotional elements of pain.[4] In both acute and chronic pain, the cognitive process underlying our appraisal of pain may sometimes become prominent perpetuating factors in the experience of pain. The success of interventions of the cognitive-behavioral type, tried in various conditions has, therefore, come to be used in the management of pain also. Briefly, specific beliefs about pain lead to emotional states of anxiety, depression, anger, and hostility. High levels of fear may lead to avoidance of activities and a withdrawal into an invalid state. Failure to cope often leads to specific cognitive patterns such as catastrophizing, which are often amenable to cognitive-behavior therapy.

OVERVIEW OF THE CHAPTER

The chapter is divided into three sections. The first section looks at interventions in the adult population and the second briefly explores the interaction of pain and other symptoms, looking at related issues. The final section examines the interventions in children. Key components of the various techniques are presented as bullet points and practical examples are given in boxes. The evidence base is examined in the increasing order of methodological rigor starting with single studies and progressing to systematic reviews. The emphasis has been on the latter whenever possible.

PSYCHOLOGICAL INTERVENTIONS IN ADULT POPULATIONS

Psycho-education

Empowerment of the patient and active participation in pain control are the key elements of psycho-education. These are intrinsically attractive as they form the cornerstones of good medical management. On a scale of psychological interventions, patient education, even though termed as "psycho-education," is at the lowest end of complexity. Typically, these interventions consist of training the patient in formalized discussions about the pharmacology of pain. The interventions are usually time-limited (15 minutes) and delivered by trained "counselors." The aim is often to ensure that medication compliance is improved and that patients adhere to the dosages and schedules that are deemed to be appropriate. Given that opioid medications still form the cornerstone of cancer pain treatment, psycho-educational efforts have an important role, as myths abound about the opioids, such as the risk of addiction (**Box 23.1**).

Box 23.1 Key components of patient education programs

- **Pain assessment**: It has been shown that pain rating scales are easily understood by patients.[5] These are usually Likert scales on a 0–10 or 0–100 basis forming reliable and clinically useful means for patient communication about pain.[6] Another tool has been pain diaries or logs that document the details of the occurrence and other features of pain throughout the day.
- **Pharmacological education**: As mentioned earlier, these are mostly centered on aspects of opioid medications such as fear of addiction, misinformation about tolerance, and side effects. There is no evidence that discussions about side effects lead to a higher perception of side effects.[7]
- **Education about nonpharmacological interventions**: Often, patients have to be informed and appropriate referral pathways pointed out with regard to nonpharmacological interventions.

EVIDENCE FOR EFFICACY OF PATIENT EDUCATION PROGRAMS

Individual studies

In 1987, Rimer and colleagues[8][III] reported on enhanced cancer pain control through patient education. Over 200 patients were divided into an experimental and control group and provided with an individual session lasting 15 minutes. It was reported that the experimental group showed a higher level of medication compliance in terms of both timing and dosage. There was a significant reduction in fears associated with opioid use, such as that of addiction, and reduced behavior of stopping medications when they were better. However, it is to be noted that although there was a trend in the experimental group to report less pain, this did not reach statistical significance.

In 1993, Ferrell and colleagues[9][III] studied the efficacy of psycho-educational intervention, albeit in a small group of 40 patients and family members. The three sessions included verbal, written, and audiotaped instructions and they found that in the experimental group there was an increase in the knowledge and use of medications and better sleep. There was also a decrease in the fear of addiction, anxiety, and pain intensity. Outcomes in the family members also reported a similar pattern.

De Wit and colleagues[10][II] evaluated the efficacy of a similar program in more than 300 patients. The intervention consisted of an individual session and two telephone contacts of an hour to an hour and a half long and the results showed, again, an increase in medication-related knowledge and a decrease in the fear of addiction and pain intensity. In this study, an interesting finding was that the reduction in pain intensity was seen purely in the group which did not receive nursing at home, suggesting that knowledge may be only one variable in affecting outcomes in the multifactorial experience that is pain.

Meta-analyses

A meta-analysis of psycho-educational care of patients with cancer in adult patients concluded that this was beneficial in relation to anxiety, depression, nausea, vomiting, pain, and knowledge.[11][I]

CONCLUSIONS – PATIENT EDUCATION PROGRAMS

There is sufficient evidence to show that patient education programs are effective. Compared to other psychological interventions, they are easier to deliver, cheaper, and should be intrinsic to any comprehensive pain management programs in oncology and palliative care.

Supportive psychotherapy

According to Werman,[12] supportive psychotherapy refers primarily, but not exclusively, to a form of treatment whose principal concern and focus is to strengthen mental functions that are acutely or chronically inadequate to cope with demands of the external world or the patient's inner psychological world. The acute deficiency or crisis occurs when the patient's life which was previously in a state of equilibrium has more or less suddenly become deeply disturbed by a stressful event (**Box 23.2**).

EVIDENCE FOR EFFICACY OF SUPPORTIVE PSYCHOTHERAPY

While a number of studies have looked at supportive psychotherapy in alleviating distress in cancer patients, only a few have looked at the efficacy in pain.

Spiegel and Bloom[13][II] looked specifically at the efficacy of supportive psychotherapy in reducing cancer pain. Therapy was delivered in a group format and outcomes assessed at four-monthly intervals. While, as could be expected, most patients in the intervention group reported improvement in psychological parameters, what was interesting is that patients in the experimental group did not report an increase in pain at the end of a year while patients in the control group reported significantly more pain.

Luborsky and others[14][I] reviewed the evidence for the relationship of a period of psychotherapy with a measure of improved physical health. They concluded that there was evidence to strongly suggest that psychotherapeutic interventions reduced pain. Of the eight studies they reviewed, three are in cancer patients and of relevance for us. Spiegel and Bloom's study, mentioned above, showed that group therapy and hypnosis reduce metastatic breast carcinoma pain. The group receiving both group therapy and hypnosis did significantly better than others. Goodwin[15][II] also reached similar conclusions in their patient group providing psychosocial supportive group intervention. Fobair et al.[16][II] offered a supportive–expressive group intervention to lesbians with early breast cancer and found similar beneficial effects. It is interesting that all three studies offered group interventions to women

---

Box 23.2 Key components of supportive psychotherapy

- Emotional support.
- Encouraging expression of emotions.
- Focusing on improving coping skills.
- Establishing achievable goals.
- Overall leading of a more meaningful life.
- Focusing on the current circumstances rather than examining the past.
- Emphasis on communication.
- Discussion of current stressors.
- Use of nonspecific techniques.
- Delivered in individual or group setting.

with breast cancers. Overall, the review found a mean effect size of 0.35. Seven out of eight studies showed a reduction in pain in relation to receiving psychotherapy.

CONCLUSIONS – SUPPORTIVE PSYCHOTHERAPY

The paucity of studies in this area make the drawing of any conclusions difficult. Studies are sparse as supportive psychotherapy is broad-based and lacks neat models which are easy to study. However, in day to day clinical practice, models such as the Problem Solving Therapy[17] offer a great deal promise.

Cognitive–behavioral therapy

CBT derives its roots from behavioral models based upon learning theory and cognitive theories. A combination of the two as CBT has been used in sufferers with non-malignant pain, particularly chronic back pain. In contrast, psychological problems in people with malignancy with or without pain have been dealt with mostly by counseling and other psychological interventions. It is only recently that cognitive-behavioral interventions have received attention in the management of malignant pain.

As with supportive psychotherapy, CBT is also delivered in individual and group formats. CBT is based on several assumptions. Maladaptive thoughts effect emotions and behaviors in a cyclical fashion. It is possible to identify recurring patterns of maladaptive thoughts. Patients are trained in recording these thoughts, subsequent feelings, and behaviors. Patients can then be taught to change the maladaptive thoughts and behaviors leading to improvements in mood and other symptoms, such as pain.

It is important to realize that the above model of CBT, with the focus perhaps more on the cognitive processes (changing maladaptive thoughts), is the model most prevalent in mainstream psychiatry, to treat a variety of disorders, such as depression and anxiety. However, perusal of the CBT literature in cancer pain clearly shows that the emphasis here has been more on the behavioral aspects and studies have focused less on changing thought processes. Loscalzo[18] reviewed the theoretical background of psychological interventions, particularly the use of cognitive-behavioral interventions in advanced cancer pain. He divided cognitive-behavioral interventions into three broad categories of cognitive, behavioral, and physical interventions. The cognitive interventions comprised of relaxation techniques, distraction, cognitive coping strategies, and thought stopping. Management of social contingencies, systematic desensitization, shaping, modeling, time outs, and stress inoculation were considered behavioral interventions. Stated task assignments, progressive muscle relaxation, and diaries were examples of physical strategies. It is interesting that many of the interventions classified below under Cognitive-behavioral techniques and coping skills, such as hypnosis and guided imagery were not included in this grouping. Over the next ten years, under the rubric of CBT, there was an explosion of studies, disproportionately focused on hypnosis and related techniques, probably due to the ease of application.

GOALS OF CBT

One of the early descriptions of CBT in pain management offered to many ill patients was by Fishman in 1992.[19] He suggested that the CBT intervention might have some or all of the following goals:

- education of the patient about pain, the relationship between pain and suffering and cognitive theories in relation to these;
- to attempt to modify specific thoughts and images associated with pain such as perception of imminent danger, guilt, shame, and other forms of cognitive distortion;
- learning of specific coping techniques, such as problem solving, relaxation, and self-control skills;
- modification of basic attitudes (beliefs, assumptions, and values) that underlie the cognitive distortions resulting in distress;
- to improve personal control (see also **Box 23.3**).

HYPNOSIS, RELAXATION, AND IMAGERY

The recent resurgence of interest in hypnosis is attributable to a growing interest in alternative cost-saving therapies and to an increasing presence of brain and neuroimaging studies in hypnosis.[20] Of all the treatment contexts in which it is used, hypnosis is best known as a pain management technique.[21]

Hypnosis is defined as a "natural state of aroused, attentive focal attention coupled with a relative suspension of the peripheral awareness" with three main components – absorption, dissociation, and suggestibility.[22] Another more sociocognitive view of hypnosis is "a social interaction in which one person designated the subject, responds to suggestion suffered by another person, designated the hypnotist, for experiences involving alterations in perception, memory, and voluntary action."[23]

Sometimes the terms relaxation training and imagery and hypnosis are used loosely and there is no formal consensus that clearly defines each of these. Syrjala et al.[24] suggest that "techniques identified as relaxation, imagery, and hypnosis do not differ empirically." Guided imagery is a related concept and involves attention to internally generated mental images without the formal use of hypnosis.

Positive mental images were a technique popularized by Simonton and colleagues,[25] which involved the person imagining his immune system fighting the cancer. This has been abandoned, quite rightly, due to lack of any evidence and potential for negative psychological sequel, such as guilt.

Box 23.3 Key components of cognitive-behavior therapy

- The use of cognitive-behavioral techniques in pain management aims at the subjective part of the pain experience, which is more defined by the patients' mood state, thoughts, and beliefs about pain and subsequent behaviors. CBT techniques would aim to modify the thoughts and behaviors so that the pain experience is altered.
- Common cognitive-behavioral strategies include:
  - progressive muscle relaxation;
  - relaxation training;
  - hypnosis;
  - guided imagery;
  - autogenic training;
  - distraction;
  - thought monitoring;
  - thought stopping;
  - coping self-statement;
  - problem solving.

Of these, the most commonly used are:

- **Hypnosis/distracting imagery**: Recent conceptualizations of hypnosis suggest that it employs classic behavioral intervention approaches such as distraction and relaxation.
- **Cognitive/attentional distraction**: This is mostly used in acute pain and involves engaging the patient in absorbing and interesting activities during invasive procedures. It is presumed to work by diverting the patient's attention or awareness of aversive stimuli by the involvement in a task. This is often used in children where storytelling, video game playing, and playing with a party blower (a paper noise maker) are used. In adults, guided imagery training has often been used.
- **Relaxation training**: Establishment of deep states of relaxation has been shown to reduce pain. Often, the training starts with a clinician and is maintained through audiotapes.
- **Cognitive restructuring**: This involves reframing stressful events as less threatening and under control. This has been used both in adults and children. Since hypnosis and related techniques are the most commonly used ones, it is worth examining these in some detail.

Physical relaxation coupled with imagery that provides a substitute focus of attention for the painful sensation is the most commonly employed technique. Depending on the degree of hypnotizabilty, this could take the form of simple distraction to feelings of floating above one's own body (see **Box 23.4**).[22]

PRACTICAL EXAMPLES OF TECHNIQUES OF HYPNOSIS IN ADULTS

A number of techniques are used depending on the individual patient characteristics, type of pain, and the illness. These can be broadly divided into dissociative, associative, and symbolic techniques.[28] In the simple forms, dissociation is achieved through diversion of awareness or focused listening, by concentrating on the body parts not experiencing any pain or by suggesting warmth or coolness. Symptom substitution is another form of dissociation in which the patient, for example, recalls the numbness felt after dental analgesia and places these pain antagonist sensations to the painful area.

Depending on the patient's hypnotic ability and rapport, this can proceed to much deeper levels of dissociation, where the patient can leave their bodies and imagine floating over.

Another of the techniques used is glove anesthesia. This is fairly easily achieved and helps build patient confidence and rapport with the therapist. Following induction of a trance state, it is suggested to the patient

---

Box 23.4 Key components of hypnosis

The therapeutic efficacy of hypnosis is differentially attributed to various components:

- Hypnotizabilty or hypnotic responsiveness or hypnotic suggestibility, a measurable and stable state, which gives an indication of an individuals potential to be hypnotized, is an important variable.[26]
- Physical relaxation and attention control. Spiegel and Moore[22] suggest that hypnotic analgesia is mediated via these two main components. This essentially involves intensification and narrowing of the focus of attention, replacing pain, which is pushed to the periphery, with a competing and pleasant sensation like warmth.
- Cognitive changes. In the social-cognitive model, hypnotic analgesia is mediated through cognitive-behavioral mechanisms, in which changes in cognition alters affective states associated with pain.[27]

that he visualizes one hand as transparent and thus be able to see the nerves which transmit the sensation from the fingertips to brain. These nerves along with other joined nerves are visualized, to reach a switchboard in the brain. The patient is instructed to turn off the pain switch for the selected hand and to notice the light over the switch to simultaneously extinguish.

At every stage the patient is encouraged to visualize the event or surroundings as fully as they can, and this ability to do so partly determines the success of the intervention. Once a patient has learned glove anesthesia the pain control can be transferred to another part of the body.[29]

EVIDENCE FOR EFFICACY OF CBT, PARTICULARLY HYPNOSIS

Up until the 1980s, research in this area was sparse and consisted mostly of case reports. A review of psychological interventions in chronic pain by Turner and Chapman[30] was skeptical of the efficacy of hypnosis and concluded that "clinical research in this area is sparse, appallingly poor, and has failed to demonstrate convincingly that hypnosis has more than a placebo effect in relieving chronic pain". Since the early 1980s, there have been a number of proper clinical trials reporting on the efficacy of hypnosis in cancer pain setting.

Randomized controlled trials are now unarguably the gold standard in primary studies, but they can vary in quality. Trials of interventions such as hypnosis can never be judged to be of top quality as double blinding is almost impossible.

Individual studies

Spiegel and Bloom's study[13][II] of efficacy of group therapy and hypnosis in metastatic breast cancer patients with pain is an often quoted study. This indeed is the first, and to our knowledge, the only study looking at the efficacy of hypnosis in persistent cancer pain in a randomized and controlled fashion and finding that group psychotherapy plus hypnosis resulted in better pain relief. Results were significant at one year and it is interesting that a combination of the two modalities resulted in better efficacy. The intervention led to significantly less pain sensation and suffering, without any difference in pain frequency or duration. The essential component of self-hypnosis is described as shift in focus from pain to a competing and alternate sensation such as cold, which is achieved under hypnotic instruction.

In two well-controlled randomized studies, Syrjala and colleagues[24, 31][II] demonstrate the efficacy of relaxation and imagery (called hypnosis in their first study) in controlling pain in a group of bone marrow transplant patients with oral mucositis pain. In the first study in 1992,[31] they reported that hypnosis appeared superior to cognitive-behavior interventions in reducing pain. The crucial component seemed to be guided imagery, which was a component of the intervention in the hypnosis group and not in the CBT group. Acceptance of hypnosis

also seemed to be higher. In the second study reported in 1995,[24] the cognitive-behavioral interventions were more limited, thereby improving patient acceptance and the terminology in the formally "hypnosis" group was clarified as relaxation, imagery, and autogenic training. This time, both the groups reported significantly less pain. The authors claim that imagery was the key component and that cognitive-behavioral intervention does not offer anything over and above hypnosis in treatment of persistent pain. The choice of the term "imagery with relaxation" instead of hypnosis sheds light not only on the patient barriers to acceptability, but also on the lack of clear definition and standardization of procedures. Apart from other things, this would also suggest the need for focusing on individual components of psychotherapeutic interventions in order to discern what is useful and what is not. Indeed, it would make sense that the various components need to be chosen to suit various patient needs and perhaps it is this matching of techniques to needs which would make the difference rather than adherence to a preconceived mode of therapy.

Sloman and colleagues[32][II] reported similar findings for the efficacy of relaxation and guided imagery in cancer pain. When progressive muscle relaxation and guided imagery were delivered either through audiotape or by nurses, this resulted in a significant reduction of pain overall. Use of medications also reduced and there was a suggestion that the live intervention was superior.

However, a study by Gaston-Johansson et al.[33][II] on breast cancer patients undergoing autologous bone marrow stem cell transplant failed to detect any significant effect on pain intensity or character when comparing a comprehensive coping skills training protocol that included guided imagery to usual care.

Anderson et al.[34][II] reported on a randomized clinical trial evaluating the efficacy of three brief cognitive-behavioral techniques – relaxation, distraction, and positive mood interventions in chronic cancer-related pain. The study was on 57 patients who were also taking opioid medications and the interventions were home-based using audiotapes. The tapes were supplemented with written instructions and followed up through telephone calls. Though patients reported pain reduction immediately after listening to the tapes, this was not maintained at two weeks. In many ways it is not surprising that simplistic interventions are not seen to produce lasting relief in complex multifaceted chronic pain situations. At the very least, interventions have to be individualized to have any chance of success. This is illustrated by the fact that over half the patients approached for the study refused to participate.

Systematic reviews/meta-analyses

Sellick and Zaza,[35][I] in a review of nonpharmacological interventions in cancer pain, conclude that there is some support for the use of hypnosis in cancer pain, although this has not been examined extensively.

Montgomery et al.,[21][I] in a meta-analysis of effectiveness of hypnosis in pain, classifies this as "well established treatment across various pain settings." They also note that the effects of hypnosis were mediated in the expected direction by measured hypnotizabilty.

Hawkins,[36][I] in a "systematic meta review," looked at published reviews of literature in this area. Specific quality guidelines and scoring systems were applied in evaluating these. There is sufficient evidence of good quality to conclude that hypnosis has demonstrable efficacy in the treatment of pain. Of the various settings considered, hypnosis in cancer pain and invasive medical procedures showed level one evidence from good quality studies.

Luebbert et al.[37][I] looked at the effectiveness of relaxation training under the rubric of CBT in adult male and female cancer patients undergoing acute treatment. They found medium to large effect sizes for pain and distress in a broad range of cancer patients.

Redd et al.[38][I] reviewed the effectiveness of behavioral intervention methods in the control of a number of aversive side effects of cancer treatment, identifying 54 published studies in the process. Redd came across 12 studies investigating the impact of behavioral interventions on cancer treatment-related pain, of which five were adverse clinical trials. Four of these five supported the efficacy of behavioral interventions. The other seven studies were of varying methodologies and all found a reduction in pain following behavioral interventions. This review found no studies of behavioral interventions in chronic cancer pain. Redd concluded that hypnotic-like methods, involving relaxation suggestion and distracting imagery, hold the greatest promise for pain management.

Mundy et al.[39][I] looked at the efficacy of behavioral interventions for a number of cancer treatment-related side effects including pain. In all, they identified 67 published studies for the review. Thirteen of the 67 studies were of behavioral interventions in cancer treatment-related pain and the behavioral components were hypnosis, distraction, relaxation training, cognitive restructuring, and rehearsal modeling. Overall, results indicated that although both behavioral training and hypnosis had equally beneficial effects on pain, hypnosis had a greater impact on treatment-related anxiety in children. In adults, it was felt that hypnosis was superior to other methods. Of the 13 studies, seven were randomized clinical trials and five of the seven supported the efficacy of behavioral intervention. The other six studies, using a variety of designs, also formed a significant reduction in pain after behavioral interventions. It is important to note that all the studies were in acute pain. Factors underlying chronic pain are obviously different, making generalization from acute pain research meaningless. Hypnotic-like methods involving relaxation, cognitive suggestions, and distraction seem to be more effective than other methods.

Graves[40][I] performed a meta-analysis of adult cancer patients and concluded that treatment packages with a larger number of "social cognitive" components had larger effect sizes. This included a number of cancer types, patients of both genders, and the outcome focused on was quality of life.

Jensen and Patterson[41] point to the continuing lack of credible control conditions and state that hypnotic analgesia is yet to demonstrate its effectiveness over and above treatment outcome expectancy in this area of research.

Tatrow and Montgomery[42][I] reported a meta-analysis of cognitive-behavioral therapy techniques for distress and pain in breast cancer patients. The review sought randomized trials comparing CBT with no treatment or standard care with the outcomes of distress and pain. A wide variety of techniques including hypnosis, imagery, and relaxation apart from cognitive-behavioral therapy were looked at. A total of 20 studies were included comprising over 1600 subjects for distress and nearly 500 for pain. Thirty effect sizes were calculated and these were by treatment rather than by study. The overall effect size was 0.31 for distress and 0.49 for pain indicating that 62 percent of patients in the treatment groups did better than those in the control groups with regards to distress and 69 percent with regard to pain. These effect sizes can be said to be in the small to medium range. Trials using individual interventions (usually smaller studies) had significantly larger effect sizes than those using group interventions (usually larger studies). As it is common for smaller studies to show larger effect sizes, one of the conclusions that could be drawn is that larger studies of individual interventions are required to prove conclusively the efficacy of CBT in cancer pain in this group of patients. The largest treatment effect size was associated with a hypnosis intervention.

Side effects of hypnotherapy

Hypnosis delivered by a skilled psychotherapist is generally considered safe. However, there have been reports of occasional adverse effects. A survey among 41 palliative care patients who used hypnosis for relaxation and coping found that 61 percent of the patients were able to cope better with their illness, whereas three reported negative psychological effects.[43]

VARIATIONS OF CBT INTERVENTIONS

Dalton and colleagues[44] reported on tailoring cognitive-behavioral treatment for cancer pain (profile-tailored CBT). Standard CBT protocols offer a similar treatment program to all patients while individualized CBT tends to tailor cognitive-behavioral interventions to patient-specific characteristics. Drawing on similar approaches in noncancer pain and alcoholism, Dalton et al.[44] attempted to match patients with cancer pain to specific CBT programs and compared it with standard CBT and usual care. The study used five weekly sessions of CBT lasting approximately an hour and had to deal with high attrition rates in a population of cancer patients undergoing chemotherapy. The resulting small sample sizes make the interpretation of the study results problematic. The profile-tailored CBT appeared to be superior to standardized CBT immediately post-therapy, but at follow up at six months, the standard CBT patients showed substantial improvement. The authors conclude by suggesting that delivery of CBT treatments by home visits, phone, or internet should be explored further.[44]

Pain was only one of 15 symptoms occurring during chemotherapy on which the effect of cognitive-behavioral intervention was studied by Given and others in 2004.[45] The study found that a ten-contact, 20-week, nurse-administered cognitive-behavioral intervention for patients receiving a first course of chemotherapy was effective for all the symptoms, including pain, for patients with higher severity of symptoms. The interaction of the cognitive-behavioral interventions with higher symptom severity baseline is interesting as well as the fact that the efficacy was sustained over and beyond the effects of supportive medications prescribed.

ACUTE VERSUS CHRONIC PAIN

In contrast to studies of acute pain in cancer, chronic cancer treatment-related pain has received less attention. Robb et al.[46] reported the findings of a preliminary study in 2006. A small sample (13 patients) received interventions including education, relaxation, exercise training, and goal setting. All patients had a positive outcome indicating promise for future better conducted studies.

MODELS FOR COGNITIVE-BEHAVIORAL INTERVENTIONS IN CANCER PAIN MANAGEMENT

Drawing on models described in healthcare literature, Kwekkeboom[47] proposed a model to predict the likelihood of success with cognitive-behavioral strategies in cancer pain. The suggested model indicated that a technique's effect on pain outcome is moderated by:

- the person's cognitive ability or skill;
- outcome expectations;
- previous use of the technique;
- perceived credibility;
- individual coping skills;
- pain outcomes.

Using this or similar models, it may be possible to match cognitive-behavioral interventions with individual factors, thereby improving effectiveness. Such models need to be tested in well-designed studies before being of practical use.

CONCLUSIONS – COGNITIVE-BEHAVIOR THERAPY

Hypnosis and other cognitive-behavioral interventions are widely used and have the strongest evidence in the management of acute procedure-related pain. In chronic pain conditions such as cancer, although the evidence is weaker, there is enough to suggest that they are useful. Well-designed studies with proper control conditions and replication of some earlier results are much needed. Equally important is the tailoring of techniques to address persistent and chronic pain. The best evidence exists for hypnosis and is most properly used as an adjunctive component of an established comprehensive pain management package.[48]

PAIN AND OTHER SYMPTOMS

Symptom clusters

Fleishman[2] points to the need for studying the efficacy of interventions for individual symptoms by looking at symptom clusters. The three symptoms that cluster in cancer are pain, depression, and fatigue.

It is clear that pain and emotional distress are intrinsically inter-related. The severity of pain increases with the severity of emotional distress.[5] It is possible that psychological interventions for pain work as essentially any psychological intervention bolsters the patient's perception of support in a situation where perceived loss of control is predominant.

The inter-relationship between psychological distress and pain is complex. Butler et al.[49][II] looked at this in a group of women with metastatic breast cancer. As part of a randomized trial of the effects of group psychotherapy, they looked at measurements of pain and distress at the time of entry into the study and looked at the progress as the patients approached death. While psychological distress remained reasonably stable between the initial measurement and the next to last point, there was significant decline from the second to last measurement until the final measurement. Group psychotherapy did not appear to have a significant role in reducing distress before death. The authors point out that this has the added implication when results of interventions in people close to death are analyzed and there seems to be a natural spike in both distress and pain before death.[49]

It is well known that pain, depression, and fatigue often cluster in patients with cancer. Fleishman[2] suggests that established treatments for one symptom may "cross over" and reduce the burden caused by other symptoms. He points out that such an approach, optimal treatment of symptom clusters, challenges the traditional model of seeing and treating symptoms individually. He suggests that the various supportive care modalities are woven together into the care plans for patients so that symptom clusters can be optimally addressed.

The study by Syrjala et al.[24] was also unique in that it looked at the efficacy of the same intervention (hypnosis) in two commonly occurring symptoms in cancer, pain and nausea/emesis. No effect was found on emesis.

An important consideration is the role of hypnosis in other symptoms that accompany cancer, such as psychological distress, insomnia, and emesis, thereby potentially offering a therapeutic intervention which reduces the overall distress of the patient.

Symptom limitations

Doorenbos et al.[50] conducted a randomized trial of problem solving cognitive-behavioral intervention on symptom limitations compared to conventional care. This approach moves away from looking at individual symptoms such as pain to the limitations imposed by a number of symptoms. They found that, on average, after ten weeks, the experimental group experienced reduced symptoms limitation and maintained this advantage over the control group.

PSYCHOLOGICAL INTERVENTIONS FOR PAIN IN CHILDREN WITH CANCER

There have been numerous advances made in the 1990s for pain research in general and specifically in pediatric pain. Many areas have been focused on, starting from the understanding of pain in children, the development of pain measures, and the use of effective strategies to control pain, both pharmacological and nonpharmacological.

In 1998, the World Health Organization published guidelines for management of pain in children with cancer for medical procedures; in all cases a combination of a psychological and a pharmacological approach was supported. Though many interventions have been applied, only two, cognitive therapy and hypnosis, qualify as empirically validated and efficacious according to the APA framework.[51]

Most of the studies carried out in pediatric pain related to cancer involve procedural pain. This has been based on previous reports on pain in children with cancer, which point out that children with cancer experience direct pain related to malignancy in only about 25 percent, while double the number (50 percent) have painful episodes due to therapy or procedures.[52] Evidence suggests that children with cancer find painful procedures to be the most difficult part of their illness and this does not get desensitized despite repeated procedures.[52] In some, distress has been seen to continue for years after treatment for cancer.[53]

Psychological interventions for procedural pain

As in adults, these could be broadly grouped into three categories:

1. education – which includes preparation and information sharing with children and parents;

2. hypnosis and imagery-based methods;
3. cognitive techniques and methods to improve coping skills.

Psycho-education

Preparation, the most common psychological intervention for children who undergo painful medical procedures, is a generic term which encompasses components like provision of information to children and their parents about the indications, need, type, and details of an impending procedure.[54] Preparatory information can be characterized as being sensory or procedural.[55] Procedural information would be those that detail the procedure, without describing the sensations, whereas sensory information would focus on the sensations that the person would experience at various stages of the procedure. A combination of both sorts of information seems to be the most effective manner.[56]

There have been several methods used to provide children with information about painful procedures such doll-play, story and coloring books, hospital tours, and cognitive strategies.[57] Video games with multimedia formats seem to have good potential.

According to a systematic review of informational interventions designed to influence knowledge among pediatric cancer patients, few conclusions can be derived and generalized, with the exception that information transfer methods which are highly interactive and individualized contribute well to health-related knowledge.[58]

Hypnosis and imagery-based methods

Hypnosis in acute and chronic pain and cancer pain has been a focus in a number of case reports and an increasing number of systematic studies.[54] As in adults, a variety of techniques, such as imagery and relaxation, are included under the term "hypnosis." Children have been found to be more responsive hypnotically than adults.[59]

PRACTICAL EXAMPLES OF TECHNIQUES OF HYPNOSIS IN CHILDREN

Direct hypnotic suggestions

Request for numbness

> We will do some strong magic now... First you have to make your low back go to sleep for a few minutes.... I'll show you how to do it... I'll just put my hand on your back and help it become sleepy and numb.... Soft and sleepy.... [60]

Indirect hypnotic suggestions using therapeutic stories and metaphors

Setting sun metaphor

> See yourself sitting on a beautiful Greek beach at sunset.... Notice the bright red sun as it descends on the far horizon... See the sun gradually sink into the sea... See the colours change from red to purple and then to blue... Enjoy the tranquillity...
>
> Adapted from Levitan[61]

Self-hypnosis techniques

The Gardner's model[62] follows a three-step method for teaching children self-hypnosis. The child is individually subjected to various induction and deepening methods usually emphasizing imagery and ideo-motor techniques. After allowing time for enjoyment of the imagery, the child is asked to count silently backward from five to one, eyes opening at three, fully alert at one.

EVIDENCE FOR EFFICACY OF HYPNOSIS IN PROCEDURAL PAIN

Individual studies of hypnosis in children

A randomized prospective controlled trial of 80 patients undergoing lumbar punctures for hematological malignancies is the most compelling study.[60][II] The children in the hypnosis group experienced significantly less pain, anxiety, and behavioral distress compared to controls. It was also noted that both direct and indirect hypnosis were equally effective, though the benefits reduced when children tried self-hypnosis. Earlier, the same group had demonstrated that when trained in hypnosis or cognitive coping skills, children undergoing bone marrow biopsy had significantly less pain.[63][III] The same study also showed that hypnosis tended to be superior to cognitive-behavioral skills training. Zeltzer and LeBaron[64][III] had also contributed to evidence establishing hypnosis being of superior value. These results reinforce findings from other studies in the same area.[65, 66]

Systematic reviews/meta-analyses of hypnosis in children

Two systematic reviews have looked into hypnosis for procedure-related pain and distress in children with cancer.

In the review carried out in 2004, nine papers were appraised, of which three studies were concluded to be well-conducted case control or cohort studies with a low risk of confounding or bias and a moderate possibility that the relationship is causal.[67][III] The rest contributed as case control or cohort studies with a high risk of confounding or bias and a significant risk that the relationship is not causal. The authors concluded that evidence to date is not robust enough to recommend hypnosis in

best-practice guidelines for procedural pain in pediatric cancer pain management, but larger scale, appropriately controlled studies are justified for the future.

The most recent systematic review analyzed the data collected from one systematic review, seven published randomized controlled trials, and one nonrandomized controlled clinical trial.[68][I] The conclusions arrived at were that research in hypnosis contributed significantly to literature, not only by narrating different, but specific, hypnotic techniques but also a foundation/framework on which future work can be built. Though hypnosis has the potential to be a clinically valuable intervention for pain in pediatric cancer patients, further research is essential to claim effectiveness and acceptability.

CONCLUSIONS – HYPNOSIS IN CHILDREN

Hypnosis has strong potential to be of clinical use to reduce pain and distress in children undergoing procedures. Additional features of these techniques which may contribute to easy acceptability and tolerance among patients are that, as such, there have been no known adverse effects or interactions. It has been noted that the hypnotic experience is enjoyable for the patients. No change has been noted in terms of other functions, especially normal mental capacity. Once learnt, the skills can be generalized to distress due to other causes, for example, nausea and vomiting. Evidence also adds that this provides the clinician with a chance to build a stronger therapeutic relationship with the patient.

COGNITIVE-BEHAVIORAL TECHNIQUES AND COPING SKILLS

According to the cognitive model, an individual's interpretation of events, not the reality of the events as such, influences behaviors and emotional reactions. For pain, the CBT model focuses on the experience being multi-dimensional and not only a sensation. A series of studies on a multicomponent CBT package have been reported on pediatric cancer patients. Jay et al.[69, 70] developed an intervention package designed to teach children effective coping skills and reduce their distress during bone marrow aspiration and lumbar puncture. The typical components have been filmed modeling, incentives, breathing exercises, emotive imagery and distraction, and behavioral rehearsal.

Efficacy of cognitive-behavioral techniques in procedural pain

INDIVIDUAL STUDIES – COGNITIVE-BEHAVIORAL TECHNIQUES IN CHILDREN

Jay et al.[69][IV] carried out a series of studies on a CBT package, comparing it with pharmacological interventions, and the combined effects of both techniques. In their first study, five children with anxiety and distress were found to have a 50 percent reduction in their distress scores after intervention. The second study was to compare the CBT package with oral diazepam and an attention control condition (30 minutes of cartoon watching before the procedure).[70][III] Overall, the pain ratings were significantly lower when CBT was compared to either the diazepam or the attention control group. Diazepam was found to reduce the anticipatory distress but not the procedural one. The next phase of this research series was to investigate the combined effects of CBT and oral diazepam in a study of 83 children. They were assigned to either a CBT package or a combined package of CBT and diazepam. Both groups were found to have decrease in pain scores from baseline to intervention; but the CBT plus diazepam group showed only one-third of the reduction compared to the CBT only group. The conclusions were that diazepam could have interfered with the learning of the CBT strategies and may have affected imagery and distraction tasks as well by affecting their concentration.[71][III]

The last project by the same set of researchers again compared CBT with general anesthesia in alleviating the distress of 18 children with cancer.[72][III] The results indicated that the children showed more behavioral distress in the CBT condition for the first minute of lying down on the treatment table. There were no significant differences in the outcome measures.

Another study using several of the same components in the CBT package compared the efficacy of conscious sedation with a combination of conscious sedation and psychological intervention.[73][III] The results showed that distress decreased over time and quality of life as well as parental stress improved concurrently. It also supported an inverse relationship between distress and age of the child.

CONCLUSIONS – COGNITIVE-BEHAVIORAL TECHNIQUES IN CHILDREN

CBT has been repeatedly shown to reduce distress in children with cancer undergoing painful medical procedures in a number of studies. However, no one intervention was distinctly more effective than another and there has been no attempt to delineate the efficacy of specific elements of each type of intervention. Many pharmacological approaches do decrease the pain and distress, the unacceptable side of this being adverse effects and medical risks whereas the risk of injury because of unrestricted movement could always occur with CBT. Other limitations also include increased staff need and recovery time.

Hypnosis and CBT are safe techniques leading to no adverse effects. They are reasonably cost effective, which may well enhance the child's compliance and reduce expensive medical input.

OVERALL CONCLUSIONS

Keefe et al.[74] reviewed the history of psychological approaches to pain focusing also on cancer pain. They point to the association between pain and psychological distress and observe that research on psychological factors has focused on the two main areas of psychological distress and coping with pain. It is interesting that they group psychosocial interventions in cancer pain into three broad categories of (1) cancer education, (2) hypnosis and imagery based methods, and (3) coping skills training. They make the following conclusions:

- The current studies provide high quality evidence that cancer pain education is practical and can improve patient outcomes.
- Hypnosis and imagery are effective at reducing acute pain in pediatric and adult cancer patients and adults undergoing bone marrow transplant. They also conclude that chronic cancer pain is likely to be responsive to hypnosis and imagery.
- There is little evidence of an added advantage of adding additional coping skills training interventions over hypnosis and guided imagery alone for patients with acute malignant pain. They suggest that coping skills training may be beneficial in chronic cancer pain, although the specific components are as yet unidentified.

CBT with the focus on cognitive restructuring has not been sufficiently explored in cancer pain management. Future research should draw from work that has already been carried out in the use of CBT in other fields.

REFERENCES

1. Abrahm JL. Management of pain and spinal cord compression in patients with advanced cancer. *Annals of Internal Medicine.* 1999; **131**: 37–46.
2. Fleishman SB. Treatment of symptom clusters: pain, depression, and fatigue. *Journal of the National Cancer Institute. Monographs.* 2004; 119–23.
3. Bond MR. Psychological issues in cancer and non-cancer conditions. *Acta Anaesthesiologica Scandinavica.* 2001; **45**: 1095–9.
4. Price DD. Psychological mechanisms of pain and analgesia. In: Anonymous. *Progress in pain research and management.* Seattle: IASP Press, 1999: 43–70.
5. Thomas EM, Weiss SM. Nonpharmacological interventions with chronic cancer pain in adults. *Cancer Control.* 2000; **7**: 157–64.
6. Syrjala KL, Chapman CR. Measurement of clinical pain: A review and integration of clinical findings. In: Benedetti C, Chapman CR, Moricca G (eds). *Advances in pain research and therapy.* New York: Raven Press, 1984.

7. Howland JS, Baker MG, Poe T. Does patient education cause side effects? A controlled clinical trial. *Journal of Family Practice.* 1990; **31**: 62–4.

8. Rimer B, Levy MH, Keintz MK. Enhancing cancer pain control regimens through patient education. *Patient Education and Counseling.* 1987; **10**: 267–77.

9. Ferrell BR, Rhiner M, Ferrell BA. Development and implementation of a pain education program. *Cancer.* 1993; **72**: 3426–32.

10. De Wit R, Van DF, Zandbelt L *et al.* A pain education program for chronic cancer pain patients: Follow-up results from a randomized controlled trial. *Pain.* 1997; **73**: 55–69.

11. Devine EC, Westlake SK. The effects of psycho educational care provided to adults with cancer: meta analysis of 116 studies. *Oncology Nursing Forum.* 1995; **22**: 1369–81.

12. Werman DS. *The practice of supportive psychotherapy.* New York: Brunner/Mazel, 1984.

* 13. Spiegel D, Bloom JR. Group therapy and hypnosis reduce metastatic breast carcinoma pain. *Psychosomatic Medicine.* 1983; **45**: 333–9.

14. Luborsky L, German RE, Diguer L *et al.* Is psychotherapy good for your health? [erratum appears in *American Journal of Psychotherapy.* 2005; **59**(1): 1 p following 81]. *American Journal of Psychotherapy.* 2004; **58**: 386–405.

15. Goodwin PJ. The effect of group psychosocial support on survival in metastatic breast cancer. *New England Journal of Medicine.* 2001; **345**: 1719–26.

16. Fobair P, Koopman C, DiMiceli S *et al.* Psychosocial interventions for lesbians with primary breast cancer. *Psycho-Oncology.* 2002; **11**: 427–38.

17. D'Zurilla T, Nezu AM. *Problem-solving therapy: a positive approach to clinical intervention,* 3rd edn. New York: Springer Publishing Co, 2006.

* 18. Loscalzo M. Psychological approaches to the management of pain in patients with advanced cancer. *Hematology – Oncology Clinics of North America.* 1996; **10**: 139–55.

19. Fishman B. The cognitive behavioral perspective on pain management in terminal illness. *Hospice Journal – Physical, Psychosocial, and Pastoral Care of the Dying.* 1992; **8**: 73–88.

20. Patterson DR, Jensen MP. Hypnosis and clinical pain. *Psychological Bulletin.* 2003; **129**: 495–521.

* 21. Montgomery GH, DuHamel KN, Redd WH. A meta-analysis of hypnotically induced analgesia: how effective is hypnosis? *International Journal of Clinical and Experimental Hypnosis.* 2000; **48**: 138–53.

22. Spiegel D, Moore R. Imagery and hypnosis in the treatment of cancer patients. *Oncology.* 1997; **11**: 1179–89.

23. Kilshtrom JF. Hypnosis. *Annual Review of Psychology.* 1985; **36**: 385–418.

24. Syrjala KL, Donaldson GW, Davis MW *et al.* Relaxation and imagery and cognitive-behavioral training reduce pain during cancer treatment: a controlled clinical trial. *Pain.* 1995; **63**: 189–98.

25. Simonton OC, Henson RM, Hamton B. *The healing journey.* New York: Bantom Books, 1994.

26. Hilgard ER, Hilgard JR. *Hypnosis in the relief of pain.* Los Altos, CA: William Kaufmann, 1975.

27. Rhue JW, Lynn SJ, Kirsch I. Hypnosis in pain management. In: Anonymous. *Handbook of clinical hypnosis.* Washington, DC: American Psychological Association, 1993: 511–32.

28. Peter B. Hypnosis in the treatment of cancer pain. *Australian Journal of Clinical and Experimental Hypnosis.* 1997; **25**: 40–52.

29. Levitan AA. The use of hypnosis with cancer patients. *Psychiatric Medicine.* 1992; **10**: 119–31.

30. Turner J, Chapman CR. Psychological interventions for chronic pain, a critical review II: Operant conditioning, hypnosis and cognitive behavioral therapy. *Pain.* 1982; **12**: 23–46.

* 31. Syrjala KL, Cummings C, Donaldson GW. Hypnosis or cognitive behavioral training for the reduction of pain and nausea during cancer treatment: a controlled clinical trial. *Pain.* 1992; **48**: 137–46.

32. Sloman R, Brown P, Aldana E, Chee E. The use of relaxation for the promotion of comfort and pain relief in persons with advanced cancer. *Contemporary Nurse.* 1994; **3**: 6–12.

33. Gaston-Johansson F, Fall-Dickson J, Nanda J *et al.* The effectiveness of the comprehensive coping strategy program on clinical outcomes in breast cancer autologous bone marrow transplantation. *Cancer Nursing.* 2000; **23**: 277–85.

34. Anderson KO, Cohen MZ, Mendoza TR *et al.* Brief cognitive-behavioral audiotape interventions for cancer-related pain: Immediate but not long-term effectiveness. *Cancer.* 2006; **107**: 207–14.

35. Sellick SM, Zaza C. Critical review of 5 nonpharmacologic strategies for managing cancer pain. *Cancer Prevention and Control.* 1998; **2**: 7–14.

* 36. Hawkins RMF. A systematic meta-review of hypnosis as an empirically supported treatment for pain. *Pain Reviews.* 2001; **8**: 47–73.

37. Luebbert K, Dahme B, Hasenbring M. The effectiveness of relaxation training in reducing treatment-related symptoms and improving emotional adjustment in acute non-surgical cancer treatment: a meta-analytical review. *Psycho-Oncology.* 2001; **10**: 490–502.

38. Redd WH, Montgomery GH, DuHamel KN. Behavioral intervention for cancer treatment side effects. *Journal of the National Cancer Institute.* 2001; **93**: 810–23.

* 39. Mundy EA, DuHamel KN, Montgomery GH. The efficacy of behavioral interventions for cancer treatment-related side effects. *Seminars in Clinical Neuropsychiatry.* 2003; **8**: 253–75.

40. Graves KD. Social cognitive theory and cancer patients' quality of life: a meta analysis of psychosocial intervention components. *Health Psychology.* 2003; **22**: 210–19.

41. Jensen MP, Patterson DR. Control conditions in hypnotic-analgesia clinical trials: Challenges and recommendations. *International Journal of Clinical and Experimental Hypnosis.* 2005; **53**: 170–97.

∗ 42. Tatrow K, Montgomery GH. Cognitive behavioral therapy techniques for distress and pain in breast cancer patients: a meta-analysis. *Journal of Behavioral Medicine.* 2006; **29**: 17–27.

43. Finlay IG, Jones OL. Hypnotherapy in palliative care. *Journal of the Royal Society of Medicine.* 1996; **89**: 493–6.

44. Dalton JA, Keefe FJ, Carlson J, Youngblood R. Tailoring cognitive-behavioral treatment for cancer pain. *Pain Management Nursing.* 2004; **5**: 3–18.

45. Given C, Given B, Rahbar M *et al.* Effect of a cognitive behavioral intervention on reducing symptom severity during chemotherapy. *Journal of Clinical Oncology.* 2004; **22**: 507–16.

46. Robb KA, Williams JE, Duvivier V, Newham DJ. A pain management program for chronic cancer-treatment-related pain: a preliminary study. *Journal of Pain.* 2006; **7**: 82–90.

47. Kwekkeboom KL. A model for cognitive-behavioral interventions in cancer pain management. *Image – the Journal of Nursing Scholarship.* 1999; **31**: 151–6.

48. King B, Nash M, Spiegel D, Kenneth J. Hypnosis as an intervention in pain management: A brief review. *International Journal of Psychiatry in Clinical Practice.* 2001; **5**: 97–101.

49. Butler LD, Koopman C, Cordova MJ *et al.* Psychological distress and pain significantly increase before death in metastatic breast cancer patients. *Psychosomatic Medicine.* 2003; **65**: 416–26.

50. Doorenbos A, Given B, Given C *et al.* Reducing symptom limitations: A cognitive behavioral intervention randomized trial. *Psycho-Oncology.* 2005; **14**: 574–84.

51. Liossi C. Psychological interventions for acute and chronic pain in children. *Pain: Clinical Updates.* 2006; **15**: 1–4.

52. Miser AW, Dothage JA, Wesley RA, Miser JS. The prevalence of pain in a pediatric and young adult population. *Pain.* 1987; **29**: 73–83.

53. Fowler-Kerry S. Adolescent oncology survivors' recollection of pain. In: Tyler D, Krane E (eds). *Pediatric pain, Advances in pain research and therapy,* 15 edn. New York: Raven Press, 1990: 365–71.

∗ 54. Liossi C. Management of paediatric procedure-related cancer pain. *Pain Reviews.* 1999; **6**: 279–302.

55. Schechter NL. Pain and pain control in children. *Current Problems in Pediatrics.* 1985; **15**: 1–67.

56. Anderson KO, Masur FT. Psychological preparation for invasive medical and dental procedures. *Behavioral Medicine.* 1983; **6**: 1–40.

57. Zeltzer L, Altman A, Cohen D *et al.* American Academy of Pediatrics Report of the Subcommittee on the Management of Pain Associated with Procedures in Children with Cancer. *Pediatrics.* 1990; **86**: 826–31.

58. Bradlyn AS, Beale IL, Kato PM. Psycho educational interventions with pediatric cancer patients: Part I Patient information and knowledge. *Journal of Child and family Studies.* 2003; **12**: 257–77.

59. Morgan A, Hilgard ER. Age differences in susceptibility to hypnosis. *International Journal of Clinical and Experimental Hypnosis.* 1973; **21**: 78–85.

60. Liossi C, Hatira P. Clinical hypnosis in the alleviation of procedure-related pain in pediatric oncology patients. *International Journal of Clinical and Experimental Hypnosis.* 2003; **51**: 4–28.

61. Levitan A. Setting sun metaphor. In: Hammond DC (ed.). *Handbook of hypnotic suggestions and metaphors.* New York: Norton, 1990.

62. Gardner GG. Teaching self-hypnosis to children. *International Journal of Clinical and Experimental Hypnosis.* 1981; **29**: 300–12.

63. Liossi C, Hatira P. Clinical hypnosis versus cognitive behavioral training for pain management with pediatric cancer patients undergoing bone marrow aspirations. *International Journal of Clinical and Experimental Hypnosis.* 1999; **47**: 104–16.

64. Zeltzer L, LeBaron S. Hypnosis and non hypnotic techniques for reduction of pain and anxiety during painful procedures in children and adolescents with cancer. *Journal of Pediatrics.* 1982; **101**: 1032–5.

65. Katz ER, Kellerman J, Ellenberg L. Hypnosis in the reduction of acute pain and distress in children with cancer. *Journal of Pediatric Psychology.* 1987; **12**: 379–94.

66. Kellerman J, Zeltzer L, Ellenberg L, Dash J. Adolescents with cancer. Hypnosis for the reduction of the acute pain and anxiety associated with medical procedures. *Journal of Adolescent Health Care.* 1983; **4**: 85–90.

∗ 67. Wild MR, Espie CA. The efficacy of hypnosis in the reduction of procedural pain and distress in pediatric oncology: a systematic review. *Journal of Developmental and Behavioral Pediatrics.* 2004; **25**: 207–13.

∗ 68. Richardson J, Smith JE, McCall G, Pilkington K. Hypnosis for procedure-related pain and distress in pediatric cancer patients: A systematic review of effectiveness and methodology related to hypnosis interventions. *Journal of Pain and Symptom Management.* 2006; **31**: 70–84.

69. Jay SM, Elliott CH, Ozolins M, Pruitt C. Behavioral management of children's distress during painful medical procedures. *Behavior Research and Therapy.* 1985; **23**: 513–20.

70. Jay SM, Elliott CH, Katz ER, Siegel SE. Cognitive behavioral and pharmacologic interventions for children undergoing painful medical procedures. *Journal of Consulting and Clinical Psychology.* 1987; **55**: 860–5.

71. Jay SM, Elliott CH, Woody PD, Siegel S. An investigation of cognitive-behavior therapy combined with oral valium for children undergoing painful medical procedures. *Health Psychology.* 1991; **10**: 317–22.

72. Jay S, Elliott CH, Fitzgibbons I *et al.* A comparative study of cognitive behavior therapy versus general anesthesia for painful medical procedures in children. *Pain.* 1995; **62**: 3–9.

73. Kazak AE, Penati B, Boyer BA *et al.* A randomized controlled prospective outcome study of a psychological and pharmacological intervention protocol for procedural distress in pediatric leukemia. *Journal of Pediatric Psychology.* 1996; **21**: 615–31.

∗ 74. Keefe FJ, Abernethy AP, Campbell C. Psychological approaches to understanding and treating disease-related pain. *Annual Review of Psychology.* 2005; **56**: 601–30.

24

Control of symptoms other than pain

EMMA HALL, NIGEL SYKES, AND VICTOR PACE

Respiratory symptoms	311	Diarrhea	324
Causes of dyspnea in cancer	311	Other symptoms	326
Drugs for palliation of dyspnea	313	Fatigue	328
Cough	314	Lymphedema	329
Hemoptysis	315	Pruritus	329
Gastrointestinal problems	316	Sweating	331
Dysphagia	317	Psychological and psychiatric problems	331
Nausea and vomiting	318	End of life care	334
Hypercalcemia	319	Conclusion	335
Small and large bowel obstruction in advanced cancer	321	References	335
Constipation	323		

KEY LEARNING POINTS

BREATHLESSNESS AND COUGH

- Treat reversible causes if possible.
- Consider nonpharmacological techniques.
- Drug treatment includes opioids and, if anxiety is a strong component, benzodiazepines.
- Nebulized drugs have a limited role in palliation.
- Oxygen and other gases should not be used without careful thought.

GASTROINTESTINAL SYMPTOMS

- Optimize dentition, manage xerostomia, and treat mucositis and candidiasis promptly.
- Dysphagia can be palliated with radiotherapy, stents, and steroids.
- Selection of antiemetics will depend on the most likely underlying cause. Hypercalcemia should be treated with bisphosphonates if appropriate.
- Stents, steroids, octreotide, and antiemetics are used in malignant bowel obstruction, while surgery has only a limited role.
- Constipation occurs more frequently than diarrhea in advanced cancer and opioids are a common cause. Laxatives should be provided whenever opioids are commenced.

- Anorexia will often respond temporarily to steroids or progestagens but improving the cachexia that occurs in many advanced cancers remains elusive.

CUTANEOUS SYMPTOMS

- Lymphedema, pruritus, and sweating: nonpharmacological and drug treatments are discussed.

PSYCHOLOGICAL SYMPTOMS

- Treatable psychiatric illness should be identified.
- Cognitive behavioral techniques are increasingly used for anxiety management.
- Reversible causes of delirium should be treated if possible. At the end of life, the use of sedative drugs may be required.

END OF LIFE CARE

- Optimal symptom management may involve changing to the subcutaneous route of administration.
- Supporting the patient's family (including bereavement) is vital.

RESPIRATORY SYMPTOMS

Breathlessness

Breathlessness (dyspnea) is defined as an uncomfortable awareness of the effort of breathing. In a recent study of 923 oncology outpatients, nearly half described breathlessness, with only about 10 percent having primary or metastatic cancer in the lungs.[1][III] The prevalence and severity rise as disease progresses and, although much can be done to ease the sensation of breathlessness, it remains a difficult symptom to control.[2][III]

PATHOPHYSIOLOGY

It appears that a respiratory effort of more than a third of that of which the individual is capable produces breathlessness.[3] Hence, any impairment of respiratory capacity will tend to bring down the point at which breathlessness will be felt, until ultimately it may be experienced even at rest. Such impairment can arise from:

- reduced ventilation of gas exchange surfaces, for example asthmatic bronchoconstriction, bronchial obstruction by tumor;
- reduced area of gas exchange surfaces, for example compression or obliteration of alveoli by tumor, pleural effusion or ascites, occupation of alveoli by fluid, bronchiectasis;
- reduced perfusion of gas exchange surfaces, for example pulmonary embolism, anemia;
- increased lung stiffness, for example pulmonary fibrosis, emphysema, pulmonary edema;
- reduced respiratory muscle capacity, for example spinal cord compression, amyotrophic lateral sclerosis, pain;
- unusual respiratory demands, for instance in diabetic ketoacidosis or in thyrotoxicosis.

The symptom of breathlessness results from cortical perception of feedback from central and peripheral receptors and the emotional response that this generates. It is a subjective sensation and is often but not always associated with tachypnea.

CAUSES OF DYSPNEA IN CANCER

In a study of 100 dyspneic cancer patients (half of whom had lung cancer), there was a median of five causes contributing to breathlessness in the study population. Nearly all patients had abnormal spirometry and the median maximal inspiratory pressure was only 16 cm of water, suggesting a hitherto unsuspected high prevalence of inspiratory muscle weakness in cancer-related breathlessness. Potentially correctable causes included bronchospasm, hypoxia and anemia.[4][III]

Clinical findings – history and examination

As with any cancer symptom, reversible causes should be excluded, as treatment may be worthwhile.

- Coexisting lung or cardiac disease should be searched for.
- Anemia, especially a hemoglobin concentration below 8 g/dL, or a recent rapid fall in hemoglobin can be associated with breathlessness, which may then respond to transfusion.
- There may be a history and signs of a chest infection or pulmonary embolus.
- Examination may reveal a pulmonary or pericardial effusion, ascites, airway obstruction, stridor, or superior vena caval obstruction.
- Hyperventilation may indicate a significant contribution of anxiety to the breathlessness-features in the history may include breathlessness that fluctuates rapidly, varies with social situations, and is poorly linked with exertion.

In making an assessment of breathlessness, the possible emotional component should not be overlooked. Breathing difficulty is frightening, and the fear that results worsens the perception of breathlessness further. Patients may worry that the dyspnea is further damaging their lungs and even that they might die in an episode of breathlessness.

Investigations

- A blood count, random blood glucose estimation, and thyroid function tests may be indicated by history and examination.
- Pulse oximetry on room air, before and after exercise and before and after oxygen may indicate the therapeutic value of oxygen.
- Spirometry may be useful to diagnose reversible airway obstruction.
- An electrocardiogram may highlight coexisting ischemic or hypertensive heart disease.
- Chest radiography may be helpful in delineating effusions, confirming cardiac failure, or revealing lymphangitis carcinomatosa, which often presents few signs on auscultation.
- Echocardiography may be indicated to identify a malignant pericardial effusion or an impaired ejection fraction.
- Pulmonary emboli are increasingly diagnosed by high resolution computed tomography (CT) scanning rather than nuclear medicine techniques. A recent retrospective review of 59 patients found to have previously unsuspected pulmonary emboli on routine cancer restaging CT scans suggested that these patients were experiencing considerable symptom

burdens from pulmonary emboli.[5][III] The inference from this study is that this condition should be actively sought, especially as pulmonary emboli may be amenable to anticoagulation.

Management

Coexisting cardiac or pulmonary disease should be treated optimally and anticoagulation considered for thromboembolism. The contribution of the cancer to the breathlessness needs to be assessed together with the possibilities of antineoplastic treatment. Supportive and interventional measures for palliation of breathlessness will be discussed.

SUPPORTIVE CARE

Aside from medical interventions, there are certain supportive approaches to breathlessness that should underpin other types of management. These include:

- understanding and, if necessary, modifying the patient and his or her family's understanding of breathlessness and its causes and consequences;
- physiotherapy assessment of aids to mobilization, and breathing retraining;
- use of a fan or open window;
- complementary therapies such as aromatherapy massage and acupuncture may be beneficial for some patients;
- attention to social isolation;
- drawing up a simple, written plan of action in case of exacerbations of breathlessness.

This approach has informed nurse-led breathlessness clinics, which have proved beneficial to cancer patients in a controlled trial.[6][II]

SPECIFIC MANAGEMENT

Airway obstruction by tumor

Chest radiography may suggest, and bronchoscopy confirm, that lung capacity is depleted by tumor obstructing a main bronchus.

- Radiotherapy can be given either by external beam or intraluminally. The external approach carries an increased risk of pulmonary fibrosis if the patient survives long enough. In a large series of breathless patients with bronchial obstruction treated with intraluminal radiotherapy, 60 percent of patients reported improvement and 46 percent of pulmonary collapses were alleviated. Retreatment for relapse provided similar rates of symptom relief, but only 7 percent of pulmonary collapses showed improvement.[7][IV]

- Laser treatment or cryotherapy via a bronchoscope can also be used for palliation.[8][V]
- As a preliminary to radiotherapy, and for those who are too ill to undergo it, a trial of steroids (dexamethasone 12–16 mg/24 h p.o. or s.c.) should be given, as reduction in peritumor edema can provide some symptomatic relief.
- In patients who are fit enough, an alternative to radiotherapy is the insertion of a metal wire stent, for which rapid symptomatic relief has been claimed.[9][IV]
- Chemotherapy may alleviate breathlessness in certain cancers, for example small-cell lung cancer.

Superior vena caval obstruction

Superior vena caval obstruction (SVCO) from mediastinal malignancy, most often lung or lymphoma, includes breathlessness among its several distressing symptoms.

- Steroids (dexamethasone 16 mg stat p.o. or s.c.) are usually given for symptom relief (or prior to radiotherapy or chemotherapy).
- Good symptom relief from radiotherapy was reported in 80 percent of a series of 125 patients with malignant SVCO.[10][IV] However, symptom relief is usually delayed seven to ten days, during which time symptoms may initially deteriorate, despite steroids.
- Radiotherapy may be less effective if the superior vena cava is thrombosed.
- Expandable wire stents have been employed in SVCO; a retrospective comparison of stents and radiotherapy found advantage in the use of stents in the magnitude and speed of onset of symptom relief.[11][IV]
- Stenting is often combined with that of thrombolytic therapy[12][IV] and has been supported by a systematic review.[13][II]

Lymphangitis carcinomatosa

This condition results from malignant infiltration of the lung lymphatic system, characteristically from a breast primary. The supposed etiology of the associated breathlessness is fluid retention in the lungs as a result of inadequate lymphatic drainage.

- Anecdotally palliation may be achieved by using dexamethasone 6–12 mg/24 hour orally on the rationale that reduction in edema around the tumor deposits may assist lymphatic function.

Malignant pleural and pericardial effusions

Malignant pleural effusions occur in approximately half of patients with metastatic cancer and short-term relief of dyspnea can be achieved with thoracocentesis. For recurrent effusions, pleurodesis with chemical sclerosants is recommended. A recent systematic review of nearly 1500 patients[14][I] concluded that:

- talc is the most effective chemical sclerosant;
- pleurodesis performed thoracoscopically was more effective than medical pleurodesis.

Pericardial effusions occur less frequently in malignancy but should be considered as a treatable cause of dyspnea. Palliation can be achieved by pericardiocentesis. Instillation of cisplatin into the pericardial space relieved symptoms and reduced recurrence rates in a series of 46 patients, particularly those patients with nonsmall cell lung cancer.[15][III] For seriously ill patients, percutaneous balloon pericardiotomy allows pericardial fluid to drain into the pleural or peritoneal space and this procedure can be performed under a local instead of a general anesthetic.[16][V]

DRUGS FOR PALLIATION OF DYSPNEA

Opioids

Despite the widespread caution exercised in the use of opioids in patients with respiratory impairment since it was established that they can cause respiratory depression,[17] these drugs are the cornerstone of palliation of breathlessness in patients with advanced cancer.

Proposed mechanisms of action include:

- reduction in the sensitivity of the respiratory center and of the awareness of breathing;
- anxiety reduction (which can have a direct impact on awareness of breathing);
- opioids are thought to reduce both preload and afterload in cardiac failure;
- although there are opioid receptors in the airways, nebulized opioids have thus far failed to demonstrate beneficial effects over and above that of saline (see below under Nebulized drugs).

Walsh[18][III] showed that morphine could safely be used for analgesia in patients with poor lung function without precipitating hypercapnia, as long as the dose was proportionate to the level of pain. A more recent study of 29 nonoxygen-dependent patients demonstrated no significant changes in end-tidal carbon dioxide during opioid titration for cancer pain.[19][III]

A small placebo-controlled single-dose trial of subcutaneous morphine in cancer patients already receiving opioids for pain and on continuous oxygen found a reduction in breathlessness and a marked patient preference for morphine over placebo (nine out of ten).[20][II] An earlier uncontrolled trial had found a similar result, but noted that the duration of relief of breathlessness was less than that of pain, beginning to diminish after 75

minutes and back to baseline after 2.5 hours.[21][III] An uncontrolled trial of oral morphine for breathlessness differed in that most of the patients were opioid naive: 5 out of 18 patients withdrew because of drowsiness or dizziness, and only one reported definite improvement.[22] [III] The starting dose used was 20 mg morphine per day.

These and other studies (most of which have been conducted in patients with nonmalignancy-related dyspnea) have been analyzed in a systematic review which concluded that there is a small but worthwhile beneficial effect of oral and injected opioids on the symptom of breathlessness.[23][I] The same review found a lack of evidence to support use of opioids by the nebulized route and no studies demonstrated an improvement in exercise tolerance. There did not appear to be a major problem with respiratory depression but this parameter was not consistently measured.

Most studies included in the review used morphine or codeine and starting doses were very variable. Further studies are required to examine:

- appropriate starting doses and whether there is a ceiling effect for dyspnea (as opposed to pain);
- long-acting versus short-acting preparations;
- as required versus regular dosing;
- comparison of efficacy of different opioids;
- effect on respiratory function (if any) when opioids are used for dyspnea as opposed to pain.

While further evidence is awaited, a pragmatic approach is as follows.

- As with pain, the preferred route is orally.
- For patients already taking opioids for pain, an increase of 25–50 percent in the analgesic dose is appropriate for persisting breathlessness.
- For those not currently taking morphine, the starting dose should be low (2.5 mg) and the preparation a short-acting one.
- Initially, morphine may be given on an as required basis or perhaps three or four times daily. Thereafter titration can occur as with pain, with the aim of moving to a long-acting preparation, if this suits the patient.
- For exercise or movement-related dyspnea, buccal or intranasal fentanyl or alfentanil has been used for a rapid onset of action but these are not usually suitable for opioid-naive patients.
- If breathlessness improves but morphine is poorly tolerated, an alternative opioid can be tried, as with pain. However, available preparations in some cases do not allow the advised low starting doses.

Anxiolytics

Given the close association between breathlessness and anxiety, it is unsurprising that anxiolytics have found a role in its management. It is less clear whether they have any other mechanism of action, in particular through the muscle relaxant properties of the benzodiazepines.

- Diazepam has not been studied in cancer-associated breathlessness, but the results from patients with chronic obstructive pulmonary disease (COPD) are predominantly negative.[24] [II] However, clinical experience indicates that daily doses much lower than the 25 mg used in COPD can improve breathlessness in cancer patients. Often, 2–5 mg t.i.d. may suffice initially and because of the long half-life of diazepam a single night-time dose may eventually be sufficient.
- Sublingual lorazepam (0.5–1.0 mg) has proved helpful in clinical experience for acute dyspneic episodes precipitated or exacerbated by anxiety.
- There is limited evidence that phenothiazines can help breathlessness: promethazine was better than placebo in COPD[25][III] and the combination of chlorpromazine and morphine reduced breathlessness caused by extensive lung metastases.[25]
- Buspirone is a nonbenzodiazepine partial 5HT1A agonist which has been found both to reduce breathlessness and to stimulate ventilation in subjects with nonmalignant lung disease.[26, 27][II] Its anxiolytic action may have a latency of onset of seven to ten days. The usual starting dose is 5 mg two or three times a day.

Medical gases

OXYGEN

Oxygen is often the first recourse of medical staff for breathless patients. Once initiated, many patients are understandably reluctant to accept its withdrawal, despite the unsightliness of the mask or nasal cannulae and the restrictions the equipment places on their freedom of movement. In a small series of severely hypoxic cancer patients, nearly all preferred oxygen to air,[28][II] but in two further randomized trials in patients with advanced cancer (with subsets of hypoxic patients) both air and oxygen appeared to confer benefit on the symptom; furthermore symptomatic benefit did not appear to be related to blood oxygen saturation.[29, 30][II]

Although oxygen should never be withheld from a patient who has previously found it useful, or one who is acutely breathless and markedly hypoxic, it is reasonable to attempt alternative approaches to the palliation of breathlessness before commencing it. Even desaturation on pulse oximetry is a poor guide to which patients will benefit, and most palliative care physicians have seen patients who have ceased to depend on oxygen once given appropriate general support and the use of morphine and an anxiolytic. A pragmatic approach can be found in Booth et al.[31][V]

HELIUM/OXYGEN AND NITROGEN/OXYGEN MIXTURES

For patients with stridulous breathing, a helium/oxygen mixture can reduce the work of breathing,[32][II] while nitrous oxide may cause pulmonary vessels to relax, as suggested in a trial with COPD patients.[33][II]

Nebulized drugs

Nebulized bronchodilators, such as salbutamol and ipratropium bromide, are indicated if there is any reversible airway obstruction. As already indicated, nebulized opioids have not demonstrated any advantage over nebulized saline.[34, 35][V] Similarly, lidocaine in nebulized form showed no benefit over saline in another small study.[36][IV] Nebulized furosemide, at a dose of 40 mg, demonstrated improvements in visual analog scores for dyspnea when compared with saline in a small randomized controlled trial of breathless COPD patients[37][II] and a small study of breathless cancer patients suggested benefit over saline.[38][III]

COUGH

Cough may be voluntary or a reflex response to mechanical and chemical receptors in the airways, mediated via the cough center in the medulla and the phrenic, intercostal, and inferior laryngeal nerves.

Clinical findings – history and examination

- Distinction should be made between productive and nonproductive cough.
- A new, recent production of yellow or green sputum accompanies lower respiratory tract infection, whereas a dry, irritating cough suggests the stimulation of airways receptors by tumor. This may result not only from bronchial carcinomas but also from cancer affecting the larynx.
- Cough occurring principally at night may indicate asthma, cardiac failure, or silent aspiration. Aspiration may also be indicated by the presence of cough during eating or drinking.
- A drug history may indicate angiotensin-converting enzyme inhibitors as the cause of cough.

Management

Chest radiography, sputum culture, and relevant antibiotic treatment may be relevant, especially if recurrent tuberculosis is a possibility.

Antineoplastic treatment

Chemotherapy, radiotherapy, and laser treatment may all relieve cough due to airway obstruction in the same way as for dyspnea. Cough caused by airway obstruction can also be relieved with the use of steroids, for example dexamethasone 4–8 mg daily but long-term side effects often preclude long-term use.

Palliative treatment of a dry cough is by suppression and for a productive cough aims to facilitate the expectoration of sputum and, if possible, reduce its production. The exception is at the end of life, when it becomes appropriate to suppress even a productive cough.

Opioids

Most cough suppressants are opioids, and there is evidence for a dose-related cough-inhibitory action of codeine, probably mediated via μ_2- and kappa receptors.[39][V] However, if morphine is already being taken for pain, it is more logical to titrate the dose further for troublesome cough rather than add a second opioid. Some patients find helpful the addition of a demulcent preparation such as simple linctus BP. If no opioid analgesia is in use, codeine, diamorphine, and methadone are all available as linctuses. The dose required to suppress cough may be less than that needed for analgesia, but nonetheless about 20 percent of cancer patients receiving dihydrocodeine for cough report drowsiness.[40][II]

Other antitussives

Pholcodine or dextromethorphan are related to the opioids, acting not via opioid receptors but on an alternative central mechanism.

Proprietary cough medicines often contain, as well as an opioid, other drugs such as antihistamines and low doses of emetic agents. Apart from sedation, any mode of antitussive action of antihistamines is unknown, and there is no evidence to support the claim that subemetic doses of drugs such as squill enhance expectoration.

Nebulized lidocaine has anecdotally been used to relieve dry cough. It can cause bronchospasm and aspiration due to loss of sensation of the protective pharyngeal reflexes.

Future potential therapeutic targets include antagonists at nociceptin, bradykinin, and vanilloid receptors.[41][V]

Mucolysis

There is some evidence that oral carbocisteine (500–750 mg t.i.d.) and nebulized N-acetylcysteine reduce the viscosity of sputum in COPD patients.[42][I] Inhalation of steam, with or without addition of aromatic substances, or nebulized saline can be helpful in aiding expectoration of sputum. A trial of a bronchodilator may also be worthwhile in case reversible airways obstruction is exacerbating sputum retention.

Bronchoalveolar carcinoma may result in unpleasant large volumes of watery sputum (bronchorrhea). Aside

from antineoplastic treatment, anecdotal success has been reported with nebulized and systemic anticholinergic drugs, nebulized nonsteroidal anti-inflammatory drugs (NSAIDs) and octreotide. The section on End of life care covers the management of retained Secretions (see below) in the terminal phase.

HEMOPTYSIS

The expectoration of blood is experienced as a particularly alarming symptom. Hemoptysis occurs in approximately 20–40 percent of lung cancers, usually through involvement of the bronchial arteries. Occasionally it is an overwhelming terminal event, particularly in association with cavitating squamous carcinomas of the bronchus.[43][IV] Massive hemoptysis (over 500 mL/24 hours) mostly causes death through asphyxia rather than blood loss. However, in the absence of lung cancer there are many nonmalignant reasons for coughing up blood and, indeed, up to 40 percent of cases remain undiagnosed. Upper or lower respiratory tract infections are by far the most common causes, followed by bronchiectasis and tuberculosis.[44]

Clinical findings – history and examination

- Distinguish between blood originating from the lungs, versus the stomach, mouth, or nose.
- Hemoptysis is generally bright red, frothy, or mixed with sputum. Blood from a gastric origin is dark and will be acidic on testing.
- The volume of blood is not necessarily helpful in diagnosis, but brief rather than prolonged episodes suggest a benign origin.
- Possible inhalation of a foreign body should be excluded.
- Accompanying symptoms of cough, pyrexia, and chest pain suggest lower respiratory tract infection or pulmonary embolism.
- Chest radiography with lateral view may identify tumor, abscess, or tuberculosis. High-resolution CT may be indicated if pulmonary embolism is suspected.

Treatment

- Cancer-related hemoptysis responds well to radiotherapy. A review of 330 patients with lung cancer receiving radiotherapy found an 83 percent response rate for hemoptysis.[45][IV] Two fractions appear to be as effective as longer treatments.[46][III]
- Hemoptysis may improve with tranexamic acid (500 mg t.i.d. to 1 g q.i.d), which is an antifibrinolytic, or the hemostatic agent ethamsylate (500 mg q.i.d.).[47][IV] A potential problem is that clots forming as a result of using these drugs may be unusually hard and, if they break loose, can in consequence be troublesome to expectorate.

GASTROINTESTINAL PROBLEMS

Oral problems

Up to 89 percent of hospice patients suffer from oral problems.[48][V]

DRY MOUTH (XEROSTOMIA)

Xerostomia may result in infection, dental caries, loss of taste, anorexia, dysphagia, and speech impairment.

The salivary glands produce 1.0–1.5 L of saliva a day. Parasympathetic stimulation makes saliva more watery, while sympathetic stimulation slows down flow, reduces its amount, and increases the organic content. Vasoactive intestinal peptide (VIP) appears to play an important role in saliva regulation. Aldosterone has a similar effect on saliva to that on the kidneys.[49]

Common causes of xerostomia are shown in **Table 24.1.**

Treatment

- Good oral hygiene, starting with meticulous mouthcare, up to two-hourly in very weak patients.
- Fluid is encouraged, and medication reviewed.[50]
- Sucking pineapple chunks is said to increase moisture and clean up furring, because fresh pineapple contains the enzyme ananase.[51][V]
- Various artificial salivas are available, to be sprayed up to several times an hour underneath the tongue and swished in the mouth for a few seconds.[52]
- A randomized trial suggested chewing sugar-free gum was at least as effective as artificial saliva and many patients preferred it, probably because of the stimulation of salivary flow.[53][II]
- Barrier preparations such as oral balance gel and gelclair may help.
- Pilocarpine (usual dose 5 mg t.i.d.) in two randomized studies demonstrated benefit in patients

Table 24.1 Common causes of dry mouth in palliative care.

Type	Cause
Reduced salivary secretion	Radiotherapy to head and neck
	Drugs: anticholinergics, tricyclic antidepressants, antihistamines, beta-blockers, diuretics, morphine
	Tumor
	Autoimmune disorders
Buccal mucosal damage	Cancer
	Chemotherapy
	Infection, e.g. herpes, *Candida*
Dehydration	
Psychological	Depression
	Anxiety

who had received head and neck radiotherapy,[54, 55] [II] especially if given concomitantly with radiotherapy and if there is residual salivary gland function. Bethanecol 25 mg t.i.d. is an alternative. Therapeutic benefit may not occur for several weeks. Systemic side effects of oral pilocarpine may be avoided by the use of the topical preparation: 4 percent pilocarpine (the eyedrop preparation) mixed with cordial to disguise the taste, two drops t.i.d.

CANDIDIASIS

Candidiasis is present in up to 89 percent of patients with terminal illness.[56] [III] Risk factors include:

- elderly patient;
- dentures;
- dry mouth;
- malnutrition;
- diabetes;
- corticosteroids;
- antibiotics;
- head and neck radiotherapy;
- human immunodeficiency virus (HIV) infection and other causes of immunosuppression.

Several species of *Candida* or other fungi may be involved; no antifungal is effective against all species. Candidal infection may be the result, rather than the cause, of mouth problems, and general oral hygiene in the terminally ill may be more important than antifungal medication.[57][V]

Candida can present as pseudomembranous stomatitis (white plaques, easily scraped off, leaving an erythematous background) or as reddened smooth mucosa – chronic atrophic candidiasis; angular cheilitis may be present. Esophageal candidiasis produces pain on swallowing and is confirmed by gastroscopy or by barium swallow showing esophageal plaques.

Treatment

The most well-known antifungal is nystatin (3–5 mL q.i.d. held in mouth and swished as mouthwash). However, many patients find it difficult to use appropriately and a recent systematic review has questioned its efficacy in both prophylaxis and treatment of candidiasis.[58][I] Its activity is impaired by chlorhexidine, which is present in many mouthwashes.

Fluconazole and itraconazole are easy to use, safe alternatives although drug interactions may be important, especially with itraconazole. Fluconazole has good oral bioavailability, so is very useful against esophageal or systemic *Candida*. Ketoconazole can be hepatotoxic, is impaired by low gastric acid (e.g. H2-blockers), and interacts with many medications. The evidence for effectiveness for various agents is stronger for prophylaxis than for treatment, but only for drugs absorbed from the gastrointestinal tract.[59, 60][I] A recent systematic review raised a potential concern about increasing resistance of some *Candida* species to fluconazole.[61][I]

Amphotericin lozenges are an alternative but appear less effective.

HERPETIC INFECTIONS

These produce excruciatingly painful vesicles and often make the patient systemically unwell. Extension into the esophagus produces much more severe pain on swallowing than does thrush. Acyclovir, started early, aborts such infections.

BACTERIAL INFECTIONS

Xerostomia and immunosuppression cause an increase in Gram-negative flora causing mixed infections. Treatment is with antibiotics and scrupulous oral hygiene. Severely dehydrated, ill patients can develop infective parotitis as a terminal event. Pus can be seen issuing from the parotid duct near the second upper molar tooth. Systemic antibiotics may be indicated, although death is usually very near and symptomatic measures are best.

Other oral problems

Mucositis may be due to chemotherapy (5-fluorouracil, methotrexate) or radiotherapy to the head and neck. It is time limited and may be reduced by benzydamine oral rinse[62][III] or sucralfate.[63][IV] Strong opioids may be required. Oropharyngeal pain may also respond to a mixture of local anesthetic and antacid. Although many treatments for mucositis have been tried, the evidence for almost all agents is very weak and further studies are suggested in a recent review.[64][I]

Taste alterations are common and arise from a multitude of causes, dry mouth, chemotherapy, infection, and medication being some of the more common ones. Treatment is directed at the underlying cause. Angular cheilitis can also be due to vitamin deficiencies and may respond to vitamin supplementation.

DYSPHAGIA

Etiology

In one series of 800 palliative care patients, dysphagia affected 12 percent of individuals.[65][IV] Some causes of dysphagia in cancer patients include:

- mucositis:
  - postradiotherapy/chemotherapy: mouth or esophagus;
  - common oral problems: sepsis, dry mouth;

- masses in the lumen:
  - head and neck tumors;
  - carcinomas of esophagus or esophagogastric junction;
  - food bolus blocking esophageal stent;
- masses in the wall:
  - esophageal neoplasms;
  - postradiotherapy or anastomotic strictures;
- extrinsic masses:
  - mediastinal tumors;
  - mediastinal lymphadenopathy;
- neurological problems:
  - cranial nerve palsies (cerebral/head and neck tumors);
  - paraneoplastic syndromes: neuropathies, myopathies e.g. Lambert–Eaton syndrome;[66]
  - perineural tumor spread into the vagus nerve or sympathetic trunk.[67][IV]

Clinical findings

Neurogenic dysphagia involves liquids initially and only later solids, whereas mechanical obstruction affects solids first. Mechanical obstruction often involves the esophageal phase; it may feel as if a lump of food refuses to go down on swallowing, or swallowing may be painful. Neurological problems are more likely to disturb the oropharyngeal phase of deglutition.[68] Patients can complain of difficulty or pain on chewing, aspiration, drooling, nasal regurgitation, and late regurgitation of undigested food.[68]

Dry mouth or insufficient mastication in edentulous patients can also cause dysphagia.

Investigation

Investigation by barium swallow, esophagogastroscopy for structural disorders, manometry, and video studies for neuromuscular disorders may be appropriate. An assessment by a skilled speech therapist can be invaluable both in elucidating pathology and in suggesting therapy.[69]

Management

- Treat xerostomia and review dentition.
- Sauces help lubricate dry food and a liquidized diet may be needed for mechanical dysphagia.
- Benign strictures can be dilated, tumors intubated or lasered.
- Patients with esophageal tubes must masticate their food thoroughly and take fizzy drinks to wash away debris. Blocked tubes can indicate displacement, a food bolus wedged in the lumen that requires endoscopic removal, or tumor overgrowth, which is sometimes amenable to laser or reintubation.

- For neurogenic dysphagia, thickeners will help if thin liquids cause aspiration and drool from the mouth easily.
- Selected patients with head and neck problems do well with appropriate orthodontic prostheses and even resuspension surgery.
- After surgery or radiotherapy to the head and neck, some patients have a temporary loss of sensation in the mouth, which results in uncoordinated swallowing; very cold or warm food may help re-educate the swallowing mechanism.[70]
- In unilateral pharyngeal palsy, turning the head to the paralyzed side forces food to go through the sound side.
- The family needs to be reeducated with the patient.
- For selected patients a nasogastric or gastrostomy feeding tube may be appropriate, particularly for patients with head and neck cancer about to undergo radical radiotherapy.

NAUSEA AND VOMITING

Prevalence, causes, and pathophysiology

In a series of 1635 cancer patients in a pain clinic, 40 percent suffered from nausea or vomiting.[71][IV] The symptom tends to be more prevalent in gynecological (a fact which may also reflect increased prevalence in women) and upper gastrointestinal cancers.

During vomiting, a complex coordinated series of events takes place, with autonomic changes, retching, and hypersalivation, followed by abdominal and diaphragmatic muscle contraction simultaneously with relaxation of sphincters and closure of the epiglottis and nasopharynx as the vomitus is expelled.[72][V] The emetic(vomiting) pattern generator (previously thought to be a more discrete structure called the vomiting center) is a diffuse collection of neurons in the brainstem which coordinates the processes involved.

Figure 24.1 demonstrates the key pathways and neurotransmitters involved while common causes are illustrated in Table 24.2.

Clinical findings

A good history should differentiate between regurgitation (from esophageal tumors or neurogenic causes) and vomiting. Nausea may or may not accompany vomiting but is often the more debilitating symptom. Certain features in the history may indicate the underlying cause, for example:

- Gastric outlet obstruction tends, at least at first, to produce large-volume vomits, free of bile if the obstruction is complete, and episodes usually occur suddenly without preceding nausea (the only other common cause of this is vomiting from raised intracranial pressure). The patient may complain of hiccups and heartburn, and will often find undigested food in the vomit from meals taken more than six hours previously.
- Squashed stomach syndrome, due to impaired gastric filling from extrinsic pressure, or from the rigid small stomach produced by linitis plastica, produces a similar picture; however, vomits are frequent and small volume as the stomach cannot fill to any appreciable extent.
- Associated features of confusion or thirst may indicate hypercalcemia as the underlying cause.
- Iatrogenic causes (from concurrent drugs and anticancer treatment) and other metabolic abnormalities such as acute renal failure should be excluded.
- Raised intracranial pressure from brain metastases may be indicated if headache, confusion, or neurological symptoms are present.
- Learned responses play an important role in anticipatory nausea and vomiting in patients who are having cytotoxics, such that even meeting persons associated with administration of treatment can bring on an attack.

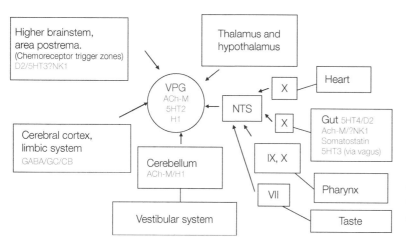

Figure 24.1 Inputs into vomiting pattern generator (VPG). Roman numerals signify the relevant cranial nerve. Script in gray denotes involved receptors/neurotransmitters: 5HT, 5 hydroxytryptamine (serotonin); ACh-M, muscarinic acetylcholine; CB, cannabinoid; D2, dopamine; GABA, gamma aminobutyric acid; GC, glucocorticoid; H, histamine; NK1, neurokinin. NTS, nucleus tractus solitarius.

Table 24.2 Common causes of nausea and vomiting in advanced cancer.

Type	Cause
Gastrointestinal	Gastritis (alcohol, nonsteroidal anti-inflammatory drugs)
	Gastric outlet obstruction (tumor, fibrosis, functional)
	Slow gastric emptying (autonomic gastropathy, functional, drugs)
	Squashed stomach syndrome (hepatomegaly, ascites, linitis plastica)
	Intestinal obstruction
	Constipation
Drugs	Opioids
	Digoxin
	Theophyllines
	Cytotoxics
	Erythromycin
Metabolic	Renal failure
	Hypercalcemia
	Hyponatremia
Neurological	Raised intracranial pressure
	Posterior fossa tumors
	Meningeal infiltration
	Skull metastases
Emotional	Anxiety
	Anticipatory vomiting with chemotherapy
Other	Severe uncontrolled pain
	Colic of any origin
	Radiotherapy: especially to L1 region, high-dose brain radiotherapy, upper hemibody radiation
	Cough, thick sputum, postnasal drip

Management

Specific treatments aimed at hypercalcemia and bowel obstruction are discussed separately below under Hypercalcemia and under Small and large bowel obstruction in advanced cancer.

NONPHARMACOLOGICAL

- Precipitating causes such as strong smells, movement, and anxiety should be addressed.
- A recent systematic review lends support to the use of acupuncture at the P6 point on the anterior wrist for acute chemotherapy-induced vomiting.[73][I]

PHARMACOLOGICAL

- Review drug causes but remember that opioid-induced nausea is usually self-limiting.

- Commonly used antiemetics, routes of administration, dosages, and sites of action are shown in **Table 24.3**.
- Pharmacological management of nausea and vomiting in advanced cancer has been discussed in a systematic review and the authors conclude that surprisingly little evidence is available to support management.[74][II]
- Suggested plans for managing common causes of nausea and vomiting are shown in **Figures 24.2, 24.3**, and **24.4**.
- Venting gastrostomy has been used to palliate large volume vomiting in mainly gastric outlet obstruction and a case series of 51 patients over a seven-year period suggested partial or complete relief of symptoms in 47.[84][IV]
- Endoscopic placement of duodenal stents has also provided symptom relief.[85][IV]

HYPERCALCEMIA

Hypercalcemia is a common cause of nausea and vomiting in late-stage cancer. It occurs in 8.5 percent of hospice patients.[86][V] It is a marker of poor prognosis, with about 80 percent of affected patients dying within a year.[87] Hypercalcemia occurs most commonly in patients with squamous cell lung carcinomas, breast and renal cancers, and myeloma (40–50 percent at some time during their illness[88]).

Bone metastases are present in the majority (approximately 80 percent) of cases, but because of other mechanisms the diagnosis must be actively sought.

An important mechanism in hypercalcemia is parathyroid hormone-related peptide (PTHrP): it is released by cancer cells and acts on endogenous PTH receptors to mobilize calcium from bone.[89][III] High PTHrP levels imply a poorer prognosis and response to treatment.[90][III]

Aside from nausea and vomiting, other symptoms include constipation, polyuria, thirst, lethargy, cardiac arrhythmias, and confusion. Later, the patient becomes unconscious; seizures may occur and eventually death. The measurement of calcium in the laboratory must be corrected for the serum albumin and associated acute renal impairment secondary to dehydration must be looked for (as patients should be well hydrated prior to definitive treatment).

Symptoms do not always correlate with the level of calcium but above 3.5 mmoL (corrected) should be considered life-threatening even if the patient is asymptomatic.

Management

- Diuretics and vitamin D and calcium supplements should be withdrawn if at all possible.

Table 24.3 Commonly used drugs in nausea and vomiting, their routes of administration and actions.

Drug	Routes of administration and doses of commonly used drugs	Receptors	Comments
Metoclopromide[74][I]	Oral, i.v., s.c., i.m. 10–20 mg t.i.d.–q.i.d	D2 and (high doses) 5HT4 antagonism	Prokinetic in gut. Can be used in continuous s.c. infusion (CSCI). Extrapyramidal side effects
Domperidone	Oral and rectal only. Doses 10–20 mg t.i.d.–q.i.d pc and 30 mg t.i.d. p.r.	D2 and (high doses) 5HT4 antagonism	Fewer extra pyramidal side effects than metoclopromide. Poor oral bioavailability
Cyclizine[75][V] Hyoscine hydrobromide	Oral, i.v., s.c., i.m. 50 mg t.i.d. p.r. Sublingual, s.c., i.m., i.v. 0.2–0.4 mg s.c.	Antihistamine/antimuscarininc Antimuscarinic	Can cause skin irritation in CSCI. Immiscible with some drugs Can be antisecretory in bowel obstruction. Generally not recommended in combination with D2 antagonist
Ondansetron/granisetron/ tropisetron/palonsetron etc.[74,76][I]	Melt, oral, i.v., s.c. Doses: see individual drugs	5HT3 antagonism	Main use in early chemotherapy/radiotherapy-induced nausea but also useful in bowel obstruction. Constipating. Expensive
Haloperidol (trials with droperidol but this is not commonly used)	Oral, s.c., i.m. 0.5–1.5 mg o.d.–b.i.d.	D2 antagonism, some antimuscarininc	Extrapyramidal side effects. Long duration of action useful for compliance. Main use in biochemical causes of nausea, especially renal failure
Levomepromazine (formerly methotrimeprazine)[77,78][V]	Oral, s.c., i.m. 2.5–6.25 mg s.c. o.d. to b.i.d.	D2, 5HT2 antagonism, antimuscarinic	Oral is half as potent as s.c. route. Long duration of action. Drowsiness and hypotension can be problematic. Skin irritation. Dose required for effective antiemesis anecdotally lower than previously thought
Olanzapine[79][III]	Melt/oral 2.5–10 mg p.o./melt o.d.	D1/D2 antagonism/modulates 5HT also	Potentially fewer extra pyramidal effects but seizure threshold stroke and diabetes more of a concern. More expensive than typical antipsychotics
Corticosteroid (usually dexamethasone)	Oral, s.c., i.v. Dexamethasone 4–8 mg o.d.	? Cerebral cortex and gut (hence use in emetogenic chemotherapy)	Systematic review (see below under Small and large bowel obstruction in advanced cancer) suggests small effect in resolving symptoms bowel obstruction. Main use in emesis due to raised intracranial pressure. Anecdotally antiemetic effect useful in intractable nausea of unknown cause. Side effects preclude prolonged use and "pulse" recommended
Aprepitant[80][II]	Oral (seek advice re. dose)	NK1 antagonism	Currently only recommended for highly emetogenic chemotherapy. Expensive
Octreotide/lanreotide	s.c. only by continuous infusion or i.m. injection fortnightly	Somatostatin analog	Will not affect nausea but can reduce intestinal secretions in bowel obstruction so reducing volume vomited (see **Figures 24.2** and **24.5** for doses)
Lorazepam	Sublingual. 0.5–1 mg 1–2 hours pretreatment	Modulates GABA (gamma aminobutyric acid)	Anticipatory nausea
Nabilone[81][I] Erythromycin[82][III], [83][V]	Oral 1 mg b.i.d. 250–500 mg q.i.d oral	? Cortical cannabinoid receptors Motilin agonism	Intractable nausea. Rarely used in view of drowsiness Mainly used in gastric statsis

Cisapride, a 5HT4 agonist which has prokinetic activity in the gut, has been discontinued in the UK because of reports of sudden cardiac death. However, newer related agents are under development.

Metoclopromide 10–20 mg t.i.d.–q.i.d. OR Domperidone 10–20 mg t.i.d.–q.i.d. p.o./30 mg pr t.i.d. Erythromycin 250 mg q.i.d. as prokinetic.

⇩

Switch route e.g. metoclopromide subcut 30–80 mg/24 hrs Consider dexamethasone 8 mg o.d. s.c./p.o. with PPI if gastric outlet obstruction

⇩

Consider adding octreotide 300–1200 µg per 24 hrs s.c.

⇩

Consider addition or replacement with: haloperidol, levomepromazine, ondansetron

⇩

Consider nasogastric tube?? Venting gastrostomy if patient fit

Figure 24.2 Suggested treatment plan for vomiting due to gastric stasis/outlet obstruction/"squashed stomach." PPI, proton pump inhibitor.

- Cyclizine 50 mg t.i.d. p.o./s.c.
- Dexamethasone 4–16 mg o.d. p.o. or s.c.
- Consider gastric cover
- Is patient fit for palliative radiotherapy?

↓

Consider addition or replacement with:
- Haloperidol, levomepromazine (NB seizure threshold with anti-psychotics)
- Ondansetron

↓

Consider s.c. route either o.d./b.d. or syringe driver

Figure 24.3 Suggested treatment plan for raised intracranial pressure nausea/vomiting.

- Special attention should be paid to patients taking digoxin – hypercalcemia increases the risk of toxicity.
- Diuretics should not be used – they worsen any preexisting dehydration.
- Rehydration via the intravenous route if the patient is unable to manage oral fluids.
- Symptomatic treatment with appropriate antiemetic (usually a D2 receptor antagonist).
- Intravenous bisphosphonates are now the mainstay of treatment. Most produce a clinical response in two to six days but it can take up to two weeks for calcium levels to return to normal.[91][II] The dose of the drug is usually titrated to the calcium level and

renal function. The response rate to bisphosphonates can be up to 70–100 percent.[92][II], [93, 94]

- The most frequently used drugs are clodronate and pamidronate but the newer, more potent bisphosphonates ibandronate and zolendronate may increase the success rate and, because of the short infusion times and longer period of normocalcemia, are probably more cost-effective.[95][I] The newer bisphosphonates are associated with greater nephrotoxicity, symptomatic hypocalcemia, and the more recently discovered problem of osteonecrosis of the jaw.[96][IV]
- Gallium nitrate has been used in resistant cases and in a recent randomized study was as effective as pamidronate.[97][II] However, it requires infusion over five days and is nephrotoxic.
- Calcitonin is very rarely used now but is another alternative – it only has a very temporary effect.
- Intravenous phosphate has been used in intensive care situations and can reduce life-threatening hypercalcemia more rapidly than anything else but its side effects of nausea, diarrhea, and ectopic calcification preclude widespread use.

SMALL AND LARGE BOWEL OBSTRUCTION IN ADVANCED CANCER

Incidence

It is difficult to assess the incidence of bowel obstruction in patients with advanced cancer. Studies involve highly selected patients at selected times of their illness. Reported figures vary from 2.5 percent in home care patients[98] [IV] to 51 percent in an autopsy study of ovarian carcinoma.[99][IV]

Pathophysiology

In advanced cancer the cause of bowel obstruction can be:[100]

- **intraluminal**, e.g. large bowel tumor;
- **intramural**, e.g. tumor spreading in the muscular layers can cause "intestinal linitis plastica," with a rigid, functionless bowel;
- **extramural**, e.g. mesenteric and omental masses and adhesions compress and kink the bowel;
- **motility disorders** – in addition to paralytic ileus (uncommon in this situation), patients can be affected by pseudo-obstruction due to infiltration of bowel muscle, mesentery, or nerve plexuses supplying the bowel, or as part of a paraneoplastic syndrome.

Other factors can also contribute, for example fecal impaction, change of bowel flora.

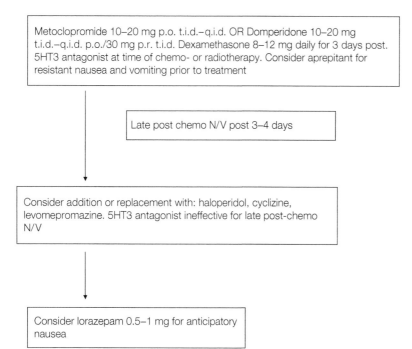

Metoclopromide 10–20 mg p.o. t.i.d.–q.i.d. OR Domperidone 10–20 mg t.i.d.–q.i.d. p.o./30 mg p.r. t.i.d. Dexamethasone 8–12 mg daily for 3 days post. 5HT3 antagonist at time of chemo- or radiotherapy. Consider aprepitant for resistant nausea and vomiting prior to treatment

Late post chemo N/V post 3–4 days

Consider addition or replacement with: haloperidol, cyclizine, levomepromazine. 5HT3 antagonist ineffective for late post-chemo N/V

Consider lorazepam 0.5–1 mg for anticipatory nausea

Figure 24.4 Suggested treatment plan for chemotherapy-induced nausea/vomiting (N/V).

Clinical features

The classical features of bowel obstruction are colicky abdominal pain, vomiting becoming progressively feculent, abdominal distension depending on the level of obstruction, and absolute constipation. However, these may be altered in advanced cancer. Onset is often insidious, the course may be intermittent, bowel distension may be absent in extensive bowel infiltration, and diarrhea is not uncommon in incomplete obstruction. A constant background abdominal pain is usually present in addition to the colic due to extensive tumor.

Management

SURGICAL INTERVENTION

Surgery needs to be considered in all cases. In approximately one-third of patients, even those with advanced disease, obstruction has a benign cause.[100] In most cases, surgery is the only definitive treatment anyway. However, this has to be balanced against an overall mortality rate for operation for acute bowel obstruction of 20 percent in advanced cancer, rising to 69 percent in patients aged over 70, and 72 percent in the malnourished.[101][IV] A more recent systematic review of surgical management of bowel obstruction in gynecological and gastrointestinal cancer highlights the wide variation in surgical practice with a large range of successful symptom relief (42–80 percent). The authors concluded that more consistent surgical procedures and improved measurement of outcomes, such as reobstruction rates and quality of life scores, were required before meaningful comparisons could be made.[102][II]

Pragmatically, surgery should be avoided if:

- there is obstruction at multiple sites (e.g. found at previous laparotomy);
- the patient is too ill for surgery;
- if the patient refuses.

Venting gastrostomy has sometimes been used to palliate large bowel obstruction, as have colonic stents. Two case series of 62 and 48 patients respectively suggest self-expanding metallic stents placed mostly in the rectum and sigmoid were feasible and safe although the risks of perforation, stent migration, and tumor overgrowth represent potential risks.[103, 104][III] [IV]

NONSURGICAL MANAGEMENT

"Drip and suck," indispensable in the short term as preparation for surgery, rarely leads to sustained symptom relief (Parker and Baines[105][V] quoting figures of 0–14 percent from various authors). Symptoms are much better managed with a combination of drugs, usually given through a syringe driver.[106][IV]

Figure 24.5 includes a management strategy for the pharmacological management of vomiting in large bowel obstruction but a strong opioid may also be required for background analgesia. Hyoscine butylbromide may have antisecretory as well as anticolic effects in this situation.[107] Octreotide has also been used to reduce gastrointestinal secretions in bowel obstruction.[108][III]

With regard to corticosteroid use, a systematic review concluded that although there was a tendency towards favoring their use, this did not achieve statistical significance.[109][II] A further study pointed out the potential

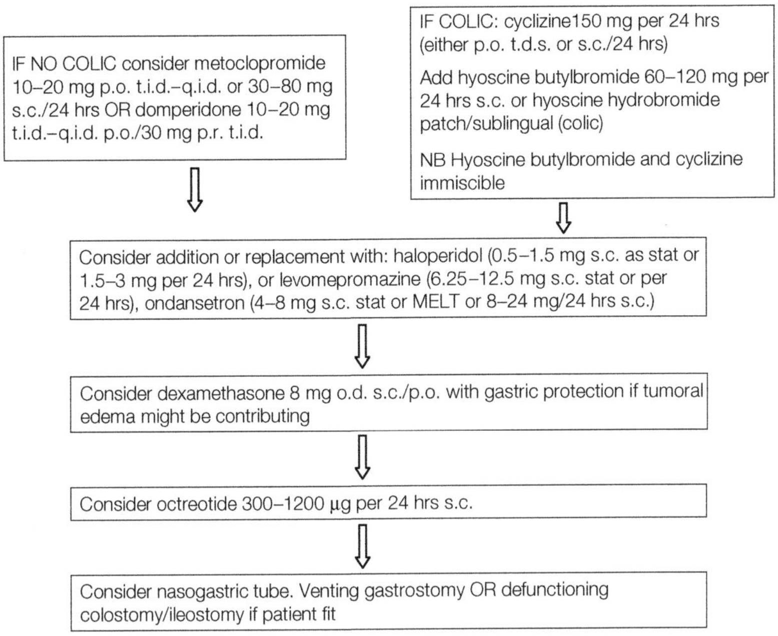

IF NO COLIC consider metoclopromide 10–20 mg p.o. t.i.d.–q.i.d. or 30–80 mg s.c./24 hrs OR domperidone 10–20 mg t.i.d.–q.i.d. p.o./30 mg p.r. t.i.d.

IF COLIC: cyclizine150 mg per 24 hrs (either p.o. t.d.s. or s.c./24 hrs)

Add hyoscine butylbromide 60–120 mg per 24 hrs s.c. or hyoscine hydrobromide patch/sublingual (colic)

NB Hyoscine butylbromide and cyclizine immiscible

Consider addition or replacement with: haloperidol (0.5–1.5 mg s.c. as stat or 1.5–3 mg per 24 hrs), or levomepromazine (6.25–12.5 mg s.c. stat or per 24 hrs), ondansetron (4–8 mg s.c. stat or MELT or 8–24 mg/24 hrs s.c.)

Consider dexamethasone 8 mg o.d. s.c./p.o. with gastric protection if tumoral edema might be contributing

Consider octreotide 300–1200 μg per 24 hrs s.c.

Consider nasogastric tube. Venting gastrostomy OR defunctioning colostomy/ileostomy if patient fit

Figure 24.5 Suggested treatment plan for nausea/vomiting due to lower gastrointestinal tract obstruction.

problems associated with placebo in palliative care with particular regard to the use of steroids in bowel obstruction.[110][II]

Nausea is often controlled but vomiting may be reduced to once or twice a day rather than totally abolished as this can at times only be done at the cost of severe drug adverse effects. Prognosis of up to seven months has been reported with this regimen, though most patients die within a few weeks.

CONSTIPATION

Constipation is a complaint of about 10 percent of the general population and 50 percent of patients with cancer admitted to palliative care units. However, 63 percent of such patients require laxatives if they are not taking opioid analgesics and 87 percent if they are.[111][III] Constipation is thus a common symptom in cancer, especially if potent analgesia is required, and has been reported as causing more distress than pain in a population with advanced disease.

Pathophysiology

The normal gut transit time is 48–72 hours in a Western population. Most of this time is spent in the colon. On a small number of occasions each day, peristaltic actions occur, which move colonic contents over considerable distances, and are associated with borborygmi and, sometimes, an urge to defecate. These mass movements are stimulated by gastric emptying and by physical activity, and in consequence the reduced food and fluid intake and the physical debility resulting from cancer are associated with constipation. In addition, drugs with anticholinergic

effects, iron, cytotoxic chemotherapy agents such as vincristine, and opioid analgesics add to the problem.

Opioids have a range of effects which are likely to exacerbate constipation markedly, as follows:

- contraction of intestinal sphincters;
- reduction in frequency of peristaltic mass movements;
- reduction in net water secretion by gut mucosa;
- impairment of rectal sensation.

Clinical findings

- Distinguish constipation from malignant intestinal obstruction and spurious diarrhea secondary to impaction.
- Enquire about the time of onset of the altered bowel habit, the stool frequency, and extent of straining at defecation, and, if there is a complaint of loose motions or fecal leakage, whether this succeeded a period of constipation. Known abdominal malignancy increases the risk of obstruction.
- Abdominal examination may reveal fecal masses in the line of the colon from tumor masses, which may be associated with obstruction. Rectal examination should reveal 90 percent of instances of fecal impaction.

Investigations

Investigations are rarely needed, but a plain abdominal radiograph may help distinguish obstruction from constipation. Constipation may precipitate vomiting, but both may be associated with hypercalcemia, which should not be overlooked.

Management

Encouragement of fluid intake and as high a dietary fiber content as is palatable, is likely to reduce the extent of constipation, although evidence is lacking. The constipating action of drugs should be anticipated and a laxative made available before the problem becomes established.

At least in advanced cancer, most patients will require a laxative but the evidence for their use derives largely from other fields.[112][I] Most British patients prefer oral administration to enemas and suppositories. Clinically, it is helpful to think of laxative agents as predominantly stool softening or predominantly gut peristalsis stimulating. Pharmacologically, the distinction is unsafe as any softening agent will increase the stool's bulk and so stretch the gut wall to cause reflex contraction, while a stimulant will reduce transit time and hence the time available for water absorption, so the stool will be softer.

However, there is evidence that in a model of constipation in human volunteers the combination of stimulant and softening drugs minimizes both medication burden and adverse effects compared with either class of agent used alone.[113][III] This is one therapeutic area where the use of combination preparations can be valid. It is vital that the laxative dose is titrated adequately against the clinical response. All too often opioid-related constipation is treated ineffectively with a single agent in a dose that is too small.

The commonly used laxatives are tabulated below (**Table 24.4**). Bulking agents, for example methyl cellulose, ispaghula, are inadvisable in cancer patients: they are relatively weak laxatives and also need to be taken with a significant volume of water, which can be intolerable to sicker patients. Reduction in the volume of water risks the formation of a viscous mass in the gut lumen, which can then precipitate or complete an obstruction.

Two peripheral opioid receptor antagonists capable of relieving opioid-induced constipation are likely to become clinically available shortly, alvimopan[114][V] and methylnaltrexone.[115][V] These agents offer the first prospect of a specific treatment for this condition.

Rectal laxatives may be needed for the clearance of fecal impaction, a sign that the oral laxative regimen requires review, or in the management of paraplegic patients who lack rectal sensation and anal sphincter tone. An alternative for the clearance of impaction is oral polyethylene glycol electrolyte solution, as long as the patient can cope with the volumes involved.[116][III]

DIARRHEA

Diarrhea is much less common than constipation in cancer care, occurring in around 10 percent of admissions for palliative care.

Pathophysiology

The bowel receives approximately 9 L of fluid daily, 2 L from oral intake and the remainder from gastric, biliary, pancreatic, and intestinal secretions. All but some 150 mL of this total is reabsorbed. The difference between constipation and diarrhea amounts to 100 mL or so of water per day, indicating a remarkably fine control of fluid balance across the gut wall. This control is exercised via the myenteric neural plexus, but is also subject to influence by luminal factors such as fatty acids and bile salts and also drugs such as opioids and some cytotoxic chemotherapy agents.[117][V]

Clinical findings

Although diarrhea is frequent evacuation of loose stool, patients may use the word to describe other situations such as an increase in frequency of any kind of stool, a single relatively loose bowel action per day, or fecal leakage or incontinence, any of which might represent constipation rather than true diarrhea. Therefore, a complaint of diarrhea must be elucidated by a careful history, including an account of drugs such as laxatives and elixir preparations, which might contain osmotically active sugars, and recent chemotherapy or radiotherapy. Abdominal and rectal examinations should also be performed, in order to exclude fecal impaction or loss of sphincter tone.

Investigations

In this patient group, investigations of diarrhea are not usually warranted because the cause emerges through history or examination, or because any infective cause is likely to be short-lived and self-limiting. However, if the patient is toxic or the diarrhea is continuing beyond about three days duration, stool samples should be taken and cultured for pathogens such as *Clostridium difficile*, *Escherichia coli*, *Salmonella*, or *Shigella*. Prolonged diarrhea should also prompt monitoring and correction of fluid and electrolyte balance.

Management

The most common cause of diarrhea in palliative medicine is an excessive laxative dose.[118] However, an unduly long suspension of laxative therapy results in a pattern of alternating constipation and diarrhea; it is usually adequate to suspend the laxatives for 24 hours and then resume a dose step down.

Specific therapies exist for certain causes of diarrhea (**Table 24.5**).

Most treatment for diarrhea is symptomatic. Available drugs are either absorbent or adsorbent, taking up water and toxins into or onto their structures, or are motility- and secretion-modifying agents (**Table 24.6**).

Table 24.4 Commonly used laxatives and their methods of action.

Mode of action	Examples	Usual dose range	Comments	Latency of action
Predominantly softening				
Osmotic agents (retain water in gut lumen)	Lactulose Magnesium hydroxide Magnesium sulfate	15–40 mL b.i.d.–t.i.d. 2–4 g daily	Active principally in the small bowel Acts throughout the bowel and may have pronounced purgative effect, possibly partly as a result of direct peristaltic stimulation	1–2 days 1–6 h (dose dependent)
	Polyethylene glycol (PEG)	1–3 sachets per day (up to eight sachets for treatment of fecal impaction)	125 mL of water required with each sachet	
Surfactant agents (increase water penetration of the stool)	Docusate sodium Poloxamer (available only in combination with danthron)	Docusate 60–300 mg b.i.d.	Probably not very effective when used alone	1–3 days
Lubricant agents	Liquid paraffin Glycerine (as suppositories) Arachis oil Olive oil (as enemas)		Paraffin is best used only in a 25% emulsion with magnesium hydroxide (Mil-Par)	
Predominantly stimulant				
Direct stimulation of myenteric nerves to induce peristalsis	Senna	7.5–30 mg b.i.d.	Anthraquinone family. Danthron available only in combination with docusate or poloxamer – stains urine red/brown	6–12 h
Reduce absorption of water from gut	Danthron	50–450 mg b.i.d.		
	Bisacodyl Sodium picosulfate	10–20 mg b.i.d. 5–20 mg b.i.d.	Polyphenolic family	6–12 h
Combination stimulant/softener preparations				
Codanthramer standard	Danthron 25 mg with poloxamer 200 mg per 5 mL or capsule Danthron not danthron		Suspension or capsule	
Codanthramer forte	Danthron 75 mg with poloxamer 1 g per 5 mL or two capsules		Suspension or capsule	
Codanthrusate	Danthron 50 mg with docusate 60 mg per 5 mL or capsule		Capsule or suspension	
Emulsion magnesium hydroxide and liquid paraffin (3:1 ratio)			Liquid only	

Table 24.5 Specific antidiarrheal therapies.

Problem	Therapy
Fat malabsorption	Pancreatic enzyme replacement
Chologenic diarrhea	Cholestyramine 4–12 g t.i.d.; calcium carbonate
Radiation-induced diarrhea	Cholestyramine 4–12 g t.i.d.; aspirin
Carcinoid syndrome	Cyproheptadine: initially 12 mg once daily (also consider octreotide; see **Table 24.6**)
Ulcerative colitis	Mesalazine 1.2–2.4 g/day; steroids
Pseudomembranous colitis	Vancomycin 125 mg q.i.d.; metronidazole 400 mg t.i.d.

Table 24.6 Symptomatic treatments for diarrhea.

Type of treatment	Example
Absorbent agents	Bulk-forming agents, e.g. methyl cellulose
	Pectin
Adsorbent agents	Kaolin
	Attapulgite
Motility- and secretion-modifying agents	Opioids
	Codeine: 10–60 mg 4-hourly
	(Morphine – usually if already in use for pain)
	Diphenoxylate (combined with atropine): 10 mg stat, then 5 mg 6-hourly
	Loperamide: 4 mg stat, then 2 mg after each loose stool up to 16 mg/24 h
	Somatostatin analogs
	Octreotide: 300 μg/24 h s.c. titrated up to 2400 μg/24 h if necessary

There is limited evidence for the efficacy of certain adsorbent and absorbent substances in acute diarrhea (e.g. pectin[119][II] or attapulgite[120][II]). The most effective general antidiarrheals are the opioids, of which loperamide is the most specific, as in adults it has an oral bioavailability close to 1 percent and hence its effects are limited almost exclusively to the gut.[121][V]

Octreotide is a somatostatin analog that has to be given by subcutaneous injection or infusion. There are clinical reports of its effectiveness in otherwise intractable diarrhea secondary to gut resection, chemotherapy, or HIV disease.[122][V] Hyoscine butylbromide has also been used anecdotally in secretory diarrhea.

OTHER SYMPTOMS

Cachexia and anorexia

Primary anorexia cachexia syndrome (ACS) involves:

- weight loss;
- weakness;
- anorexia;
- fatigue;
- chronic nausea.[123]

An unintentional weight loss of more than 10 percent (some would say 5 percent) over six months compared with pre-morbid weight loss defines it quantitatively.[124][V]

ACS is extremely common in some cancers (esophagus, stomach, pancreas, small-cell carcinoma of the bronchus) but not in others (breast cancer, ovarian cancer, sarcomas, testicular tumors). ACS also occurs with a number of noncancer illnesses (e.g. acquired immunodeficiency syndrome (AIDS), heart failure). Its presence in both malignant and nonmalignant conditions implies a poor prognosis.[124, 125][III] Cachexia becomes more common with disease progression.[126] However, marked cachexia can be present at diagnosis[127][III] or even before, and the relationship with tumor bulk is unclear. It is probably the primary cause of death in 20–30 percent of cancer patients, due to irreversible metabolic damage and loss of energy production.[128][V]

PATHOPHYSIOLOGY

The key pathophysiological processes involved are:

- changes in protein, lipid and carbohydrate metabolism;
- changes in anabolic hormones;

- neurohormonal mechanisms (which have their predominant effect on appetite via the gut and hypothalamus) – the latter are shown in more detail in **Figure 24.6**;
- some of the changes are thought to be mediated by inflammatory cytokines.[129][V]

The key to understanding ACS is that it represents an entirely different state to starvation: in starvation there is lack of substrates for energy production, so starvation is a low-output state aimed at conserving energy, while in ACS the metabolic rate is artificially raised and there is marked skeletal muscle loss (much more so than in starvation) and some fat loss. Although cytokines produced by the patient are partly responsible, increasing emphasis is currently being placed on tumoral factors: lipid-mobilizing factors (LMFs) and protein-mobilizing factors (PMFs) and the pathways involved in proteolysis, particularly the ubiquitin-dependent protesome pathway.[124, 128]

CLINICAL FINDINGS AND INVESTIGATIONS

Patients lose considerable weight, with both adipose tissue and muscle being affected. Fatigue, anemia and dyspnea (due to loss of intercostal muscle), and edema may also be present. There may be evidence of specific nutritional deficiencies, although this should lead one to look for particular causes. Hepatic synthesis of acute-phase proteins (e.g. C-reactive protein (CRP)) is increased, but that of functional proteins such as albumin and transferrin is reduced. Cachectic patients therefore often develop hypertriglyceridemia, hypoalbuminemia, hypoproteinemia, glucose intolerance, anemia, and lactic acidosis.

MANAGEMENT

Secondary or reversible causes should be sought and treated wherever possible, for example:

- treating the underlying disease;
- controlling nausea, or other uncontrolled symptoms;
- excluding depression;
- adequate mouthcare.

Nonpharmacological interventions include:

- gentle exercise programmes;[130][V]
- nutritional advice and supplements, although the latter in a systematic review neither increased weight nor survival.[131][II] The two possible exceptions to nutritional interventions are fish oil derivatives and supplements containing branched chain amino acids (see below under Eicosapentaenoic acid and Other potential treatments);
- support for the patient and family using the skills of the multiprofessional team. One study reported higher levels of distress caused by anorexia in carers than patients, despite reasonable agreement in reporting the symptom between carers and patients.[132][IV]

PHARMACOLOGICAL TREATMENTS

Corticosteroids

Corticosteroids (e.g. dexamethasone 3–6 mg, methylprednisolone 30–125 mg daily) are effective in stimulating appetite and providing a sense of well-being.[133][V] There is, however, no weight gain or increase in survival, and the effect disappears after a few weeks. This benefit has to be weighed against the often serious adverse effects of steroid

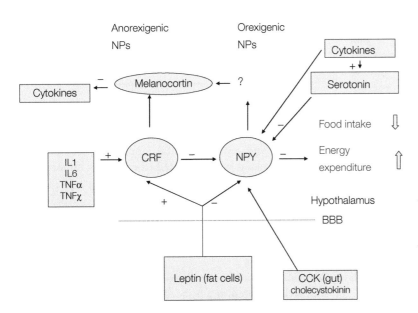

Figure 24.6 Neurohormonal mechanisms in cancer anorexia/cachexia. Il, interleukin; NP, neuropeptides; TNF, tumor necrosis factor; NPY, neuropeptide Y; CRF, corticotrophin-releasing factor, BBB, blood–brain barrier. Adapted and simplified from: Inui A. Cancer anorexia–cachexia syndrome: are neuropeptides the key? *Cancer Research.* 1999; **52**: 4493–501.

use, including that of proximal myopathy. Steroids should therefore be tried for a week, and if not clearly helping they should be stopped. Discontinuing dexamethasone 6 mg abruptly after a week's treatment is safe, though this is not the case for higher doses or longer courses. If there is benefit, the patient should be left on the lowest effective dose; once no longer effective, steroids should be stopped.[134][V] Corticosteroids can precipitate or exacerbate diabetes, and it is good practice to check blood or urine sugars over the first few days of the steroid course until it is clear whether hypoglycemic treatment will be required.

Progestogens (megestrol acetate and medroxyprogesterone)

The results of two systematic reviews on the use of megestrol acetate[135, 136][I] demonstrated the following:

- Megestrol acetate is significantly superior to placebo in increasing appetite, producing weight gain, and increasing patients' sense of well-being.
- Weight gain is dose related (160–1600 mg in various trials).
- Weight gain is mainly due to fat and fluid retention – there is no increase in muscle mass (lean body mass).
- Megestrol has an antinauseant effect.
- Quality of life improvements were generally poorly measured in the reviewed trials and there was no effect on survival.

Mechanisms of action are still being elucidated, but progestogens appear to inhibit the production of cachexia-producing cytokines.[137][IV]
   The main side effects of progestagens are:

- fluid retention;
- venous thromboembolism;
- hyperglycemia.

Cannabinoids

Delta 9-tetrahydrocannabinol (THC) has been shown in open and retrospective studies to produce weight gain and improved appetite varying from "slight" in one study of patients with advanced cancer to a weight gain of 0.6 kg/month in a small group of AIDS patients. A recent study showed THC to be less effective than megestrol in producing appetite improvement and weight gain, and the addition of THC to megestrol conferred no additional benefit.[138][II] In addition, a further study of approximately 200 patients with advanced cancer randomly assigned to two cannabis derivatives and placebo showed no demonstrable difference in appetite gain or quality of life scores between the three groups.[139][II]

NSAIDs

NSAIDs reduce resting energy expenditure and serum CRP levels in pancreatic cancer patients,[140][II] although their side effects may preclude prolonged use.

Eicosapentaenoic acid

The mechanism of action of this polyunsaturated fatty acid derived from fish oil appears to be the inhibition of proteolysis and reduction in the metabolic rate. One study of weight-losing pancreatic cancer patients appeared to show beneficial effects on weight gain compared with standard nutritional supplements.[141][II] Unfortunately, large numbers of capsules or liquid supplement have to be taken to have any benefit and another study demonstrated poor compliance with treatment.[142] [II] A recent systematic review of trials involving over 500 patients concluded that there is insufficient evidence of efficacy of eicosapentaenoic acid (EPA) over placebo.[143][I]

OTHER POTENTIAL TREATMENTS

- Branched chain amino acids (BCAA) have demonstrated some promise experimentally[144][V] (the profile of amino acids is altered in ACS, away from BCAA) although delivering them to the patient by a convenient route may be a challenge.
- Thalidomide appears to have beneficial effects on appetite and weight gain independent of its anticancer effects and has been used in HIV-AIDS ACS.
- Melatonin (20 mg given in the hours of darkness) in one retrospective survey appeared to improve appetite and weight gain[145][III] but more studies are needed.
- Much interest has been focused on ghrelin, a stomach hormone, and finding synthetic analogs.[146][V]
- Orexin has been used experimentally in a mouse model to improve food intake – the mechanism appears to be via cholecystokinin, a gut hormone.[147][III]

Despite being logical in their site of action, the following drugs have not demonstrated sufficient efficacy to warrant their continued use in ACS: cyproheptadine, hydrazine sulphate, and pentoxifylline.[148][I]

FATIGUE

This is a common and debilitating symptom in advanced cancer with up to 40 percent of patients reporting fatigue at diagnosis.[149][V] It encompasses weakness, low exercise capacity, and reduced mental functioning and becomes more prevalent with advanced disease. It is important to exclude treatable causes:

- anemia;
- metabolic abnormalities such as diabetes, hypothyroidism, or hypoadrenalism;
- depression;
- side effects of preexisting drugs(which may not be so well tolerated in advanced cancer).

Management includes:

- Supervised exercise programmes – several studies have demonstrated beneficial effects on fatigue for example, in breast cancer patients and survivors.[150] [I]
- The erythropoietin analogs (erythropoietin alpha or darbopoetin) may have beneficial effects on fatigue independent of their effects in hemoglobin, especially during chemotherapy,[151][V] although a small recent study suggested that pre-erythropoietin psychological factors may have an important effect on the response to treatment.[152][III]
- Amphetamines such as methylphenidate (5 mg once to twice daily as starting dose) have appeared to confer benefit on fatigued cancer patients in small open-label studies but a recent double-blind, randomized controlled trial of 112 patients showed no benefit over placebo at one week (although placebo and active drug both conferred benefit).[153][II]

LYMPHEDEMA

This results from impaired lymphatic drainage, usually from a limb, from the affected part of the body. It can be secondary to lymph node dissection or radiotherapy performed as part of cancer treatment or it can occur due to lymph node metastases. The true incidence is difficult to quantify as studies vary widely with definitions: for example, reported figures range from 2 to 56 percent for breast cancer patients.[154]

Management

- It is important to distinguish lymphedema in a limb from deep vein thrombosis or from inferior or superior vena cava obstruction which may be amenable to stenting. It is also important to exclude cardiac failure as an underlying cause.
- If the lymphedema is disease-related, radiotherapy or chemotherapy may be beneficial.
- The patient should be counseled on careful care of the skin including avoiding trauma, blood tests, etc. on the affected area. They should be alerted to seek prompt attention should any signs of cellulitis occur.
- A number of physical techniques are used to try and reduce swelling: bandaging, manual lymphatic drainage, and compression pumps.[154][I]
- Various drugs have been tried, for example benzo-pyrones, but a systematic review concluded that there was insufficient evidence at present to support their use.[155][I]
- If the prognosis is very short, some relief may be gained by use of a closed-system subcutaneous

drainage using a reasonable-sized needle. This method is described in a small case series of eight patients, seven of whom described the technique as helpful.[156]

PRURITUS

Pruritus, or itch, occurs in 5 percent of patients overall with advanced cancer. The prevalence is much higher in Hodgkin's lymphoma and in Sezary syndrome. Cholestasis is very often associated with itch, whatever the cause.

Pathology

Pruritus is mediated by a subset of peripheral C-fibers that are functionally, although not anatomically, distinct from those transmitting pain.[157] Itch can be central or peripheral in origin and be associated with nerve damage or intact nerves. Mast cell release of histamine or direct stimulation of peripheral nerves are the mechanisms by which endogenous pruritogens such as opioids, cytokines, and eicosanoids can act. Damage to nervous tissue can lead to the "neuropathic itch" seen in postherpetic neuralgia, multiple sclerosis and, rarely, cerebral tumors.

Other endogenous chemicals involved in transmission or modulation include: substance P, cytokines, serotonin, prostaglandin E_2, opioids at μ-receptors (especially important in cholestasis), and, possibly, VIP. Pruritus is suggestible, revealing a contribution of central neural processing.

Causes

- Age-related "senile pruritus" usually associated with drying of skin.
- Morphine: intrathecally/epidurally (10–90 percent). Rarely orally (1 percent).
- Uremia.
- Cholestatic jaundice.
- Hodgkin's disease or Sezary syndrome as presenting symptom.
- Postherpetic neuralgia.
- General medical/dermatological causes.

Clinical findings

- Generalized pruritus should be distinguished from local, and itching should be distinguished from related sensations that could represent neuropathic pain.
- Associated conditions and potential allergens should be excluded.
- Anemia or renal failure should be looked for clinically and with appropriate blood tests.

- Examination will reveal the extent of skin excoriation caused by scratching, and areas of local itching should be checked for evidence of fungal or mite infestation.
- The presence, distribution, and form of any rash will help distinguish between general allergic reactions, eczema, and locally provoked dermatoses.

Management

General measures should be undertaken (**Box 24.1**). Specific treatments aimed at underlying cause:

- if related to oral morphine, consider switching opioid;
- bile duct stenting for malignant obstructive jaundice or nephrostomies/ureteric stents for malignant ureteric obstruction.

Topical treatments

- Counterirritants and local anesthetics, for example phenol 0.5–2 percent, menthol 0.25–2 percent, camphor 1–3 percent, provide anesthesia of cutaneous nerve endings or a cooling sensation. However, crotamiton, often used in this way, has been shown to be ineffective.[158][II]
- Capsaicin 0.025 percent causes depletion of substance P in peripheral nerves and blocks C-fiber conduction but also gives rise to local burning sensations, which may need local anesthetics for their relief. It can also take up to two weeks to have an effect. Capsaicin has been found to be effective in relieving renal failure-associated itch.[159][II]
- Transcutaneous electrical nerve stimulation (TENS) provides an electrical equivalent of counterirritation to produce surround inhibition of transmission of pruritic stimuli. There are case reports of its successful clinical use.[160]
- Topical 5 percent sodium cromoglycate has been reported to be effective in Hodgkin's lymphoma itching after the failure of other therapies.[161]

Box 24.1 General measures for pruritus

- Avoid friction from clothing, towels, and bed linen
- Avoid excessive heat
- Use emulsifying ointment rather than soap for washing
- Avoid vasodilators (which for some will include coffee and alcohol)
- Allow gentle rubbing but discourage scratching
- Topical steroids to inflamed areas
- Diversion
- Control of other symptoms

s0475
p1710
p1715
p1720
p1725
p1730
p1735
p1740
p1745

Systemic treatments

Some systemic treatments for pruritus are general and others are associated with particular diseases.

GENERAL

- H1 antihistamines are most effective when there is evidence of a local histamine involvement in itching but are also often used in other conditions. It appears that efficacy is related to the degree of sedation caused, for example chlorpheniramine 4 mg four-hourly.
- Approximately 30 percent of those with generalized pruritus have evidence of depression, but the claimed effectiveness of doxepin,[162] paroxetine[163] and mirtazepine[164] in pruritus of a range of etiologies is attributed to their modulation of histamine and serotonin systems.
- Ultraviolet light has been used in itch from cutaneous metastases[165][IV] and in other types of pruritus.[166][III]
- Gabapentin has been used anecdotally for a variety of causes of pruritus.
- Thalidomide has also been used but it is difficult to prescribe and potential side effects of neuropathy have limited its use.

SPECIFIC

Cholestasis

- Opioid receptor antagonists such as methylnaltrexone have been successfully used, particularly in nonmalignant liver disease.[167][II] The mechanism is thought to involve modulation of the enhanced opioidergic tone associated with intrahepatic cholestasis. Clearly there is a concern about precipitating pain in patients taking exogenous opioids. A topical preparation of methylnaltrexone has also been used in itch associated with dermatological conditions[168][II] and it may have a therapeutic role in cholestasis.
- Rifampicin has also been used in cholestasis and there are a number of trials supporting its use[169][I] but its drug interactions may limit its use.
- Ondansetron has been found to be ineffective in cholestatic itch.[170][II]
- Cholestyramine binds bile salts in the gut and is used occasionally. It can be very unpalatable to take.
- NOTE: The anabolic steroid stanozolol which was previously used for this situation was discontinued in 2002.

Uremic itch

- Parathyroidectomy has relieved itch due to secondary hyperparathyroidism.
- Ondansetron has not shown consistent efficacy.

- Nalfurafine, a novel kappa opioid agonist demonstrated benefit over placebo in 144 patients with uremic itch.[171] [II] It is thought that there is imbalance between kappa and mu opioid receptors in uremic itch
- Erythropoietin[172] [II] may have a beneficial effect independent of its effect on anemia.

Others

- Pruritus associated with lymphoma may respond to cimetidine[173] or plasma exchange.
- Ondansetron has been reported to be effective in a randomized controlled trial in epidural morphine-induced pruritus.[174][II]

SWEATING

Excessive sweating occurs widely in cancer but is reported particularly by patients with lymphomas, leukemia, or liver metastases. It is not necessarily associated with fever or with infection and may be worse at night.

Pathology

Human body temperature control is accurate and complex. It appears that the anterior hypothalamus integrates information from temperature sensors in the skin, central nervous system (CNS), and viscera to stimulate autonomic and behavioral thermoregulatory mechanisms in order to maintain the body temperature at a set point. This set point can be altered in a number of circumstances, including malignancy, sepsis, and dehydration. Blood transfusion, cytotoxics (such as bleomycin), and changes in estrogen balance can also induce fever.

Clinical findings and investigations

The principal aim is to identify any infection, but hormone-related sweating ("hot flushes") will be suggested by a menopausal history or hormonal manipulation for breast or prostate cancers.

Management

General measures are important:

- use of cotton rather than artificial fibers;
- availability of regular changes of clothing;
- provision of a fan;
- regular tepid sponging;
- regular washing;
- encouragement of oral fluids.

Specific measures are as follows.

- Infections causing systemic toxicity should be treated.
- Megestrol acetate starting at 40 mg/24 hours is effective for hot flushes ("flashes") in both breast and prostate cancer, and does not appear to impair tumor control. In a randomized controlled trial, megestrol acetate was significantly better than placebo for hot flushes and the accompanying sweating in patients with breast or prostate cancer.[175][II]
- Paracetamol (acetaminophen) is worth using initially, although its effectiveness is said to be reduced in neoplastic fevers.
- NSAIDs can be effective in malignancy-related sweating, with particular value being claimed for naproxen.[176][II] However, if loss of efficacy occurs, a change to another NSAID may recover it.
- There is case history evidence for the use of thioridazine, the limiting factor being sedation. It is rarely used now because of its association with sudden cardiac death.
- Anticholinergic drugs and beta blockers have also been used.
- Thalidomide has also been used but its side effects and complexity of prescribing it may limit its use.
- Steroids may be helpful in leukemia or lymphoma.

PSYCHOLOGICAL AND PSYCHIATRIC PROBLEMS

Depression

Depression is more common in cancer patients than in the general population though no more so than in patients with other physical illnesses.[177][V] It can precede diagnosis.[178] Both depression and suicide risk are increased in the early stages of cancer[179][IV] and are higher in some cancers, for example head and neck tumors,[180] and if pain or severe symptoms are present.[181, 182][V] Disease progression and recurrence are again associated with increased psychiatric morbidity.

DIAGNOSIS AND PREVALENCE

Adjustment reactions and appropriate sadness have to be distinguished from true depression. Somatic features of depression (e.g. loss of interest in normal activities, psychomotor retardation, anorexia, and weight loss) in advanced cancer can be due entirely to the physical deterioration. This has led to attempts to replace the somatic criteria in the Diagnostic and Statistical Manual (DSM) classification with nonsomatic ones with greater discriminative power for cancer patients.[183, 184][V] Alternatively, Cohen-Cole *et al.*[184] proposed ignoring anorexia and fatigue in the DSM criteria and using only the remaining criteria.

It has also been suggested that the simple question "Are you depressed?" carries a higher sensitivity and specificity[185][III] than formal questionnaires, and doubt has been cast on the applicability of the Hospital Anxiety and Depression Scale in hospice patients,[186, 187] though others dispute this.[188][III]

With all these provisos in mind, the prevalence of depression has been reported as varying between 1 percent for acute leukemia and 50 percent for pancreatic cancer.[189][V] Most experts agree an overall prevalence of 10–25 percent for patients with terminal illness.[190]

Ideas of worthlessness, hopelessness, guilt, and suicidal ideation need to be explored.

MANAGEMENT

Nonpharmacological

Psychotherapy (individual or group) and cognitive-behavioral therapy have important roles to play in treating depression in cancer patients. Fawzy *et al.*[191][V] and Sellick and Crooks[192][V] produce evidence for the effectiveness of various forms of psychotherapy in cancer patients.

Pharmacological

A systematic review of antidepressant drug treatment showed that just over four patients with physical illness would have to be treated to produce one recovery that would not have occurred using placebo (number needed to treat (NNT) of 4.2) (95 percent confidence interval 3.2–6.4).[193][I]

- Tricyclic antidepressants are highly effective but cause troublesome adverse effects such as postural hypotension, cardiac arrhythmias, and anticholinergic effects.
- Selective serotonin reuptake inhibitors (SSRIs) are an alternative – the main adverse effects are nausea, diarrhea, and insomnia. Different SSRIs also inhibit different hepatic enzymes, increasing the potential for drug interactions.[194][V] However, SSRIs can usually be started at a therapeutic dose, unlike the tricyclics, which have to be built up over time.
- Most antidepressants require two to three weeks or longer to work. Mirtazepine, a newer antidepressant, may be an exception – it is claimed to have a faster onset of action.[195][II]
- Amphetamines have been used anecdotally in combination with antidepressants – they may improve mood more rapidly than antidepressants.

Suicide risk

Roth and Breitbart[196] list the following risk factors for suicide in cancer patients:

- advanced illness;
- concurrent psychiatric morbidity (major depression, delirium, adjustment disorder);
- uncontrolled pain;
- sense of helplessness and loss of control;
- fatigue of resources, physical, psychosocial, and spiritual;
- lack of a good support system;
- suicidal ideation or prior attempts.

The suicidal patient should be managed in an appropriate setting – a psychiatric unit may not be required provided there is support from the psychiatric team. Occasionally patients will require detention against their will and in so doing a formal assessment of mental capacity will be required.

Anxiety

Anxiety severe enough to disrupt day-to-day activity can be a feature of adjustment disorder or a condition in its own right. Again, DSM-IV somatic diagnostic criteria (muscle tension, aches or soreness; easy fatiguability; shortness of breath or smothering sensations; dry mouth, dizziness, or diarrhea; trouble falling or staying asleep and irritability) can equally well be due to the cancer itself. Psychological symptoms have to be relied on more heavily than the somatic in making decisions about such patients anxiety levels.

PREVALENCE

This depends on the cut-off points one chooses to make the diagnosis. Anxiety is about twice as common in persons with chronic medical conditions as in those with no physical illness, though whether it is more common in cancer than in other illnesses is unclear. Noyes *et al.*,[197] reviewing various studies, quote a prevalence of 9–19 percent for cancer patients. Mixed anxiety–depression is common. Once again, anxiety symptoms and panic attacks can be premonitors of cancer.[198]

ETIOLOGY

Factors increasing risk of severe anxiety include:

- premorbid personality;
- more advanced disease;
- active treatment with surgery, chemotherapy, or radiotherapy;
- poorly controlled pain;

- physical factors, for example sepsis, hypoxia;
- medication: corticosteroids, phenothiazines or derivatives, such as metoclopramide (e.g. akathisia), sudden alcohol or smoking cessation.

Sex, age, marital status, and other demographic variables are less useful predictors for anxiety than in the normal population. In the last weeks of life, patients who wanted more information than they had been given scored significantly higher on anxiety scales than those whose information needs were satisfied.[199]

MANAGEMENT

Nonpharmacological

There is evidence that concurrent psychotherapy and drug treatment is superior to either modality alone in treating anxiety or depression.[200][V] Exploration of a patient's fears in a psychotherapeutic environment can reduce psychological distress and improve coping.

Cognitive-behavioral therapy (CBT) is effective in reducing anxiety in both early and late stage cancer patients, and the effect may persist for 12 months.[201][II] Moorey et al.[202][II] found CBT to be superior to supportive nondirective psychotherapy in relieving anxiety, improving adjustment to cancer, and improving coping strategies; this effect remained at four months' follow-up.

A further study demonstrated feasibility of training staff in CBT techniques with a brief educational intervention,[203][III] while preliminary results from a randomized controlled trial in a specialist palliative care setting lends further support to this intervention.[204] Anxiety reduction was the main beneficial outcome in a systematic review of effectiveness of aromatherapy massage in advanced cancer patients.[205][I]

Pharmacological

A recent systematic review[206][II] found that the evidence for drug treatment for anxiety in cancer was very poor and that further studies were needed. Antidepressants can be effective and are perhaps overlooked. Buspirone may be useful if there is associated dyspnea but it can take several weeks to take effect.

Benzodiazepines reduce anxiety; in some situations (e.g. acute frightening exacerbations of breathlessness) the amnesic properties of these drugs also come in useful.

Delirium

Acute confusional states, sometimes superimposed on background dementia, occur in 15–20 percent of palliative care patients,[207] though figures of up to 85 percent have been reported.[208]

CLINICAL FEATURES

Delirium is often preceded by prodromal restlessness, anxiety, sleep disturbance, and irritability. It follows a highly fluctuant course, with disturbances of attention, perception, psychomotor activity, orientation, memory, and thinking.

Causes of confusion in terminally ill patients

These include:

- drugs, e.g. opioids, anticholinergics, steroids, cytotoxics;
- biochemical, e.g. hyponatremia, hypercalcemia, hypoglycemia; dehydration;
- neoplastic, e.g. brain primary or secondary tumor;
- paraneoplastic, e.g. nonmetastatic cerebral syndromes in small-cell lung cancer;
- organ failure: hepatic, renal, respiratory, cardiac;
- infection, e.g. chest, urinary;
- pain;
- alcohol or nicotine withdrawal;
- fear and extreme anxiety.

MANAGEMENT

Environmental manipulation can reduce the prevalence of delirium.[209][III] Medication is needed only if the patient is distressed or a danger to self or others. Happily confused patients should be treated if the underlying cause is reversible or they have a good prognosis.

- Reduce risk to the patient:
  - ensure a safe environment (e.g. patient not isolated, not easily able to inflict self-injury);
  - use medication if necessary (see below);
  - very occasionally use physical restraint.
- Defuse sense of threat experienced by the patient:
  - quiet, well-lit room;
  - familiar objects and persons, e.g. family;
  - reduce the number of persons the patient sees;
  - take an empathic approach (sit on same level as patient, touch, keep calm).
- Assess, and if possible treat, the underlying cause:
  - but this is often not amenable to treatment in this patient group.
- Try to ground the patient into reality:
  - gently point out misperceptions.
- Work out management plan for future events.

MEDICATION

- In general, drugs should be used sparingly, as they may worsen confusion, and adequate time should be given for them to work.

- There is little evidence to guide practice: a Cochrane review identified only one eligible trial and this compared haloperidol with chlorpromazine and lorazepam in terminally ill AIDS patients, with the finding that haloperidol was the most effective with fewer side effects.[210][I] Small doses (0.5–1 mg) used every 45–60 minutes are very effective; the dose can be increased if necessary.
- The new antipsychotic agents (e.g. risperidone, olanzapine) have been used at low doses with success to treat delirium, but evidence for their effectiveness is still being built up. They have fewer extrapyramidal effects but the risk of seizures and stroke is greater than older drugs.
- Benzodiazepines are another option (at low doses) but they may cause disinhibition and worsen confusion or behavioral problems.[211][V] However, they are the drugs of choice in substance withdrawal or if the patient is prone to fit, when major tranquilizers may further lower seizure threshold.
- In addition, short-acting benzodiazepines, for example midazolam, have found a definite place in palliative care, for example in controlling terminal agitated delirium.[212][V]

END OF LIFE CARE

Death is not necessarily seen as unwelcome by patients in the late stages of cancer. It can be a consolation to patients to be told that their condition will not go on for much longer.

Some professionals find it very difficult to be asked by patients for an estimate of prognosis, not only because any attempt at accuracy is likely to be misplaced, but also because they fear that the answer will cause the person to give up. Relatives are even more likely to take this view. However, there is evidence that the grounds for hope change as illness progresses,[213][IV] from the hope that cure may be achieved to one that the disease may be slowed in its progression, to the achievement of particular practical goals, and ultimately to hope for relief of discomfort and for a peaceful end to life.

Prior involvement of a multiprofessional palliative care team with 24-hour availability can facilitate the continuing care of the patient at home, where most terminally ill people wish to be.[214] As life becomes more difficult, the proportion wishing to stay at home diminishes but still remains at about 50 percent.[215][IV] For a significant number of families there comes a point when they feel they can no longer look after the patient at home, despite practical assistance. In this the patient may agree, or there may be divergence of opinion.

Even if all are in agreement that admission is needed, family members may still be left with a sense of failure and of guilt that they have let their relative down. It is important for their response in bereavement that families receive reassurance about the quality of their caring efforts prior to the admission, and the appropriateness of seeking inpatient care now. It is also important that there are the facilities and encouragement to enable relatives to remain with the patient as death approaches, if that would be helpful to them.

Most bereaved people do not need specific bereavement care. For a minority, perhaps up to 25 percent, adjustment can be facilitated by specialist bereavement support. This is increasingly widely available, and in Britain can be accessed through CRUSE, the local hospice, or the social service department.

Symptom control

Good symptom control at the end of life requires preparedness. It is a wholly inadequate response to the onset of a distressing symptom if control has to wait on a doctor's order or the pharmacist's acquisition of the medication required. The following categories of drug are most often required:

- opioids and other analgesics;
- sedatives;
- antiemetics;
- anticholinergic agents.

Pain relief

Pain is not generally a problem at the end of life if it has been adequately controlled previously. In patients who can no longer indicate their feelings, carers interpret nonverbal signs of distress – for instance groaning, grimacing, or restlessness. Before increasing medication, it should be checked whether there are remediable causes of discomfort, particularly a full bladder or rectum.

Opioid and nonopioid analgesia

- Many patients will require a change of route from oral to parenteral, although often only in the last 48 hours of life.
- Regular subcutaneous injections (made less uncomfortable if a plastic cannula is left in place to avoid repeated needle sticks) or, more conveniently, continuous subcutaneous infusion delivered by a portable syringe driver, are commonly used.
- Alfentanil or fentanyl are better tolerated in renal failure than morphine or diamorphine.
- Alternative routes include transdermal (fentanyl or buprenorphine), sublingual, and rectal (morphine and oxycodone). The transdermal patches are not ideal for rapidly changing pain.[216][III]
- Conversion ratios should be checked when converting from oral to other routes.

- Other analgesics: NSAIDs or paracetamol can be given by suppository (diclofenac or ketoprofen) or by continuous s.c. infusion (diclofenac or ketorolac). Via the s.c. route, NSAIDs usually require a separate pump.

Agitation

- Exclude and treat uncontrolled pain, a full bladder or rectum as a cause of agitation.
- Myoclonic jerks may be worsened by opioids, especially in the presence of phenothiazines.
- Benzodiazepines are the usual "first-line" drugs used to manage agitation (especially in the frightened, breathless patient): diazepam suppositories rectally or liquid via a gastrostomy, given p.r.n. or b.i.d.–t.i.d., or midazolam s.c.
- Midazolam combines satisfactorily with morphine or anticholinergic agents in a syringe driver. An initial midazolam dose is 2.5 mg stat or 10 mg/24 hours. Up to 120 mg per 24 hours has been given but tolerance can occur.
- Antipsychotics suitable for s.c. use are haloperidol (0.5–1.5 mg s.c. stat, 1.5–5 mg per 24 hours infusion) or the more sedating levomepromazine (6.25–25 mg stat, s.c. infusion 12.5–200 mg per 24 hours). Both have an antiemetic effect, if this is important.
- Sometimes a combination of benzodiazepine and antipsychotic is required.
- For intractable agitation, phenobarbital (100–200 mg s.c. stat, followed by s.c. infusion 600–2400 mg in a separate pump) or propofol (intravenous route only so unsuitable for many patients) may sometimes help.
- Pragmatic guidelines on the use of sedation at the end of life have been drawn up by an international panel of palliative care experts.[217][V]

Secretions

Any severely ill patient with reduced ability to cough can accumulate secretions in the upper airways, resulting in noisy breathing, which even if not distressing to the patient may well upset attending relatives. At the end of life this problem is one that is best anticipated, as it is not easy to get rid of secretions which have already gathered.

A chest infection may be present, producing purulent exudates; this cannot be prevented by anticholinergics so that it is not possible to stop rattly breathing altogether.

- Explain to the patient's family the mechanism of the noisy breathing, what is being done, and what its limitations are, and to reassure them that by this stage of their illness the dying person is unlikely to be nearly as aware of the sounds as they are themselves.

- Addition of an anticholinergic drug to an opioid and an anxiolytic in a subcutaneous infusion can help and the three widely used drugs and doses are shown below. Any of these can be given subcutaneously by syringe driver in combination with opioid and midazolam or levomepromazine.
  - hyoscine butylbromide: 20 mg stat s.c., 60–240 mg/24 hours by s.c. infusion;
  - glycopyrronium bromide: 0.2–0.4 mg stat s.c., 0.6–1.2 mg/24 hours by s.c. infusion;
  - hyoscine hydrobromide: 0.4 mg stat s.c., 1.2–2.4 mg/24 hours by s.c. infusion. (More sedating but faster onset of action and more expensive than the first two drugs.)

CONCLUSION

Care at the end of life is crucial because it provides some of the most powerful memories for those who are left behind. The future attitudes of the patient's family and friends toward severe illness in themselves or others, and toward death itself, will be molded by it. Good symptom control and good communication with the patient as long as this is possible, and with the family, are crucial not only for their direct benefit to the dying patient but also as a public health measure for the bereaved.

REFERENCES

1. Dudgeon DJ, Kristjanson L, Sloan JA, Lertzman M, Clement K. Dyspnea in cancer patients: prevalence and associated factors. *Journal of Pain and Symptom Management.* 2001; **21**: 95–102.

∗ 2. Higginson I, McCarthy M. Measuring symptoms in terminal cancer: are pain and dyspnoea controlled? *Journal of the Royal Society of Medicine.* 1989; **82**: 264–7.

3. Ganong WF. *Review of medical physiology*, 6th edn. Los Altos, CA: Lange, 1973: 500.

4. Dudgeon DJ, Lertzman M. Dyspnea in the advanced cancer patient. *Journal of Pain and Symptom Management.* 1998; **16**: 212–19.

5. O'Connell CL, Boswell WD, Duddalwar V et al. Unsuspected pulmonary emboli in cancer patients: clinical correlates and relevance. *Journal of Clinical Oncology.* 2006; **24**: 4928–32.

6. Bredin M, Corner J, Krishnasamy M et al. Multicentre randomized controlled trial of nursing intervention for breathlessness in patients with lung cancer. *British Medical Journal.* 1999; **318**: 901–04.

7. Gollins SW, Burt PA, Barber PV, Stout R. High dose rate intraluminal radiotherapy for carcinoma of the bronchus: outcome of treatment of 406 patients. *Radiotherapy and Oncology.* 1994; **33**: 31–40.

* 8. Detterbeck FC, Jones DR, Morris DE. Palliative treatment of lung cancer. In: Detterbeck FC, Rivera MP, Socinski MA, Rosenman JG (eds). *Diagnosis and treatment of lung cancer: An evidence-based guide for the practicing clinician.* 29, Philadelphia: W.B. Saunders, 2001: 419–36.

9. de Souza AC, Keal R, Hudson NM *et al.* Use of expandable wire stents for malignant airway obstruction. *Annals of Thoracic Surgery.* 1994; **57**: 1573–7.

10. Armstrong BA, Perez CA, Simpson JR, Hederman MA. Role of irradiation in the management of superior vena cava syndrome. *International Journal of Radiation Oncology, Biology, Physics.* 1987; **13**: 531–9.

11. Nicholson AA, Ettles DF, Arnold A *et al.* Treatment of malignant superior vena cava obstruction: metal stents or radiation therapy. *Journal of Vascular and Interventional Radiology.* 1997; **8**: 781–8.

12. Kee ST, Kinoshita L, Razavi MK *et al.* Superior vena cava syndrome: treatment with catheter-directed thrombolysis and endovascular stent placement. *Radiology.* 1998; **206**: 187–93.

* 13. Rowell NP. Gleeson FVSteroids, radiotherapy, chemotherapy and stents for superior vena caval obstruction in carcinoma of the bronchus: a systematic review. *Clinical oncology (Royal College of Radiologists (Great Britain)).* 2002; **14**: 338–51.

* 14. Shaw P Agarwal R. Pleurodesis for malignant pleural effusions. *Cochrane Database of Systematic Reviews.* 2004; **CD002916**.

15. Tomkowski WZ, Wisniewska J, Szturmowicz M *et al.* Evaluation of intrapericardial cisplatin administration in cases with recurrent malignant pericardial effusion and cardiac tamponade. *Supportive Care in Cancer.* 2004; **12**: 53–7. Epub 2003 Sep 23.

16. Galli M, Politi A, Pedretti F *et al.* Percutaneous balloon pericardiotomy for malignant pericardial tamponade. *Chest.* 1995; **108**: 1499–501.

17. Wilson RH, Hoseth W, Dempsey ME. Respiratory acidosis. I. Effects of decreasing respiratory minute volume with specific reference to oxygen, morphine and barbiturates. *American Journal of Medicine.* 1954; **17**: 464.

18. Walsh TD. Opiates and respiratory function in advanced cancer. *Recent Results in Cancer Research.* 1984; **89**: 115–17.

* 19. Estfan B, Mahmoud F, Shaheen P *et al.* Respiratory function during parenteral opioid titration for cancer pain. *Palliative Medicine.* 2007; **21**: 81–6.

20. Bruera E, MacEachern T, Ripamonti C, Hanson J. Subcutaneous morphine for dyspnea in cancer patients. *Annals of Internal Medicine.* 1993; **119**: 906–7.

21. Bruera E, Macmillan K, Pither J, MacDonald RN. Effects of morphine on dyspnea of terminal cancer patients. *Journal of Pain and Symptom Management.* 1990; **5**: 83–93.

22. Boyd KJ, Kelly M. Oral morphine as symptomatic treatment of dyspnoea in patients with advanced cancer. *Palliative Medicine.* 1997; **11**: 277–81.

* 23. Jennings AL, Davies AN, Higgins JP, Broadley K. Opioids for the palliation of breathlessness in terminal illness.

Cochrane Database of Systematic Reviews. 2001; **CD002066**.

24. Woodcock AA, Gross ER, Geddes DM. Drug treatment of breathlessness: contrasting effects of diazepam and promethazine in pink puffers. *British Medical Journal.* 1981; **283**: 343–6.

25. Ventafridda V, Spoldi E, De Conno F. Control of dyspnoea in advanced cancer patients. *Chest.* 1990; **6**: 1544–5.

26. Craven J, Sutherland A. Buspirone for anxiety disorders in patients with severe lung disease. *Lancet.* 1991; **338**: 249.

27. Argyropoulou P, Patakas D, Koukou A *et al.* Buspirone effect on breathlessness and exercise performance in patients with chronic obstructive pulmonary disease. *Respiration.* 1993; **60**: 216–20.

28. Bruera E, de Stoutz N, Velasco-Leiva A *et al.* Effects of oxygen on dyspnoea in hypoxaemic terminal cancer patients. *Lancet.* 1993; **342**: 13–14.

* 29. Booth S, Kelly MJ, Cox NP *et al.* Does oxygen help dyspnea in patients with cancer. *American Journal of Respiratory and Critical Care Medicine.* 1996; **153**: 1515–18.

30. Philip J, Gold M, Milner A *et al.* A randomised, double-blind, crossover trial of the effect of oxygen on dyspnea in patients with advanced cancer. *Journal of Pain and Symptom Managementment.* 2006; **32**: 541–50.

* 31. Booth S, Wade R, Johnson M *et al.* Expert Working Group of the Scientific Committee of the Association of Palliative Medicine. The use of oxygen in the palliation of breathlessness. A report of the expert working group of the Scientific Committee of the Association of Palliative Medicine. *Respiratory Medicine.* 2004; **98**: 66–77. Erratum in: Respiratory Medicine. 2004; **98**: 476.

32. Ahmedzai SH, Laude E, Robertson A *et al.* A double-blind, randomised, controlled Phase II trial of Heliox28 gas mixture in lung cancer patients with dyspnoea on exertion. *British Journal of Cancer.* 2004; **90**: 366–71.

33. Vonbank K, Ziesche R, Higenbottam TW *et al.* Controlled prospective randomised trial on the effects on pulmonary haemodynamics of the ambulatory long term use of nitric oxide and oxygen in patients with severe COPD. *Thorax.* 2003; **58**: 289–93.

* 34. Davis C. The role of nebulized drugs in palliating respiratory symptoms of malignant disease. *European Journal of Palliative Care.* 1995; **2**: 9–15.

35. Ahmedzai S, Davis C. Nebulised drugs in palliative care. *Thorax.* 1997; **52**: S75–7.

36. Wilcock A, Corcoran R, Tattersfield AE. Safety and efficacy of nebulized lignocaine in patients with cancer and breathlessness. *Palliative Medicine.* 1994; **8**: 35–8.

37. Ong KC, Kor AC, Chong WF *et al.* Effects of inhaled furosemide on exertional dyspnea in chronic obstructive pulmonary disease. *American Journal of Respiratory and Critical Care Medicine.* 2004; **169**: 1028–33. Epub 2004 Feb 20.

38. Kohara H, Ueoka H, Aoe K *et al.* Effect of nebulized furosemide in terminally ill cancer patients with dyspnea. *Journal of Pain and Symptom Management.* 2003; **26**: 962–7.

39. Kamei J. Role of opioidergic and serotonergic mechanisms in cough and antitussives. *Pulmonary Pharmacology.* 1996; **9**: 349–56.

40. Luporini G, Barni S, Marchi E, Daffonchio L. Efficacy and safety of levodropizine and dihydrocodeine on nonproductive cough in primary and metastatic lung cancer. *European Respiratory Journal.* 1998; **12**: 97–101.

✱ 41. Chung KF. Current and future prospects for drugs to suppress cough. *IDrugs.* 2003; **6**: 781–6.

✱ 42. Poole PJ, Black PN. Mucolytic agents for chronic bronchitis or chronic obstructive pulmonary disease. *Cochrane Database of Systematic Reviews.* 2006; **CD001287.**

43. Miller RR, McGregor DH. Hemorrhage from carcinoma of the lung. *Cancer.* 1980; **46**: 200–5.

44. Cooke N. Hemoptysis. In: Walsh TD (ed.). *Symptom control.* Oxford: Blackwell Scientific Publications, 1989: 235–9.

45. Slawson RG, Scott RM. Radiation therapy in bronchogenic carcinoma. *Radiology.* 1979; **132**: 175–6.

✱ 46. Rees GJ, Devrell CE, Barley VL, Newman HF. Palliative radiotherapy for lung cancer: two versus five fractions. *Clinical Oncology.* 1997; **9**: 90–5.

47. Dean A, Tuffin P. Fibrinolytic inhibitors for cancer-associated bleeding problems. *Journal of Pain and Symptom Management.* 1997; **13**: 20–4.

48. Jobbins J, Bagg J, Finlay IG *et al.* Oral and dental disease in terminally ill cancer patients. *British Medical Journal.* 1992; **304**: 1612.

49. Ganong WM. *Review of medical physiology,* 19th edn. Stamford, CT: Appleton and Lange, 1999: 467–8.

50. Ventafridda V, Ripamonti C, Sbanotto A, De Conno F. Mouth care. In: Doyle D, Hanks GWC, MacDonald N (eds). *Oxford textbook of palliative medicine,* 2nd edn. Oxford: Oxford Medical Publications, 1998: 693.

51. Grad H, Grushka M, Yanover L. Drug-induced xerostomia. *Journal of the Canadian Dental Association.* 1985; **4**: 296–300.

52. Twycross RG. *Symptom management in advanced cancer.* Oxford: Radcliffe Medical Press, 1997: 146.

53. Davies AN. A comparison of artificial saliva and chewing gum in the management of xerostomia in patients with advanced cancer. *Palliative Medicine.* 2000; **14**: 197–203.

54. Johnson JT, Ferretti GA, Nethery WJ *et al.* Oral pilocarpine for post-irradiation xerostomia in patients with head and neck cancer. *New England Journal of Medicine.* 1993; **329**: 390–5.

✱ 55. Nyarady Z, Nemeth A, Ban A *et al.* A randomized study to assess the effectiveness of orally administered pilocarpine during and after radiotherapy of head and neck cancer. *Anticancer Research.* 2006; **26**: 1557–62.

56. Finlay I. Oral symptoms and candida in the terminally ill. *British Medical Journal.* 1986; **292**: 592–3.

✱ 57. Finlay I. Oral fungal infections. *European Journal of Palliative Care.* 1995, 24.

✱ 58. Gotzsche PC, Johansen HK. Nystatin prophylaxis and treatment in severely immunodepressed patients. *Cochrane Database of Systematic Reviews.* 2002; **CD002033.**

✱ 59. Clarkson JE, Worthington HV, Eden OB. Interventions for preventing oral candidiasis for patients with cancer receiving treatment. *Cochrane Database of Systematic Reviews.* 2007; **CD003807.**

✱ 60. Worthington H, Clarkson J, Eden O. Interventions for treating oral candidiasis for patients with cancer receiving treatment. *Cochrane Database of Systematic Reviews.* 2007; **CD001972.**

61. Brion LP, Uko SE, Goldman DL. Risk of resistance associated with fluconazole prophylaxis: systematic review. *Journal of Infection.* 2007; **54**: 521–9. Epub 2007 Jan 18.

62. Epstein EB, Stevenson-Moore P, Jackson S *et al.* Prevention of oral mucositis in radiation therapy: a controlled study with benzydamine hydrochloride rinse. *International Journal of Radiation Oncology, Biology, Physics.* 1989; **16**: 1571–5.

63. Solomon MA. Oral sucralfate suspension for mucositis. *New England Journal of Medicine.* 1986; **315**: 459–60.

✱ 64. Clarkson J, Worthington H, Eden O. Interventions for treating oral mucositis for patients with cancer receiving treatment. *Cochrane Database of Systematic Reviews.* 2007; **CD001973.**

65. Sykes NP, Baines M, Carter RL. Clinical and pathological study of dysphagia conservatively managed in patients with advanced malignant disease. *Lancet.* 1988; **2**: 726–8.

66. Elrington G. The Lambert Eaton myasthenic syndrome. *Palliative Medicine.* 1992; **6**: 9–17.

67. Carter RL, Pittam MR, Tanner NSB. Pain and dysphagia in patients with squamous carcinomas of the head and neck: the role of perineural spread. *Journal of the Royal Society of Medicine.* 1982; **75**: 598–606.

68. Mattioli S. Dysphagia. In: Bianchi-Porro G, Cremer M, Kreis G *et al.* (eds). *Gastroenterology and hepatology.* London: McGraw Hill, 1999: 20.

69. Leonard R, Kendall K. *Dysphagia assessment and planning: a team approach.* San Diego, CA: Singular Publishing Group, 1997.

70. Boyle JO, Kraus DH. Functional rehabilitation. In: Close LG, Larson DL, Shah JP (eds). *Essentials of head and neck oncology.* New York, NY: Thieme, 1998: 369–78.

71. Grond S, Zech D, Diefenbach C, Bischoff A. Prevalence and pattern of symptoms in patients with cancer pain: a prospective evaluation of 1635 patients referred to a pain clinic. *Journal of Pain and Symptom Management.* 1994; **9**: 372–82.

✱ 72. Hornby PJ. Central neurocircuitry associated with emesis. *American Journal of Medicine.* 2001; **111**: 106S–12.

✱ 73. Ezzo JM, Richardson MA, Vickers A *et al.* Acupuncture-point stimulation for chemotherapy-induced nausea or vomiting. *Cochrane Database of Systematic Reviews.* 2006; **CD002285.**

✱ 74. Glare P, Pereira G, Kristjanson LJ *et al.* Systematic review of the efficacy of antiemetics in the treatment of nausea in patients with far-advanced cancer. *Supportive Care in Cancer.* 2004; **12**: 432–40. Epub 2004 Apr 24.

75. Dundee JW, Jones PO. The prevention of analgesic-induced nausea and vomiting by cyclizine. *British Journal of Clinical Practice.* 1968; **22**: 379–82.

76. Tramer MR, Reynolds DJM, Stoner NS *et al.* Efficacy of 5-HT3 receptor antagonists in radiotherapy-induced nausea and vomiting: a quantitative systematic review. *European Journal of Cancer.* 1998; **34**: 1836–44.

77. Higi M, Niederle N, Bierbaum W *et al.* Pronounced antiemetic activity of the antipsychotic drug levomepromazine (L) in patients receiving cancer chemotherapy. *Journal of Cancer Research and Clinical Oncology.* 1980; **97**: 81–6.

* 78. Twycross RG, Barkby GD, Hallwood PM. The use of low dose levomepromazine (methotrimeprazine) in the management of nausea and vomiting. *Progress in Palliative Care.* 1997; **5**: 49–53.

79. Navari RM, Einhorn LH, Passik SD *et al.* A phase II trial of olanzapine for the prevention of chemotherapy-induced nausea and vomiting: a Hoosier Oncology Group study. *Supportive Care in Cancer.* 2005; **13**: 529–34. Epub 2005 Feb 8.

* 80. de Wit R, Herrstedt J, Rapoport B *et al.* The oral NK(1) antagonist, aprepitant, given with standard antiemetics provides protection against nausea and vomiting over multiple cycles of cisplatin-based chemotherapy: a combined analysis of two randomised, placebo-controlled phase III clinical trials. *European Journal of Cancer.* 2004; **40**: 403–10.

81. Tramèr MR, Carroll D, Campbell FA *et al.* Cannabinoids for control of chemotherapy induced nausea and vomiting: quantitative systematic review. *British Medical Journal.* 2001; **323**: 16–21.

82. Hill ADK, Walsh TN, Hamilton D *et al.* Erythromycin improves emptying of the denervated stomach after oesophagectomy. *British Journal of Surgery.* 1993; **80**: 879–81.

83. Catnach SM, Fairclough PD. Erythromycin and the gut. *Gut.* 1992; **33**: 397–401.

84. Brooksbank MA, Game PA, Ashby MA. Palliative venting gastrostomy in malignant intestinal obstruction. *Palliative Medicine.* 2002; **16**: 520–6.

85. Nassif T, Prat F, Meduri B *et al.* Endoscopic palliation of malignant gastric outlet obstruction using self-expandable metallic stents: results of a multicenter study. *Endoscopy.* 2003; **35**: 483–9.

86. Kaye PM, Oliver DJ. Hypercalcaemia in advanced malignancy. *Lancet.* 1985i; **1**: 512.

87. Heath DA. Hypercalcaemia in malignancy: fluids and bisphosphonates are best when life is threatened. *British Medical Journal.* 1989; **298**: 1468–9.

88. Warrell RP. Metabolic emergencies. In: De Vita *et al.* (eds). *Cancer: principles and practice of oncology,* 4th edn. Philadelphia, PA: Lippincott, 1993: 2128.

89. Ratcliffe WA, Hutchesson ACJ, Bundred NJ, Ratcliffe JG. Role of assays for parathyroid-hormone-related-protein in investigation of hypercalcaemia. *Lancet.* 1992; **339**: 164–7.

90. Wimalawansa SJ. Significance of plasma PTH-rp in patients with hypercalcaemia of malignancy treated with bisphosphonate. *Cancer.* 1994; **73**: 2223–30.

91. Bilezikian JP. Management of acute hypercalcemia. *New England Journal of Medicine.* 1992; **326**: 1196–203.

92. Purohit OP, Radstone CR, Anthony C *et al.* A randomized double-blind comparison of intravenous pamidronate and clodronate in the hypercalcaemia of malignancy. *British Journal of Cancer.* 1995; **72**: 1289–93.

93. Plosker GL, Goa KL. Clodronate: a review of its pharmacological properties and therapeutic efficacy in resorptive bone disease. *Drugs.* 1994; **47**: 945–82.

94. Judson I, Booth F, Gore M, McElwain T. Chronic high dose pamidronate in refractory malignant hypercalcaemia. *Lancet.* 1990; **335**: 802.

* 95. Ross JR, Saunders Y, Edmonds PM *et al.* A systematic review of the role of bisphosphonates in metastatic disease. *Health Technology Assessment.* 2004; **8**: 1–176.

* 96. Bamias A, Kastritis E, Bamia C *et al.* Osteonecrosis of the jaw in cancer after treatment with bisphosphonates: incidence and risk factors. *Journal of Clinical Oncology.* 2005; **23**: 8580–7.

97. Cvitkovic F, Armand JP, Tubiana-Hulin M *et al.* Randomized, double-blind, phase II trial of gallium nitrate compared with pamidronate for acute control of cancer-related hypercalcemia. *Cancer Journal.* 2006; **12**: 47–53.

98. Mercadante S. Bowel obstruction in home care patients: 4 years' experience. *Supportive Care in Cancer.* 1995; **3**: 190–3.

99. Dvoretsky PM, Richards KA, Angel C *et al.* Survival time, causes of death, and tumor/treatment-related morbidity in 100 women with ovarian cancer. *Human Pathology.* 1988; **19**: 1273–9.

*100. Baines MJ. The pathophysiology and management of malignant intestinal obstruction. In: Doyle D, Hanks GW, MacDonald N (eds). *Oxford textbook of palliative medicine.* Oxford: Oxford University Press, 1998: 526.

101. Walsh HPJ, Schofield PF. Is laparotomy for small bowel obstruction justified in patients with previously treated malignancy? *British Journal of Surgery.* 1984; **71**: 933–5.

*102. Feuer DJ, Broadley KE, Shepherd JH, Barton DP. Surgery for the resolution of symptoms in malignant bowel obstruction in advanced gynaecological and gastrointestinal cancer. *Cochrane Database of Systematic Reviews.* 2000; CD002764.

103. Soto S, Lopez-Roses L, Gonzalez-Ramirez A *et al.* Endoscopic treatment of acute colorectal obstruction with self-expandable metallic stents: experience in a community hospital. *Surgical Endoscopy.* 2006; **20**: 1072–6. Epub 2006 May 13.

104. Ptok H, Meyer F, Marusch F *et al.* Palliative stent implantation in the treatment of malignant colorectal obstruction. *Surgical Endoscopy.* 2006; **20**: 909–14. Epub 2006 May 11.

*105. Parker MC, Baines MJ. Intestinal obstruction in patients with advanced cancer. *British Journal of Surgery.* 1996; **83**: 1–2.

*106. Baines MJ, Oliver DJ, Carter RL. Medical management of intestinal obstruction in patients with advanced malignant disease: a clinical and pathological study. *Lancet.* 1985; **2**: 990–3.

107. De Conno F, Caraceni A, Zecca E *et al.* Continuous subcutaneous infusion of hyoscine butylbromide reduces secretions in patients with gastrointestinal obstruction. *Journal of Pain and Symptom Management.* 1991; **6**: 484–6.

108. Mercadante S, Ripamonti C, Casuccio A *et al.* Comparison of octreotide and hyoscine butylbromide in controlling gastrointestinal symptoms due to malignant inoperable bowel obstruction. *Supportive Care in Cancer.* 2000; **8**: 188–91.

*109. Feuer DJ, Broadley KE. Corticosteroids for the resolution of malignant bowel obstruction in advanced gynaecological and gastrointestinal cancer. *Cochrane Database of Systematic Reviews.* 2000; **CD001219**.

110. Hardy J, Ling J, Mansi J *et al.* Pitfalls in placebo-controlled trials in palliative care: dexamethasone for the palliation of malignant bowel obstruction. *Palliative Medicine.* 1998; **12**: 437–42.

111. Sykes NP. The relationship between opioid use and laxative use in terminally ill cancer patients. *Palliative Medicine.* 1998; **12**: 375–82.

*112. Miles CL, Fellowes D, Goodman ML, Wilkinson S. Laxatives for the management of constipation in palliative care patients. *Cochrane Database of Systematic Reviews.* 2006; **CD003448**.

113. Sykes NP. A volunteer model for the comparison of laxatives in opioid-induced constipation. *Journal of Pain and Symptom Management.* 1997; **11**: 363–9.

114. Schmidt WK. Alvimopan* (ADL 8-2698) is a novel peripheral opioid antagonist. *American Journal of Surgery.* 2001; **18**: 227S–38.

115. Yuan CS, Israel RJ. Methylnaltrexone, a novel peripheral opioid receptor antagonist for the treatment of opioid side effects. *Expert Opinion on Investigational Drugs.* 2006; **15**: 541–52.

116. Culbert P, Gillett H, Ferguson A. Highly effective oral therapy (polyethylene glycol/electrolyte solution) for faecal impaction and severe constipation. *British Journal of General Practice.* 1998; **481**: 599–600.

*117. Ippoliti C. Antidiarrheal agents for the management of treatment-related diarrhea in cancer patients. *American Journal of Health-System Pharmacy.* 1998; **55**: 1573–80.

118. Twycross RG, Lack SA. Diarrhoea. In: *Control of alimentary symptoms in far advanced cancer.* London: Churchill Livingstone, 1986: 208–9.

119. de la Motte S, Bose-O'Reilly S, Heinisch M, Harrison F. Double-blind comparison of an apple pectin–chamomile extract preparation [in German]. *Arzneimittel-Forschung.* 1997; **47**: 1247–9.

120. DuPont HL, Ericsson CD, DuPont MW *et al.* A randomized, open-label comparison of non-prescription loperamide and attapulgite in the symptomatic treatment of acute diarrhea. *American Journal of Medicine.* 1990; **88**: 20S–3.

*121. Ruppin H. Review: loperamide – a potent antidiarrhoeal drug with actions along the alimentary tract. *Alimentary Pharmacology and Therapeutics.* 1987; **1**: 179–90.

122. Harris AG, O'Dorisio TM, Woltering EA *et al.* Consensus statement: octreotide dose titration in secretory diarrhea: Diarrhea Management Consensus Panel. *Digestive Diseases and Sciences.* 1995; **40**: 1464–73.

123. Billingsley KG, Alexander HR. The pathophysiology of cachexia in advanced cancer and AIDS. In: Bruera E, Higginson I (eds). *Cachexia-anorexia in cancer patients.* Oxford: Oxford University Press, 1996: 1–22.

*124. Inui A. Cancer anorexia-cachexia syndrome: current issues in research and management. *CA: A Cancer Journal for Clinicians.* 2002; **52**: 72–91.

125. Anker SD, Ponikowski P, Varney S *et al.* Wasting as independent risk factor for mortality in chronic heart failure. *Lancet.* 1997; **349**: 1050–3.

126. Bruera E, MacDonald N. Nutrition in cancer patients: an update and review of our experience. *Journal of Pain and Symptom Management.* 1988; **3**: 133–40.

127. Wigmore SJ, Plester CE, Richardson RA, Fearon KC. Changes in nutritional status associated with unresectable pancreatic cancer. *British Journal of Cancer.* 1997; **75**: 106–9.

*128. Tisdale MJ. Cachexia in cancer patients. *Nature Reviews. Cancer.* 2002; **2**: 862–71.

129. Dunlop RJ, Campbell CW. Cytokines and advanced cancer. *Journal of Pain and Symptom Management.* 2000; **20**: 214–32.

*130. Zinna EM, Yarasheski KE. Exercise treatment to counteract protein wasting of chronic diseases. *Current Opinion in Clinical Nutrition and Metabolic Care.* 2003; **6**: 87–93.

*131. Brown JK. A systematic review of the evidence on symptom management of cancer-related anorexia and cachexia. *Oncology Nursing Forum.* 2002; **29**: 517–32.

132. Hawkins C. Anorexia and anxiety in advanced malignancy: the relative problem. *Journal of Human Nutrition and Dietetics.* 2000; **13**: 113–17.

*133. Fainsinger R. Pharmacological approach to cancer anorexia and cachexia. In: Bruera E, Higginson I (eds). *Cachexia-anorexia in cancer patients.* Oxford: Oxford University Press, 1996: 128–40.

134. Twycross R. Corticosteroids in advanced cancer. *British Medical Journal.* 1992; **305**: 969–70.

*135. Berenstein EG, Ortiz Z. Megestrol acetate for the treatment of anorexia-cachexia syndrome. *Cochrane Database of Systematic Reviews.* 2005; **CD004310**.

*136. Pascual Lopez A, Roque i Figuls M, Urrutia Cuchi G *et al.* Systematic review of megestrol acetate in the treatment of anorexia-cachexia syndrome. *Journal of Pain and Symptom Management.* 2004; **27**: 360–9.

137. Mantovani G, Maccio A, Esu S *et al.* Medroxyprogesterone acetate reduces the in vitro production of cytokines and serotonin involved in anorexia/cachexia and emesis by

peripheral blood mononuclear cells of cancer patients. *European Journal of Cancer.* 1997; **33**: 602–7.

*138. Jatoi A, Windschitl HE, Loprinzi CL et al. Dronabinol versus megestrol acetate versus combination therapy for cancer-associated anorexia: a North Central Cancer Treatment Group study. *Journal of Clinical Oncology.* 2002; **20**: 567–73.

139. Cannabis-In-Cachexia-Study-Group, Strasser F, Luftner D, Possinger K et al. Comparison of orally administered cannabis extract and delta-9-tetrahydrocannabinol in treating patients with cancer-related anorexia-cachexia syndrome: a multicenter, phase III, randomized, double-blind, placebo-controlled clinical trial from the Cannabis-In-Cachexia-Study-Group. *Journal of Clinical Oncology.* 2006; **24**: 3394–400.

140. Wigmore SJ, Falconer JS, Plester CE et al. Ibuprofen reduces energy expenditure and acute-phase protein production compared with placebo in pancreatic cancer patients. *British Journal of Cancer.* 1995; **72**: 185–8.

*141. Fearon KC, Von Meyenfeldt MF, Moses AG et al. Effect of a protein and energy dense N-3 fatty acid enriched oral supplement on loss of weight and lean tissue in cancer cachexia: a randomised double blind trial. *Gut.* 2003; **52**: 1479–86.

*142. Bruera E, Strasser F, Palmer JL et al. Effect of fish oil on appetite and other symptoms in patients with advanced cancer and anorexia/cachexia: a double-blind, placebo-controlled study. *Journal of Clinical Oncology.* 2003; **21**: 129–34.

*143. Dewey A, Baughan C, Dean T et al. Eicosapentaenoic acid (EPA, an omega-3 fatty acid from fish oils) for the treatment of cancer cachexia. *Cochrane Database of Systematic Reviews.* 2007; **CD004597**.

144. Laviano A, Muscaritoli M, Cascino A et al. Branched-chain amino acids: the best compromise to achieve anabolism? *Current Opinion in Clinical Nutrition and Metabolic Care.* 2005; **8**: 408–14.

145. Lissoni P. Is there a role for melatonin in supportive care? *Supportive Care in Cancer.* 2002; **10**: 110–6. Epub 2001 Nov 13.

146. De Vriese C, Delporte C. Influence of ghrelin on food intake and energy homeostasis. *Current Opinion in Clinical Nutrition and Metabolic Care.* 2007; **10**: 615–9.

147. Asakawa A, Inui A, Inui T et al. Orexin reverses cholecystokinin-induced reduction in feeding. *Diabetes, Obesity and Metabolism.* 2002; **4**: 399–401.

*148. Yavuzsen T, Davis MP, Walsh D et al. Systematic review of the treatment of cancer-associated anorexia and weight loss. *Journal of Clinical Oncology.* 2005; **23**: 8500–11.

149. Hofman M, Ryan JL, Figueroa-Moseley CD et al. Cancer-related fatigue: the scale of the problem. *Oncologist.* 2007; **12**: 4–10.

*150. McNeely ML, Campbell KL, Rowe BH et al. Effects of exercise on breast cancer patients and survivors: a systematic review and meta-analysis. *Canadian Medical Association Journal.* 2006; **175**: 34–41.

*151. Djulbegovic B. Erythropoietin use in oncology: a summary of the evidence and practice guidelines comparing efforts of the Cochrane Review group and Blue Cross/Blue Shield to set up the ASCO/ASH guidelines. *Best Practice and Research. Clinical Haematology.* 2005; **18**: 455–66.

152. Geiser F, Hahn C, Conrad R et al. Interaction of psychological factors and the effect of epoetin-alfa treatment in cancer patients on hemoglobin and fatigue. *Supportive Care in Cancer.* 2007; **15**: 273–8. Epub 2006 Aug 25.

*153. Bruera E, Valero V, Driver L et al. Patient-controlled methylphenidate for cancer fatigue: a double-blind, randomized, placebo-controlled trial. *Journal of Clinical Oncology.* 2006; **24**: 2073–8.

*154. Badger C, Preston N, Seers K, Mortimer P. Physical therapies for reducing and controlling lymphoedema of the limbs. *Cochrane Database of Systematic Reviews.* 2004; **CD003141**.

*155. Badger C, Preston N, Seers K, Mortimer P. Benzo-pyrones for reducing and controlling lymphoedema of the limbs. *Cochrane Database of Systematic Reviews.* 2004; **CD003140**.

156. Clein LJ, Pugachev E. Reduction of edema of lower extremities by subcutaneous, controlled drainage:eight cases. *American Journal of Hospice and Palliative Care.* 2004; **21**: 228–32.

157. Twycross R, Greaves MW, Handwerker H et al. Itch: scratching more than the surface. *Q JM.* 2003; **96**: 7–26.

158. Smith EB, King CA, Baker MD. Crotamiton lotion in pruritus. *International Journal of Dermatology.* 1984; **23**: 684–5.

159. Tarng DC, Cho YL, Liu HN, Huang TP. Hemodialysis-related pruritus: a double-blind, placebo-controlled, crossover study of capsaicin 0.025% cream. *Nephron.* 1996; **72**: 617–22.

160. Monk BE. Transcutaneous electronic nerve stimulation in the treatment of generalised pruritus. *Clinical and Experimental Dermatology.* 1993; **18**: 67–8.

161. Leven A, Naysmith A, Pickens S, Pottage A. Sodium cromoglycate and Hodgkin's disease. *British Medical Journal.* 1997; **2**: 896.

162. Smith PF, Corelli RL. Doxepin in the management of pruritus associated with allergic cutaneous reactions. *Annals of Pharmacotherapy.* 1997; **31**: 633–5.

163. Zylicz Z, Smits C, Krajnik M. Paroxetine for pruritus in advanced cancer. *Journal of Pain and Symptom Management.* 1998; **16**: 121–4.

164. Davis MP, Frandsen JL, Walsh D et al. Mirtazapine for pruritus. *Journal of Pain and Symptom Management.* 2003; **25**: 288–91.

*165. Holme SA, Mills CM. Crotamiton and narrow-band UVB phototherapy: novel approaches to alleviate pruritus of breast carcinoma skin infiltration. *Journal of Pain and Symptom Management.* 2001; **22**: 803–5.

166. Seckin D, Demircay Z, Akin O. Generalized pruritus treated with narrowband UVB. *International Journal of Dermatology.* 2007; **46**: 367–70.

167. Wolfhagen FH, Sternieri E, Hop WC et al. Oral naltrexone treatment for cholestatic pruritus: a double-blind,placebo-controlled study. Gastroenterology. 1997; **113**: 1264–9.

168. Bigliardi PL, Stammer H, Jost G et al. Treatment of pruritus with topically applied opiate receptor antagonist. Journal of the American Academy of Dermatology. 2007; **56**: 979–88. Epub 2007 Feb 22.

∗169. Khurana S, Singh P. Rifampin is safe for treatment of pruritus due to chronic cholestasis: a meta-analysis of prospective randomized-controlled trials. Liver International. 2006; **26**: 943–8.

170. O'Donohue JW, Pereira SP, Ashdown AC et al. A controlled trial of ondansetron in the pruritus of cholestasis. Alimentary Pharmacology and Therapeutics. 2005; **21**: 1041–5.

171. Wikstrom B, Gellert R, Ladefoged SD et al. Kappa-opioid system in uremic pruritus: multicenter, randomized, double-blind, placebo-controlled clinical studies. Journal of the American Society of Nephrology. 2005; **16**: 3742–7. Epub 2005 Oct 26.

172. Marchi S, Cecchin E, Villalta D et al. Relief of pruritus and decreases in plasma histamine concentrations during erythropoietin therapy in patients with uremia. New England Journal of Medicine. 1992; **326**: 969–74.

173. Aymard JP, Lederlin P, Witz F et al. Cimetidine for pruritus in Hodgkin's disease. British Medical Journal. 1980; **280**: 151–2.

∗174. Borgeat A, Stirnemann HR. Ondansetron is effective to treat spinal or epidural morphine-induced pruritus. Anesthesiology. 1999; **90**: 432–6.

175. Loprinzi CL, Michalak JC, Quella SK et al. Megestrol acetate for the prevention of hot flashes. New England Journal of Medicine. 1994; **331**: 347–52.

∗176. Tsavaris N, Zinelis A, Karabelis A et al. A randomised trial of the effects of three non-steroidal anti-inflammatory agents in ameliorating cancer induced fever. Journal of Internal Medicine. 1990; **228**: 451–5.

∗177. Harrison J, Maguire P. Predictors of psychiatric morbidity in cancer patients. British Journal of Psychiatry. 1994; **165**: 593–8.

178. Lishman WA. Organic psychiatry: the psychological consequences of cerebral disorder, 3rd edn. Oxford: Blackwell Science, 1997: 744.

179. Harris EC, Barraclough BM. Suicide as an outcome for medical disorders. Medicine. 1994; **73**: 281–96.

180. Moadel AB, Ostroff JS, Schanz SP. Head and neck cancer. In: Holland JC (ed.). Psycho-oncology. New York: Oxford University Press, 1998: 314–23.

181. Spiegel D. Health caring: psychosocial support for patients with cancer. Cancer. 1994; **74**: 1453–7.

182. McDaniel JS, Musselman DL, Porter MR et al. Depression in patients with cancer. Archives of General Psychiatry. 1995; **52**: 89–99.

∗183. Endicott J. Measurement of depression in patients with cancer. Cancer. 1984; **53**: 2243–8.

∗184. Cohen-Cole SA, Brown FW, McDaniel JS. Diagnostic assessment of depression in the medically ill.

In: Stoudemire A, Fogel B (eds). Psychiatric care of the medical patient. New York: Oxford University Press, 1993: 199–212.

185. Chochinov HM, Wilson KG, Enns M, Lander S. "Are you depressed?" Screening for depression in the terminally ill. American Journal of Psychiatry. 1997; **154**: 674–6.

186. Faull CM, Johnson IS, Butler TJ. The hospital anxiety and depression (HAD) scale: its validity in patients with terminal malignant disease. Palliative Medicine. 1994; **8**: 69.

187. Urch CE, Chamberlain J, Field G. The drawback of the Hospital Anxiety and Depression Scale in the assessment of depression in hospice inpatients. Palliative Medicine. 1998; **12**: 395–6.

188. Le Fevre P, Devereux J, Smith S et al. Screening for psychiatric illness in the palliative care inpatient setting: a comparison between the Hospital Anxiety and Depression Scale and the General Health Questionnaire-12. Palliative Medicine. 1999; **13**: 399–407.

189. Porter MR, Musselman DL, McDaniel JS, Nemeroff CB. From sadness to major depression: assessment and management in patients with cancer. In: Portenoy RK, Bruera E (eds). Topics in Palliative Care. vol. 3. New York: Oxford University Press, 1998: 193.

∗190. Breitbart W, Chochinov HM, Passik S. Psychiatric aspects of palliative care. In: Doyle D, Hanks GWC, MacDonald N (eds). Oxford textbook of palliative medicine, 2nd edn. Oxford: Oxford Medical Publications, 1998: 937.

∗191. Fawzy IF, Fawzy NW, Arndt LA, Pasnau RO. Critical review of psychosocial intervention in cancer care. Archives of General Psychiatry. 1995; **52**: 100–13.

∗192. Sellick SM, Crooks DL. Depression and cancer: an appraisal of the literature for prevalence, detection, and practical guideline development for psychological interventions. Psycho-Oncology. 1999; **8**: 315–33.

∗193. Gill D, Hatcher S. Antidepressants for depression in medical illness. Cochrane Database of Systematic Reviews. 2000; **CD001312**.

∗194. Kalash GR. Psychotropic drug metabolism in the cancer patient: clinical aspects of management of potential drug interactions. Psycho-Oncology. 1998; **7**: 307–20.

∗195. Quitkin FM, Taylor BP, Kremer C. Does mirtazapine have a more rapid onset than SSRIs? Journal of Clinical Psychiatry. 2001; **62**: 358–61.

196. Roth AJ, Breitbart W. Psychiatric emergencies in terminally ill cancer patients. Haematology/Oncology Clinics of North America. 1996; **10**: 235–59.

∗197. Noyes R, Holt CS, Massie MJ. Anxiety disorders. In: Holland JC (ed.). Psycho-oncology. New York: Oxford University Press, 1998: 551.

198. Passik SD, Roth AJ. Anxiety symptoms and panic attacks preceding pancreatic cancer diagnosis. Psycho-Oncology. 1999; **8**: 268–72.

199. Lloyd-Williams M, Friedman T, Rudd N. Information needs and levels of anxiety and depression in last weeks of life. Psycho-Oncology. 1998; **7**. abstract no. 304.

*200. Twillman RK, Manetto C. Concurrent psychotherapy and pharmacotherapy in the treatment of depression and anxiety in cancer patients. *Psycho-Oncology.* 1998; **7**: 285–90.

*201. Moorey S, Greer S, Watson M *et al.* Adjuvant psychological therapy for patients with cancer: outcome at 1 year. *Psycho-Oncology.* 1994; **3**: 39–46.

202. Moorey S, Greer S, Bliss J, Law M. A comparison of adjuvant psychological therapy and supportive counselling in patients with cancer. *Psycho-Oncology.* 1998; **7**: 218–28.

203. Mannix KA, Blackburn IM, Garland A *et al.* Effectiveness of brief training in cognitive behaviour therapy techniques for palliative care practitioners. *Palliative Medicine.* 2006; **20**: 579–84.

204. Monroe B, Moorey S, Cort E *et al.* A randomised controlled trial of Cognitive Behaviour Therapy (CBT) for common mental disorders in patients with advanced disease under the care of a specialist palliative care team. Abstract: 10th Congress of the European Association for Palliative Care, Budapest, Hungary, 7–9 June 2007.

*205. Fellowes D, Barnes K, Wilkinson S. Aromatherapy and massage for symptom relief in patients with cancer. *Cochrane Database of Systematic Reviews.* 2004; **CD002287**.

*206. Jackson KC, Lipman AG. Drug therapy for anxiety in palliative care. *Cochrane Database of Systematic Reviews.* 2004; **CD004596**.

207. Gelder M, Gath D, Mayou R, Cowen P. *Oxford textbook of psychiatry*, 3rd edn. Oxford: Oxford University Press, 1996: 169.

*208. Breitbart W, Cohen CR. Delirium. In: Holland JC (ed.). *Psycho-oncology.* New York: Oxford University Press, 1998: 564.

*209. Inouye SK, Bogardus ST, Charpentier PA *et al.* A multicomponent intervention to prevent delirium in hospitalised older patients. *New England Journal of Medicine.* 1999; **340**: 669–76.

210. Jackson KC, Lipman AG. Drug therapy for delirium in terminally ill patients. *Cochrane Database of Systematic Reviews.* 2004; **CD004770**.

*211. American Psychiatric Association Practice Guidelines: practice guideline for the treatment of patients with delirium. *American Journal of Psychiatry.* 1999; **156**: 1–20.

212. McNamara P, Minton M, Twycross RG. Use of midazolam in palliative care. *Palliative Medicine.* 1991; **5**: 244–9.

213. Herth K. Fostering hope in terminally ill people. *Journal of Advanced Nursing.* 1990; **15**: 1250–9.

214. Dunlop RJ, Hockley JM, Davies RJ. Preferred versus actual place of death – a Hospital Terminal Care Support Team experience. *Palliative Medicine.* 1989; **3**: 197–201.

*215. Hinton J. Which patients with terminal cancer are admitted from home care? *Palliative Medicine.* 1994; **8**: 197–210.

*216. Portenoy RK, Southam MA, Gupta SK *et al.* Transdermal fentanyl for cancer pain. *Anesthesiology.* 1993; **78**: 36–43.

*217. de Graeff A, Dean M. Palliative sedation therapy in the last weeks of life: a literature review and recommendations for standards. *Journal of Palliative Medicine.* 2007; **10**: 67–85.

PART **IV**

CLINICAL MANAGEMENT OF PAIN IN SPECIAL SITUATIONS

25   Pediatric cancer pain   345
     John J Collins, Michael M Stevens, and Charles B Berde

26   Cancer pain in older people   359
     Margot Gosney

27   Cancer pain management in the context of substance abuse   379
     Sharon M Weinstein

28   Pain in the dying person   389
     Kate Skinner and Steven Z Pantilat

29   Pain in cancer survivors   399
     W Paul Farquhar-Smith

30   Cancer pain management in the community setting   411
     Margaret Gibbs, Vicky Robinson, Nigel Sykes, and Christine Miaskowski

25

Pediatric cancer pain

JOHN J COLLINS, MICHAEL M STEVENS, AND CHARLES B BERDE

Introduction	345	Pharmacological management of cancer pain in children	347
The etiology of tumor-related pain	345	Anesthetic approaches to pain management	354
The epidemiology of cancer pain in pediatrics	346	Terminal sedation	354
Breakthrough cancer pain in children	346	Tolerance, physical dependence, addiction	354
Nonpharmacological methods of pain control in children with cancer	346	References	355

KEY LEARNING POINTS

- Pain is a common symptom in children with cancer.
- Pediatric cancer pain management should follow the logical, simple guidelines produced by the World Health Organization in combination with knowledge of the individual child and her or his family and an open mind about individual responses to analgesics.
- Most cancer pain in children is due to treatment. Tumor-related pain occurs at diagnosis, at the time of tumor recurrence, and when tumors become

treatment resistant. Breakthrough cancer pain in children is usually of sudden onset, severe, and short-lived.
- Most cancer pain in children can be adequately treated.
- A small percentage of children develop intractable pain which is more common in children with solid tumors metastatic to the spinal cord, spinal nerve roots, or large peripheral nerves. In these circumstances, consideration for a rapid opioid dose escalation or nerve block should be given.

INTRODUCTION

The World Health Organization (WHO) developed guidelines for the global application of the principles of pain management and palliative care for children with cancer.[1, 2] The guidelines contain information on pain assessment, the administration of analgesics and adjuvant analgesics, and the application of nonpharmacologic pain interventions as applicable to children with cancer pain.[1, 2] In effect, the WHO has established the principles of pain management and palliative care as a required standard of care for all children with cancer, irrespective of geographic location.

THE ETIOLOGY OF TUMOR-RELATED PAIN

Nociceptors are nerves which receive and transmit painful stimuli. Nociceptors use a diversity of signal transduction mechanisms to detect noxious physiological stimuli, and several of these mechanisms may be involved in driving cancer pain.[3] When nociceptors are exposed to products of tumor cells, tissue injury or inflammation, their excitability is altered and this information is relayed to the spinal cord and then to higher centers in the brain.[3] Some of the mechanisms that appear to be involved in generating and maintaining cancer pain include activation of nociceptors by factors such as extracellular protons, endothelin-1, interleukins, prostaglandins, and tumor necrosis factor.[3]

THE EPIDEMIOLOGY OF CANCER PAIN IN PEDIATRICS

Pain is a common symptom experienced by children with cancer. As part of the validation study of the Memorial Symptom Assessment Scale 10–18 (MSAS 10–18),[4][V] detailed information was acquired about symptom characteristics from a heterogeneous population of children with cancer aged 10–18 years at Memorial Sloan Kettering Cancer Center, New York. The MSAS 10-18 is a 30-item multidimensional symptom assessment scale that records the prevalence and characteristics of a broad range of physical and psychological symptoms. Children were asked about their symptoms during the preceding week. Pain was the most prevalent symptom in the inpatient group (84.4 percent) and was rated as moderate to severe by 86.8 percent and highly distressing ("quite a bit to very much") by 52.8 percent of these children. Pain was experienced by 35.1 percent of the outpatient group, of whom 75 percent rated it as being moderate to severe and 26.3 percent rated distress as "quite a bit to very much."

A study of children with noncentral nervous system (CNS) malignancies at the National Cancer Institute found that 62 percent presented to their practitioners with complaints of pain prior to the diagnosis of cancer.[5] [V] Pain was present for a median of 74 days before definitive treatment was begun. The duration of pain experienced by patients with metastatic disease was not longer than that for patients without distant spread. The majority of children had resolution of pain following the initiation of therapy directed at their cancer. Children with hematological malignancy had a shorter duration of pain following the institution of cancer treatment than those with solid tumor.[5]

Children with brain tumors often present to their practitioners with either symptoms consistent with raised intracranial pressure or abnormal neurological signs.[6] A retrospective review of children with spinal cord tumors showed that most children with spinal cord tumors present with a complaint of pain.[7] Back pain is more common than abnormal neurological signs as a sign of spinal cord compression in children[8] and spinal cord compression due to metastatic disease is more likely to occur late in a child's illness.[8]

Tumor-related pain predominates at diagnosis and during the early phase of treatment for childhood cancer and may recur at the time of relapse or when tumors become resistant to treatment. As multimodality cancer treatment protocols evolve for each patient, treatment-related, rather than tumor-related, causes of pain predominate.[9] Causes of treatment-related pain include mucositis, phantom limb pain, infection, antineoplastic therapy-related pain, postoperative pain, and procedure-related pain (e.g. needle puncture, bone marrow aspiration, lumbar puncture, removal of central venous line).

Tumor-related pain frequently recurs in patients at the time of relapse and during the terminal phase of an illness. Palliative chemotherapy and radiation therapy, depending on tumor type and sensitivity, are sometimes instituted as modalities of pain control in terminal pediatric malignancy. Severe pain in terminal pediatric malignancy occurs more commonly in patients with solid tumors metastatic to spinal nerve roots, nerve plexi, large peripheral nerve, or spinal cord compression.[10]

A variety of chronic pain conditions have been encountered in young adult survivors of childhood cancer as a consequence of cancer treatment.[11] These conditions include chronic regional pain syndrome of the lower extremity, phantom limb pain, avascular necrosis of multiple joints, mechanical pain due to failure of bony union after tumor resection, and postherpetic neuralgia. A proportion of these patients require opioids for the management of their nonmalignant pain.

BREAKTHROUGH CANCER PAIN IN CHILDREN

The prevalence, characteristics, and impact of breakthrough pain in children with cancer have only recently been characterized.[12][V] Twenty-seven pediatric in- and outpatients with cancer (aged 7–18 years) who had severe pain requiring treatment with opioids and who received care in the Oncology Unit at the Children's Hospital at Westmead, Sydney, Australia participated in this study. The children responded to a structured interview designed to characterize breakthrough pain in children. Measures of pain, anxiety, and depressed mood were completed. Fifty-seven percent experienced one or more episodes of breakthrough pain during the preceding 24 hours, each episode lasted seconds to minutes, occurred three to four times per day, and most commonly was characterized as "sharp" and "shooting" by the children. Younger children (7–12 years) had a significantly higher risk of experiencing breakthrough pain compared to teenagers. Although no statistical difference could be shown between children with and without breakthrough pain in regard to anxiety and depression, children with breakthrough pain reported significantly more interpersonal problems on the Child Depression Inventory subtest. The most effective treatment of an episode of breakthrough pain was a patient-controlled analgesia (PCA) opioid bolus dose.

NONPHARMACOLOGICAL METHODS OF PAIN CONTROL IN CHILDREN WITH CANCER

Nonpharmacological methods of pain control in children include a variety of techniques categorized as physical (e.g. massage, heat and cold stimulation, electrical nerve stimulation, acupuncture), behavioral (e.g. exercise, operant conditioning, relaxation, biofeedback, modeling, desensitization, art and play therapy), or cognitive (e.g. distraction, attention, imagery, thought stopping, hypnosis, music therapy, psychotherapy), according to whether the intervention is focused on modifying an individual's sensory perception, behaviors, or thoughts and coping abilities.[13]

A quiet, calm environment conducive to reducing stress and anxiety, in a location separate from the child's room, is a nonpharmacological strategy arranged prior to performing a medical procedure in a child. Providing a combination of a description of the steps of a given procedure and of the sensations experienced is perhaps the most common intervention for the preparation of children about to undergo invasive medical procedures. Unexpected stress is more anxiety provoking than anticipated or predictable stress.[14]

The choice of which nonpharmacological method to use is based on factors such as the child's age, behavioral factors, coping ability, fear and anxiety, and the type of pain experienced.[13] Cognitive-behavioral techniques are most commonly used in the pediatric cancer patient to decrease distress and enhance a child's ability to cope with medical procedures. The decision to use a psychologic or pharmacologic approach or both depends on the knowledge of the procedure, the skill of the practitioner, the understanding of the child, and the expectations of pain and anxiety for that child undergoing that procedure.[14]

Similarly, the role of distraction techniques in reducing children's distress during procedures has been examined by several investigators and shown to be generally effective. Distraction was less effective for younger children in one study.[15] Another study enlisted the support of parents, and showed not only a reduction in the children's behavioral distress but also lowering of the parent's anxiety.[16] Several investigators have examined and shown the effectiveness of cognitive-behavioral interventions comprising of multiple components, which have included preparatory information, relaxation, imagery, positive coping statements, modeling, and/or behavioral rehearsal.[13, 17, 18] The effectiveness of hypnosis in the reduction of pain and anxiety during bone marrow aspiration and lumbar puncture in children has been confirmed by several reports.[19, 20, 21, 22][V]

PHARMACOLOGICAL MANAGEMENT OF CANCER PAIN IN CHILDREN

Analgesic studies

The need to improve pain management in children with cancer is demonstrated by data which indicate that pain is often not adequately assessed and treated effectively in this population.[23] Improvement in pain management will be dependent not only on advances in pediatric analgesic therapeutics but also on strategies to correct barriers to the adequate treatment of pain in these children. Few analgesic studies have been performed in children with cancer.

The major difficulty in performing analgesic studies in children with cancer relates to the heterogeneous nature of pain in this population. Solid tumors are less common in children than in the adult population and it is less likely that children will have chronic cancer pain due to their tumor. Children often receive therapies directed at the control of their tumors until late in the course of their illnesses. These epidemiological and treatment variables make it less likely that a subpopulation of children with cancer exists that has a chronic stable pattern of pain amenable to evaluation in an analgesic drug trial.

Most analgesic studies performed in children with cancer had small patient numbers, few were controlled studies, and only recently has self-report been used as an outcome measure for the effectiveness of analgesia. There have been no controlled clinical trials of adjuvant analgesic agents in pediatrics. Given the difficulties of performing analgesic studies in children with cancer, pediatric analgesic studies have usually been performed using a postoperative pain model. Although the pharmacokinetic and the major pharmacodynamic properties (analgesia and sedation) of most opioids have been studied in this manner in pediatrics, little information is available about oral bioavailability, potency ratios, and other pharmacodynamic properties.

Analgesics for the management of tumor or treatment-related cancer pain

Analgesics can be divided into three groups of drugs: (1) nonopioid analgesics, (2) opioid analgesics, (3) adjuvant analgesics. The prescription of these drugs for children with cancer pain is based on the WHO analgesic ladder which emphasizes pain intensity as the guide to choice of analgesic, rather than etiologic factors. In other words, the prescription of analgesics should be according to pain severity, ranging from acetaminophen and nonsteroidal anti-inflammatory drugs (NSAID) for mild pain to opioids for moderate to severe pain. The choice of analgesics is individualized to achieve an optimum balance between analgesia and side effects (see Part II, Drug therapies for cancer pain).

PARACETAMOL (ACETAMINOPHEN)

Paracetamol is one of the most commonly used non-opioid analgesics in children with cancer. It has a potential for hepatic and renal injury[24] but this is uncommon in therapeutic doses. Unlike aspirin, paracetamol does not have an association with Reye syndrome. The antipyretic action of paracetamol may be contraindicated in neutropenic patients in whom it is important to monitor fever. Pediatric dosing of paracetamol has been based on the antipyretic dose–response. Oral dosing of 15 mg/kg every four to six hours is recommended, with a maximum daily dose of 60 mg/kg/day for patients of normal or average build.

No data are available on the safety of chronic paracetamol administration in children. In Australia, New South Wales Health Policy mandates that paracetamol should not be administered to children for more than 48 hours without a medical review.[25][V] Intravenous paracetamol is available as a therapeutic analgesic option in some countries. Its use has been documented in the context of pediatric postoperative pain management[26] and practice guidelines are evolving.[27]

ACETYLSALICYLIC ACID (ASPIRIN) AND NSAIDS

Acetylsalicylic acid and NSAIDs are frequently contraindicated in pediatric oncology patients who are often at risk from bleeding due to thrombocytopenia. In a comparative study of acetylsalicylic acid and ibuprofen in children with juvenile rheumatoid arthritis, the drugs were equally efficacious, but the drop-out rate caused by side effects was significantly higher in the aspirin group.

Choline magnesium trisalicylate (Trilisate®) has been widely recommended because of reports in adults of minimal effects on platelet function *in vitro* and experimental studies showing minimal gastric irritation in rats, in contrast to acetylsalicylic acid.[28] The studies do not include medically frail patients with thrombocytopenia or other morbidities.

The cyclooxygenase-2 (COX-2) inhibitors target a specific isoenzyme involved in the generation of prostanoids, which contribute to pain and inflammation. Whilst celecoxib and meloxicam have undergone some limited trials in children with rheumatoid arthritis and postoperative pain,[29, 30] their role in pediatric pain management is unclear. Rofecoxib was removed from the international market because of increased risk of cardiovascular events in adults.[31]

CODEINE

In pediatrics, codeine is commonly administered via the oral route and often administered in combination with paracetamol. It is prescribed for mild to moderate pain. Codeine is typically administered in pediatrics in oral doses of 0.5–1 mg/kg every four hours for children over six months of age. Pharmacogenetic studies have demonstrated that 4–14 percent of the population lack the hepatic enzyme responsible for the conversion of codeine to morphine. A pediatric study has shown that 35 percent of children showed inadequate conversion of codeine to morphine.[32] The prescription of codeine as an analgesic in pediatrics is declining.

TRAMADOL

Tramadol may be a useful analgesic for the management of moderate cancer pain and is thought to cause less respiratory depression than morphine. Few data exist on the safety and efficacy of tramadol in patients less than 16 years of age.

OXYCODONE

Oxycodone is used for moderate to severe pain in children with cancer. Oxycodone may be available only as an oral preparation in combination with paracetamol in some countries. The total daily paracetamol dose may be the limiting factor in dose escalation of these products. Oxycodone has a higher clearance value and a shorter elimination half-life ($t_{1/2}$) in children aged 2–20 years than adults.[33, 34] Oxycodone is available as a long-acting preparation in some countries.

MORPHINE

Morphine is one of the most widely used opioids for moderate to severe cancer pain in children. Evolving data indicate that a variable human analgesic response to morphine may be explained, in part, by genetic variation and different μ-opioid receptor neurotransmitter responses.[35]

The binding of morphine to plasma protein is age-dependent. In premature infants, less than 20 percent is bound to plasma proteins.[36, 37] Within the neonatal period for term infants, the volume of distribution is linearly related to age and body surface area,[36, 37, 38] but after the neonatal period the values are approximately the same as adults.[39, 40]

Morphine clearance is delayed in the first one to three months of life. The half-life of morphine ($t_{1/2}$) changes from values of 10–20 hours in preterm infants to values of one to two hours in preschool children.[39, 40] Therefore, starting doses in very young infants should be reduced to approximately 25–30 percent on a per kilogram basis relative to dosing recommended for older children.

Following oral dosing, morphine has a significant first pass metabolism in the liver. An oral to parenteral potency ratio of approximately 3:1 is commonly encountered during chronic administration.[41] A typical starting dose for immediate release oral morphine in opioid-naive children is 0.3 mg/kg every four hours. Typical starting intravenous infusion rates are 0.02–0.03 mg/kg per hour beyond the first three months of life, and 0.015 mg/kg per hour in younger infants. Sustained release preparations of morphine are available for children and permit oral dosing at intervals of either twice or three times daily. Crushing sustained released tablets produces immediate release of morphine. This limits their use in children who must chew tablets.

HYDROMORPHONE

Hydromorphone is an alternative opioid when the dose escalation of morphine is limited by side effects. Hydromorphone is available for oral, intravenous, subcutaneous, epidural, and intrathecal administration. Adult studies indicate that intravenous hydromorphone is five to eight times as potent as morphine. A double-blinded randomized cross-over comparison of morphine to hydromorphone using PCA in children and adolescents with mucositis following bone marrow transplantation showed that hydromorphone was well tolerated and had a potency ratio of approximately 6:1 relative to morphine in this setting.[42][II] Because of its high potency and aqueous solubility, hydromorphone is convenient for subcutaneous infusion. Little is known about the pharmacokinetics of hydromorphone in infants.

FENTANYL

Fentanyl is a synthetic opioid which is approximately 50–100 times more potent than morphine during acute intravenous administration. The half-life of this opioid is prolonged in preterm infants undergoing cardiac surgery,[43] but comparable values with those of adults are reached within the first months of life.[44, 45, 46, 47] The clearance of fentanyl appears to be higher in infants and young children than in adults.[46, 47] Fentanyl may also be used for continuous infusion for selected patients with dose-limiting side effects from morphine. Rapid administration of high doses of intravenous (i.v.) fentanyl may result in chest wall rigidity and severe ventilatory difficulty.

Oral transmucosal fentanyl produces a rapid onset of effect and escapes first-pass hepatic clearance. Schechter et al.[48][V] described the use of oral transmucosal fentanyl for sedation/analgesia during bone marrow biopsy/aspiration and lumbar puncture. This formulation was safe and effective, although the frequency of vomiting may be a limiting factor in its tolerability. Its use for breakthrough cancer pain in adults has been described.[49]

In a small study utilizing a clinical protocol, the utility, feasibility, and tolerability of transdermal fentanyl was demonstrated in children with cancer pain.[50][V] The mean clearance and volume of distribution of transdermal fentanyl are the same for both adults and children, but the variability is higher in adults.[50] A subsequent larger study confirmed the effectiveness of this analgesic for children.[51][V]

PETHIDINE (MEPERIDINE)

Pethidine has been used for procedural and postoperative pain in children. It is a short half-life synthetic opioid. Neonates have a slower elimination of pethidine than children and young infants.[52, 53, 54, 55, 56] Normeperidine is the major metabolite of pethidine. This can cause CNS excitatory effects, including tremors and convulsions,[57] particularly in patients with impaired renal clearance. Pethidine is therefore not generally recommended for children with chronic pain, but may be an acceptable alternative to fentanyl for short painful procedures.

METHADONE

Methadone is a synthetic opioid which has a long and variable half-life. Following single parenteral doses, its potency is similar to that of morphine. In children receiving postoperative analgesia, methadone produced more prolonged analgesia than morphine.[58, 59] Due to its prolonged half-life, methadone has a risk of delayed sedation and over-dosage occurring several days after initiating treatment.

The oral:parenteral potency ratio is approximately 2:1. Frequent patient assessment is the key to safe and effective use of methadone. If a patient becomes comfortable after initial doses, the dose should be reduced or the interval extended to reduce the likelihood of subsequent somnolence. If a patient becomes oversedated early in dose escalation, it is recommended to stop dosing, not just reduce the dose, and to observe the patient until there is increased alertness. Although "as needed" dosing is discouraged for most patients with cancer pain, some clinicians find this approach a useful way to establish a dosing schedule for methadone.[58, 59] Methadone remains a long-acting agent when administered either as an elixir or as crushed tablets.

Routes and methods of analgesic administration

ORAL

Oral administration of analgesics is the first choice for the majority of children and young patients. Analgesics should generally be administered to children by the simplest, safest, most effective, and least painful route. Oral dosing is generally predictable, inexpensive, and does not require invasive procedures or technologies.

TOPICAL

The eutectic mixture of local anesthetics (EMLA®) is a topical preparation which provides local anesthesia to the skin, dermis, and subcutaneous tissues if applied under an occlusive dressing for at least one hour. It has been shown to be useful for procedural pain, including lumbar puncture[60] and central venous port access[61] in children with cancer. Preliminary studies of topical amethocaine for percutaneous analgesia prior to venous cannulation in children have demonstrated promising safety and efficacy data.[62] The newer generation of topical local anesthetics promise a quicker onset of action and are currently being reviewed.[63]

INTRAVENOUS

Intravenous administration has the advantage of rapid onset of analgesia, easier opioid dose titration, bio-availability, and continuous effect when infusions are used. The intravenous route of administration is often an option in children with cancer since many have indwelling intravenous access.

SUBCUTANEOUS

The subcutaneous route is an alternative route of administration for children with either no or poor intravenous access. Solutions are generally concentrated so that infusion rates do not exceed 1–3 mL/hour.[64] An application of a topical local anestheic agent is recommended prior to the placement of a subcutaneous needle. A small catheter or butterfly needle (27 gauge) may be placed under the skin of the thorax, abdomen, or thigh and sites changed approximately every three days.

INTRAMUSCULAR

Intramuscular administration is painful and may lead to the underreporting of pain. This route of administration does not permit easy dose titration or infusion and should be avoided.

RECTAL

Rectal administration is discouraged in the pediatric cancer population because of concern regarding infection and because of the great variability of rectal absorption of morphine.[65] Nevertheless, this route of administration may be useful in the home care of the dying child when no other route is available. Slow release morphine tablets can be administered via the rectum.

PCA

PCA is a method of opioid administration that permits the patient to self-administer small bolus doses of opioid within set time limits. PCA caters to an individual's variation in pharmacokinetics, pharmacodynamics, and pain intensity. PCA allows appropriate children to have control over their analgesia and allows them to choose a balance between the benefits of analgesia versus the side effects of opioids. In patients with severe mucositis, for example, opioid dosing can be timed with routine mouth care and other causes of incidental mouth pain. In postoperative use, PCA is widely used successfully by children aged six to seven and above.

PCA has been used successfully for the management of prolonged oropharyngeal mucositis pain following bone marrow transplantation in children and adolescents.[42, 66, 67][II] A controlled comparison of staff-controlled continuous infusion (CI) of morphine and PCA in adolescents with severe oropharyngeal mucositis found that the PCA group had equivalent analgesia but less sedation and less difficulty concentrating.[66][II]

Opioid dose schedules

Unless a child's episodes of pain are truly incidental and unpredictable, analgesics should be administered at regular times to prevent breakthrough pain. "Rescues" are supplemental "as needed" doses of opioid incorporated into the analgesic regimen to allow a patient to have additional analgesia should breakthrough pain occur. Rescue doses of opioid may be calculated as approximately 5–10 percent of the total daily opioid requirement and may be administered every hour.[41]

Opioid dose escalation may be required after opioid administration begins and periodically thereafter. The size of a dose increment may be calculated as follows.

- If greater than approximately six "rescue" doses of opioid are given in a 24-hour period, then the total daily opioid dose should be increased by the total of opioid given as "rescue" medication. For example, the hourly average of the total daily rescue opioid should be added to the baseline opioid infusion. An alternative to this method would be to increase the baseline infusion by 50 percent.[41]
- "Rescue" doses are kept as a proportion of the baseline opioid dose. This dose can be 5–10 percent of the total daily dose.[41] An alternative guideline for opioid infusions is between 50 and 200 percent of the hourly basal infusion rate (see **Box 25.1**).[41]

Opioid switching

The usual indication for switching to an alternative opioid is dose-limiting toxicity. This approach is recommended by the observation that a switch from one opioid to another is often accompanied by change in the balance between analgesia and side effects.[68] A favorable change in opioid analgesia to side effect profile may be experienced if there is less cross-tolerance at the opioid receptors mediating analgesia than at those mediating adverse effects.[69]

Following a prolonged period of regular dosing with one opioid, equivalent analgesia may be attained with a dose of a second opioid that is smaller than that calculated from an equianalgesic table, as shown in **Table 25.1**.[69] An opioid switch is usually accompanied by a reduction in the equianalgesic dose (approximately 50

Box 25.1 Case examples for opioid dose calculation and dose escalation

A four-year-old girl, weighing 20 kg has severe continuous pain related to metastatic neuroblastoma. What is an appropriate opioid dose schedule?

Due to the continuous nature of this patient's pain, an appropriate schedule would be to provide either regular dosing via the oral route, or, alternatively, a continuous intravenous infusion should be started. In addition, to account for additional or "breakthrough" pain, the regime should have supplementary opioid to be given when required.

OPTIONS

The oral dose of morphine is 0.3 mg/kg every four hours (i.e. 6 mg po every four hours) using immediate release morphine (IRM). An appropriate "breakthrough" dose would be 3.5 mg IRM every hour (i.e. the total daily opioid dose is 36 mg, 10 percent of this dose is approximately 3.5 mg morphine). If this regime seems satisfactory with time, it may be reasonable to switch from IRM to slow release morphine (SRM). An appropriate regime would be 15 mg SRM twice a day. The "breakthrough" IRM dose remains the same.

As an alternative, a loading dose of intravenous morphine (0.1 mg/kg) could be given, followed by starting a morphine infusion of 0.02 mg/kg per hour (= 0.4 mg per hour morphine). An appropriate "breakthrough" dose could be 0.4 mg i.v. every hour.

During the next 24 hours, six additional "breakthrough" doses of oral morphine were given. How should the opioid regime be changed?

An additional 21 mg of oral morphine was given as "breakthrough" dosing (i.e. 6 × 3.5 mg = 21 mg). This dose could be divided and be given as additional SRM. An appropriate new regime could be 25 mg SRM twice a day. The total daily dose of morphine is now 50 mg, an appropriate "breakthrough" dose of IRM would now be 5 mg.

used short half-life opioid. A protocol for methadone dose conversion and titration has been documented for adults.[70] The basis of this dose reduction is because of the d-methadone effect as an antagonist at the N-methyl-D-aspartic acid (NMDA) receptor.

A retrospective study was performed to determine the therapeutic value of opioid rotation in a large pediatric oncology center.[71][V] Fourteen percent of children receiving opioid therapy had 30 opioid rotations. Mucositis was the major cause of pain. The opioid was rotated either for excessive side effects with adequate analgesia (70 percent), excessive side effects with inadequate analgesia (16.7 percent), or tolerance (6.7 percent). Adverse opioid effects were resolved in 90 percent of cases, all failures occurred when morphine was rotated to fentanyl. There was no significant loss of pain control or increase in mean morphine equivalent dose requirements. Opioid rotation had a positive impact on managing dose-limiting side effects of, or tolerance to, opioid therapy during cancer pain treatment in children. This was accomplished without loss of pain control or having to significantly increase the dose of opioid therapy.[71]

Opioid side effects

All opioids can potentially cause the same constellation of side effects. Children do not necessarily report side effects voluntarily (e.g. constipation, pruritus, dreams) and should be asked specifically about these problems. An assessment of opioid side effects is included in an assessment of analgesic effectiveness. If opioid side effects limit opioid dose escalation, then consideration should be given to an opioid switch. Tolerance to some opioid side effects (e.g. sedation, nausea and vomiting, pruritus) often develops within the first week of starting opioids. Children do not develop tolerance to constipation as an opioid side effect and concurrent treatment with laxatives should always be considered (see **Table 25.2**).

Adjuvant analgesics

Adjuvant analgesics are a heterogeneous group of drugs that have a primary indication other than pain but are analgesic in some painful conditions.[72] Adjuvant analgesics are commonly, but not always, prescribed with primary analgesic drugs. Common classes of these agents include antidepressants, anticonvulsants, neuroleptics, psychostimulants, antihistamines, corticosteroids, and centrally acting skeletal muscle relaxants.

ANTIDEPRESSANTS

Data from adult studies have guided the use of antidepressants as adjuvant analgesics in pediatrics. Tricyclic antidepressants have been used for a variety of pain conditions in adults, including postherpetic neuralgia,[73]

percent for short half-life opioids). In contrast to short half-life opioids, the doses of methadone required for equivalent analgesia after switching may be of the order of 10–20 percent of the equianalgesic dose of the previously

Table 25.1 Opioid analgesic initial dosage guidelines.

Drug	Equianalgesic doses		Usual starting i.v. or s.c. doses and intervals		Parenteral/oral dose ratio	Usual starting oral doses and intervals	
	Parenteral	Oral	Child <50 kg	Child >50 kg		Child <50 kg	Child >50 kg
Codeine	120 mg	200 mg	NR	NR	1:2	0.5–1.0 mg/kg q 3–4	30–60 mg q 3–4
Morphine	10 mg	30 mg (chronic)	Bolus: 0.1 mg/kg q 2–4 h Infusion 0.03 mg/kg/h	Bolus 5–8 mg q 2–4 h Infusion 1 mg/h	1:3 (chronic) 1:6 (single dose)	Immediate release: 0.3 mg/kg q 3–4 h Sustained release: 20–35 kg: 10–15 mg q 8–12 h 35–50 kg: 15–30 mg q 8–12 h	Immediate release: 15–20 mg q 3–4 h Sustained release: 30–45 mg q 8–12 h
Oxycodone	NA	15 mg	NA	NA	NA	0.1–0.2 mg/kg q 3–3 h	5–10 mg q 3–4 h
Methadone[a]	10 mg	10 mg	0.1 mg/kg q 4–8 h	1:2	1:1.5–1:2	0.15–0.2 mg/kg q 4–8 h	7–10 mg q 4–8 h
Fentanyl	100 µg (0.1 mg)	NA	Bolus: 0.5–1.0 µg/kg q 1–2 h Infusion: 0.5–2.0 µg/kg/h	Bolus: 25–50 µg q 1–2 h Infusion 25–100 µg/h	NA	NA	NA
Hydromorphone	1.5–2.0 mg	6–8 mg	Bolus: 0.02 mg q 2–4 h Infusion: 0.06 mg/kg/h	Bolus: 1 mg q 2–4 h Infusion: 0.3 mg/h	1:4	0.04–0.09 mg/kg q 3–4 h	2–4 mg q 3–4 h
Meperidine[b] (pethidine)	75–100 mg	300 mg	Bolus: 0.8–1.0 mg/kg q 2–3 h	Bolus: 50–75 mg q 2–3 h	1:4	2–3 mg/kg q 3–4 h	100–150 mg q 3–4 h

[a]Methadone requires additional vigilance, because it can accumulate and produce delayed sedation. If sedation occurs, doses should be withheld until sedation resolves. Thereafter, doses should be substantially reduced or the dosing interval should be extended to 8–12 hours (or both).

[b]Meperidine should be generally avoided if other opioids are available, especially with chronic use, because its metabolite can cause seizures.

NA, not available; NR, not recommended.

Note: Doses refer to patients older than six months. In infants younger than six months, initial doses per kilogram should begin at approximately 25 percent of the doses per kilogram recommended here. All doses are approximate and should be adjusted according to clinical circumstances. Reprinted from Berde CB, Billett AL, Collins JJ. Symptom management in supportive care. In: Pizzo PA, Poplack DG (eds). *Principles and practice of pediatric oncology*, 5th edn. 2006, with permission from Lippincott Williams and Wilkins.

Table 25.2 Management of opioid side effects.

Side effect	Treatment
Constipation	1. Regular use of stimulant and stool softener laxatives (fiber, fruit juices are often insufficient)
	2. Ensure adequate water intake
Sedation	1. If analgesia is adequate, try dose reduction
	2. Unless contraindicated, add nonsedating analgesics, such as acetaminophen or NSAIDs, and reduce opioid dosing as tolerated
	3. If sedation persists, try methylphenidate or dextroamphetamine 0.05–0.2 mg/kg po b.i.d. in early am and midday
	4. Consider an opioid switch
Nausea	1. Exclude disease processes (e.g. bowel obstruction, increased intracranial pressure)
	2. Antiemetics (phenothiazines, ondansetron, hydroxyzine)
	3. Consider an opioid switch
Urinary retention	1. Exclude disease processes (e.g. bladder neck obstruction by tumor, impending cord compression, hypovolemia, renal failure, etc.)
	2. Avoid other drugs with anticholinergic effects (e.g. tricyclics, antihistamines)
	3. Consider short-term use of bethanechol or Crede maneuver
	4. Consider short-term catheterization
	5. Consider opioid dose reduction if analgesia adequate or an opioid switch if analgesia inadequate
Pruritus	1. Exclude other causes (e.g. drug allergy, cholestasis)
	2. Antihistamines (e.g. diphenhydramine hydroxyzine)
	3. Consider an opioid dose reduction if analgesia adequate, or an opioid switch. Fentanyl causes less histamine release
Respiratory depression:	
Mild–moderate	1. Awaken, encourage to breathe
	2. Apply oxygen
	3. Withhold opioid dosing until breathing improves, reduce subsequent dosing by at least 25%
Severe	1. Awaken if possible, apply oxygen, assist respiration by bag and mask as needed
	2. Titrate small doses of naloxone (0.02 mg/kg increments as needed), stop when respiratory rate increases to 8–10/min in older children or 12–16/min in infants, do not try to awaken fully with naloxone
	∗∗Do not give a bolus dose of naloxone as severe pain and symptoms of opioid withdrawal may ensue∗∗
	3. Consider a low-dose naloxone infusion or repeated incremental dosing
	4. Consider short-term intubation in occasional cases where risk of aspiration is high
Dysphoria/confusion/ hallucinations	1. Exclude other pathology as a cause for these symptoms before attributing them to opioids
	2. When other causes excluded, change to another opioid
	3. Consider adding a neuroleptic such as haloperidol (0.01–0.1 mg/kg po/i.v. every 8 hours to a maximum dose of 30 mg/day)
Myoclonus	1. Usually seen in the setting of high-dose opioids, or alternatively, rapid dose escalation
	2. No treatment may be warranted, if this is infrequent and not distressing to the child
	3. Consider an opioid switch or treat with clonezepam (0.01 mg/kg po every 12 hours to a maximum dose of 0.5 mg/dose) or a parenteral benzodiazepine (e.g. diazepam) if the oral route is not tolerated

Reprinted from Berde CB, Billett AL, Collins JJ. Symptom management in supportive care. In: Pizzo PA, Poplack DG (eds). *Principles and Practice of Pediatric Oncology*, 5th edn. 2006, with permission from Lippincott Williams and Wilkins.

[II] diabetic neuropathy,[74][II] tension headache,[75] migraine headache,[76] rheumatoid arthritis,[77] chronic low back pain,[78] and cancer pain.[79] Antidepressants are effective in relieving neuropathic pain. With very similar results for anticonvulsants it is still unclear which drug class should be the first choice.[80]

Baseline hematology and biochemistry tests (including liver function tests) and an electrocardiogram (ECG) to exclude Wolff–Parkinson–White syndrome or other cardiac conduction defects have been recommended prior to starting treatment with tricyclic antidepressants.[81] The

measurement of antidepressant plasma concentration allows confirmation of compliance and ensures that optimization of dosage has occurred before discontinuing. An ECG is recommended periodically during long-term use, or if standard milligrams per kilogram dosages are exceeded.[82]

PSYCHOSTIMULANTS

Dextroamphetamine potentiates opioid analgesia in postoperative adult patients[83] and methylphenidate counteracts opioid-induced sedation[84] and cognitive dysfunction[85] in advanced cancer patients. Psychostimulants may allow dose escalation of opioids in patients who have somnolence as a dose-limiting side effect.[72] The potential side effects of methylphenidate include anorexia, insomnia, and dysphoria. The use of dexamfetamine (dextroamphetamine) and methylphenidate was reported in a retrospective survey of 11 children receiving opioids for a variety of indications, including cancer pain.[86] Somnolence was reduced in these patients without significant adverse side effects.

CORTICOSTEROIDS

Corticosteroids may produce analgesia by a variety of mechanisms, including anti-inflammatory effects, reduction of tumor edema, and, potentially by a reduction of spontaneous discharge in injured nerves.[87] Dexamethasone tends to be used most frequently because of its high potency, longer duration of action, and minimal mineralocorticoid effect. Corticosteroids may have a role in bone pain due to metastatic bone disease,[88] cerebral edema due to either primary or metastatic tumor,[89] or epidural spinal cord compression.[90]

ANTICONVULSANTS

The mechanism of action of anticonvulsants in controlling lancinating pain is not known but is probably related to reducing paroxysmal discharges of central and peripheral neurons. Anticonvulsants are effective in relieving neuropathic pain. With very similar results for antidepressants, it is still unclear which drug class should be the first choice.[80] The use of phenytoin, carbamazepine, and valproate may be problematic in the pediatric cancer population due to their potential adverse effects on the hematological profile. Gabapentin is well tolerated and appears to have a benign efficacy to toxicity ratio in children[91] and may be useful for the treatment of neuropathic pain.

RADIONUCLIDES

The use of other radionuclides for painful osseous metastases has been reported in the adult literature.[92] One pediatric case report indicates the potential role of [131]iodine-metaiodobenylguanidine ([131I]MIBG) for painful metastatic bone disease due to neuroblastoma.[93] The side effects of [131I]MIBG were thrombocytopenia and cystitis.

NEUROLEPTICS

Methotrimeprazine, a phenothiazine, has been reported as being analgesic in the setting of adult cancer pain.[94]

Methotrimeprazine is not considered to be a substitute for opioid analgesia. The mechanism by which methotrimeprazine produces analgesia and its role as an adjuvant agent in pediatric cancer pain is unclear. It may be useful as an adjuvant analgesic in a patient with disseminated cancer who experiences pain associated with anxiety, restlessness, or nausea.[72]

ANESTHETIC APPROACHES TO PAIN MANAGEMENT

The use of epidural or subarachnoid infusion in children for cancer pain management is rare, since the majority of pediatric cancer pain is well managed by the methods outlined above.[95] Frequently, by the time these modalities of pain control are considered, relative or absolute contraindications to their use have occurred (e.g. infection or thrombocytopenia, etc.). Anesthetic approaches are usually confined to patients who have pain not responsive to the more common methods of pain control. Anesthetic approaches are more likely to be successful for patients with their most severe pain in a specific region of the body below the neck. Specialists with experience in pediatric regional anesthesia and cancer pain management should be consulted if anesthetic techniques are being considered.[11]

TERMINAL SEDATION

The use of sedation to reduce conscious awareness in the setting of intractable symptom management is rare in pediatrics.[10] Guidelines for the evaluation and treatment of patients with intractable symptoms has been described previously.[96] There is no consensus regarding best practice for sedative prescription in this setting, which should be only considered in the setting of intractable pain or other symptom management. The prescription of terminal sedation should only be made by senior clinicains highly skilled in the symptom management of children.

Although the NMDA antagonist ketamine is commonly administered as a sedative or anesthetic agent, it has been used in a lower dose range as an analgesic for patients with refractory pain. Infusions in a dose range up to 0.2 mg/kg per hour can provide helpful analgesia and generally do not produce dissociation or unconsciousness.

TOLERANCE, PHYSICAL DEPENDENCE, ADDICTION

Analgesic tolerance refers to the progressive decline in potency of an opioid with continued use, so that increasingly higher doses are required to achieve the same analgesic effect. Patients and parents are often reluctant to increase dosing because of a fear that tolerance will make opioids ineffective at a later date. Parents should be reassured that tolerance in the majority of cases can be managed by simple dose escalation, use of adjunctive medications, or perhaps by opioid switching in the setting of dose-limiting side effects. Clinically relevant pharmacological tolerance is not usually an issue in cancer pain management.

There are some data to suggest that younger patients may be more prone to develop analgesic tolerance. This has been verified in rat studies, indicating that morphine tolerance occurs in younger rats. The notion has been verified in adult studies, indicating that age is an important variable in opioid dose escalation.[97, 98]

Physical dependence is a physiologic state induced after dose reduction or discontinuation of an opioid, or administration of an opioid antagonist. Initial manifestations of withdrawal include yawning, diaphoresis, lacrimation, coryza, and tachycardia. Patients with cancer who have received opioids over a long period of time and in whom it is appropriate to either stop or reduce opioids, should have the opioid dose reduced slowly.

Addiction is a psychological and behavioral syndrome characterized by drug craving and aberrant drug use. Some parents may fear that an exposure to opioids will result in their child subsequently becoming a drug addict. The incidence of opioid addiction was examined prospectively in 12,000 hospitalized adult patients who received at least one dose of a strong opioid.[99] There were only four documented cases of subsequent addiction in patients without a prior history of drug abuse. These data suggest that iatrogenic opioid addiction is an exceedingly uncommon problem, an observation consistent with a large worldwide experience with opioid treatment of cancer pain.

REFERENCES

1. McGrath PA. Development of the World Health Organization Guidelines on cancer pain relief and palliative care in children. *Journal of Pain and Symptom Management.* 1996; **12**: 87–92.

* 2. World Health Organization. *Cancer pain relief and palliative care in children.* Geneva: WHO, 1998.

3. Mantyh PW. Cancer pain: causes, consequences and therapeutic opportunities. In: McMahon SB, Koltzenburg M (eds). *Wall and Melzack's textbook of pain.* London: Elsevier Churchill Livingstone, 2006: 1087–97.

* 4. Collins JJ, Byrnes ME, Dunkel I *et al.* The Memorial Symptom Assessment Scale (MSAS): validation study in children aged 10–18. *Journal of Pain and Symptom Management.* 2000; **19**: 363–7.

* 5. Miser AW, McCalla J, Dothage P *et al.* Pain as a presenting symptom in children and young adults with newly diagnosed malignancy. *Pain.* 1987; **29**: 363–77.

6. Blaney SM, Kun LE, Hunter J *et al.* Tumors of the central nervous system. In: Pizzo PA, Poplack DG (eds). *Principles and practice of pediatric oncology,* 5th edn. Philadelphia: Lippincott Williams and Wilkins, 2006: 786–864.

7. Hahn YS, McLone DG. Pain in children with spinal cord tumors. *Child's Brain.* 1984; **11**: 36–46.

8. Lewis D, Packer R, Raney B *et al.* Incidence, presentation, and outcome of spinal cord disease in children with systemic cancer. *Pediatrics.* 1986; **78**: 438–43.

9. Miser AW, Dothage P, Wesley RA *et al.* The prevalence of pain in a pediatric and young adult population. *Pain.* 1987; **29**: 265–6.

* 10. Collins JJ, Grier HE, Kinney HC, Berde CB. Control of severe pain in terminal pediatric malignancy. *Journal of Pediatrics.* 1995; **126**: 653–7.

11. Berde CB, Billett A, Collins JJ. Symptom management in supportive care. In: Pizzo PA, Poplack DG (eds). *Principles and practice of pediatric oncology,* 5th edn. Philadelphia: Lippincott Williams and Wilkins, 2006: 1348–79.

12. Friedrichsdorf S, Finney D, Bergin M *et al.* Breakthrough pain in children with cancer. *Journal of Pain and Symptom Management.* 2007; **34**: 209–16.

13. McGrath PA, DeVeber LL. The management of acute pain evoked by medical procedures in children with cancer. *Journal of Pain and Symptom Management.* 1986; **1**: 145–50.

14. Zeltzer L, Jay S, Fisher D. The management of pain associated with pediatric procedures. In: Schechter NL (ed.). *The pediatric clinics of North America.* Philadelphia: W.B. Saunder Company, 1989: 914–64.

15. Kuttner L, Bowman M, Teasdale M. Psychological treatment of distress, pain and anxiety for children with cancer. *Journal of Developmental and Behavioral Pediatrics.* 1988; **9**: 374–81.

16. Manne SL, Redd WH, Jacobsen P *et al.* Behavioral intervention to reduce child and parent distress during venipuncture. *Journal of Consulting and Clinical Psychology.* 1990; **58**: 565–72.

17. Manne SL, Bakeman R, Jacobsen P *et al.* Adult and child interaction during invasive medical procedures: sequential analysis. *Health Psychology.* 1992; **11**: 241–9.

18. Jay SM, Elliott C, Ozolins M *et al.* Behavioral management of children's distress during painful medical procedures. *Behaviour Research and Therapy.* 1985; **5**: 513–20.

19. Katz E, Kellerman J, Ellenberg L. Hypnosis in the reduction of acute pain and distress in children with cancer. *Journal of Pediatric Psychology.* 1987; **12**: 379–94.

20. Hilgard J, LeBaron S. Relief of anxiety and pain in children and adolescents with cancer: quantitative measures and clinical observations. *International Journal of Clinical and Experimental Hypnosis.* 1982; **30**: 417–42.

21. Kellerman J, Zeltzer L, Ellenberg L, Dash J. Adolescents with cancer: hypnosis for the reduction of the acute pain and anxiety associated with medical procedures. *Journal of Adolescent Health Care.* 1983; **4**: 85–90.

22. Zeltzer L, LeBaron S. Hypnosis and nonhypnotic techniques for reduction of pain and anxiety during painful

procedures in children and adolescents with cancer. *Journal of Pediatrics*. 1982; **101**: 1032–5.

∗ 23. Ljungman G, Kreugar A, Gordh T *et al.* Treatment of pain in pediatric oncology: a Swedish nationwide survey. *Pain*. 1996; **68**: 385–94.

24. Sandler DP, Smith JC, Weinberg CR *et al.* Analgesic use and chronic renal disease. *New England Journal of Medicine*. 1989; **320**: 1238–43.

25. NSW Health. Paracetamol use. 2006. Available from: www.health.nsw.gov.au/policies/pd/2006/PD2006_004.html.

∗ 26. Wurthwein G, Koling S, Reich A *et al.* Pharmacokinetics of intravenous paracetamol in children and adolescents under major surgery. *European Journal of Clinical Pharmacology*. 2005; **60**: 883–8.

27. NSW Therapeutic Advisory Group Inc. IV paracetamol – where does it sit in hospital practice? 2005. NSW, Australia. Current Opinion. Available from: www.ciap.health.nsw.gov.au/nswtag/publications/posstats/ivparacetamol.pdf

28. Stuart JJ, Pisko EJ. Choline magnesium trisalicylate does not impair platelet aggregation. *Pharnatheraoeutica*. 1981; **2**: 547.

29. Foeldvari I, Burgos-Varos R, Thon A, Tuerck D. High response rate in the phase 1/11study of meloxicam in juvenile rheumatoid arthritis. *Journal of Rheumatology*. 2002; **29**: 1079–83.

30. Stempak D, Gammon J, Klein J *et al.* Single-dose and steady-state pharmacokinetics of celecoxib in children. *Clinical Pharmacology and Therapeutics*. 2002; **72**: 490–7.

31. Mukherjee D, Nissen SE, Topol EJ. Risk of cardiovascular events associated with selectiev COX -2 inhibitors. *Journal of the American Medical Association*. 2001; **286**: 954–9.

32. Williams D, Patel A, Howard R. Pharmacogenetics of codeine metabolism in an urban population of children and its implication for analgesic reliability. *British Journal of Anaesthesia*. 2002; **89**: 839–45.

33. Poyhia R, Seppala T. Lipid solubility and protein binding of oxycodone in vitro. *Pharmacology and Toxicology*. 1994; **74**: 23–7.

34. Pelkonen O, Kaltiala EH, Larmi TKL *et al.* Comparison of activities of drug metabolizing enzymes in human fetal and adult liver. *Clinical Pharmacology and Therapeutics*. 1973; **14**: 840–6.

35. Ross J, Riley J, Welsh K. Genetic variation in the catechol-o-methyl-transferase gene is associated with response to morphine in cancer patients. In: Flor H, Kalso E, Dostrovsky JO (eds). *Proceedings of the 11th World Congress on Pain*. Seattle: IASP Press, 2006: 461–7.

36. McRorie TI, Lynn A, Nespeca MK *et al.* The maturation of morphine clearance and metabolism. *American Journal of Diseases of Children*. 1992; **146**: 972–6.

37. Bhat R, Chari G, Gulati A *et al.* Pharmacokinetics of a single dose of morphine in pre-term infants during the first week of life. *Jounal of Pediatrics*. 1990; **117**: 477–81.

38. Pokela ML, Olkkala KT, Seppala T *et al.* Age-related morphine kinetics in infants. *Developmental Pharmacology and Therapeutics*. 1993; **20**: 26–34.

39. Stanski DR, Greenblatt DJ, Lowenstein E. Kinetics of intravenous and intramuscular morphine. *Clinical Pharmacology and Therapeutics*. 1978; **24**: 52–9.

40. Olkkola KT, Maunuksela EL, Korpela R, Rosenberg PH. Kinetics and dynamics of postoperative intravenous morphine in children. *Clinical Pharmacology and Therapeutics*. 1988; **44**: 128–36.

∗ 41. Cherny NI, Foley KM. Nonopioid and opioid analgesic pharmacotherapy of cancer pain. *Hematology/Oncology Clinics of North America*. 1996; **10**: 79–102.

∗ 42. Collins JJ, Geake J, Grier HE *et al.* Patient-controlled analgesia for mucositis pain in children: a three-period crossover study comparing morphine and hydromorphone. *Jounal of Pediatrics*. 1996; **129**: 722–8.

43. Collins C, Koren G, Crean P *et al.* Fentanyl pharmacokinetics and hemodynamic effects in preterm infants during ligation of patent ductus arteriosus. *Anesthesia and Analgesia*. 1985; **64**: 1078–80.

44. Koren G, Goresky G, Crean P *et al.* Unexpected alterations in fentanyl pharmacokinetics in children undergoing cardiac surgery: age related or disease related? *Developmental Pharmacology and Therapeutics*. 1986; **9**: 183–91.

45. Koren G, Goresky G, Crean P *et al.* Pediatric fentanyl dosing based on pharmacokinetics during cardiac surgery. *Anesthesia and Analgesia*. 1984; **63**: 577–82.

46. Johnson K, Erickson J, Holley F, Scott J. Fentanyl pharmacokinetics in the pediatric population. *Anesthesiology*. 1984; **61**: A441.

47. Gauntlett IS, Fisher DM, Hertzka RE *et al.* Pharmacokinetics of fentanyl in neonatal humans and lambs: effects of age. *Anesthesiology*. 1988; **69**: 683–7.

∗ 48. Schechter NL, Weisman SJ, Rosenblum M *et al.* The use of oral transmucosal fentanyl citrate for painful procedures in children. *Pediatrics*. 1995; **95**: 335–9.

49. Payne R, Coluzzi P, Hart L *et al.* Long-term safety of oral transmucosal fentanyl citrate for breakthrough cancer pain. *Journal of Pain and Symptom Management*. 2001; **22**: 575–83.

50. Collins JJ, Dunkel I, Gupta SK *et al.* Transdermal fentanyl in children with cancer: feasibility, tolerability, and pharmacokinetic correlates. *Journal of Pediatrics*. 1999; **134**: 319–23.

51. Hunt A, Goldman A, Devine T, Phillips M. Transdermal fentanyl for pain relief in a paediatric palliative care population. *Palliative Medicine*. 2001; **15**: 405–12.

52. Tamsen A, Hartvig P, Fagerlund C *et al.* Patient-controlled analgesic therapy, part 1: pharmacokinetics of pethidine in the pre- and postoperative periods. *Clinical Pharmacokinetics*. 1982; **7**: 149–63.

53. Hamunen K, Maunuksela EL, Seppala T *et al.* Pharmacokinetics of iv and rectal pethidine in children undergoing ophthalmic surgery. *British Journal of Anaesthesia*. 1993; **71**: 823–6.

54. Koska AJ, Kramer WG, Romagnoli A *et al.* Pharmacokinetics of high dose meperidine in surgical patients. *Anesthesia and Analgesia.* 1981; **60**: 8–11.

55. Pokela ML, Olkkala KT, Koivisto M *et al.* Pharmacokinetics and pharmacodynamics of intravenous meperidine in neonates and infants. *Clinical Pharmacology and Therapeutics.* 1992; **52**: 342–9.

56. Mather LE, Tucker GT, Pflug AE *et al.* Meperidine kinetics in man: intravenous injection in surgical patients and volunteers. *Clinical Pharmacology and Therapeutics.* 1975; **17**: 21–30.

57. Kaiko RF, Foley KM, Grabinsky PY *et al.* Central nervous system excitatory effects of meperidine in cancer patients. *Annals of Neurology.* 1983; **13**: 180–5.

58. Berde CB, Sethna NF, Holzman RS *et al.* Pharmacokinetics of methadone in children and adolescents in the perioperative period. *Anesthesiology.* 1987; **67**: A519.

∗ 59. Berde CB, Beyer JE, Bournaki MC *et al.* Comparison of morphine and methadone for prevention of postoperative pain in 3- to 7-year-old children. *Jounal of Pediatrics.* 1991; **119**: 136–41.

60. Kapelushnik J, Koren G, Solh H *et al.* Evaluating the efficacy of EMLA in alleviating pain associated with lumbar puncture: comparison of open and double-blinded protocols in children. *Pain.* 1990; **42**: 31–4.

∗ 61. Miser AW, Goh TS, Dose AM *et al.* Trial of a topically administered local anesthetic (EMLA cream) for pain relief during central venous port accesses in children with cancer. *Journal of Pain and Symptom Management.* 1994; **9**: 259–64.

62. Van Kan HJM, Egberts ACG, Rijnvos WPM *et al.* Tetracaine versus lidocaine-prilocaine for preventing venipuncture-induced pain in children. *American Journal of Health-system Pharmacy.* 1997; **54**: 388–92.

∗ 63. Houck CS, Sethna NF. Transdermal analgesia with local anesthetics in children: review, update and future directions. *Expert Review of Neurotherapeutics.* 2005; **5**: 625–34.

64. Bruera E, Brenneis C, Michaud M *et al.* Use of the subcutaneous route for the administration of narcotics in patients with cancer pain. *Cancer.* 1988; **62**: 407–11.

65. Gourlay G, Boas RA. Fatal outcome with use of rectal morphine for postoperative pain control in an infant. *British Medical Journal.* 1992; **304**: 766–7.

∗ 66. Mackie AM, Coda BC, Hill HF. Adolescents use patient controlled analgesia effectively for relief for relief from prolonged oropharyngeal mucositis pain. *Pain.* 1991; **46**: 265–9.

67. Dunbar PJ, Buckley P, Gavrin JR *et al.* Use of patient-controlled analgesia for pain control for children receiving bone marrow transplants. *Journal of Pain and Symptom Management.* 1995; **10**: 604–11.

∗ 68. Galer BS, Coyle N, Pasternak GW *et al.* Individual variability in the response to different opioids: report of five cases. *Pain.* 1992; **49**: 87–91.

69. Portenoy RK. Opioid tolerance and responsiveness: research findings and clinical observations. In: Gebhart GF, Hammond DI, Jensen TS (eds). *Progress in pain research and management.* Seattle: IASP Press, 1994: 615–19.

∗ 70. Inturrisi CE, Portenoy RK, Max M *et al.* Pharmacokinetic-pharmacodynamic relationships of methadone infusions in patients with cancer pain. *Clinical Pharmacology and Therapeutics.* 1990; **47**: 565–77.

∗ 71. Drake R, Longworth J, Collins JJ. Opioid rotation in children with cancer. *Journal of Palliative Medicine.* 2004; **7**: 419–22.

∗ 72. Lussier D, Portenoy RK. Adjuvant analgesics in pain management. In: Doyle D, Hanks GWC, Cherny N, Calman K (eds). *Oxford textbook of palliative medicine.* Oxford: Oxford University Press, 2004: 349–78.

73. Watson C, Evans R, Reed K *et al.* Amitriptyline versus placebo in postherpetic neuralgia. *Neurology.* 1982; **32**: 671–3.

∗ 74. Max MB. Antidepressants as analgesics. In: Fields HL, Liebeskind JC (eds). *Progress in pain research and pain management.* Seattle: IASP Press, 1994: 229–46.

75. Diamond S, Baltes B. Chronic tension headache treatment with amitriptyline – a double blind study. *Headache.* 1971; **11**: 110–16.

76. Couch J, Ziegler D, Hassanein R. Amitriptyline in the prophylaxis of migraine: effectiveness and relationship of antimigraine and antidepressant effects. *Neurology.* 1976; **26**: 121–7.

77. Frank R, Kashani J, Parker J *et al.* Antidepressant analgesia in rheumatoid arthritis. *Journal of Rheumatology.* 1988; **15**: 1632–8.

78. Ward NG. Tricyclic antidepressants for chronic low back pain: mechanisms of action and predictors of response. *Spine.* 1986; **11**: 661–5.

∗ 79. Magni G. The use of antidepressants in the treatment of chronic pain. *Drugs.* 1991; **42**: 730–48.

∗ 80. McQuay HJ, Tramer M, Nye BA *et al.* A systematic review of antidepressants in neuropathic pain. *Pain.* 1996; **68**: 217–27.

81. Heiligenstein E, Gerrity S. Psychotropics as adjuvant analgesics. In: Schechter NL, Berde CB, Yaster M (eds). *Pain in infants, children, and adolescents.* Baltimore: Williams & Wilkins, 1993: 173–7.

82. Biederman J, Baldessarini RJ, Wright V *et al.* A double-blind placebo controlled study of desipramine in the treatment of ADD: II. Serum drug levels and cardiovascular findings. *Journal of the American Academy of Child and Adolescent Psychiatry.* 1989; **28**: 903–11.

83. Forrest WH, Brown BW, Brown CR *et al.* Dextroamphetamine with morphine for the treatment of postoperative pain. *New England Journal of Medicine.* 1977; **296**: 712–15.

84. Bruera E, Miller MJ, Macmillan K, Kuehn N. Neuropsychological effects of methylphenidate in patients receiving a continuous infusion of narcotics for cancer pain. *Pain.* 1992; **48**: 163–6.

85. Bruera E, Faisinger R, MacEachern T, Hanson J. The use of methylphenidate in pateints with incident pain receiving regular opiates: a preliminary report. *Pain.* 1992; **50**: 75–7.

86. Yee JD, Berde CB. Dextroamphetamine or methylphenidate as adjuvants to opioid analgesia for adolescents with cancer. *Journal of Pain and Symptom Managment.* 1994; **9**: 122–5.

87. Watanabe S, Bruera E. Corticosteroids as adjuvant analgesics. *Journal of Pain and Symptom Managment.* 1994; **9**: 442–5.

88. Tannock I, Gospodarowicz M, Meakin W *et al.* Treatment of metastatic prostatic cancer with low-dose prednisone: evaluation of pain and quality of life as pragmatic indices of response. *Journal of Clinical Oncology.* 1989; **7**: 590–7.

89. Weinstein JD, Toy FJ, Jaffe ME, Goldberg HI. The effect of dexamethasone on brain edema in patients with metastatic brain tumors. *Neurology.* 1973; **23**: 121–9.

90. Greenberg HS, Kim J, Posner JB. Epidural spinal cord compression from metastatic tumor: results with a new treatment protocol. *Annals of Neurology.* 1980; **8**: 361–6.

91. Khurana DS, Riviello J, Helmers S *et al.* Efficacy of gabapentin therapy in children with refractory partial seizures. *Jounal of Pediatrics.* 1996; **128**: 829–33.

92. Silberstein EB, Williams C. Strontium-89 therapy for painful osseous metastases. *Journal of Nuclear Medicine.* 1985; **26**: 345–8.

93. Westlin JE, Letocha H, Jakobson S *et al.* Rapid, reproducible pain relief with [131I]iodine-meta-iodobenzylguanidine in a boy with disseminated neuroblastoma. *Pain.* 1995; **60**: 111–14.

94. Beaver WT, Wallenstein S, Houde RW, Rogers A. A comparison of the analgesic effects of methotrimeprazine and morphine in patients with cancer. *Clinical Pharmacology and Therapeutics.* 1966; **7**: 436–46.

95. Collins JJ, Grier HE, Sethna NF, Berde CB. Regional anesthesia for pain associated with terminal malignancy. *Pain.* 1996; **65**: 63–9.

96. Cherny NI, Portenoy RK. Sedation in the management of refractory symptoms: guidelines for evaluation and treatment. *Journal of Palliative Care.* 1994; **10**: 31–8.

97. Wang Y, Mitchell J, Moriyama K *et al.* Age-dependent morphine tolerance development in the rat. *Anesthesia and Analgesia.* 2005; **100**: 1733–9.

98. Buntin-Mushock C, Phillip L, Moriyama K, Palmer PP. Age-dependent opioid escalation in chronic pain patients. *Anesthesia and Analgesia.* 2005; **100**: 1740–5.

99. Porter J, Jick H. Addiction is rare in patients treated with narcotics. *New England Journal of Medicine.* 1980; **302**: 123.

26

Cancer pain in older people

MARGOT GOSNEY

Introduction	359	Patient knowledge and experience	364
Is pain different in older people?	360	Pharmacokinetics and pharmacodynamics	364
Pain assessment	361	Simple analgesics	365
Pain control	362	Opioids	366
Misconceptions about analgesics	363	Additional analgesia	368
Quality of life issues	363	Specific problems of later life	370
Carer knowledge and experience	363	References	372

KEY LEARNING POINTS

- Older people with pain are often not diagnosed or managed in a timely fashion.
- Cognitive impairment and communication difficulties result in difficulties in the detection and quantification of pain.
- Pain assessment scales are generally not developed specifically for older people and are therefore difficult to use and lack validation in an elderly population.

- Pharmacological agents are more likely to cause side effects in older patients, due to alterations in pharmacodynamics and pharmacokinetics.
- Drug side effects may worsen older people's functioning and result in impaired quality of life.
- Research into the meaning of pain, its detection, and management in older individuals is still sparse, often conflicting in results, and lacking in scientific rigor.

INTRODUCTION

There are many definitions of pain.[1, 2] Pain is the most common symptom associated with cancer and often the most distressing one[3] and the meaning of pain is influenced by the individual's personal, social, and cultural experiences.[4]

Although most studies on pain are exclusively from the perspective of the patient, it is important in older patients to consider the meaning of pain from the perspective of the patient, family, caregiver, and healthcare professionals caring for the patient with cancer.[5]

Although acute and chronic pain are defined by their duration, the traditional dichotomy between acute pain,

with its recent onset and short duration, and chronic pain, which persists after an injury has healed, is increasingly untenable.[6] Acute pain associated with a new tissue injury might last for less than one month but, at times, for longer than six months.[7] Older people are more likely to suffer both acute and chronic pain[8, 9] and, although cancer pain in older sufferers may be considered to last for short periods because of limited survival, some authors never consider it to be chronic in nature.[10]

In older people it may be difficult to distinguish between pain from unrelated pathology and pain due to malignant disease. However, pain, discomfort and suffering must not be equated with the process of normal aging.[11]

Pain is a frequent complaint of elderly people,[12] and researchers have developed conceptual models of the impact of pain on the dimensions of quality of life.[13] This model depicts four domains of pain: physical well-being and symptoms, psychological well-being, social well-being, and spiritual well-being. The models fail to address many factors that are specific to older people, and this must be considered when analyzing response to therapy in this age group. Perhaps the most helpful definition of pain is that of McCaffery,[14] which, although not specific to pain in the elderly, states, "Pain is whatever the patient says it is and exists when he says it does." This concept needs to be borne in mind when dealing with older patients.

Worldwide, seven million new cases of cancer are diagnosed annually, with over 50 percent in patients aged 70 years or above. Between 50 and 80 percent of patients with cancer cite pain as a significant problem that disturbs overall quality of life,[15] with some studies suggesting that more than 50 percent of patients, many of whom are elderly, suffer unrelieved pain.[16, 17, 18, 19, 20, 21][III] A working party from the UK Royal College of Surgeons and College of Anaesthetists[22] reported that healthcare professionals working in acute pain management are ineffectual in suppression of this distressing symptom, with a study by Lynn et al.[23][III] of 3357 seriously ill and elderly patients reporting that 40 percent of the study subjects complained of being in severe pain in the last three days of life.

Ageist attitudes exist in clinical practice, and oncology and palliative care are no exception. Patients and physicians often dismiss many symptoms attributable to cancer as being the normal consequence of aging. Bone pain is attributed to arthritis, abdominal pain to diverticulitis, and confusion is invariably considered to be the result of dementia.

Pain is related to the primary site of the tumor, to disease progression, and to the treatment that the patient receives. These facts are particularly pertinent in older patients, who have more advanced disease at presentation,[24][II] are less likely to receive active treatment,[25, 26, 27] and, in many cases, lack a definitive diagnosis, thus preventing definitive treatment.[28][IV]

Breast and lung cancers are more likely to be associated with pain, and these are tumors that are predominantly found in older people. Although as many as 85 percent of patients with a primary bone tumor (common in young people) experience pain, there are few data on bony metastases, which are especially common in patients with primary breast, lung, or prostate cancers.

Uncontrollable pain is a reason for hospital admission and, when admitted, older patients spend more time in hospital.[29] Unfortunately, despite the fact that over half of all terminally ill patients say they would prefer to die at home, 63 percent actually died in hospital.[30] In a study of 434 patients, including individuals up to the age of 93 years with incurable malignant disease, palliative care intervention, including pain control, enabled more patients than controls to die at home (25 versus 15 percent, $p < 0.05$).[31] Older patients with cancer are more likely to die in hospital for a variety of reasons. Firstly, the diagnosis of cancer is often made after an older patient presents in an atypical fashion. Thus, the older man who has "gone off his legs" actually has lung cancer with hypercalcemia, constipation, spurious diarrhea, and urinary retention. It may be during this admission that the patient dies from the new diagnosis of lung cancer. Secondly, older people have a prolonged active life expectancy, with the resultant onset of terminal dependency being postponed and also have a duration of terminal dependency that increases. Thus, it may be during this period of terminal dependency that the patient dies, with cancer being one of many diagnoses active at the time.[32]

Although it is easy to extrapolate that with increasing age, irrespective of diagnosis, older people are more likely to be admitted to hospital in the last year of their lives, very elderly subjects, i.e. 85 years or older, are the least likely to be admitted to hospital in the last year of their lives, and generalizations must be avoided.[33]

In a Swedish study of 4357 elderly individuals in residential care of whom 55 percent had cognitive impairment, staff judged 2111 residents (56.7 percent) to be suffering from pain, although 27.9 percent of these residents were not receiving any regular analgesic drugs. Staff considered that more patients were actually being prescribed regular analgesics than were actually receiving it, suggesting a lack of communication.[34]

IS PAIN DIFFERENT IN OLDER PEOPLE?

Older people complain less about pain than younger subjects do. This may be because they attribute pain to normal aging or are more stoical about pain, but there is also evidence that older people have altered tolerance to pain from various stimuli. Harkins[35] found that deep pain tends to become less frequent and less intense with age, although superficial pain does not alter with increasing age. In postoperative pain control, older patients achieve the same degree of pain control with less analgesic medication than younger patients,[36] suggesting reduced pain experience in this group.

There may be difficulties in determining the etiology of pain in older people. Brochet et al.[37] found the prevalence of pain to be over 70 percent among community-living subjects over the age of 65 years. Although the etiology was unstated, the most commonly affected sites were limb joints and the back.

Of more concern is the finding by Vigano et al.[38] that cancer patients aged 75 years or older, when compared with younger adults, received significantly lower amounts of opioid analgesia.

In the case of renal dysfunction, due either to aging or to disease, there is evidence of increased potency of opioids.[39, 40] Older patients with pain are often not studied in a controlled and prospective fashion. Although some information may be obtained from extrapolating existing knowledge, it may lead to suboptimal or dangerous therapy for older people.

Experience of pain at night is particularly troublesome for older people. A correlation exists between the severity of pain and the number of nights of troubled sleep. When combined with other causes of impaired sleep, such as nocturia, an elderly person's quality of life may be particularly impacted.[41]

Older patients may choose quantity over quality of life, and this may not be predictable from the person's clinical diagnosis. In a study by Tsevat et al.,[42][III] 414 hospitalized patients aged 80–98 years were asked whether they would prefer to live for one year in their current state of health or less time in excellent health. They found that 69 percent of patients were unwilling to exchange 12 months of life in their present state of health for one month in excellent health. Thus, although we strive for quality of pain control, older people may have different goals to the physician.

PAIN ASSESSMENT

It is vital to use instruments that are reliable, valid, and feasible in day-to-day clinical practice. There are three major areas for the assessment of pain. The first is a linear analog scale (LAS) or visual analog scale (VAS),[43, 44] the second a verbal rating scale (VRS) or categorical-rated scale (CRS),[45] and the third method is a patient daily diary card. It has been suggested that it is easier to explain to elderly patients verbal scales rather than the more abstract analog scales, but this remains to be formally tested[46][IV] and impaired vision and/or manual dexterity and cognition may make diary cards more difficult.

Although it is clear that no one scale will be suitable for all patients, and particularly for older patients, it has been recommended that there is a universal adoption of a scale for clinical assessment of pain intensity in adults who are capable of responding to simple queries. This may be particularly valuable in the management of older patients with cancer pain.[47] It must be remembered that with all tools designed for use with younger adults, their appropriateness for older people remains preliminary.[48]

Pain assessment in older people may be complicated by a number of factors, which are often associated with normal aging. These are barriers to pain assessment,[49] coexistent medical conditions and concurrent medication,[50] cognitive impairment,[51] communication difficulties,[52] sensory impairment,[53] and motor loss.[54]

In pain assessment, the use of a core questionnaire covering areas such as physical, psychological, and social well-being as well as a specific module relating to the primary tumor or topic under study is required. One example is the approach of the European Organization for Research and Treatment of Cancer (EORTC).[55] This does little to cover the spiritual aspect of palliative care and does not take account of other diseases that occur coincidentally with the primary cancer, as seen especially in older patients.

Pain affects social functioning, and in elderly patients this can be measured by the Katz Activities of Daily Living score, which is a standard instrument, validated for use in elderly patients with cancer.[56]

Although many of the effects of pain in elderly patients are also seen in younger patients, including depression, disrupted sleep, and impaired mobility, there are additional consequences that specifically affect older patients. For example, elderly patients experience an increased number of falls, one of the "giants of geriatric medicine," which may occur as a result of impaired mobility, cognitive dysfunction, or polypharmacy.[57, 58] The risk of malnutrition is increased when pain is poorly controlled, and poor nutrition in older patients is well described in both cancer and noncancer literature.[59, 60][IV] Delirium (acute confusion) may result from pain per se or occur as a result of drug therapy. In many older patients, polypharmacy is often a problem prior to the introduction of analgesic drugs with such drugs adding to an already complex list.

A parallel recording of activity level and pain scale may show subtle changes in activities of daily living, with no perceived alteration in pain level. This is particularly important during medication alterations and when both mobility and pain relief are primary outcome measures.[61]

Measurement of pain relief is important in older patients, although the true benefit of the prescribed medication may not be fully apparent due to coexisting morbidity or as a consequence of the newly prescribed drug. For example, the use of steroids may reduce pain but cause immobility due to muscle wasting, metabolic disturbances, or vertebral collapse as a result of osteoporosis. Thus, physical function or some global aspects of quality of life may not improve and the added frustration of pain relief in the absence of improved mobility may worsen the patient's quality of life. Although pain assessment scales may be difficult to administer and interpret, it is important not to abandon these in favor of easily recorded data such as analgesic consumption. This may be poorly recalled and the poor compliance and undertreatment that occurs in older patients makes these data meaningless.

Although the McGill Pain Questionnaire is well validated,[62] it is important that other self-reported measures of patients' ability to engage in functional activities are taken into account.[63] While older patients can identify pain intensity on a VAS or a numerical rating scale (NRS), it has been found that nurses may be unable to identify patients in pain or choose an appropriate treatment.[64] [IV] Increasing age has also been associated with a higher frequency of incorrect responses to VAS,[65] but this is not a consistent finding.[66] The use of body charts has been well validated in younger people; however, there are few data on their use in older patients with cancer.[67]

Pain assessment scoring systems developed for diseases other than cancer may be particularly appropriate in older patients with existing comorbidity. A pain management inventory (PMI) was developed to measure 17 independent self-management methods used by patients experiencing chronic pain due to arthritis. The PMI found valid and viable pain management methods, including prescribed medication, but also relaxation methods, stress control methods, and distracting techniques.[68] Such studies require replication in older patients with cancer, but may form an important framework for pain management. I would recommend the McGill Pain Questionnaire for those elderly patients with no cognitive impairment. However, for those with an abbreviated mental test score of seven or less, nurse observation of behavior in combination with the use of body charts provides a level of basic pain assessment.

PAIN CONTROL

Pain control is poorly achieved for a variety of reasons, which can be subdivided into patient and/or carer attitudes.[69, 70]

Patients' attitudes

Patients of all ages with cancer have a reluctance to report pain.[71] Yates et al.[72] demonstrated that older people were more reluctant to express their pain and that the cause of such reluctance was multifactorial:[73, 74]

- not wishing to be a nuisance;
- a belief that pain is a judgment and must be borne;
- a belief that pain is an inevitable part of cancer;
- not wishing to distract the doctor or nurse from treating the cancer;
- considering that nothing can be done to relieve pain.

Attitudes of healthcare professionals

DOCTORS

Studies of the management of cancer pain by doctors exist but, although doctors from a wide variety of specialist areas are represented, most are hospital based. These studies may help understand general principles, but fail to address the beliefs of doctors most likely to encounter patients with cancer, i.e. primary care physicians and medical oncologists.[75, 76][IV] Larue et al.[77][IV] studied 600 primary care physicians and 300 medical oncologists in France. A 12-minute interview included both multiple choice and closed-ended questions on pain assessment, as well as problems associated with morphine usage, and included an assessment of the physicians training in cancer pain management. Seventy-three percent of primary care physicians (PCPs) and 61 percent of medical oncologists (ONCs) reported never having received training in cancer pain management, and both PCPs (88 percent) and ONCs (90 percent) reported that they relied on their patients' claims to assess pain. Less than half of the 900 doctors studied prescribed morphine frequently or very frequently, and 30 percent of ONCs and 20 percent of PCPs reported problems with pharmacists when attempting to have morphine prescriptions filled. Only 27 percent of PCPs and 42 percent of ONCs knew that oral morphine could be prescribed daily to an adult without any upper limitation in dosage and 76 and 50.3 percent, respectively, expressed reluctance to prescribe morphine, with 40.2 percent of PCPs and 26.7 percent of ONCs citing fear of side effects as a reason. Almost one-fifth of doctors said that they would hesitate to prescribe morphine because there were other drugs as effective as morphine available. Women doctors prescribed morphine less frequently than male physicians and increasing doctor age resulted in less frequent prescription of morphine. The doctors who prescribed less frequently perceived the barriers to be risk of tolerance, availability of drugs as effective as morphine, constraints of the prescribing forms, and poor image of morphine in public opinion. The doctors who prescribed morphine more frequently reported a higher prevalence of pain among their patients, were more likely to rely on their patients to assess the pain, agreed that morphine could be prescribed at any stage of the disease, and perceived respiratory depression as a low concern.[77][IV] Thus, education of doctors is essential to ensure that patients are not undertreated with opioids, particularly in the case of older patients, who complain less frequently.

NURSES

In 1983, McCaffery[78] reported that nurses seem to be responsible for controlling patients' expression of pain and that this may be accomplished by ignoring the patients' manifestations of pain. Ferrell et al.[79] stated that nurses performed pain assessment rarely, poorly, or inconsistently. There is little information available that identifies nurses' experiences and skills in managing pain specifically in older people with malignant disease, although Closs,[58] in her study of four clinical areas (cardiothoracic surgery, orthopedic surgery, general surgery, and care of the elderly wards), attempted to address this. Of the 55 percent of nurses who returned questionnaires, almost 84 percent reported that elderly people suffered more chronic pain than younger people. Although there is no evidence that pain and discomfort are unavoidable consequences of aging, more than half of the nurses in the sample felt this to be the case. Nurses from care of the elderly areas correctly believed that there are differences in response to painful stimuli with age. In contrast, nurses from acute surgical areas were more likely to identify that older patients were less likely to request pain relief. Some nurses were unaware that the duration of analgesic effect from a given medication differs between elderly and young patients, although higher grade nurses and those working on acute surgical wards more commonly answered this question correctly.

Nurses should ask patients how the pain feels rather than whether they need anything for pain. The latter allows the patient to decline help regardless of how they actually feel whereas the former gives patients "permission" to ask for help to manage their pain.[58]

MISCONCEPTIONS ABOUT ANALGESICS

Anxiety about the administration of opioids is exhibited by healthcare professionals, patients, and carers.[80] The proper use of opioids does not cause addiction,[81] and although elderly people do experience higher peaks and a longer duration of action when given opioids, they do not experience the respiratory depression that many doctors and nurses predict.[82] Such inaccurate and widespread perceptions could undoubtedly lead to undermedication and ineffective pain control[58] when respiratory depression is in fact a rare occurrence and should present no problem when effective patient monitoring is in progress.[83, 84]

QUALITY OF LIFE ISSUES

The assessment of quality of life in older patients with cancer differs in many ways. Clinicians must be aware that in the management of older patients with cancer there is often acceptance of potentially toxic treatment for a seemingly small survival benefit.[85]

The older patient with cancer may be at risk of suicide due to pain, helplessness, and exhaustion or poor contact with the healthcare system. In an Italian study of cancer patients cared for at home, the five patients who committed suicide had a mean age of 55 years (range 50–76) and, despite their age and the apparent easy availability of drugs, only one took an overdose of morphine.[86]

In younger patients with pain, significant associations are found between interference with activities of daily living due to pain and mood or anxiety. Anxiety and depression were positively correlated with different interferences, i.e. walking ability, relations with other people, etc. Although these studies have excluded older people, they may help to determine the true impact of advanced cancer pain in old age.[87] When chronic pain was assessed in elderly patients in the pain clinic setting, two themes emerged, the desire for independence and control and the adaptation to a life with chronic pain.[88]

CARER KNOWLEDGE AND EXPERIENCE

Many elderly patients with cancer are cared for at home surrounded by family members. Although family members play an important role,[89, 90, 91] it is fortunate that they can provide effective pain management despite not understanding the basic mechanisms of pain.[92] If caregivers deny that the patient is in pain to avoid accepting that the disease process is progressing and the patient is close to death, this may result in the underadministration of analgesia. Many family members, in the absence of formal teaching of caregiving skills by healthcare providers, are left to administer pain relief by a process of trial and error.[93] Although previous studies have identified pain as a major source of concern, there has been very little focused research on caregivers and pain management. Ferrell et al.[80] identified the diversity of mean rating of patients' pain as assessed independently by caregivers and patients. Caregivers overrated the pain; using a scale from 0 (no pain) to 100 (severe pain), the patients' mean rating of their pain was 45, whereas caregivers' mean rating of the patients' pain was 70.

Ferrell et al.[94] developed and implemented a pain education program for patients and family caregivers. Information was delivered in a variety of formats. The booklet developed was reasonably short in length and printed in larger typeface and included illustrations. In addition, audiocassette tapes were produced and left with the patients at the conclusion of each of the first two education sessions. After education, the patients experienced a decrease in pain intensity and severity, a decrease in fear of addiction, and a subsequent increase in use of pain medication. The caregiver was also found to have an improved knowledge and a reduced fear of addiction or respiratory depression when using strong analgesia.

Ferrell et al.[13] assessed caregivers' knowledge in the care of 80 patients with cancer. Of a 14-item scale assessing carer knowledge and attitudes about pain, ten items improved on retest as a result of educational intervention.

Ferrell et al.[95] suggested that caregivers' knowledge about pain management differed according to the settings where patients received care – an important consideration when elderly patients with cancer are likely to be treated in the hospital rather than the community.

If caregivers are to feel positive about their role, they must have positive experiences. When comparing scores obtained by caregivers and patients, family caregivers showed more positive scores in the domain of physical well-being. These included feelings of usefulness, strength, and appetite, and were in contrast to patients, who showed more positive results in the emotional aspects such as worry and sense of control.[13] In five areas patients were more positive than their caregivers. These included patients being more likely to believe that pain could be relieved and that family members were useful helpers in pain management. The study also showed that family caregivers of elderly patients were less optimistic and more distressed by the pain experience than the patients themselves.[13] Similarly, Yeager et al.[91] found that significantly higher levels of patient pain and patient distress were reported by family caregivers than by patients themselves, and family caregivers experienced significantly more distress as a result of the patient's pain than the patient believed to be the case.

It is essential that we consider the demographics of such caregivers. In a study of caregivers by Ferrell et al.,[13] the median age of caregivers was 63.5 years; 76 percent were female, 66 percent were the spouse, and 22 percent were the child of the index patient. Thus, older patients requiring informal care may be reliant on elderly spouses or daughters who are combining this caregiving with child care and paid employment. In the study, although 92 percent of caregivers lived with the patient, 22 percent were also employed outside the home, and 10 percent were older than 74 years of age.

Clotfelter[96][IV] studied 36 subjects over 65 years of age with a diagnosis of cancer. The randomized study group watched a 14-minute video on managing cancer pain and also received written information. A follow-up assessment found that the study group had significantly less pain than the control group, and the author concluded that pain education is a central component in preventing and managing cancer pain in elderly people.

This highlights the need for close monitoring of both patient and caregiver, particularly with regard to education and false beliefs. If patients and caregivers interpret the pain experience differently, then management is based on inappropriate estimates of pain intensity.[97]

Nurses

Clinical research must be relevant to everyday clinical practice. This is particularly the case in nursing research, and problems such as lack of replication, lack of organizational structure to support its integration, and lack of interest and understanding of research on the part of practicing nurses may be of paramount importance.[98] In order to avoid this problem, practicing nurse clinicians must identify a nursing practice problem, which is then studied by researchers. Dufault et al.[99] found that nurses who identified and participated in key research-based areas, improved their attitudes towards research and their competency in research utilization.

Although most studies show that nurses generally underestimate patients' pain, Jandelli[100] found that the six nurses in her study overestimated the patient's pain in the majority of cases. In contrast to other studies, in which oncology patients' pain was found to be underestimated, studies of medical inpatients[101] and surgical inpatients[102] found pain to be overestimated. However, these patients were younger and had no communication problems. The nurses in Jandelli's study had all received Oncology or Care of the Dying Patient certificates, which may at least

partly explain the fact that pain is usually underestimated by nurses not experienced in or trained about pain management. Wakefield[103] found that nurses tend to categorize patients according to symptoms or overt pain behavior and their knowledge influenced the way in which they managed postoperative pain.

Nurses attribute significantly less pain to a patient with no physical pathology and more pain to a patient with symptoms of depression.[104] Patient age influences pain management as nurses may be more willing to believe the reports given by older patients than younger patients,[105] but less willing to administer opioid analgesia to such patients.[106]

DOCTORS

In a prospective study of patients with prostate cancer undergoing palliative therapy, symptoms were measured by means of patient- and physician-completed assessments. Although all patients were male and elderly, the data were not analyzed by age bands. Doctors tended to underestimate both nausea and pain and attributed a decreased performance status to the patient compared with the person's own self-assessments.[107]

In a study in Italy of 148 physicians and 182 general practitioners, two-thirds of the sample agreed that, if more attention was paid to quality of life issues and pain control, euthanasia and physician-assisted suicide would be eliminated.[108][V]

PATIENT KNOWLEDGE AND EXPERIENCE

In 1984, Jones et al.[109] studied 82 patients with cancer to assess their knowledge about pain management. Although the compliance seen in these patients was high, patients were unaware of common side effects of their drugs, and 11 of the 54 patients took medication as required even when it was prescribed on a regular basis. Patients' attitudes to cancer pain may also be affected by public attitudes: in a telephone survey of 496 adults, 57 percent felt that patients with cancer usually died a painful death and almost 50 percent viewed cancer pain to be severe.[110]

Eighty patients with a median age of 67 years were recruited and received three education and two evaluation visits. Throughout the period of evaluation, patients reported improvement in pain intensity and distress and an increase in pain relief. Both patients and healthcare providers found the pain education program to be beneficial and reported that it improved all aspects of quality of life.[111]

PHARMACOKINETICS AND PHARMACODYNAMICS

Pharmacokinetics encompasses the movement of drugs through the body, including absorption, distribution, metabolism, and excretion. Thus, pharmacokinetics determines drug concentrations in plasma and tissues, in contrast to pharmacodynamics, which is the process that determines the body's response to a given tissue or plasma concentration of a drug. Aging can affect either pharmacokinetics or pharmacodynamics, and on occasions will affect both.

Pharmacokinetics

Although there are now abundant data on the effect of age or aging on pharmacokinetics, most studies have been performed on healthy volunteers, with little reference to the frail elderly patient with multiple pathology. In older people, acid secretion is reduced and gastric emptying impaired, and the absorptive capacity of the small bowel and blood flow to the intestine are also reduced. The first-pass metabolism of some drugs declines significantly with age, and both the liver volume and hepatic blood flow are reduced with increasing age. Thus, the systemic concentration of drugs that undergoes significant first-pass metabolism may be greatly increased in elderly subjects.

DISTRIBUTION

In normal aging, both total body water and lean body mass decrease, resulting in a relative increase in body fat. The lipid solubility of a drug therefore determines the serum level with advancing age. Drugs that are water soluble, such as morphine, will tend to have a smaller volume of distribution, which results in a higher serum level. In older people, drugs such as benzodiazepines or barbiturates, which are lipid soluble, have a larger volume distribution and prolonged half-life.

Protein binding determines the levels of free drug available to cross plasma membranes. Acidic compounds bind principally to albumin. Thus, in older patients who have a reduced level of serum albumin and hence reduced acid drug-binding capacity, the levels of free salicylic acid and benzodiazepines will be higher than in younger subjects for a given dose. In addition, α_1-acid glycoprotein, which binds to basic drugs, is increased by intercurrent illness, resulting in a higher level of plasma protein binding and reduced levels of free basic drugs.

Clearance of drugs from the body is primarily dependent on whether the compound is polar or nonpolar. Polar compounds are water soluble and thus are usually excreted unchanged through the kidneys. Normal aging is associated with a reduction in glomerular filtration rate, renal plasma flow, and tubular function, and thus renal excretion of drugs such as nonsteroidal anti-inflammatory drugs (NSAID) is reduced in older patients. Drugs that are nonpolar are poorly soluble in water and must be metabolized before excretion. Hepatic clearance is reduced in the normal older person and this, together with alterations

in conjugation, results in reduced clearance of paracetamol (acetaminophen) and lorazepam.[112, 113]

Although one may postulate that metastatic liver disease, particularly in older patients, would result in a reduction in liver metabolism, this has not been a consistent finding,[114] perhaps because normal hepatic parenchyma is preserved as a result of hepatic enlargement.[115]

Pharmacodynamics

The effect of drugs on the body is in essence pharmacodynamics. Although some clear-cut pharmacodynamics data in older patients exist, there is a paucity in sick frail older people. Drugs of particular relevance in the management of pain in older patients include benzodiazepines, which may produce increased sedation and confusion and impaired postural righting reflexes,[116, 117] and neuroleptics, which, used either for sedation or for their antiemetic effect, may result in tardive dyskinesia and parkinsonism.[118, 119] Drugs such as prochlorperazine are prescribed to older people with dizziness and nausea although such agents increase postural sway and impair balance.

SIMPLE ANALGESICS

Paracetamol does not cause gastric irritation and is more effective when used in combination with a NSAID than when given alone. It is the nonopioid analgesic of choice, particularly in elderly people.[12] Paracetamol may enhance the effect of warfarin in prolonged use, whereas the coadministration of metoclopramide increases the absorption and therefore the effectiveness of paracetamol.[120] Paracetamol should be avoided in known liver dysfunction and alcohol dependence.[121]

Aspirin causes irreversible inactivation of both cyclooxygenase (COX)-1 and COX-2. It displaces a number of drugs from protein binding sites in the blood, and is of particular relevance in older patients taking tolbutamide, chlorpropamide, and phenytoin. Coadministration of aspirin and warfarin results in an increased anticoagulant effect, partly by displacement of warfarin from protein binding sites and partly through a direct effect of aspirin on platelets. Recently, there has been an increase in the prescription of spironolactone for congestive cardiac failure among older patients. Aspirin reduces the pharmacological activity of spironolactone and may worsen cardiac failure.[122]

Mild to moderate pain warrants the prescription of NSAIDs. NSAIDs are weak acids and are thus well absorbed in the stomach. In the bloodstream, most NSAIDs are protein bound, and a quarter of the drug is excreted in the urine unchanged, the remainder is oxidized or conjugated. Urinary excretion of NSAIDs is higher when the urine is acid and may be affected by the coadministration of other drugs. As renal function declines with age, the urinary excretion of NSAIDs must be carefully considered.

NSAIDs are responsible for almost one-quarter of all adverse drug reactions reported in the UK.[122] Every year, 0.5–2 percent of people administered a NSAID have a serious gastrointestinal event, including both perforation or bleeding.[123] These complications cause an estimated 2000 deaths per year in the UK.[124] Mucosal erosions, ulceration, or bleeding may be detected if the patient is symptomatic; however, slowly developing anemia may present atypically in the older patient. In a meta-analysis, ibuprofen was associated with the lowest incidence of gastrointestinal side effects and piroxicam and ketoprofen with the highest incidence of gastric adverse effects.[125]

NSAIDs cause both salt and water retention, resulting in hypertension and edema. As all NSAIDs are highly protein bound, the free fraction of NSAIDs is increased in patients with hypoalbuminemia, and such subjects have a propensity to increasing peripheral edema. Poor mobility, pressure area instability, and falls may result from inability to wear footwear over edematous feet.

Although NSAIDs are well absorbed, an age-related decrease in gastric absorption may result in sub-therapeutic levels. Alteration of hepatic enzymes with increasing age may also result in decreased levels of active agents such as fenbufen, a propionate that must be metabolized by the liver to yield active metabolites.

NSAIDs may cause renal toxicity as a result of papillary necrosis or interstitial nephritis.

Naproxen accumulates in patients with renal impairment, and its half-life is prolonged. Thus, older patients may need smaller doses and, as underpins all drug prescribing in older patients, drugs with a short half-life may be safer on the whole and prodrugs may be less nephrotoxic.[126] Careful monitoring of renal function is essential in all elderly patients receiving long-term treatment with NSAIDs. Naproxen undergoes enterohepatic recycling, and any alterations in the gut flora due to aging changes may affect its excretion.

Proton pump inhibitors are particularly useful for suppressing acid secretion in patients requiring regular NSAIDs. The ASTRONAUT study[127][II] found omeprazole to be significantly more effective than ranitidine ($p < 0.001$) and, although many patients with cancer receive NSAIDs for only short periods of time, the finding of this study was that after six months treatment, omeprazole was also more effective than ranitidine in preventing ulcer formation.

Rofecoxib is well absorbed after oral administration, with a plasma peak concentration at two to four hours. The plasma half-life is approximately 16–18 hours and elimination is almost entirely by metabolism by non-cytochrome enzymes in the liver, resulting in inactive derivatives which are excreted in the urine. Studies of patients with osteoarthritis or rheumatoid arthritis have shown rofecoxib to have similar efficacy to diclofenac and naproxen, respectively.[128, 129]

Celecoxib has an earlier peak plasma concentration of two to three hours, with an elimination half-life of 8–12 hours. Celecoxib is metabolized to inactive derivatives in the liver, chiefly by the cytochrome P450 2C9, with only small amounts of unchanged drug appearing in the urine and feces. Its efficacy in rheumatoid arthritis is superior to placebo, but in a longer double-blind study, it had a similar efficacy to diclofenac slow-release.[130]

Whilst both rofecoxib and celecoxib have good gastrointestinal safety, recent evidence has cast doubt on other aspects of its safety.[131] The Multinational Etoricoxib and Diclofenac Arthritis Long-term (MEDAL) program studied 34,701 patients with arthritis who were randomized to two different treatment arms. After an average treatment duration of 18 months, subsequent follow up noted that upper gastrointestinal events were lower with etoricoxib than diclofenac, when comparing perforation, bleeding, obstruction, and ulcer formation, and etoricoxib yielded 1.24 thrombotic cardiovascular events versus 1.30 per 100 patient-years in the diclofenac group. This study therefore concluded similar rates of thrombotic cardiovascular events in patients with arthritis on etoricoxib and diclofenac, with long-term use. Whilst this goes someway towards reassuring those prescribing COX-2 selective inhibitors, further data are awaited.[132][II]

A recent review found NSAIDs were more effective than placebo for cancer pain, but with no clear evidence to support the seniority of one. The combination of a NSAID with an opioid showed no statistically significant trend towards superiority when comparing the NSAID, plus an opioid versus either drug alone. Thus the routine coadministration of a NSAID and an opioid should not be recommended, particularly in older people at risk of drug interactions.[133][I]

OPIOIDS

Opioids are particularly useful in the management of moderate to severe pain.[134] A further advantage of opioids in older patients is the variety of possible methods of delivery.

There are, however, problems associated with the introduction of opioids. A recent public poll found that 74 percent felt that morphine was dangerous and addictive, and a survey of general practitioners (GPs) found that patients were specifically concerned about addiction and dependency with morphine use, with 36 percent of GPs believing that the prescription of morphine signals that death is imminent. Although opioids are beneficial in the treatment of pain, psychological support must be provided to patients when they are first administered.[135]

Weak opioids include codeine, dihydrocodeine, and dextropropoxyphene. However, cimetidine and fluoxetine, which may be co-prescribed in older patients, have both been reported to inhibit the enzyme that converts codeine into morphine, and thus their co-prescription may block the analgesic effect. Problems commonly seen with dextropropoxyphene are the enhancement of blood levels of carbamazepine, resulting in drowsiness and increased anticoagulant effects of warfarin.

Drug combinations should, on the whole, be avoided in elderly patients. Although codeine causes confusion and constipation in older subjects,[136] Moore et al.[137][I] found that the combination of codeine 60 mg and acet-aminophen 600/650 mg is a more effective analgesic than acetaminophen 600/650 mg alone. The addition of codeine to paracetamol increased the number of patients achieving at least 50 percent pain relief by 12 percent. The Cochrane Systematic Review concluded that paracetamol is an effective analgesic, associated with a low incidence of side effects. The addition of codeine 60 mg to paracetamol produces additional pain relief even in single oral doses but may be accompanied by an increase in drowsiness and dizziness.[138][I] Coproxamol, once the drug of choice combining paracetamol and dextropropoxyphene, became unpopular after a large number of successful suicide attempts and may cause confusion and drowsiness in older people because of its long elimination half-life.[139] The Cochrane Systematic Review of dextropropoxyphene alone and in combination with paracetamol focused on the effectiveness of the combination in relieving post-operative pain. It found that single-dose dextropropoxyphene and paracetamol were as effective as tramadol in postoperative pain and were associated with a lower incidence of adverse effects. Although it concluded that the same dose of paracetamol combined with codeine appeared to be more effective than paracetamol alone, there was an overlap in the 95 percent confidence intervals, allowing room for this conclusion to be challenged. This review also found that the number needed to treat was lower for ibuprofen than for either the combination of dextropropoxyphene plus paracetamol or tramadol.[140]

Strong opioids include morphine as well as some synthetic drugs, such as fentanyl. Tramadol and bupre-norphine do not provide better analgesia than morphine but may cause fewer gastrointestinal side effects, respira-tory problems, and urinary difficulties, than in older people receiving opioids.[141] In humans, morphine is metabolized extensively to M3G and M6G. These are both excreted predominantly into the urine,[142] and the requirements for morphine are lowered in patients with renal failure.[143] More recent experimental work has sug-gested that the nonrenal elimination of M3G becomes more important during renal failure.[144][III] Care, how-ever, must be maintained when administering morphine to older patients with physiological or pathologically impaired renal function.

In a randomized crossover study comparing trans-dermal fentanyl with sustained-release oral morphine, a significantly higher number of patients up to the age of 89 years preferred fentanyl patches,[145] despite the fact that WHO performance status and EORTC Global Quality of Life scores indicated that there were significant differences in pain relief between groups.

Morphine, particularly if administered intrathecally, will inhibit detrusor contractions. Although published data are lacking, terminally ill elderly patients with an overactive bladder may respond well to the administra-tion of morphine. This may in part explain the urinary retention frequently encountered in patients receiving morphine; although this effect traditionally is blamed on the coexistence of constipation, inhibition of detrusor contractions is a plausible alternative explanation.

The analgesic effect of opioids increases with increas-ing age. There is an inverse relationship between self-administered morphine consumption and age.[146, 147][III] This is fortunate as older people are four times as sensi-tive to opioid analgesia as younger ones, a finding that has been attributed to slower metabolism and elimination of these drugs in elderly subjects.[148] Mercadante et al.[149] found that patients aged 75 years or over were no more likely to be sensitive to opioid effects during titration of dose than individuals less than 65 years of age. Whilst the older group were receiving lower doses than the younger group, this study of 100 consecutive patients with cancer pain suggests that careful titration should be based on the individual response, rather than guided by age alone.

Constipation is a major problem associated with opioid administration. In older people, opioid use results in a decrease in peristalsis and secretion, thus a combi-nation of a softener and stimulant such as codanthrusate is the most appropriate approach. Gastric stasis is com-mon and dose related and, together with nausea, is most frequently an initial side effect of morphine. Campara et al.[150] reported an incidence of opioid-induced emesis of 28 percent.

Renal impairment may reduce the clearance of active metabolites of propoxyphene and morphine and, although morphine clearance is only minimally affected by mild or moderate hepatic impairment, it may be sig-nificantly reduced in patients with advanced disease.[151]

Many cancer patients continue to suffer pain and, even in cancer centers, documented evidence of morphine efficacy may be lacking.[152]

Cherny et al.[153] found that patients up to the age of 86 years referred to a pain service received a median of two different opioid drugs (range 1–8 different drugs), administered by a median of two different routes (range 1–4 routes), prior to their referral. Factors considered to be most important for selection of a specific opioid were that the drug had been used previously by the patient and was effective and well tolerated, or that the drug had been used without adverse effects or had not previously been tried. Thus, even patients with pain that is difficult to control often remain on oral opioid following referral to a specialist pain service. Unfortunately, a systematic review of different formulations of morphine failed to provide clear advice about sustained release morphine versus immediate release morphine.[154][I]

Many older people wish to return to the community for their palliative care. The use of implantable ports and catheter systems permits ambulatory delivery of drugs when combined with electronic pumps, and may be particularly useful for older patients who wish to remain in either their own homes or in nursing homes.[155] Whilst breakthrough pain has a negative impact on both patient and carer, the role of supplemental analgesia (rescue medication) has not been well studied. There is some evidence that transmucosal fentanyl is useful in the management of breakthrough pain and may be more effective than morphine, however, trials have been small in both terms of recruitment and number.[156][I]

Hydromorphone is a µ-selective full opioid agonist. It exerts similar pharmacological actions to morphine, and the oral analgesic potency ratio of hydromorphone to morphine is approximately 7.5:1. In a study including patients up to the age of 81 years, sedation, constipation, and nausea were reduced with hydromorphone compared with morphine.[157] Those patients who were switched from morphine to hydromorphone because of uncontrollable side effects experienced a 73 percent reduction in side effects and an improvement in pain control on a VAS.[158] Therefore, patients with uncontrolled pain who develop side effects with increasing doses of morphine may respond to conversion to hydromorphone.[159]

Oxycodone is a semisynthetic opioid derived from the naturally occurring opium alkaloid thebaine. The suggested oral potency ratio between oxycodone and morphine is between 2:3 and 3:4. However, because of the high oral bioavailability of oxycodone (up to 87 percent), a conservative approach to dose conversion is recommended, particularly in older people.[160] Other advantages of oxycodone are its short half-life[161] and it causes less nausea, hallucinations, and disturbed sleep than morphine sulfate tablets (MST).[162] Modified release oxycodone releases active drug in two distinct phases, leading to two apparent absorption half-lives of 0.6 and 6.9 hours.[163] It has good efficacy and is well tolerated in the management of cancer pain.[164]

Transdermal buprenorphine has superior safety when considering respiratory depression, renal impairment, and immunological deficit when compared with other WHO Step III opioids. It is well tolerated in older individuals with cancer pain.[165] Buprenorphine is beneficial in patients with reduced renal function, including those on hemodialysis and many of the problems of "rebound" of metabolites between dialysis sessions and the reduced dosage of morphine and codeine secondary to decreased renal clearance is avoided, due to its main excretion through the liver.[166] Therefore, in older individuals with impaired renal function, buprenorphine should be considered.

Fentanyl is a strong µ-agonist with potent analgesic action. Its delivery via a transdermal therapeutic system is particularly useful in older people. Although the usual dosing interval is 72 hours, individual pharmacokinetic variability is large, and some patients may require dosing intervals of 48 hours. Transdermal drug delivery is particularly beneficial in older patients who are unable to swallow because of impaired consciousness, severe mucositis, intractable nausea and vomiting, or dysphagia, and in those who experience unacceptable side effects with morphine preparations. The weight of evidence suggests that constipation is less common with fentanyl than with morphine. However, older patients with chronic skin disorders and limited dexterity are not ideal candidates for fentanyl patches.[167]

Much of the research about fentanyl has been in nonmalignant pain. Transdermal fentanyl has been found in chronic pain in AIDS patients, chronic low back pain, painful chronic pancreatitis and nonmalignant neuropathic pain to be both efficacious and to improve functional measures.[168, 169, 170, 171] A series of case reports of patients with chronic nonmalignant pain serve to indicate side effects of erythema at the application site, nausea, severe sweating, and pruritus.[172][IV] A large study comparing transdermal fentanyl and sustained relief oral morphine in a randomized crossover design, studied 256 patients (up to the age of 82 years) with chronic noncancer pain. Sixty-five percent of the patients preferred transdermal fentanyl, whereas 28 percent preferred sustained release oral morphine. Constipation was more common with morphine, than with fentanyl (48 versus 29 percent, $p < 0.001$). More patients withdrew due to adverse events whilst on fentanyl (10 versus 5 percent) with mild or moderate cutaneous problems being experienced by 41 percent of patients. Whilst this study did not include patients with malignant disease, the lower incidence of constipation is clearly an important consideration in the management of older patients.[173][III]

Swallowing impairment in many elderly patients may be a consequence of frailty, intercurrent disease such as stroke, motor neuron disease, or Parkinson's disease or tumor. Continuous infusion has the advantage that it can be used to administer not only analgesics but also drugs to manage nausea. The addition of anxiolytic agents may be particularly helpful in older patients who are agitated as a consequence of an acute confusional state. Although neuroleptics may be administered in younger patients, their use in older people may precipitate parkinsonian side effects, which impair mobility, feeding, and other activities of daily living.

ADDITIONAL ANALGESIA

Anesthetic agents

Whilst controlled trials are lacking, there is moderate evidence that ketamine is an effective analgesic, especially when used in combination with opioids,[174] including morphine.[175]

Antidepressants

Up to 12–15 percent of community-dwelling older people are diagnosed with depression.[176] The relationship between depression and pain in patients with cancer is well known, although the influence of one upon the other is still poorly understood. In a study by Spiegel et al.[177] that included older patients, the prevalence of depressive disorders was significantly higher among patients in the high-pain than among those in the low-pain group. The authors concluded that pain might play a causal role in producing depression, but their data could also have supported the opposite conclusion. Amitriptyline, a tricyclic antidepressant, is useful in treating neuropathic pain.[178][III] Many older patients with pain also have depression and difficulty sleeping. There is evidence of the analgesic efficacy of amitriptyline in older patients with trigeminal neuralgia and diabetic neuropathy,[179] although data in older patients with pain are lacking. The analgesic action of tricyclic antidepressants in neuropathic pain appears to be independent of their antidepressant effects as the speed of onset is faster and the effective dose is lower than for depression.[178][III] However, tricyclic antidepressants are difficult drugs to administer in older patients as they can result in postural hypotension, urinary hesitancy, and glaucoma.

Drugs affecting bone metabolism

Primary or secondary bone tumors are very painful and commonly found in older individuals. This is particularly the case with metastases spread from primary breast, lung, and prostate tumors. The hormone calcitonin not only has the potential to relieve pain, but also retains bone density. Whilst few studies looked predominantly at the treatment of bone pain from metastases with calcitonin, papers showed a nonsignificant effect of calcitonin on total pain and no evidence of calcitonin reducing analgesia consumption. A greater number of adverse effects were also observed in the group given calcitonin.[180][I]

In contrast to the role of calcitonin, bisphosphonates have been shown to be efficacious in providing some pain relief for bone metastases. After extrapolation of data from a systematic review, the number needed to treat to obtain pain relief at 4 weeks was 11 and at 12 weeks was 7. Unfortunately adverse drug reactions were high, with nausea and vomiting being reported in 24 studies. As with other studies, elderly patients were not analyzed separately and the small studies show only a trend to support the effectiveness of bisphosphonates in providing pain relief and they should therefore be considered when analgesics and/or radiotherapy are inadequate, rather than as a first line therapy.[181][I] The pain from metastatic prostate cancer has been shown to reduce from 27.9 to 21.1 percent, which was statistically significant. Further studies are needed because systematic reviews so far have included studies with different pain assessment tools and different bisphosphonates. The evidence so far is, however, suggestive that this particular group of patients may benefit more than others from bisphosphonates.[182][I] In contrast, patients with multiple myeloma, have been shown to have an amelioration of pain (OR = 0.59) (95 percent CI = 0.46 to 0.76) with bisphosphonates. The number needed to treat (NNT) was 11 to prevent one patient experiencing pain, and the recommended agents were clodronate or pamidronate.[183][I]

Anticonvulsant drugs

Like tricyclic antidepressants, anticonvulsants such as carbamazepine and phenytoin are useful in the management of neuropathic pain. Unfortunately, phenytoin may result in sedation or confusion as well as dizziness and unsteadiness, particularly on standing. Similarly, carbamazepine may cause sedation and nausea, which results in a poor oral intake. Neutropenia and thrombocytopenia as well as aplastic anemia have been reported in patients receiving carbamazepine, and thus repeated full blood counts are necessary in older patients, especially those with bone marrow involvement or who have recently undergone chemotherapy or radiotherapy. Hepatotoxicity and congestive cardiac failure have also been reported, and older patients may be particularly at risk of hyponatremia due to inappropriate secretion of antidiuretic hormone (ADH). Clonazepam may cause ataxia, and for this reason must be cautiously used in an elderly person in whom mobility is already impaired and/or who is liable to falls. Extreme care must be exercised when withdrawing benzodiazepines because of the risk of seizures, which are troublesome in their own right but often lead to falls and bony injury in older people.[184]

Evidence for the efficacy of anticonvulsant drugs in relieving acute and chronic pain is lacking. Wiffen et al.[185][I],[186] investigated trials of anticonvulsant use in patients with acute and chronic pain but could find no trials comparing different anticonvulsants and only one study specifically of cancer pain. In addition, there is no evidence that anticonvulsants are effective in relieving acute pain, although carbamazepine has been shown to be effective in chronic noncancer pain.[187][I] Similarly, gabapentin has been used in cancer-related neuropathic pain, with limited benefit.[188]

Nonpharmacological

Nonpharmacological analgesia in the form of imagery, relaxation training, and hypnosis has been used to treat procedure pain and many guidelines for the management of acute pain mention relaxation and cognitive approaches. Complementary and alternative medicine (CAM) is now considered to be an important form of care in both patients with cancer and chronic pain. A US study of the veterans attending oncology and chronic pain clinics, found a prevalence of 27.3 percent of individuals reporting CAM use within the past 12 months. The users had higher levels of education, higher income, and a belief that lifestyle contributes to illness. There was no difference in prevalence of CAM usage in those individuals with chronic pain versus those with cancer.[189] A study of 241 patients aged 18–92 years undergoing percutaneous vascular and renal procedures found that, although pain increased linearly with procedure time in the standard and the structured attention group, among the 82 patients in the hypnosis group (mean age 45, range 19–82 years) pain remained constant over time. Drug use in the standard treatment group was significantly higher than in either the structured attention or hypnosis group. With benefits for both economic considerations and patient comfort, the procedure times were significantly shorter in the hypnosis group than in the standard group.[190] A systematic review evaluated 27 papers, including one randomized controlled trial, and 24 case studies concluded that whilst hypnotherapy was used to treat a variety of symptoms, including pain, the heterogeneity and poor quality of the studies resulted in a call for further research to validate its efficacy.[191]

Ferrell et al.[111] found that, before entering a pain management program, older patients rarely used nondrug interventions. On a scale of 0–4 (0 = not helpful, 4 = very helpful) heat was used by 68 percent of patients, with a mean effectiveness of 3.2, cold was used by 19 percent of patients, with a mean effectiveness of 2.9, massage was used by 64 percent of patients, with a mean effectiveness of 2.9, and distraction was used by 47 percent of patients, with a mean effectiveness of 3.3. Auricular acupuncture has been used in older individuals with acute hip fracture in an attempt to reduce pain level. Those patients treated at three auricular acupuncture points had reduced anxiety level, reduced pain, and a lower heart rate on arrival at hospital than the placebo group. This may therefore guide research in older individuals with localized cancer pain.[192]

MASSAGE

There is a lack of sound research regarding the effectiveness of massage for pain relief among older people. Although Fraser and Kerr[193] found that back massage reduced anxiety scores, the groups studied were small. A study by Ferrell-Torry and Glick[194] of male patients up to the age of 77 found an average 60 percent reduction in the level of pain perception and a 24 percent fall in anxiety after two consecutive evenings of 30 minutes of therapeutic massage. Further research is needed to determine the benefit of massage as training is expensive and may at best provide no benefit and at worst have adverse effects if used inappropriately.[195] A Cochrane Systematic Review studied aromatherapy massage and found a reduction in

anxiety with both massage or aromatherapy, although three studies containing 117 patients of whom a large proportion were elderly found a reduction in pain following the intervention.[196]

TRANSCUTANEOUS ELECTRICAL NERVE STIMULATION

In transcutaneous electrical nerve stimulation (TENS), surface electrodes connected to a small portable battery are used to stimulate large-diameter nerves in the skin and subcutaneous tissues. The advantages of the use of TENS in older patients are that the machine is compact, lightweight, easily portable and, if patients wish to purchase one, relatively inexpensive. It is difficult to predict which patients will respond to TENS, but it is effective in some patients. Many elderly patients may already be familiar with TENS for the treatment of noncancer pain.

Although skin irritation, burns, and allergy to the gel applied to the skin are rare, it is important that TENS should not be used in the area of the carotid sinus and the larynx as there is a risk of hypotension or laryngeal spasm and TENS is not appropriate in patients who have a cardiac pacemaker in situ.[197]

RADIOTHERAPY

Radiotherapy for the palliation of painful bone metastases has been widely studied in a variety of age groups. On the whole, radiotherapy produces complete pain relief at one month in approximately 25 percent of patients and at least 50 percent relief in almost half of patients. Radioisotopes alone produce equivalent relief with a similar onset and duration to radiotherapy. However, following radioisotope treatment, patients report significantly fewer new sites of pain compared with control subjects who receive external irradiation alone.[198] A systematic review found little discernible difference in efficacy between fractionation schedules and different doses of the same schedule, although the data were not subanalyzed by age.[199] Cerebral metastases often cause intractable pain, and patients of all ages can be treated with radiotherapy.[200]

SPECIFIC PROBLEMS OF LATER LIFE

Dealing with patients who cannot respond verbally

Many elderly patients are unable to respond to questioning. These patients may have communication problems and be cognitively intact, or they may have cognitive impairment with no language barriers. Other communication difficulties may be exacerbated by distorted facial expression, such as occurs after a stroke, in patients with advanced Parkinson's disease, or as a result of facial dystonic movements. Communicating with such patients about food and drink or the need to be toileted is problematic, but determining patients' needs in these areas requires only crude levels of communication, whereas pain management is more complex and involves identification of pain and an assessment of response to treatment. Marzinski[201] devised methods of assessing pain using nonverbal behavior but found none to be entirely suitable. Most documented pain behaviors have been described in patients with acute pain aged 65 or younger, and research on chronic pain is usually conducted in alert elderly people. The difficulty of developing such scales was highlighted by Hurley et al.[202] who, after devising a scale to measure discomfort based on nursing observation of patients with advanced Alzheimer's disease, found that only nine items from an original 26-item scale remained after reliability testing.

Simons and Malabar,[203] in a study of three elderly care wards, used a combination of data sheet, pain assessment chart, and menu of observable pain behavior to identify those patients who were experiencing pain. They studied those patients who were able to communicate to validate nurses' observations. Although some nurses experienced difficulties using such a schema, it took about eight minutes to carry out the initial assessment and three minutes for each reassessment. The authors concluded that pain management in the verbally unresponsive older patient was improved by the schema and that the combined documentation was both effective and easy to administer.

Many ill or older people are silent when questioned about pain. This may not indicate the absence of pain but simply that the older person is trying to process the information that has been given.[204] There are guidelines "Responding to patients who are silent" which include elucidating the meanings of silence, its variability across cultures, and other factors that may be learned by patient observation.[205]

Many nursing home residents are cognitively impaired. In a US study of community nursing homes, the mean Folstein mini-mental state exam score was 12.1 ± 7.9 in the 217 subjects assessed. Of those able to take part in the study, 62 percent complained of pain, although this was not consistently documented in their records.[206]

A systematic review of papers assessing the diagnosis and management of pain in patients with cognitive impairment showed a pain prevalence of between 45 and 80 percent, with the prevalence of cognitive impairment being 50 percent. They highlighted the need for good VASs, and with limited success, used the colored analog scale (CAS), facial affective scale (FAS), and the faces pain scale (FPS), although they pointed out that many patients with dementia failed to fully comprehend them.[207]

The pain assessment in advanced dementia (PAINAD) scale, was validated in 88 nursing home residents with moderate and severe dementia. The PAINAD correlated with a nurse-reported pain score (NRPS), but poorly with a self-reported pain score (SRPS). When residents were found to be depressed using the Cornell scale for depression in dementia (CSDD), there was a difference between the SRPS and the NRPS. However, where no depression existed, there was no difference found. They concluded that PAINAD was a new and useful scoring system, although it failed to add much to assessments already reported by the nursing staff.[208][IV]

Patients with Down syndrome express pain or discomfort more slowly and in a less precise fashion than the general population. This study of 26 individuals lends further evidence that medical teams managing patients with communication problems should use pain control procedures even in the absence of obvious pain manifestations.[209]

People who are profoundly cognitively impaired cannot express their pain verbally, and behavior and physiological indices may provide the only indications that they are in pain.[210]

Nursing or residential home patients

Many older people with cancer may be living in residential or nursing homes. These patients are often frail and have multiple pathology, are being treated with numerous drugs, and, in many cases, have impaired cerebral function or communication problems, which compound the management of pain. The quality of pain management within this setting has been identified as an issue of concern.[211]

Although most authors do not study cancer pain exclusively, a high level of pain is seen in these patients. Over half of all nursing home residents report pain on a regular basis irrespective of cause, and a study of 49,971 nursing home residents found that 26 percent experienced pain daily.[212] In 25 percent of those with daily pain, no analgesia is prescribed.[213] In many residents, pain was associated with impairment in activities of daily living and mood. Even when pain was recognized, men, members of the racial minorities, and cognitively impaired patients had a higher risk of undertreatment. Indeed, only 25 percent of the residents experiencing daily pain were on appropriate medication.[214][IV] In a US study of 13,625 patients with cancer aged 65 or older, only 16 percent of those reporting pain received simple analgesia; 32 and 26 percent were given weak opioids and morphine, respectively. Of particular concern is the fact that patients older than 85 who were in pain were about 50 percent less likely to receive analgesia than those aged 65–74, and this group are likely to be overrepresented in a nursing home population. This study also confirmed that people from ethnic minority groups were less likely to receive analgesia, and for about 50 percent of the time there was a level of cognitive impairment in patients that made communication about pain difficult.[215]

Yates *et al.*[72] conducted interviews over three months in five large residential care settings in Australia. The ten focus groups included people aged 65 or older. Three key areas emerged: first, a resignation to pain, i.e. pain is common in chronic and long-term elderly people; second, ambivalence about the benefit of action, i.e. that pain-relieving medication and other pain management strategies provide only limited pain relief; and, finally, a reluctance to express pain, with participants indicating that one should not bother others with one's pain, that staff are too busy to help, and that the willingness of staff to help varied.

Pain is a common and underdiagnosed feature in older patients with cancer. Its management is poorly studied and, where evidence exists, undertreatment is often exposed. Old patients pose particular problems and until evidence exists, best practice will be lacking.

REFERENCES

1. IASP Subcommittee on Taxonomy. Pain terms: a list with definitions and notes on usage. *Pain.* 1980; **8**: 249–52.
2. Federation of State Medical Boards of the United States. *Model guidelines for the use of controlled substances for the treatment of pain.* Euless, TX: Federation of State Medical Boards of the United States, 1998.
3. Portenoy RK, Lesage P. Management of cancer pain. *Lancet.* 1999; **353**: 1695–700.
4. Ferrell BR, Dean G. The meaning of cancer pain. *Seminars in Oncology Nursing.* 1995; **11**: 17–22.
* 5. Ferrell BR, Taylor EJ, Sattler GR *et al.* Searching for the meaning of pain: cancer patients', caregivers' and nurses' perspectives. *Cancer Practice.* 1993; **1**: 185–94.
6. Carr DB, Goudas LC. Acute pain. *Lancet.* 1999; **353**: 2051–8.
7. Katz B, Helme RD. Pain problems in old age. In: Tallis RC, Fillit HM, Brocklehurst JC (eds). *Brocklehurst's textbook of geriatric medicine and gerontology*, 5th edn. London: Churchill Livingstone, 1998: 1423–30.
* 8. Ferrell BA, Ferrell BR, Osterweil D. Pain in the nursing home. *Journal of the American Geriatrics Society.* 1990; **38**: 409–14.
9. Bowling A, Browne PD. Social networks, health, and emotional well-being among the oldest old in London. *Journal of Gerontology.* 1991; **46**: S20–32.
10. Merskey H, Bogduk N (eds). *Classification of chronic pain: descriptions of chronic pain syndromes and definition of pain terms. Report by the International Association for the Study of Pain Task Force on Taxonomy*, 2nd edn. Seattle, WA: IASP Press, 1994.
11. Harkins SW, Kwentus J, Price DD. Pain and suffering in the elderly. In: Bonica JJ (ed.). *The management of pain*, 2nd edn. Philadelphia, PA: Lea & Febiger, 1990: 552–9.
* 12. Brockopp D, Warden S, Colclough G, Brockopp G. Elderly people's knowledge of and attitudes to pain management. *British Journal of Nursing.* 1996; **5**: 556–62.
* 13. Ferrell BR, Grant M, Chan J *et al.* The impact of cancer pain education on family caregivers of elderly patients. *Oncology Nursing Forum.* 1995; **22**: 1211–18.
14. McCaffery M. *Nursing the patient in pain.* Philadelphia, PA: JB Lippincott, 1972.
15. Anon. *Guideline No. 9.* Rockville, MD: Agency for Healthcare Policy and Research, 1994.
16. Bonica JJ. Treatment of cancer pain: current status and future needs. In: Fields JL, Dubner R, Cervero J (eds). *Advances in pain research and therapy.* New York: Raven Press, 1985: 589–616.
17. World Health Organization. *Cancer pain relief.* Geneva: WHO, 1986.
18. Portenoy RK. Cancer pain, epidemiology and syndromes. *Cancer.* 1989; **63**: 2298–307.
19. Bonica JJ, Loeser JD. Medical evaluation of the patient with pain. In: Bonica JJ, Loeser JD, Chapman CR, Fordyce WE (eds). *The management of pain*, 2nd edn. Philadelphia, PA: Lea & Febiger, 1990: 563–80.
20. World Health Organization. *Cancer pain relief and palliative care.* Geneva: WHO, 1990.
21. Cleeland CS, Gonin R, Hatfield AK *et al.* Pain and its treatment in outpatients with metastatic cancer. *New England Journal of Medicine.* 1994; **330**: 592–6.
22. Royal College of Surgeons and College of Anaesthetists Working Party (1990). *Commission on the provision of surgical services. Report of the Working Party on Pain after Surgery.* London: Royal College of Surgeons and College of Anaesthetists, 1990.
23. Lynn J, Teno JM, Phillips RS *et al.* Perceptions by family members of the dying experience of older and seriously ill patients. SUPPORT investigators. Study to understand prognoses and preferences for outcomes and risks of treatments. *Annals of Internal Medicine.* 1997; **126**: 97–106.
24. Goodwin JS, Samet JM, Key CR *et al.* Stage at diagnosis of cancer varies with age of the patient. *Journal of the American Geriatrics Society.* 1986; **34**: 20–6.
25. Samet JM, Hunt WC, Key CR *et al.* Choice of cancer therapy varies with age of patient. *Journal of the American Medical Association.* 1986; **255**: 3385–90.
* 26. Greenfield S, Blanco DM, Elashoff RM, Ganz PA. Patterns of care related to age of breast cancer patients. *Journal of the American Medical Association.* 1987; **257**: 2766–70.
* 27. Markman M, Lewis JL, Saigo P *et al.* Epithelial ovarian cancer in the elderly: the Memorial Sloan-Kettering Cancer Center experience. *Cancer.* 1993; **71**: 634–7.
28. Watkin SW, Hayhurst GK, Green JA. Time trends in the outcome of lung cancer management: a study of 9,090 cases diagnosed in the Mersey Region, 1974–1986. *British Journal of Cancer.* 1990; **61**: 590–6.
29. Henderson J, Goldacre MJ, Griffith M. Hospital care of the elderly in the final year of life: a population based study. *British Medical Journal.* 1990; **301**: 17–19.
30. Dunlop RJ, Davies RJ, Hockley JM. Preferred vs actual place of death: a hospital palliative care support team experience. *Palliative Medicine.* 1989; **3**: 197–201.

31. Jordhøy MS, Fayers P, Saltnes T *et al.* A palliative-care intervention and death at home: a cluster randomised trial. *Lancet.* 2000; **356**: 888–93.

32. Stout RW, Crawford V. Active-life expectancy and terminal dependency: trends in long-term geriatric care over 33 years. *Lancet.* 1988; **1**: 281–3.

33. Cartwright A. The role of hospitals in caring for people in the last year of their lives. *Age and Ageing.* 1991; **20**: 271–4.

34. Lövheim H, Sandman PO-laf, Kallin K *et al.* Poor staff awareness of analgesic treatment jeopardises adequate pain control in the care of older people. *Age and Ageing.* 2006; **35**: 257–61.

35. Harkins SW. Geriatric pain. Pain perceptions in the old. *Clinics in Geriatric Medicine.* 1996; **12**: 435–59.

∗ 36. Bellville J, Forrest WH, Miller E, Brown BW. Influence of age on pain relief from analgesics: a study of post operative patients. *Journal of the American Medical Association.* 1971; **217**: 1835–41.

∗ 37. Brochet B, Michel P, Barberger-Gateau P, Dartigues JF. Population-based study of pain in elderly people: a descriptive survey. *Age and Ageing.* 1998; **27**: 279–84.

∗ 38. Vigano A, Bruera E, Suarez-Almazor ME. Age, pain intensity, and opioid dose in patients with advanced cancer. *Cancer.* 1998; **83**: 1244–50.

∗ 39. Milne RW, McLean CF, Mather LE *et al.* Influence of renal failure on disposition of morphine, morphine-3-glucuronide and morphine-6 glucurinide in sheep during intravenous infusion with morphine. *Journal of Pharmacology and Experimental Therapeutics.* 1997; **282**: 779–86.

∗ 40. Davies G, Kingswood C, Street M. Pharmacokinetics of opioids in renal dysfunction. *Clinical Pharmacokinetics.* 1996; **31**: 410–22.

41. Dickson J. Night-time pain: the hidden problem. *Prescriber.* Supplement 1997; 3–6.

42. Tsevat J, Dawson NV, Wu AW *et al.* Health values of hospitalized patients 80 years or older. HELP Investigators. Hospitalized elderly longitudinal project. *Journal of the American Medical Association.* 1998; **279**: 371–5.

43. Scott J, Huskisson EC. Graphic representation of pain. *Pain.* 1976; **2**: 175–84.

44. Carlsson AM. Assessment of chronic pain. Aspects of the reliability and validity of the Visual Analogue Scale. *Pain.* 1983; **16**: 87–101.

45. Dalton J, Twomey T, Workman M. Pain relief for cancer patients. *Cancer Nursing.* 1988; **11**: 322–8.

46. Ahmedzai S. Palliative and terminal care. In: Fentiman IS, Monfardini S (eds). *Cancer in the elderly: treatment and research.* Oxford: Oxford Medical Publications, 1994: 152–68.

47. Dalton JA, McNaull F. A call for standardizing the clinical rating of pain intensity using a 0 to 10 rating scale. *Cancer Nursing.* 1998; **21**: 46–9.

48. Gagliese L, Melzack R. Chronic pain in elderly people. *Pain.* 1997; **70**: 3–14.

49. Baier RR, Gifford DR, Patry G *et al.* Ameliorating pain in nursing homes: a collaborative quality-improvement project. *Journal of the American Geriatrics Society.* 2004; **52**: 1988–95.

50. Gloth 3rd FM. Geriatric pain. Factors that limit pain relief and increase complications. *Geriatrics.* 2000; **55**: 46–8.

51. Cohen-Mansfield J. Nursing staff members' assessments of pain in cognitively impaired nursing home residents. *Pain Management Nursing.* 2005; **6**: 68–75.

52. Weiner DK, Rudy TE. Attitudinal barriers to effective treatment of persistent pain in nursing home residents. *Journal of the American Geriatrics Society.* 2002; **50**: 2035–40.

53. Bird J. Assessing pain in older people. *Nursing Standard.* 2005; **19**: 45–52.

54. Cowan DT, Fitzpatrick JM, Roberts JD *et al.* The assessment and management of pain among older people in care homes: current status and future directions. *International Journal of Nursing Studies.* 2003; **40**: 291–8.

∗ 55. Aaronson NK, Bullinger M, Ahmedzai S. A modular approach to quality of life assessment in cancer clinical trials. *Recent Results in Cancer Research.* 1988; **111**: 231–49.

56. Beck-Friis B, Strang P, Eklund G. Physical dependence of cancer patients at home. *Palliative Medicine.* 1989; **3**: 281–6.

57. Ferrell BA. Pain management in elderly people. *Journal of the American Geriatrics Society.* 1991; **39**: 64–73.

∗ 58. Closs SJ. Pain and elderly patients: a survey of nurses' knowledge and experiences. *Journal of Advanced Nursing.* 1996; **23**: 237–42.

59. Hardy C, Wallace C, Khansur T *et al.* Nutrition, cancer, and aging: an annotated review. II. Cancer cachexia and aging. *Journal of the American Geriatrics Society.* 1986; **34**: 219–28.

60. McWhirter JP, Pennington CR. Incidence and recognition of malnutrition in hospital. *British Medical Journal.* 1994; **308**: 945–8.

61. Murray N. Use of pain charts to optimise pain control in patients with multiple myeloma. *Palliative Care Today.* 1993: 54–55.

62. Melzack R. The McGill Pain Questionnaire: major properties and scoring methods. *Pain.* 1975; **1**: 277–99.

63. Turk DC, Okifuji A. Assessment of patients' reporting of pain: an integrated perspective. *Lancet.* 1999; **353**: 1784–8.

64. Carpenter JS, Brockopp D. Comparison of patients' ratings and examination of nurses' responses to pain intensity rating scales. *Cancer Nursing.* 1995; **18**: 292–8.

65. Jensen MP, Karoly P, Braver S. The measurement of clinical pain intensity: a comparison of six methods. *Pain.* 1986; **27**: 117–26.

66. Herr KA, Mobily PR. Comparison of selected pain assessment tools for use with the elderly. *Applied Nursing Research.* 1993; **6**: 39–46.

67. Latham J. Assessment and measurement of pain. *Palliative Care.* 1994; **3**: 75–8.

68. Davis GC, Atwood JR. The development of the Pain Management Inventory for patients with arthritis. *Journal of Advanced Nursing.* 1996; **24**: 236–43.

69. Cleary JF. Cancer pain in the elderly. In: Balducci L, Lyman GH, Ershler WB (eds). *Comprehensive geriatric oncology.* Amsterdam: Harwood Academic Publishers, 1998: 753–64.

70. Forbes K. Management of cancer pain in elderly patients. *Prescriber.* 1998; June: 21–8.

∗ 71. Ward SE, Goldberg N, Miller-McCauley V *et al.* Patient-related barriers to management of cancer pain. *Pain.* 1993; **52**: 319–24.

∗ 72. Yates P, Dewar A, Fentiman B. Pain: the views of elderly people living in long-term residential care settings. *Journal of Advanced Nursing.* 1995; **21**: 667–74.

73. Cherny NI, Catane R. Professional negligence in the management of cancer pain. *Cancer.* 1995; **76**: 2181–5.

74. Redmond K, Aapro MS. The nursing care of the elderly with cancer. In: Redmond K, Aapro MS (eds). *Cancer in the elderly. A nursing and medical perspective.* Scientific Updates, No. 2. Amsterdam: Elsevier, 1997: 63–78.

∗ 75. Cleeland CS, Cleeland LM, Dar R, Rinehardt LC. Factors influencing physician management of cancer pain. *Cancer.* 1986; **58**: 796–800.

76. Von Roenn JH, Cleeland CS, Gonin R *et al.* Physician attitudes and practice in cancer pain management: a survey from the Eastern Cooperative Oncology Group. *Annals of Internal Medicine.* 1993; **119**: 121–6.

77. Larue F, Colleau SM, Fontaine A *et al.* Oncologists and primary care physicians' attitudes towards pain control and morphine prescribing in France. *Cancer.* 1995; **76**: 2375–82.

78. McCaffery M. *Nursing the patient in pain*, 2nd edn. London: Harper and Row, 1983.

79. Ferrell BR, McGuire DV, Donovan MI. Knowledge and beliefs regarding pain in a sample of nursing faculty. *Journal of Professional Nursing.* 1993; **9**: 79–88.

80. Ferrell BR, Ferrell BA, Rhiner M, Grant M. Family factors influencing cancer pain management. *Postgraduate Medical Journal.* 1991; **67**: S64–9.

81. Porter J, Jick H. Addiction is rare in patients treated with narcotics. *New England Journal of Medicine.* 1980; **302**: 123.

82. Kaiko RF. Age and morphine analgesia in cancer patients with postoperative pain. *Clinical Pharmacology and Therapeutics.* 1980; **28**: 823–6.

83. Watt-Watson JH. Nurses' knowledge of pain issues: a survey. *Journal of Pain and Symptom Management.* 1987; **2**: 207–11.

∗ 84. McCaffery M, Ferrell B, O'Neil-Page E *et al.* Nurses' knowledge of opioid analgesic drugs and psychological dependence. *Cancer Nursing.* 1990; **13**: 21–7.

∗ 85. Slevin ML, Stubbs L, Plant JH *et al.* Attitudes to chemotherapy: comparing views of patients with cancer with those of doctors, nurses, and general public. *British Medical Journal.* 1990; **300**: 1458–60.

∗ 86. Ripamonti C, Filiberti A, Totis A *et al.* Suicide among patients with cancer cared for at home by palliative-care teams. *Lancet.* 1999; **354**: 1877–8.

87. Mystakidou K, Tsilika E, Parpa E *et al.* Psychological distress of patients with advanced cancer: Influence and contribution of pain severity and pain interference. *Cancer Nursing.* 2006; **29**: 400–5.

88. Sofaer B, Moore AP, Holloway I *et al.* Chronic pain as perceived by older people: a qualitative study. *Age and Ageing.* 2005; **34**: 462–6.

89. Given B, Given CW. Cancer nursing for the elderly. A target for research. *Cancer Nursing.* 1989; **12**: 71–7.

90. Woods NF, Lewis FM, Ellison ES. Living with cancer. Family experiences. *Cancer Nursing.* 1989; **12**: 28–33.

∗ 91. Yeager KA, Miaskowski C, Dibble SL, Wallhagen M. Differences in pain knowledge and perception of the pain experience between out-patients with cancer and their family caregivers. *Oncology Nursing Forum.* 1995; **22**: 1235–41.

∗ 92. Ferrell BR, Taylor EJ, Grant M *et al.* Pain management at home: struggle, comfort, and mission. *Cancer Nursing.* 1993; **16**: 169–78.

93. Grobe ME, Ilstrup DM, Ahmann DL. Skills needed by family members to maintain the care of an advanced cancer patient. *Cancer Nursing.* 1981; **4**: 371–5.

∗ 94. Ferrell BR, Rhiner M, Ferrell BA. Development and implementation of a pain education program. *Cancer.* 1993; **72**: 3426–32.

95. Ferrell BR, Rhiner M, Cohen MZ, Grant M. Pain as a metaphor for illness. Part 1: Impact of cancer pain on family caregivers. *Oncology Nursing Forum.* 1991; **18**: 1303–09.

96. Clotfelter CE. The effect of an educational intervention on decreasing pain intensity in elderly people with cancer. *Oncology Nursing Forum.* 1999; **26**: 27–33.

97. Rousseau P. Pain management in the terminally ill. *Journal of the American Geriatrics Society.* 1994; **42**: 1217–21.

98. Stetler C. Research utilization: defining the concept. *Image – The Journal of Nursing Scholarship.* 1985; **17**: 40–4.

99. Dufault MA, Bielecki C, Collins E, Willey C. Changing nurses' pain assessment practice: a collaborative research utilization approach. *Journal of Advanced Nursing.* 1995; **21**: 634–45.

100. Jandelli K. A comparative study of patients' and nurses' perceptions of pain relief. *International Journal of Palliative Nursing.* 1995; **1**: 74–80.

101. Marks RM, Sachar EJ. Under treatment of medical in-patients with narcotic analgesics. *Annals of Internal Medicine.* 1973; **78**: 173–81.

∗102. Cohen FL. Postsurgical pain relief: patients' status and nurses' medication choices. *Pain.* 1980; **9**: 265–74.

103. Wakefield AB. Pain: an account of nurses' talk. *Journal of Advanced Nursing.* 1995; **21**: 905–10.

104. Morrison P. Psychology of pain. *Surgical Nursing.* 1991; **4**: 18–20.

105. Woodward S. Nurse and patient perceptions of pain. *Professional Nurse.* 1995; **10**: 415–16.

106. Short LM, Burnett ML, Egbert AM, Parks LH. Nurse and patient perceptions of pain. Medicating the postoperative elderly: how do nurses make their decisions? *Journal of Gerontology Nursing.* 1990; **16**: 12–17.

∗107. Fossa SD, Aaronson NK, Newling D *et al.* Quality of life and treatment of hormone resistant metastatic prostatic cancer. *European Journal of Cancer.* 1990; **26**: 1133–6.

∗108. Grassi L, Agostini M, Magnani K. Attitudes of Italian doctors to euthanasia and assisted suicide for terminally ill patients. *Lancet.* 1999; **354**: 1876–7.

109. Jones WL, Rimer BK, Levy MH, Kinman JL. Cancer patients' knowledge, beliefs, and behaviour regarding pain control regimens: implications for education programmes. *Patient Education and Counseling.* 1984; **5**: 159–64.

∗110. Levin DN, Cleeland CS, Dar R. Public attitudes towards cancer pain. *Cancer.* 1985; **56**: 2337–9.

∗111. Ferrell BR, Ferrell BA, Ahn C, Tran K. Pain management for elderly patients with cancer at home. *Cancer.* 1994; **74**: 2139–46.

∗112. Greenblatt D, Allen MD, Locniskar A *et al.* Lorazepam kinetics in the elderly. *Clinical Pharmacology and Therapeutics.* 1979; **26**: 103–13.

∗113. Wynne HA, Cope LH, Herd B *et al.* The association of age and frailty with paracetamol conjugation in man. *Age and Ageing.* 1990; **19**: 419–24.

114. Preiss R, Matthias M, Sohr R *et al.* Pharmacokinetics of adriamycin, adriamycinol and antipyrine in patients with moderate tumour involvement of the liver. *Journal of Cancer Research and Clinical Oncology.* 1987; **113**: 593–8.

∗115. Robertz-Vaupel GM, Lindecken KD, Edeki T *et al.* Disposition of antipyrine in patients with extensive metastatic liver disease. *European Journal of Clinical Pharmacology.* 1992; **42**: 465–9.

∗116. Castleden CM, George CF, Marcer D, Hallett C. Increased sensitivity to nitrazepam in old age. *British Medical Journal.* 1977; **1**: 10–12.

∗117. Cook PJ, Flanagan R, James IM. Diazepam tolerance: effect of age, regular sedation, and alcohol. *British Medical Journal.* 1984; **289**: 351–3.

118. Smith JM, Baldessarini RJ. Changes in prevalence, severity and recovery in tardive dyskinesia with age. *Archives of General Psychiatry.* 1980; **37**: 1368–73.

∗119. Bateman DN, Darling DW, Boys R, Rawlins MD. Extrapyramidal reactions to metoclopramide and prochlorperazine. *Quarterly Journal of Medicine.* 1989; **71**: 307–11.

120. Cox S, Tookman A. Management of cancer and neuropathic pain. *Prescriber.* 1998; March: 85–8.

121. Campbell W. Appropriate drug treatment of mild-to-moderate pain. *Prescriber.* 2004: 36–48.

122. Beaulieu J. Recommended analgesics in acute and chronic pain. *Prescriber.* 2000; September: 63–74.

123. Singh G, Rosen Ramey D. NSAID induced gastrointestinal complications: the ARAMIS perspective – 1997. Arthritis, Rheumatism, and Aging Medical Information System. *Journal of Rheumatology.* Supplement. 1998; **51**: 8–16.

124. Tramer MR, Moore RA, Reynolds DJ *et al.* Quantitative estimation of rare adverse events which follow a biological progression: a new model applied to chronic NSAID use. *Pain.* 2000; **85**: 169–82.

∗125. Henry D, Lim LL, Garcia-Rodrigues LA *et al.* Variability in risk of gastrointestinal complications with individual non-steroidal anti-inflammatory drugs: results of a collaborative meta-analysis. *British Medical Journal.* 1996; **312**: 1563–6.

126. McCallion J, McLaren B, Blech JJF, Erwin L. Effects of fenbufen and indomethacin on renal function and prostaglandin synthesis in elderly patients. *Journal of Clinical and Experimental Gerontology.* 1989; **11**: 97–105.

127. Yeomans ND, Tulassay Z, Juhasz L *et al.* A comparison of omeprazole with ranitidine for ulcers associated with nonsteroidal anti-inflammatory drugs. Acid Suppression Trial: Ranitidine versus Omeprazole for NSAID-associated Ulcer Treatment (ASTRONAUT) Study Group. *New England Journal of Medicine.* 1998; **338**: 719–26.

∗128. Cannon GW. Rofecoxib: a specific cyclooxygenase inhibitor. *Drugs of Today.* 2000; **36**: 255–62.

∗129. Schnitzer TJ, Truitt K, Fleischmann R *et al.* The safety profile, tolerability, and effective dose range of rofecoxib in the treatment of rheumatoid arthritis. Phase II Rofecoxib Rheumatoid Arthritis Study Group. *Clinical Therapeutics.* 1999; **21**: 1688–702.

130. Emery P, Zeidler H, Kvien TK *et al.* Celecoxib versus diclofenac in long-term management of rheumatoid arthritis: randomised double-blind comparison. *Lancet.* 1999; **354**: 2106–11.

131. Are rofecoxib and celecoxib safer NSAIDs? *Drug and Therapeutics Bulletin.* 2000; **38**: 81–86.

132. Cannon CP, Curtis SP, Fitzgerald GA *et al.* Cardiovascular outcomes with etoricoxib and diclofenac in patients with osteoarthritis and rheumatoid arthritis in the Multinational Etoricoxib and Diclofenac Arthritis Long-term (MEDAL) programme: a randomised comparison. *Lancet.* 2006; **368**: 1771–81.

133. McNicol E, Strassels SA, Goudas L *et al.* NSAIDS or paracetamol, alone or combined with opioids, for cancer pain. *Cochrane Database of Systematic Reviews.* 2005; CD005180.

134. Field GB, Parry J. Pain control: some aspects of day-to-day management. *Palliative Care.* 1994; **3**: 79–86.

135. Tookman A. Myths of morphine. *Palliative Care Today.* 1996; **13**.

∗136. de Craen AJ, di Giulio G, Lampe-Schoenmaeckers JE *et al.* Analgesic efficacy and safety of paracetamol/codeine combinations versus paracetamol alone: a systematic review. *British Medical Journal.* 1996; **313**: 321–5.

137. Moore A, Collins S, Carroll D, McQuay H. Paracetamol with and without codeine in acute pain: a quantitative systemic review. *Pain.* 1997; **70**: 193–201.

138. Moore A, Collins S, Carroll D, McQuay H. Single dose paracetamol (acetaminophen), with and without codeine,

for postoperative pain. *Cochrane Database of Systematic Reviews.* 2000; **CD001547**.

*139. Flanagan RJ, Johnston A, White AS, Crome P. Pharmacokinetics of dextropropoxyphene and nordextropropoxyphene in young and elderly volunteers after single and multiple dextropropoxyphene dosage. *British Journal of Clinical Pharmacology.* 1989; **28**: 463–9.

*140. Collins SL, Edwards JE, Moore RA, McQuay HJ. Single dose dextropropoxyphene, alone and with paracetamol (acetaminophen), for postoperative pain. *Cochrane Database of Systematic Reviews.* 2000; **CD001440**.

141. Livingstone H, Young J. Morphine. Appropriate use in older people. *Geriatric Medicine.* 2000; February: 33–6.

142. Osborne R, Joel S, Trew D, Slevin M. Morphine and metabolite behaviour after different routes of morphine administration: demonstration of the importance of the active metabolite morphine-6-glucuronide. *Clinical Pharmacology and Therapeutics.* 1990; **47**: 12–19.

143. Regnard CF, Twycross RG. Metabolism of narcotics. *British Medical Journal (Clinical Research Edition).* 1984: **288**: 860.

144. Milne RW, McLean CF, Mather LE *et al.* Influence of renal failure on the disposition of morphine, morphine-3-glucuronide and morphine-6-glucuronide in sheep during intravenous infusion with morphine. *Journal of Pharmacology and Experimental Therapeutics.* 1997; **282**: 779–86.

145. Ahmedzai S, Brooks D. Transdermal fentanyl versus sustained-release oral morphine in cancer pain: preference, efficacy, and quality of life. *Journal of Pain and Symptom Management.* 1997; **13**: 254–61.

*146. Burns JW, Hodsman NB, McLintock TT *et al.* The influence of patient characteristics on the requirements for post operative analgesia. *Anaesthesia.* 1989; **44**: 2–6.

147. Zacharias M, Pfeifer MV, Herbison P. Comparison of two methods of intravenous administration of morphine for post-operative pain relief. *Anaesthesia and Intensive Care.* 1990; **18**: 205–09.

*148. Kaiko RF, Wallenstein SL, Rodgers AE *et al.* Narcotics in the elderly. *Medical Clinics of North America.* 1982; **66**: 1079–89.

149. Mercadante S, Ferrera P, Villari P, Casuccio A. Opioid escalation in patients with cancer pain: the effect of age. *Journal of Pain and Symptom Management.* 2006; **32**: 413–9.

150. Campara E, Merlin L, Pace M. The incidence of narcotic induced emesis. *Journal of Pain and Symptom Management.* 1991; **6**: 428–30.

151. Cherny NI, Portenoy RK. Cancer pain management. Current strategy. *Cancer.* 1993; **72**: 3393–415.

*152. Zenz T. Palliative pain relief. *Lancet.* 2000; **356**: 1273–4.

*153. Cherny NJ, Chang V, Frager G *et al.* Opioid pharmacotherapy in the management of cancer pain. *Cancer.* 1995; **76**: 1283–93.

154. Wiffen PJ, Edwards JE, Barden J, McQuay HJ. Oral morphine for cancer pain. *Cochrane Database of Systematic Reviews.* 2003; **CD003868**.

155. Shaw HL. Treatment of intractable cancer pain by electronically controlled parenteral infusion of analgesic drugs. *Cancer.* 1993; **72**: 3416–25.

156. Zeppetella G, Ribeiro MD. Opioids for the management of breakthrough (episodic) pain in cancer patients. *Cochrane Database of Systematic Reviews.* 2006; **CD004311**.

157. MacDonald CJ, Smith AT, Smith KJ *et al.* Opioid rotation: a place for hydromorphone. *Poster Presentation, Pain Society of Great Britain and Ireland.* 1997.

*158. De Stoutz ND, Bruera E, Suarez-Almazor M. Opioid rotation for toxicity reduction in terminal cancer patients. *Journal of Pain and Symptom Management.* 1995; **10**: 378–84.

159. Ellershaw J. Hydromorphone: a new alternative to morphine. *Prescriber.* 1998; February: 21–4.

160. Jones B, Finlay I. Oxycodone: alternative to morphine in cancer pain. *Prescriber.* 2000; October: 43–50.

161. Leng M. Oxycodone's place in pain in malignancy. *Prescriber.* Supplement. 2000; (Suppl): 9–12.

*162. Kalso E, Vainio A. Morphine and oxycodone hydrochloride in the management of cancer pain. *Clinical Pharmacology and Therapeutics.* 1990; **47**: 639–46.

163. O'Brien A. Oxycodone. *Palliative Care Today.* 2000: 54–5.

164. Kaplan R, Parris WC, Citron ML *et al.* Comparison of controlled-release and immediate-release oxycodone tablets in patients with cancer pain. *Journal of Clinical Oncology.* 1998; **16**: 3230–7.

165. Sittl R. Transdermal buprenorphine in cancer pain and palliative care. *Palliative Medicine.* 2006; **20**: s25–30.

166. Böger RH. Renal impairment: a challenge for opiod treatment? The role of buprenorphine. *Palliative Medicine.* 2006; **20**: s17–23.

167. Edmonds P, Davies C. New approaches to the pharmacological management of pain. *Palliative Care Today.* 1995: 32–4.

168. Newshan G, Lefkowitz M. Transdermal fentanyl for chronic pain in AIDS: a pilot study. *Journal of Pain and Symptom Management.* 2001; **21**: 69–77.

169. Niemann T, Madsen LG, Larsen S, Thorsgaard N. Opioid treatment of painful chronic pancreatitis. *International Journal of Pancreatology.* 2000; **27**: 235–40.

170. Simpson Jr RK, Edmondson EA, Constant CF, Collier Jr C. Transdermal fentanyl as treatment for chronic low back pain. *Journal of Pain and Symptom Management.* 1997; **14**: 218–24.

171. Dellemijn PL, van Duijn H, Vanneste JA. Prolonged treatment with transdermal fentanyl in neuropathic pain. *Journal of Pain and Symptom Management.* 1998; **16**: 220–9.

172. Milligan KA, Campbell C. Transdermal fentanyl in patients with chronic, nonmalignant pain: a case study series. *Advances in Therapy.* 1999; **16**: 73–7.

173. Allan L, Hays H, Jensen NH *et al.* Randomised crossover trial of transdermal fentanyl and sustained release oral morphine for treating chronic non-cancer pain. *British Medical Journal.* 2001; **322**: 1154–8.

174. Legge J, Ball N, Elliott DP. The potential role of ketamine in hospice analgesia: a literature review. *Consultant Pharmacist.* 2006; **21**: 51-7.

175. Bell RF, Eccleston C, Kalso E. Ketamine as adjuvant to opioids for cancer pain. A qualitative systematic review. *Journal of Pain and Symptom Management.* 2003; **26**: 867-75.

176. Beekman ATF, Copeland JRM, Prince MJ. Review of community prevalence of depression in late life. *British Journal of Psychiatry.* 1999; **174**: 307-11.

*177. Speigel D, Sands S, Koopman C. Pain and depression in patients with cancer. *Cancer.* 1994; **74**: 2570-8.

178. McQuay HJ, Tramer M, Nye BA et al. A systematic review of antidepressants in neuropathic pain. *Pain.* 1996; **68**: 217-27.

179. Portenoy RK. Adjuvant analgesics in pain management. In: Doyle D, Hanks GWC MacDonald N (eds). *Oxford textbook of palliative medicine.* Oxford: Oxford University Press, 1993: 187-203.

180. Martinez-Zapata MJ, Roque M, Alonso-Coello P, Catala E. Calcitonin for metastatic bone pain. *Cochrane Database of Systematic Reviews.* 2006; **CD003223**.

181. Wong R, Wiffen PJ. Bisphosphonates for the relief of pain secondary to bone metastases. *Cochrane Database of Systematic Reviews.* 2002; **CD002068**.

182. Yuen KK, Shelley M, Sze WM et al. Bisphosphonates for advanced prostate cancer. *Cochrane Database of Systematic Reviews.* 2006; **CD006250**.

183. Djulbegovic B, Wheatley K, Ross J et al. Bisphosphonates in multiple myeloma. *Cochrane Database of Systematic Reviews.* 2002; **CD003188**.

184. Anon. Drug treatment of neuropathic pain. *Drugs and Therapeutics Bulletin.* 2000; **38**: 89-93.

185. Wiffen P, Collins S, McQuay H et al. Anticonvulsant drugs for acute and chronic pain. *Cochrane Database of Systematic Reviews.* 2000; **CD001133**.

186. Wiffen P, Collins S, McQuay H et al. Anticonvulsant drugs for acute and chronic pain. *Cochrane Database of Systematic Reviews.* 2005; **CD001133**.

187. Wiffen PJ, McQuay HJ, Moore RA. Carbamazepine for acute and chronic pain. *Cochrane Database of Systematic Reviews.* 2005; **CD005451**.

188. Wiffen PJ, McQuay HJ, Edwards JE, Moore RA. Gabapentin for acute and chronic pain. *Cochrane Database of Systematic Reviews.* 2005; **CD005452**.

189. McEachrane-Gross FP, Liebschutz JM, Berlowitz D. Use of selected complementary and alternative medicine (CAM) treatments in veterans with cancer or chronic pain: a cross-sectional survey. *BMC Complementary and Alternative Medicine.* 2006; **6**: 34.

*190. Lang EV, Benotsch EG, Fick LJ et al. Adjunctive non-pharmacological analgesia for invasive medical procedures: a randomised trial. *Lancet.* 2000; **355**: 1486-90.

191. Rajasekaran M, Edmonds PM, Higginson IL. Systematic review of hypnotherapy for treating symptoms in terminally ill adult cancer patients. *Palliative Medicine.* 2005; **19**: 418-26.

192. Barker R, Kober A, Howerauf K et al. Out-of-hospital auricular acupressure in elder patients with hip fracture: a randomized double-blinded trial. *Academic Emergency Medicine.* 2006; **13**: 19-23.

*193. Fraser J, Kerr JR. Psychophysiological effects of back massage on elderly institutionalised patients. *Journal of Advanced Nursing.* 1993; **18**: 238-45.

*194. Ferrell-Torry AT, Glick OJ. The use of therapeutic massage as a nursing intervention to modify anxiety and the perception of cancer pain. *Cancer Nursing.* 1993; **16**: 93-101.

195. Closs SJ. Pain in elderly patients: a neglected phenomenon? *Journal of Advanced Nursing.* 1994; **19**: 1072-81.

196. Fellowes D, Barnes K, Wilkinson S. Aromatherapy and massage for symptom relief in patients with cancer. *Cochrane Database of Systematic Reviews.* 2004; **CD002287**.

197. Sharma K. TENS and sensibility. *Health and Ageing.* 2001; April: 28-9.

*198. Porter AT, McEwan AJ. Strontium-89 as an adjuvant to external beam radiation improves pain relief and delays the disease progression in advanced prostate cancer: results of a randomised controlled trial. *Seminars in Oncology.* 1993; **20**: 38-43.

199. McQuay HJ, Collins SL, Carroll D, Moore RA. Radiotherapy for the palliation of painful bone metastases. *Cochrane Database of Systematic Reviews.* 2000; **CD001793**.

200. Coia LR. The role of radiotherapy in the treatment of brain metastases. *International Journal of Radiation Oncology, Biology, Physics.* 1992; **23**: 229-38.

201. Marzinski LR. The tragedy of dementia: assessing pain in the confused non-verbal elderly. *Journal of Gerontology Nursing.* 1991; **17**: 25-8.

*202. Hurley AC, Volicer BJ, Hanrahan PA et al. Assessment of discomfort in advanced Alzheimer patients. *Research in Nursing and Health.* 1992; **15**: 369-77.

*203. Simons W, Malabar R. Assessing pain in elderly patients who cannot respond verbally. *Journal of Advanced Nursing.* 1995; **22**: 663-9.

204. Murray R, Hueskoetter M. *Psychiatric/mental health nursing.* Norwalk, CT: Appleton and Lange, 1987.

205. Davidhizar R, Giger-Newman J. When your patient is silent. *Journal of Advanced Nursing.* 1994; **20**: 703-06.

206. Ferrell BA, Ferrell BR, Rivera L. Pain in congnitively impaired nursing home patients. *Journal of Pain and Symptom Management.* 1995; **10**: 591-8.

207. Frampton M. Experience assessment and management of pain in people with dementia. *Age and Ageing.* 2003; **32**: 248-51.

208. Leong IY, Chong MS, Gibson SJ. The use of a self-reported pain measure, a nurse-reported pain measure and the PAINAD in nursing home residents with moderate and severe dementia: a validation study. *Age and Ageing.* 2006; **35**: 252-6.

*209. Hennequin M, Morin C, Feine JS. Pain expression and stimulus localization in individuals with Down's syndrome. *Lancet.* 2000; **356**: 1882–7.

210. Abu-Saad HH. Challenge of pain in the cognitively impaired. *Lancet.* 2000; **356**: 1867–8.

211. Hutt E, Pepper GA, Vojir C *et al.* Assessing the apprpriateness of pain medication prescribing practices in nursing homes. *Journal of the American Geriatrics Society.* 2006; **54**: 231–9.

212. Ferrell BR, Ferrell BA. Easing the pain. *Geriatric Nursing.* 1990; **11**: 175–8.

213. Won AB, Lapane KL, Vallow S *et al.* Persistent nonmalignant pain and analgesic prescribing patterns in elderly nursing home residents. *Journal of the American Geriatrics Society.* 2004; **52**: 867–74.

214. Won A, Lapane K, Gambassi G *et al.* on behalf of the SAGE Study Group. Correlates and management of nonmalignant pain in the nursing home. *Journal of the American Geriatrics Society.* 1999; **47**: 936–42.

*215. Bernabei R, Gambassi G, Lapane K *et al.* for the SAGE Study Group Management of pain in elderly patients with cancer. *Journal of the American Medical Association.* 1998; **279**: 1877–82.

Cancer pain management in the context of substance abuse

SHARON M WEINSTEIN

Introduction   379
The impact of substance abuse on cancer pain
   management   380
Patient assessment   381
Management guidelines   381
Case example   385
Medicolegal issues   386
Research directions   386
Conclusions   386
References   387

KEY LEARNING POINTS

- The care of cancer pain patients with substance abuse is complex.
- Multidisciplinary management of cancer pain patients with substance abuse is often necessary.
- Cancer pain patients with substance abuse may be treated with psychoactive medications, including opioid analgesics.
- Body fluid screening and written care agreements may be useful in the management of cancer pain patients with substance abuse.

- Oncologists should be familiar with general guidelines for the management of pain patients with substance abuse.
- Pain medicine and palliative care specialists may be best suited to coordinate the multidisciplinary care of cancer pain patients with substance abuse.

INTRODUCTION

Among the most challenging problems in all of medicine is the management of cancer patients with pain and substance abuse disorder (substance use despite harm or addiction). A concurrent diagnosis of a substance abuse (SA) disorder complicates clinical pain management. Significant medicolegal and ethical considerations may arise.

The use of certain substances (alcohol and nicotine) is known to increase the risk of cancer, and so patients with concurrent SA may be overrepresented in the cancer population. Although a minority of all patients with cancer-related pain, this subpopulation requires careful management. Clinicians providing pain management and palliative care should be prepared for complex presentations. Patients with cancer-related pain and SA require closer supervision than patients without such dual diagnoses and they generally utilize more health care resources. Unscheduled outpatient and emergency visits occur often. Frequent multidisciplinary staff meetings and family conferences may be required. When also socially disadvantaged, patients may require financial assistance, transportation arrangements, housing, and legal aid. It is important to remember, however, that SA is not restricted to the lower socioeconomic stratum.

Although clinical reports and formal research in this area are limited, there is extensive literature on pertinent subjects, which include guidelines for the therapeutic use of opioid analgesics; definitions and conceptualizations of addiction and related phenomena; treatment of chemical dependency; psycho-oncology; and quality of life.[1, 2, 3]

Clinicians treating patients with cancer-related pain should be thoroughly familiar with the general principles of pain management. The proper prescribing of opioid analgesics requires a thorough understanding of their physiological effects, including analgesia. The analgesic effect of opioid agonists is due to the interaction of exogenously administered drug with complex neural networks that transmit and interpret nociceptive messages, through reversible binding to endogenous opioid receptors of several subtypes. Marked interindividual variability of opioid responsiveness is well recognized. The benefit-to-risk ratio of opioid therapy relates to various factors, foremost of which is the clinical condition with which pain is associated. Opioids are the mainstay of therapy for acute pain, cancer-related pain, and chronic pain associated with other life-limiting illnesses. The first United States federal guidelines for the treatment of cancer-related pain were released by the Agency for Health Care Policy and Research in 1994.[4] The majority of cancer patients will obtain adequate pain control using oral opioids according to the World Health Organization three-step analgesic ladder.[5] In contrast to persons without pain who are seeking mood-altering effects of psychoactive substances, cancer patients with pain report dysphoria more commonly than euphoria as a side effect of opioids. The risk of iatrogenic addiction in the setting of pain treatment is extremely low.

In recent decades, understanding of SA and addiction has evolved considerably, although the interplay between heredity and environment is not fully understood. Neurotransmitter systems involved in reward circuits in the human brain have been identified.[6] It is noted that there is overlap between the physiologic systems that mediate reward and analgesia although they are clearly distinct in many aspects. The two key components of the syndrome of substance abuse are: (1) use of a substance for its psychoactive effects despite the presence or potential for detrimental results ("use despite harm"), and (2) inability to control substance use or behavior ("compulsive use"). The Diagnostic and Statistical Manual (DSM) IV definition of substance dependence specifies physical dependence as a criterion. It is essential to recognize however, that physical dependence is not as useful a criterion in the setting of pain treatment with opioid analgesics. Patients maintained on chronic opioid therapy will generally develop physical dependence, but that is rarely associated with psychological dependence and is not usually clinically problematic. The DSM IV criteria for substance abuse emphasize the kinds of harm a patient may experience as a result of a maladaptive pattern of drug use.[7] Other authors have proposed a new nomenclature to

be used in the settings of pain management and palliative care.[8]

It has been noted that healthcare professionals' knowledge deficits, fear of scrutiny by regulatory agencies, and exaggerated fear of patient addiction result in underprescribing of opioid analgesics.[9][IV] Cancer pain patients with concurrent SA are at elevated risk of undertreatment of their pain, due to practitioner inexperience and the complexity of clinical issues. The treatment of SA in other settings usually includes psychological interventions and abstinence from the drug of abuse. There are limited data on which to base a nonabstinence model of treatment for the cancer pain patient with SA. It is difficult to find programs for patients needing both treatment for psychological dependence and ongoing medical therapy with psychoactive drugs, especially opioids.

Advances in the field of psycho-oncology have helped define the nature of psychological and psychiatric issues experienced by cancer patients. Contemporary psycho-oncology offers specific strategies for the provision of psychological support and psychiatric treatment of common diagnoses, such as depression, anxiety, and delirium. Quality of life research has emphasized the different components of distress or suffering in the cancer population, which include unrelieved physical symptoms, psychological and family concerns. Regardless of prognosis, when managing pain with opioid analgesics it is essential to distinguish worsening function from pain relief with improved function as outcomes of treatment. However, for patients with very advanced cancer, functional goals must be carefully established as physical capabilities can be expected to decline due to disease progression. When patients are approaching death, there may not be sufficient time to offer in-depth psychotherapy for the treatment of SA, and psychological interventions may be mainly supportive to the patient and family as they face end of life issues.[10][V]

The objectives of this chapter are to describe the impact of concurrent SA on cancer pain management, detail methods of patient assessment, describe a multidisciplinary approach to enhance compliance with pain treatment in cancer patients with SA, and outline issues for future investigation.

THE IMPACT OF SUBSTANCE ABUSE ON CANCER PAIN MANAGEMENT

The management of pain in the cancer patient is complicated by concurrent SA in several ways:

- assessment is based on trust, which may be eroded;
- patients may not always be able to distinguish analgesia from other psychoactive effects;
- patients lack personal behavioral controls;
- patients often live in "dysfunctional" settings;
- medicolegal and ethical issues arise.

Firstly, trust is the basis of any therapeutic relationship. Trust is easily eroded when clinicians are expecting manipulative behavior from patients and patients have long-term experience with reluctant care providers.[11] Pain assessment is difficult if it is assumed that patients cannot make distinctions between pain, anxiety, and other kinds of psychological distress. Patients with SA are more likely to have poor family and social support systems. They may be living with persons who also have SA. The lack of control over use of a potentially addictive substance characterizes SA, and this can interfere directly with the implementation of effective pharmacologic therapy for pain. Overt illegal behaviors may further limit the prescription and use of controlled substances. Under these circumstances, patients' pain may be left untreated resulting in increased suffering, worsening psychological distress, and an ensuing vicious cycle. Care becomes chaotic as patients make erratic, ineffective use of healthcare resources.

PATIENT ASSESSMENT

Early identification of patients with SA is important, since patients with this diagnosis are thought to be at increased risk for aberrant drug taking during medical therapy with abusable drugs. Early identification also allows the coordinated engagement of clinical professionals who bring specific expertise to the management plan. Suggested multidisciplinary care team members are as follows:

- physicians:
  - pain specialist;
  - psychiatrist;
  - addiction specialist;
- nurses:
  - pain specialist;
  - psychiatric clinician;
  - addiction specialist;
- social workers:
  - mental health specialist;
  - addiction specialist;
- psychologists:
  - pain specialist;
  - addiction specialist;
- clinical pharmacists:
  - pain specialist;
  - addiction specialist.

There are several ways in which SA may be recognized in the clinical practice setting:

- history:
  - medical history;
  - psychiatric history;
  - substance use history;
  - psychosocial history;

- examination:
  - physical examination;
  - psychiatric examination;
- family interviews.

Methods of prospective identification of patients with SA include routine medical history taking, physical examination, interviews of family members, and the use of self-administered questionnaires or more extensive structured interview tools. A simple yet specific method of screening for alcohol abuse may be easily incorporated in routine practice.[12][IV] In the absence of a complete history, provider observations of patient behaviors may lead to the diagnosis. Body fluids' screening is used more commonly after the clinical index of suspicion has been raised, or as part of the care plan after diagnosis (see below under Drug testing in pain management). Complete neuropsychological and psychiatric assessment is recommended when questions of cognitive dysfunction and psychiatric comorbidity are raised.

It is useful to characterize different types of aberrant drug-taking behavior.[13] Some medication requests ("drug-seeking" behavior) may reflect undertreatment of pain with "pseudo-addiction"[14] while other behaviors may reflect true SA. Pseudo-addiction may be associated with increasing pain, inadequate pain management, or logistical problems such as lack of access to prescribed medications and nonpharmacologic therapies. Other more problematic behaviors demand immediate attention from the provider, such as confirmed criminal activity. A format for categorizing clinical problems is shown in **Table 27.1**. It is suggested that this be used to organize the clinical problem list for multidisciplinary team discussion and treatment planning.

The diagnosis of SA is made in the context of a thorough evaluation of the patient, including full characterization of the underlying pathophysiology of the pain complaint(s). Clinicians should remember that many cancer patients experience neuropathic pain for which there may be no confirmatory diagnostic tests and that often require complex pharmacotherapy with several psychoactive medications, i.e. rational polypharmacy. Careful physical examination with detailed neurologic testing will often reveal neurologic dysfunction that is supportive of the clinical diagnosis of neuropathic pain. It is also important for clinicians to keep in mind that pain is only one of several symptoms that are likely to be present.

MANAGEMENT GUIDELINES

At one busy tertiary cancer center, the University of Texas MD Anderson Cancer Center (MDACC), a program was instituted in 1992 to address the special needs of cancer pain patients with SA while endeavoring to conserve clinical resources. This multidisciplinary program included

Table 27.1 Spectrums of active clinical problems – apply to individual patient.

Type of substance[a]	Current use (Y/N)	In recovery (Y/N)	Functional impairment[b] (Y/N)	Legal issue[c] (Y/N)
Alcohol				
Prescription drugs				
Illicit drugs				
Methadone maintenance				

[a]Tobacco deliberately excluded.
[b]Examples: "use despite harm," no gainful employment, marital discord.
[c]Examples: Driving under influence (DUI), drug trafficking, probation, incarceration.

institutional policy development, screening to identify patients at risk for aberrant drug-taking behavior, a multimodal approach to pain therapy, and incorporation of written agreements to facilitate outpatient treatment with opioids and other psychoactive drugs (**Table 27.2**). A broad institutional policy was first presented to and endorsed by the center's administration. A multidisciplinary core management team and clinical resources in the community were identified. Rules for prescribing and documentation were established. Controlled prescribing was necessary at times and written agreements were utilized when routine written clinic guidelines were insufficient (see below under Written care agreements).[15][IV]

The program personnel were interested in establishing screening procedures to identify patients at risk of aberrant drug use. When possible, patients with concurrent SA were identified on the first clinic evaluation by routine screening questions in the medical history, although at times diagnosis was delayed until a "crisis" situation arose. When the index of suspicion for concurrent SA was high, psychiatric and neuropsychological evaluations were instituted in order to more effectively diagnose comorbid conditions.

At MDACC, and currently at the University of Utah Huntsman Cancer Institute, routine pain management practice utilizes an individual case-by-case determination of the necessity and potential contraindications to opioid therapy. Initial comprehensive evaluation includes the use of standard pain assessment tools. The World Health Organization and other guidelines for pharmacotherapy of cancer pain are followed. Cancer pain patients with concurrent SA are closely monitored for abuse behaviors and prescribing schedules are modified accordingly. Nonpharmacologic approaches are utilized in conjunction with medications. Psychotherapy and cognitive/behavioral strategies are employed along with involvement of the patient's family and support systems. The use of social support services may be extensive at times.

Table 27.2 Elements of a multidisciplinary program for cancer pain patients with concurrent substance abuse disorders.

Elements of a multidisciplinary program		
Institutional policy development	Hospital administration	
	Physician-in-chief	
	Pharmacy	
	Emergency department	
	Risk management	
	Ethics committee	
Patient identification methods	Medical history	
	Self-report tool	
	Structured interview	
	Observation of behaviors	
	Body fluids screening	
Pain clinic program	Multidisciplinary team structure	
	Community resources	
	Treatment program	Psychiatric/neuropsychological evaluation
		Rules for prescribing controlled substances
		Monitoring of behaviors
		Body fluids screening
		Written care agreements

In 1992, a retrospective review of 2100 MDACC Pain Clinic patient records revealed less than a 5 percent incidence of SA, although it is clear that some patients with SA were not identified in the course of usual clinical practice. Of the 84 patients noted to have concurrent SA, most were between the ages of 20 and 60, and the majority was male. Almost all patients had a diagnosis of cancer-related pain, and nearly all were prescribed opioids. Polysubstance abuse was noted in 33 percent, alcohol abuse alone in 14 percent; 9 percent had a positive family history of SA, and unsanctioned dose escalation occurred in 9 percent. There was a known criminal history in 5 percent, and other prescription drug abuse in 2 percent. Two or more of these problems occurred in 28 percent. The majority had undergone a psychiatric evaluation, rendering additional diagnoses of depression in 28 percent, anxiety in 11 percent, and personality disorder in 6 percent. Seventeen of these patients were managed with written care agreements. Overall, less than 5 percent of pain clinic patients were managed with written care agreements.[16][IV] The case series is described in **Tables 27.3** and **27.4**.

Unfortunately, the medical literature does not adequately address the impact of SA on the outcome of cancer treatment. In a retrospective review of a long-term cohort of 132 MDACC patients with genitourinary cancers and SA, survival was noted to be unaffected compared to patients without SA (personal communication). At presentation, information regarding prior substance use was gathered via a structured interview tool as part of a comprehensive psychosocial assessment. Specific drugs used, amount and frequency of use, duration of use, and prior discontinuation or concurrent use at time of interview were recorded along with family history and the impact of substance use on personal relationships and job or school performance. This review revealed that while SA may complicate pain assessment and treatment, it may not significantly limit survival from cancer. Mortality, medical complications, time to disease recurrence, number of cancer relapses, and treatment courses to remission were similar in the sample identified with SA compared to the remainder of the study population.[16]

Psychosocial support groups

Individual counseling and a pilot psychosocial support group were incorporated in the previously described nonabstinence model program for SA patients at MDACC. Clinical impressions were that these interventions facilitated pain treatment and enhanced compliance in patients with psychosocial problems, psychiatric diagnoses, and/or illicit behaviors. It was determined that patients with SA can often make distinctions between analgesia and other psychoactive effects of their medicines. Group therapy assisted them in coping with the many stresses of chronic pain, complex cancer treatment

Table 27.3 Case series: University of Texas MD Anderson Cancer Center 1992.

Factor	Detail	%
Age	0–20	1
	20–40	47
	40–60	47
	>60	5
Gender	F	42
	M	58
Pain diagnosis	Cancer-related	>97
Pain medications	Opioids	>98
Identification methods	Polysubstance use	33
Alcohol	Abuse	14
	Family issues	9
	Dose escalation	9
	Criminal activity	5
	Prescription abuse	2
	2 or more	28
Written contracts	17	20
Psychiatric diagnosis	Not evaluated/uncertain	44
	Depression	28
	Anxiety	11
	No diagnosis	11
	Personality disorder	6

$n = 84$.

Table 27.4 Outcomes of written care agreements.

Outcomes	n
Compliant, kept on contract	5
Compliant, went off contract	4
Dismissed	4
"Lost to follow-up"	2
Referred for substance abuse treatment	1
Noncompliant/referred to hospice	1

$n = 17$.

decisions, the threat of tumor progression or recurrence, and personal losses in many domains. Some patients responded positively to a strictly structured approach to their pain management.[16] Based on this favorable experience, it was recommended that institutions consider establishing such groups and facilitating their functioning independently as peer support groups (see **Box 27.1**).

Written care agreements

A written care agreement between patient and provider may be indicated when SA complicates pain management.[15] The written care agreement documents a detailed individualized agreement between patient and provider, clearly setting out rules and expectations for both

---

Box 27.1 Structure of pilot program – University of Texas MD Anderson Cancer Center 1992

- Structure of pilot program
- Patient assessment
- Group, individual, family therapy
- Staff development
- Multidisciplinary staff meetings for treatment planning
- Documentation, including written care agreements
- Prescription scheduling
- Community interface
- Monitoring of efficacy of program

Box 27.2 Samples content for written care agreement

- I understand that my pain treatment will consist of the following: _____.
- I agree to take medications at the dose and frequency prescribed. Any changes in the dose will be only at the direction of _____ or her/his designee _____.
- I will receive my prescriptions at the following interval: _____.
- I agree to come to all scheduled appointments. My next appointment is _____.
- I understand that prescriptions will only be supplied at my clinic visit. I will not request prescriptions by telephone.
- I consent to random urine and blood drug tests.
- I will safeguard my medications. I will not give my medications to any other person.
- I understand that lost or stolen medications may not be replaced. I agree to report stolen medications to the police.
- I understand that if I have questions regarding my pain or side effects of medications, I am to call (*telephone number*) during regular business hours (*specify*).
- I understand that a copy of this agreement is placed on my medical record.
- I understand that a copy of this agreement is being sent to (*name of primary physician*).
- I understand that my failure to comply with this agreement may result in termination of my pain treatment.

Patient (*signature*) Date _____
Physician (*signature*) Date _____
Other team clinician(s) (*signature*) Date _____
Renewal Date _____

---

parties.[17, 18, 19][V] Suggested criteria for initiating a written agreement are summarized below:

- enrollment in a methadone maintenance program;
- evidence of excessive alcohol use;
- evidence of ongoing illicit drug use;
- repeated acts of noncompliance with pain treatment;
- history of conviction or incarceration for a drug-related offense.

The minimum information in the agreement includes expectations for patient compliance with medication schedules and appointments for prescription refills; a medication replacement policy; and permission to randomly screen body fluids for drugs (**Box 27.2**). Such instructions are most useful when the consequence of noncompliance are outlined and may include a statement describing the likelihood of termination of medical treatment in the event of continued noncompliance. Written agreements serve as a communication tool for patient and provider, as well as a guide for different providers within the team and institution. This type of formally structured agreement also ideally addresses patients' problem behaviors such as poor impulse control and "splitting" of staff. Copies of the signed written agreement should be given to the patient and included in the record. Clear documentation is then assured in the event that a patient must be dismissed from care. It should be noted that the written care agreement is neither an informed consent document nor a legal contract. To date, there is no evidence that written agreements improve clinical outcomes, yet the use of such "contracts" has been promoted as a part of general pain management practice.

Although most pain specialists practicing in the cancer setting will encounter patients with cancer-related pain and concurrent SA, dismissal from pain treatment is an infrequent outcome. In such cases, clinicians and their institutions must adequately document that the benefit of continued pain treatment is outweighed by its risk. In most cases, consultation with clinical peers and institutional risk managers is highly recommended. For the most difficult circumstances, the practicing clinician may wish to consult with an institutional ethics committee.[20]

Analgesic therapy

There is no clinical evidence that any given opioid agonist analgesic is more or less "addictive" than others in clinical use. Any drug preparation may be misused and/or diverted for illicit purposes. Controlled-release preparations of opioids may facilitate patients' compliance with medication schedules and may lessen the reinforcing aspects of pill-taking behavior. However, noting that pain intensity fluctuates, it is customary to prescribe immediate-release or short-acting medication for breakthrough pain when prescribing controlled-release preparations. Some patients with SA cannot maintain complicated medication schedules successfully and are less confused with immediate-release medication. For these patients, short-acting medications alone may be the safest treatment.

For SA patients on methadone maintenance therapy, Passik et al.[21] suggest that methadone being given for opioid dependency can be titrated to analgesia. It is the authors' preference to avoid disturbing the established use of the methadone, regarding it as if it were an endogenous opioid, and to use a different opioid drug as the analgesic. Although this approach may be more pharmacologically complicated, it respects the legal restrictions on prescribing methadone for opioid maintenance, i.e. the requirement for special registration as a methadone clinic. It also allows for dosage titration of the analgesic without having to involve the methadone maintenance program in dosage changes. The need for repeated communication regarding analgesic titration is reduced when using an alternative to methadone for analgesia in this setting. However, periodic communication between the pain clinician and the methadone clinic staff is still strongly recommended to confirm the specific agents prescribed and to discuss concerning behaviors.

It is essential that psychiatric conditions such as depression and anxiety be treated as distinct clinical problems. Psychoactive medications prescribed for these indications may interact with analgesics. It is important that regular communication between prescribers occur and periodic team conferences are recommended whenever possible.

Comprehensive pain management includes nonpharmacologic as well as pharmacologic interventions. All nonpharmacologic means of controlling symptoms should be explored with cancer patients with pain and concurrent SA. Anesthetic or neurosurgical procedures to alleviate pain may reduce the need for analgesic medications, thus potentially simplifying drug therapy. Psychological and behavioral techniques should also be incorporated, although patients with high levels of distress and personality disorders may be less able to utilize these techniques successfully.

Drug testing in pain management

Body fluid screening with urine and serum tests is useful to confirm the presence or absence of prescribed controlled substances and nonprescribed substances (licit or illicit).[22, 23, 24, 25, 26, 27, 28][V] Patients must give consent for clinical tests, which are unethical to perform without the patient's knowledge. The limitations of most routine drug screening tests require that pain clinicians and laboratory staff collaborate to assure that the drugs of interest are screened. One must also confirm that detection thresholds for specific drugs are adequate in the tests performed. Generally, urine screening will be most readily available and is preferable for routine clinical purposes. However, commonly prescribed opioids are not included in many urine screening test panels. Substance detection depends on many variables, such as the drug, dose, frequency of use, route of administration, individual metabolism, body weight, hydration status, and sensitivity of the detection method used. In addition, it should be recognized that there is poor correlation between analgesic dose and serum levels.[29] Given these variables and the possibility of laboratory error, it is advisable to obtain more than one urine test with serum confirmation testing before results are incorporated in clinical decision making.

Test results should be discussed with the patient. The clinician's interpretation of test results should be clearly communicated with specific reference to the pain management plan. If the screening test results cause significant changes in the management plan, these should be documented and if there is a written agreement in place, it should be updated (see **Tables 27.5** and **27.6**).

CASE EXAMPLE

A 54-year-old female with malignant melanoma of the lower extremity was referred for pain and symptom management due to persistent thigh pain after groin tumor excision and femoral node dissection. Initial consultation revealed neuropathic pain with femoral deafferentation; chronic headaches; chronic pancreatitis; chronic obstructive pulmonary disease; anxiety disorder; history of tobacco, alcohol, and prescription drug abuse; a physically abusive alcoholic husband; chaotic family circumstances; and children with active illicit drug use. The patient was treated with antidepressant, benzodiazepine, and opioid analgesic medications. She was counseled by a psychiatric nurse clinician and social worker with credentials in substance abuse treatment. She was referred to Alcoholics Anonymous. Repeated acts of noncompliance with the general pain clinic rules led to strict prescribing and written care agreements. Nevertheless, at outpatient visits, the patient was unable to account for her medications and several urine screenings failed to detect her prescribed drugs. During a subsequent hospitalization, a strong suspicion arose that her opioid and benzodiazepine medications were being diverted. The patient's daughter had obtained the patient's outpatient prescriptions and was found unresponsive in the patient's hospital bathroom. On search of the hospital room, the patient's prescribed opioid was found in the daughter's purse with a syringe inserted. Under advisement from institutional risk management staff, the police were informed. The

Table 27.5 Interpretations of drug tests in pain management.

Urine drug test result	Clinical decision making
Prescribed drug present	Repeat as indicated to document compliance
Prescribed drug absent	Serum quantitative level; if negative, consider termination
Nonprescribed drug present	Confirm source; if not legitimate, counsel/refer for SA treatment, consider termination
Alcohol present	Counsel/refer for SA treatment, consider termination
Illicit substance present	Counsel/refer for SA treatment, consider termination

SA, substance abuse.

Table 27.6 Body fluid tests for substances.

Patient communication	Laboratory communication
Specify test(s) to be done	Specify substances to be screened
Explain purpose of test(s) and use of information to be obtained from test	Consider lowering thresholds of detection for substances of interest
Patient consent for testing	Work with laboratory staff to improve efficiency of testing and reporting
Repeat testing for confirmation	

patient was dismissed from the pain clinic with an explanation that it had been determined that she was not taking her medications and there was concern that her medications were being diverted to others. The pain specialists remained available for inpatient consultation for the management of painful procedures or cancer treatment, and for outpatient reevaluation of changes in clinical condition.

MEDICOLEGAL ISSUES

There are medicolegal considerations that arise in the management of patients with cancer pain and concurrent SA that are largely beyond the scope of this chapter. Federal statues, state laws, and state regulations recognize that the medical treatment of pain with opioid analgesics is essential, falling within the scope of good medical practice. The documentation of diagnosis, treatment plan and follow-up care should be every prescriber's routine.[30] [V] Clinicians should consider obtaining legal counsel to address the use of information regarding a patient's illicit activities. When overt illicit behaviors are viewed as a contraindication to the prescribing of controlled substances, patient complaints of pain may be untreated. Prescribers' obligations and patients' rights may then come into conflict, resulting in ethical dilemmas that may be difficult to resolve.

RESEARCH DIRECTIONS

Many scientific and clinical questions remain. Can we differentiate distinct brain regions mediating analgesia versus reward using currently available functional brain imaging techniques? Do patients with pain and SA respond differently to opioid analgesics than pain patients without SA? What is the relationship between analgesic and mood effects of opioids in patients with SA compared to those without SA? What is the role of psychological analgesic intervention for pain patients with SA? How does SA impact analgesic therapy and outcome from cancer treatment? Can we better define the clinical issues in treating pain in patients with SA? Do multidisciplinary programs for pain patients with SA improve clinical outcomes and are they cost-effective? How can we balance individual rights and societal concerns in an ethical manner?

CONCLUSIONS

The majority of cancer patients will experience significant pain during their illness and opioid analgesics are integral to cancer care. The prevalence of SA disorders in the United States, for example, may be as great as 15 percent. The prevalence of SA in the cancer pain population may be even greater. Patients with a history of SA and those with active abuse may engage in behaviors that complicate the assessment of pain as a subjective reported experience. The efficacy of therapeutic interventions may be difficult to measure in the patient using medications for unintended psychoactive effects. In short, the therapeutic alliance is easily eroded making pain treatment stressful for patients and providers alike. Legal problems may arise for the practitioner and institutions, yet the standard approach to chemical dependency (detoxification and abstinence) may be inappropriate for those patients with severe, persistent cancer-related pain.

Working with patients with cancer-related pain and SA provokes consideration of fundamental clinical and ethical questions. In the broad perspective, the relationship between the medical use of opioids and the problem of SA is still clouded in controversy, but meaningful dialogue has progressed.[31, 32, 33] We must remain mindful of our assumptions and make efforts to structure clinical approaches for different practice settings. Cancer patients without pain who require treatment solely for substance abuse are best referred to dedicated substance abuse treatment if their cancer-related prognosis is sufficiently long.

It is important to recognize the exceptional care that patients with cancer pain and substance abuse require.[34] In the oncology setting, pain medicine and palliative care specialists may be best suited to coordinate necessary multidisciplinary treatment. Our aim should be to maintain the therapeutic alliance to the degree possible, by reestablishing trust and thus furthering the goals of pain relief and improved quality of life. Patients who are multiply afflicted with cancer, pain, and SA suffer greatly, and they deserve compassionate, professional attention despite the challenges involved.

REFERENCES

1. Passik SD, Kirsh KL. Opioid therapy in patients with a history of substance abuse. *CNS Drugs*. 2004; **18**: 13–25.
2. Whitcomb LA, Kirsh KL, Passik SD. Substance abuse issues in cancer pain. *Current Pain and Headache Reports*. 2002; **6**: 183–90.
3. Ballantyne JC. Chronic pain following treatment for cancer: the role of opioids. *Oncologist*. 2003; **8**: 567–75.
4. Agency for Health Care Policy and Research, U.S. Dept of Health and Human Services. *Clinical Practice Guideline Number 9: Management of Cancer Pain*. Washington, DC: U.S. Dept of Health and Human Services, 1994.
5. World Health Organization. *Cancer pain relief and palliative care*. Geneva: World Health Organization, 1990.
6. O'Brien CP, Gardner EL. Critical assessment of how to study addiction and its treatment: human and non-human animal models. *Pharmacology and Therapeutics*. 2005; **108**: 18–58.
7. American Psychiatric Association. *Diagnostic and statistical manual for mental disorders – IV*. Washington, DC: American Psychiatric Association, 1994: 175–272.
8. Passik SD, Kirsh MS, Portenoy RK. Understanding aberrant drug-taking behavior: Addiction redefined for palliative care and pain management settings. In: Berger A, Levy MH, Portenoy RK, Weissman DE (eds). *Principles and practice of supportive oncology*, Vol. 2. Philadelphia, PA: Lippincott, Williams, & Wilkins, 1999: 1–12.

9. Weinstein SM, Laux LF, Thornby JI *et al.* Physicians' attitudes toward pain and the use of opioid analgesics: Results of a survey from the Texas Cancer Pain Initiative. *Southern Medical Journal*. 2000; **93**: 479–87.
10. Kirsh KL, Passik SD. Palliative care of the terminally ill drug addict. *Cancer Investigation*. 2006; **24**: 425–31.
11. Penson RT, Nunn C, Younger J *et al.* Trust violated: analgesics for addicts. *Oncologist*. 2003; **8**: 199–209.
12. Ewing JA. Detecting alcoholism: the CAGE questionnaire. *Journal of the American Medical Association*. 1984; **252**: 1905–07.
∗ 13. Passik SD, Kirsh KL, Donaghy KB, Portenoy RK. Pain and aberrant drug-related behaviors in medically ill patients with and without histories of substance abuse. *Clinical Journal of Pain*. 2006; **22**: 173–81.
14. Weissman DE, Haddox JD. Opioid psuedoaddiction – an iatrogenic syndrome. *Pain*. 1989; **36**: 363–6.
15. Weinstein SM. Written contracts facilitate cancer pain treatment in the patient with substance use disorder. Proceedings of the Thirteenth Annual Scientific Meeting American Pain Society. Miami Beach, Florida, November, 1994.
16. Weinstein SM, Cunningham M, Edwards J. A multidisciplinary program for cancer pain patients with substance use disorder. Proceedings of the Twelfth Annual Scientific Meeting, American Pain Society. Orlando, Florida, November, 1993.
17. Doleys DM, Rickman L. Other benefits of an opioid "agreement." *Journal of Pain and Symptom Management*. 2003; **25**: 402–03.
18. Fishman SM, Kreis PG. The opioid contract. *Clinical Journal of Pain*. 2002; **18**: S70–5.
19. Fishman SM, Bandman TB, Edwards A, Borsook D. The opioid contract in the management of chronic pain. *Journal of Pain and Symptom Management*. 1999; **18**: 27–37.
20. Cohen MJ, Jasser S, Herron PD, Margolis CG. Ethical perspectives: opioid treatment of chronic pain in the context of addiction. *Clinical Journal of Pain*. 2002; **18**: S99–107.
21. Passik SD, Portenoy RK, Ricketts PL. Substance abuse issues in cancer patients. Part 2: Evaluation and treatment. *Oncology*. 1998; **12**: 729–34.
22. Vaglienti RM, Huber SJ, Noel KR, Johnstone RE. Misuse of prescribed controlled substances defined by urinalysis. *West Virginia Medical Journal*. 2003; **99**: 67–70.
23. Manchikanti L, Manchukonda R, Pampati V *et al.* Does random urine drug testing reduce illicit drug use in chronic pain patients receiving opioids? *Pain Physician*. 2006; **9**: 123–9.
24. Heit HA, Gourlay DL. Urine drug testing in pain medicine. *Journal of Pain and Symptom Management*. 2004; **27**: 260–7.
25. Swanson J. Urine drug screening for opioids. *Journal of Pain and Palliative Care Pharmacotherapy*. 2002; **16**: 111–14.
26. Katz NP, Sherburne S, Beach M *et al.* Behavioral monitoring and urine toxicology testing in patients

receiving long-term opioid therapy. *Anesthesia and Analgesia.* 2003; **97**: 1097–102.

27. Hickey K, Seliem R, Shields J *et al.* A positive drug test in the pain management patient: deception or herbal cross-reactivity? *Clinical Chemistry.* 2002; **48**: 958–60.

28. Robinson RC, Gatchel, Polatin P *et al.* Screening for problematic prescription opioid use. *Clinical Journal of Pain.* 2001; **17**: 220–8.

29. Cunningham M. Pain management in individuals with dual diagnosis: pain and substance use disorder. In: Kingdon RT, Stanley KJ, Kizior RJ (eds). *Handbook for pain management.* St Louis: VC Mosby, 1997: 249–93.

30. Weinstein SM, Thorpe DM. McCrory L: What the new board rules mean for your practice. *Texas Medicine.* 1995; **91**: 36.

∗ 31. Joranson DE, Portenoy RK. Pain medicine and drug law enforcement: an important step toward balance. *Journal of Pain and Palliative Care Pharmacotherapy.* 2005; **19**: 3–5.

32. Savage SR, Joranson DE, Covington EC *et al.* Definitions related to the medical use of opioids: evolution towards universal agreement. *Journal of Pain and Symptom Management.* 2003; **26**: 655–67.

33. Portenoy RK, Payne R. Acute and Chronic Pain. In: Lowinson JH, Millman JG (eds). *Substance abuse: a comprehensive textbook.* Baltimore: Williams & Wilkins, 1997: 691–721.

34. Hoffman M, Provatas A, Lyver A, Kanner R. Pain management in the opioid-addicted patient with cancer. *Cancer.* 1991; **68**: 1121–2.

28

Pain in the dying person

KATE SKINNER AND STEVEN Z PANTILAT

What is unique about care of the dying person?	389	Treatment choices for pain in the dying adult are diverse	393
Special challenges must be considered in treating pain at the end of life	391	Summary	395
		Acknowledgments	395
Assessment of pain in the dying is critical for supporting appropriate treatment decisions	392	References	395
Opioids are the mainstay of pharmacological treatment for severe cancer pain	392		

KEY LEARNING POINTS

- Pain is a common and feared symptom among the dying.
- Pain in the dying person may arise not only from physiologic causes, but also from emotional, psychological, and spiritual distress.
- Effective management of pain in the dying person requires the involvement of a team of clinicians with expertise in addressing the myriad issues and sources of pain and suffering experienced by the dying person.
- Management of pain in the dying person poses certain challenges, including the fact that very often the patient is unable to communicate.

- Opioids are the mainstay of pharmacologic management of pain in the dying person, although very often multiple medications and modalities are needed to relieve pain.
- The presence of many other symptoms including dyspnea, fatigue, and nausea can contribute to pain and suffering in the dying person and require treatment.
- The skillful clinician may derive enormous personal satisfaction from caring for patients and their families at this important time of life.

WHAT IS UNIQUE ABOUT CARE OF THE DYING PERSON?

First we must understand of whom we are speaking when we refer to the dying person. Although there is little consensus in the medical literature on the terminology,[1, 2] we define the dying state as one in which death is expected, and curative or supportive treatment cannot prevent it. The dying state is most easily recognized when death is imminent within hours, days, or weeks. In this period, it is more appropriate to focus on patient function and

preference for treatments as evidence of the dying state rather than on a particular time-frame since predictions of prognosis are fraught with challenges.[3] Patients with diminished functioning, who are primarily bed bound, have limited ability to perform activities of daily living, and who often no longer prefer to pursue curative or disease-modifying therapy, can be considered as dying and the approach to pain control outlined in this chapter would apply. In these patients, a focus on palliation gradually replaces cure as the primary goal of care and the dying person receives progressively less disease-modifying therapy and more symptom-oriented therapy. Because of a change in the focus of care, a more aggressive approach to pain management in which relief of suffering is the primary objective may be more appropriate (**Figure 28.1**).

The common belief that dying, particularly from cancer, is inevitably painful is belied by an observation that as many as a quarter to half of patients dying of cancer had no pain or analgesic use.[4, 5][III] Nevertheless, moderate to severe pain predominates in terminally ill patients[6] and in both cancer and noncancer patients.[7] The dying trajectory with cancer is relatively predictable and most cancer patients function quite well until approximately the last two months of life (**Figure 28.2**).[8] Performance status, rather than pain *per se*, is the best prognostic factor. In patients with metastatic cancer, a Karnofsky performance scale score of less than 50 percent correlates with life expectancy of less than eight weeks.[9] Good pain management is important at any point in illness with cancer, but as the ability to alter the course of the disease and the patient's desire for disease-modifying therapy diminish, the focus on pain and symptom relief becomes primary. At that point it would be appropriate to discontinue all medications not essential for the patient's comfort,[10] as well as all assessments and treatments that do not promote comfort, for example blood pressure monitoring.

Although not all patients dying from cancer have pain, pain is very common in people who are dying from cancer. Studies have shown that in the last week of life up to 99 percent of patients with cancer experience pain.[11] In the one study that assessed pain directly from patients, 71 percent reported having pain and pain was the most common symptom.[12] In addition, patients with cancer can have many sources and types of physical pain and pain can occur in the absence of physically definable lesions. It is important to understand that pain and the suffering associated with it, the "total pain" concept

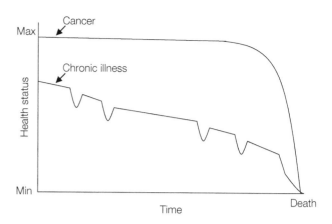

Figure 28.2 Dying trajectories. Functional changes and trajectory to death are more predictable in the long term in cancer than in other chronic, terminal illnesses such as heart failure, chronic pulmonary disease, or cirrhosis. In cancer, a typical course is that functional status is preserved until late in the illness and death follows predictably within months. With chronic illness, repeated exacerbations are common and death can occur suddenly and less predictably as the result of an exacerbation.

described by Dame Cicely Saunders, who founded the modern hospice and palliative care movement,[13] come from many sources.[14, 15] The components of total pain can be as follows:

- physical;
- psychological;
- emotional;
- social;
- spiritual.

The etiologic sources of pain in the dying person are diverse and best addressed through comprehensive assessment and management by an interdisciplinary palliative care team. The patient who reports pain "everywhere" requires careful evaluation for these multiple sources of suffering, ideally by an interdisciplinary team coordinated by a palliative care specialist. Such a team brings to bear expertise in multiple areas that allows a comprehensive evaluation of the patient's pain and suffering and can relieve suffering not only from physiologic sources, but also from spiritual, emotional, and psychological pain. The team approach to palliative care provides higher quality care at the end of life including better pain control, increased patient and caregiver satisfaction, and improvements in other health outcomes.[16][I], [17, 18][I], [19]

Unfortunately, there are few randomized controlled trials supporting efficacy of clinical interventions in the dying. There are even fewer randomized controlled studies to guide management of pain in dying infants and children, and therefore we will focus our discussion on what is known about dying adults. There are few studies partly because of the difficulties in diagnosing the dying state,

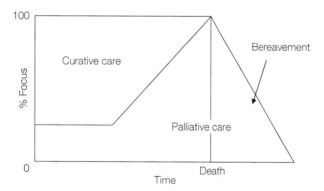

Figure 28.1 Current model of palliative care. Palliative care plays a role in the care of the patient from the time of diagnosis until death and is provided simultaneously with all other appropriate medical treatments. As the disease progresses, palliative care may play a larger role, either because cure is no longer possible and/or the patient's goals of care change and the patient no longer desires attempts at curative treatment.

and thus knowing who to include, and partly because there is reluctance to use dying patients as subjects since it might increase suffering and pose an undue burden.[20] Thus much of the published literature uses surrogate endpoints, such as family caregiver perception of pain control. Such reports found that in 40–54 percent of cases of patients dying in the hospital, family members remembered pain in their loved one as being moderate to severe.[21, 22, 23] A recent study of factors considered important to patients and caregivers (including families and physicians) at the end of life showed good concordance and ranked pain control as most important.[24] When caregivers have discordant perceptions from patients, caregivers report greater pain and physical suffering.[25] Interestingly, in studies where both patients and caregivers are interviewed, and the pain assessments of bereaved caregivers are collected, retrospective caregiver assessment showed poor correlation with patient assessment, with pain described as more severe in retrospect.[26, 27]

There is no evidence in the primary literature to suggest that the sensory aspect of pain differs for the dying person. Somewhat surprisingly, there is evidence of both decreases[11, 28] as well as increases[29] in pain perception during the terminal phase. Both results could be due to movement-related pain or the lack of it, or another non-pain symptom. For example, terminal delirium could be difficult to differentiate from pain or could make reporting of pain less likely. However imprecise the measurement or whoever is pondering the assessment, it is clear that too often symptom control for the dying patient is inadequate. The SUPPORT study documented that for 50 percent of conscious patients who died in the hospital, family members reported moderate to severe pain at least half of the time, and often in conditions not usually associated with pain, such as congestive heart failure.[30] The losses inherent in dying can exacerbate or even produce pain. A major source of suffering for dying people is loss of control or autonomy. Therefore it is essential to assess the goals of care of the dying person and to provide therapy tailored to those wishes.[31]

Improved quality of life and pain control are often primary goals.[32] In one study,[33] patients with acquired immunodeficiency syndrome (AIDS) were particularly focused on pain control as a goal, whereas cancer patients tended to value maintaining hope more highly. It is important to realize that many patients wish to remain alert at the end of life and will tolerate a degree of pain in order to accomplish this goal. Others will prefer complete relief of pain even if that means that they will be sedated and unresponsive. Skillful discussion[34] between medical personnel, the patient, and the family about the patient's values and goals can improve symptom control, increase family satisfaction, and demonstrate respect for patient wishes.[35][IV] Often the ideal goal is to provide appropriate symptom control to allow for peaceful awareness until the time of death. Patients who had described themselves as at peace had better quality of death

outcomes and their caregivers had better bereavement outcomes in a recent prospective study.[36][II]

SPECIAL CHALLENGES MUST BE CONSIDERED IN TREATING PAIN AT THE END OF LIFE

Pain is prevalent and often under-treated at the end of life. Fear of pain in cancer patients at end of life correlates with euthanasia requests,[37, 38] although recent studies suggest that factors other than pain, such as loss of dignity or wish for control over time or manner of death, are prime motivations in requests for assisted suicide and euthanasia.[39, 40, 41] Such requests are typically withdrawn when clinicians provide patients with pain management and other substantive interventions including referral to hospice.[42] Aggressive treatment of pain, even to the point of suppressing respirations, and withdrawal of life-sustaining interventions, including artificial feeding and hydration, are morally and ethically acceptable if carried out with palliative intent.[43] By the ethical principle of double effect, treatment of pain is legally and morally acceptable, as long as the primary intent is to provide relief from suffering, and hastening death is a known but unintended consequence.[44] Likewise, terminal sedation, the controlled use of medication to produce unconsciousness when that is the only way to relieve pain,[45] is legally and ethically justified in cases of otherwise uncontrollable suffering.[46, 47, 48] Due to the emotional and psychological stress for patients, families, and staff, it is particularly important to educate and provide ongoing support for all concerned when there is a request for palliative sedation.[48] Concerns about causing death through palliative treatments are common, but such events are rare in clinical practice. Effective communication with patients and families about the emotionally charged issues at the end of life (fear of abandonment, expectation of pain or debility, defining hope as the patient's belief in what is still possible) is an essential prelude to effective symptom management.[49] Questions you might ask include:

- Do you have any concerns about pain or suffering?
- When you think about the future, what do you hope for?
- When you look ahead, what worries you the most?
- How are you coping with your illness?
- How are you feeling within yourself?
- How would you hope to be remembered?
- Is there anything in your relationships with family or friends that needs healing?
- Do you still have important things to say to the special people in your life?
- If you were to die soon, would there be anything left undone in your life?
- How can I help you to deal with all that you are going through?
- Are you a religious or a spiritual person?

These questions may open avenues of meaningful communication and lead the dying person toward resolution of some sources of suffering at the end of life.

ASSESSMENT OF PAIN IN THE DYING IS CRITICAL FOR SUPPORTING APPROPRIATE TREATMENT DECISIONS

The dying person is often cognitively impaired, whether from debility or dementia, and assessment methods must reflect this reality as the end of life approaches. The best way to know if a patient is in pain is to ask,[50] since there are no objective measures for pain. Even impaired individuals can often acknowledge pain,[51] but communication with the patient may be aided by the use of pain scales that quantify pain and provide the data for ongoing adjustments of therapy. Hospitalized elders with mild to moderate cognitive impairment can reliably report their worst and usual pain retrospectively, though they have difficulty with retrospective ratings of "least pain."[52] That said, it is not always necessary or possible to try to involve the critically ill person in symptom assessment when such attempts could cause additional pain or suffering (**Figure 28.3**).[53]

A person who cannot speak can still have pain. Signs such as tachycardia, tachypnea, diaphoresis, and elevated blood pressure can provide evidence of pain, but the clinician should be aware that patients with chronic pain frequently do not show these classic physiologic signs of acute pain. In addition, in dying patients these signs may reflect physiologic changes other than pain, such as dehydration or fever, or exist as the side effects of medications used to treat other symptoms. Other signs that may indicate pain include facial expressions such as grimacing, verbalization such as moaning, body movements such as repeatedly touching a particular part of the body, and changes in activity level.[51] Direct observation of behaviors can provide meaningful information about the dying person's pain experience and can be used to guide adjustments in pain management. Pain-related behaviors could include:

- tachycardia;
- tachypnea;
- diaphoresis;
- facial expressions/grimacing;
- verbalizations/moaning;
- changes in activity;
- irritability;
- withdrawal, sleeping;
- body movements, particularly during transfers or movement;
- poor appetite;
- resistance to personal care.

New instruments for formal assessment of pain in cognitively impaired older adults include the Checklist of

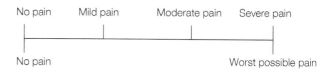

Figure 28.3 Simple pain scales. Simple assessment instruments may be helpful when cognitive ability is impaired, as it often is at the end of life.

Nonverbal Pain Indicators, which measures six pain-related behaviors.[54] This instrument modified an existing scale to eliminate items requiring ambulation, making it potentially suitable for pain assessment at the end of life, although it has not yet been validated in this patient population.

Because the focus of care in the actively dying patient centers on quality of life, patients need to have the space and time to explore spiritual concerns, consolidate relationships, and consider meaning in their life and death.[55] Good symptom control makes this type of life review and closure possible, and adequate assessment is essential. However, it is also important to minimize the "medicalization" of care in the actively dying in order to avoid creating iatrogenic burdens and increasing suffering. For example, clinicians need to make case by case decisions about whether the benefits of performing a complete skin examination, or asking the patient to quantify their pain every time, outweigh the risks of what might be excessively intrusive assessments for the dying person. Still, assessment must be ongoing to avoid missing potentially treatable causes of pain. Comprehensive assessment in one population of 276 cancer pain patients found previously undiagnosed sources of pain in 64 percent of patients.[56]

Pain in hospice patients with cancer is intimately associated with other physical symptoms as well as with the critical psychological tasks of the dying. This kind of "total pain" experience is reflected in patients' language and typically includes few (31 percent) of the standard words used to describe pain found in commonly used pain assessment tools.[50] Thus the standardized assessment tools may not fully reflect the patients' pain experience and might provide inadequate data for changes in treatment. One study found that of all the standard descriptions of pain used in assessment tools, the descriptors of the Visual Analog Scale, "no pain" and "pain as bad as it can be," best reflected the language of elderly hospice patients with cancer.[50]

OPIOIDS ARE THE MAINSTAY OF PHARMACOLOGICAL TREATMENT FOR SEVERE CANCER PAIN

After adequate and complete assessment, appropriate pharmacological management is the mainstay for treatment of pain in the dying person.[57] As in any other clinical situation, choice of analgesics depends on the type, etiology, and degree of pain. Mild pain may be alleviated by paracetamol, aspirin, or nonsteroidal anti-inflammatory drugs (NSAIDs). Moderate to severe pain often requires opioids used in the stepwise fashion recommended in the WHO three-step analgesic ladder.[58] Retrospective studies have documented the safety and efficacy of this approach in advanced cancer patients.[5] [III], [59][III]

For pain that is poorly controlled, the opioid dose should be rapidly titrated upward, by the subcutaneous or intravenous route if possible, to provide the most rapid relief. For unrelieved moderate pain, increase the dose by 25 to 50 percent; for severe pain, by 50 to 100 percent.[60] Continual administration with repeated boluses and breakthrough dosing administered by nurses skilled in palliative care can quickly control pain. Assessments and adjustments should be frequent enough and based on the pharmacokinetics of the medication to ensure quick and adequate relief. Intravenous patient-controlled analgesia (PCA) may be useful for patients who are cognitively intact and not too debilitated. Unfortunately, at the very end of life, the actively dying are often too ill to properly use PCAs.

At any time in the course of a painful illness, commonly held myths and fears about the dangers of opioid use must be recognized and addressed so that patients and their families and caregivers can accept appropriate treatment.[61] Fear of addiction, misunderstanding of tolerance and dependence, and worries about over-sedation all contribute to under-treatment of pain.[62] The perception that opioids will hasten death is common, but while higher opioid doses are associated with shortened survival in one large cohort, multivariate analysis shows that this association does not explain the variance in time until death.[63][III] Other hospice studies do not show an association of high-dose opioid treatment and shortened survival.[64] In fact, opioids may improve functioning as measured by Karnofsky performance scores.[65][III] Adequate doses of opioids should never be withheld out of fear of shortened survival.

Most dying patients will require long-acting opioids for pain control, in addition to short-acting medications for breakthrough pain. The principles of titration, equianalgesic dosing, and opioid rotation are the same for dying patients as for other patients in pain. Regarding long-acting opioids, there were no significant differences in efficacy or constipation severity among sustained-release oxycodone, sustained-release morphine, or transdermal fentanyl in one retrospective study of 12,000 terminally ill patients admitted to hospice,[66][III] and therefore no inherent reason to choose one over the others. The transdermal route is clearly useful for patients who cannot take oral medication. Although patches are less easily titrated because of their extended time to steady-state delivery, they are associated with good pain control in the hospice or cancer pain setting.[67, 68] Pure opioid agonists have no ceiling effect. Large doses may be needed and should never be withheld if they are necessary for adequate pain control because they are safe and may be necessary to be effective. Occasionally, side effects such as nausea or myoclonus require reductions in dose or rotation to another opioid.

Although it may be best known for its use in maintenance programs for heroin withdrawal, methadone has several properties that make it a very useful opioid analgesic for dying patients and in the hospice setting. First, methadone has efficacy similar to morphine[69][I] but, unlike morphine, methadone is very lipophilic so it is rapidly absorbed by multiple routes and is effective within three minutes after absorption in the gastrointestinal tract. Second, the long half-life of methadone permits twice daily dosing after titration. Third, methadone is inexpensive compared to long-acting opioid preparations and thus offers an advantage for patients and providers. Fourth, unlike morphine, it has no active metabolites and so can be used in renal or hepatic failure. Finally, there is evidence at the case history level that it causes less constipation than morphine.[70] Because of N-methyl-D-aspartate receptor blockade and norepinephrine and seratonin reuptake inhibition, methadone is theoretically useful in neuropathic pain states. A recent Cochrane review of eight randomized controlled trials in patients with cancer pain found that the studies that evaluated methadone for treatment of neuropathic pain were too brief to accurately reflect clinical practice and therefore concluded that there is no trial evidence to support a role for methadone in treating neuropathic pain from cancer.[69][I] A recent long-term case series of noncancer patients for whom other opioids had failed suggested that methadone can be useful in this setting and that randomized controlled trials are indicated.[71]

There are potential problems with methadone that must be addressed for safe use in dying patients. The association with heroin withdrawal programs may make it unacceptable to some patients and families without adequate counseling. The prolonged elimination half-life makes quick titration impossible and increases risk of overdosing. Converting doses from other opioids is complex because of patient variability in pharmacokinetics, again predisposing to toxicities common to most opioids, including sedation and respiratory depression.[72] Methadone can also produce local erythema and induration when given subcutaneously.[73] Nevertheless, it can be a useful medication in this setting as well as for opioid rotation and possibly for neuropathic pain.[74]

TREATMENT CHOICES FOR PAIN IN THE DYING ADULT ARE DIVERSE

As with treating any chronic pain, long-acting formulations are preferred. Breakthrough doses must be available[75] and ongoing pain assessment pursued because pain in the dying person, and cancer pain in particular, is usually progressive due to advancing inanition or to tumor growth into bone, nerves, or viscera. The oral route is preferred as long as the dying person can swallow safely. In the terminal stages, decreased gut motility, vomiting, or bowel obstruction can make absorption of all oral medication unreliable. High-dose therapy may impose an unacceptable "pill burden." Intravenous or subcutaneous administration,[76, 77] although there is some discomfort involved, offers the considerable advantages of prompt analgesia and facilitated titration. Whatever the initial route, when pain control is achieved, an alternate medication route can be selected that is appropriate to the patient's progressive clinical course. At the very end of life when patients can no longer take oral medications, subcutaneous, intravenous, transdermal, and rectal routes are most useful. Intramuscular injection is painful and not indicated in the dying. Rectal administration is underutilized[78] but may be unacceptable to some patients or family members unused to such intimate forms of caregiving. The rectal route is useful in the dying, because some oral medications can be delivered rectally in lubricated gelatin capsules, although absorption can be variable. Polypharmacy is almost universal and is appropriate, both because there are often multiple etiologies of pain and because different pharmacological mechanisms can work synergistically. Useful adjuvants may include multiple analgesics such as opioids, acetaminophen, salicylates, and NSAIDs; antidepressants; anticonvulsants; sedatives; anxiolytics; bisphosphonates for pain from bony metastases; antibiotics for relief of pain from closed space infections, such as sinusitis; and corticosteroids. Case studies have suggested a role for low-dose intravenous ketamine[79][V] and intravenous lidocaine[80][V] for intractable pain at the end of life. Furthermore, addition of adjuvant medications may be needed in order to decrease the dose of opioid in the setting of intolerable side effects.

Corticosteroids are useful for a number of pain conditions at the end of life. They are anti-inflammatory, provide resistance to stressors, and affect fluid balance.[81] Corticosteroids are frequently used at the end of life for spinal cord compression and cerebral edema. They are also useful for pain, particularly where there is tissue damage or compression, as in metastatic bone pain or nerve infiltration, and can improve appetite and mood.[82] [V], [83][V] A Cochrane review of three unpublished randomized, double-blind, placebo-controlled trials and seven prospective and retrospective studies revealed a trend for resolution of malignant bowel obstruction and no difference in survival data with corticosteroid use.[84][I] Unfortunately, there are no high quality trials of corticosteroids for treatment of pain in the dying, and use is empirical. Dexamethasone (4–8 mg/day) is useful because it can be given by mouth, intravenously, subcutaneously, or by rectum. Corticosteroids are usually given for short courses, even in large doses, without difficulty in the dying due to the typical short duration of usage, but if adverse effects arise, such as stomach pain, or steroid-induced psychosis, they should be quickly tapered or simply stopped.

Managing symptoms other than pain is essential for adequate pain control. A challenging aspect of care of the dying is that the moribund patient may not be able to verbalize these sensations. Dyspnea, anxiety, fatigue, vomiting, and myoclonic jerking can all exacerbate pain. Urinary retention, dry mouth, and nausea can become painful, and one must have a high index of suspicion for these etiologies of worsened pain. One management strategy, for example, is to use a Foley catheter in the setting of retention. Such an intervention will likely be acceptable to most patients if the benefits are explained. Fever can also be uncomfortable and paracetamol can be appropriately used, orally or as a suppository, to suppress fever in the actively dying. Because it can be administered intramuscularly or intravenously, the NSAID ketorolac may be useful for fever unresponsive to paracetamol.

There is no *a priori* reason not to use other modalities such as intrathecal,[85] epidural[86] or peripheral nerve blocks, radiation,[87] or chemotherapy for palliative intent if the expected lifespan is enough to justify the discomfort of the intervention. However, many patients feel the burdens of these treatments outweigh the benefits. One advantage of these modalities is that by allowing for reduced systemic doses of opioids, they can help relieve intolerable side effects from high-dose opioids, such as constipation or sedation. When considering such interventions, consultation with an anesthesiologist or pain medicine specialist with expertise in these modalities can be helpful. In general, these interventions are used earlier in the course of illness.

Nonpharmacological, complementary, or alternative treatments such as acupuncture, transcutaneous electrical nerve stimulation, massage, group or brief psychotherapy, herbal preparations, and music therapy may be helpful in subsets of patients.[88][V], [89][III], [90][I], [91][II] Simple cutaneous techniques such as superficial massage, providing heat or cool stimuli, and gentle movement can be taught to family caregivers, providing an adjunct to pharmacological control of pain and encouraging the active participation of family in terminal care.[92][V]

The clinician should remain alert for adverse effects of treatment. Elderly patients in particular are at increased risk for medication side effects.[93] For example, the anti-inflammatory properties of aspirin and NSAIDs provide primary or adjunctive help for the pain of bony metastases. However, these drugs can precipitate an exacerbation of congestive heart failure by causing renally mediated fluid retention, so should be used with care in patients with heart disease.[94] At stable doses, most side effects of opioids resolve within a week, but patients do not become tolerant to the constipating effects of opioids.[95] Both a stool softener and a stimulant laxative must be provided to prevent constipation, and the doses titrated to produce regular soft stools. One caveat is that in the last hours to days of life it may not make sense to continue to promote daily bowel movements, especially if the patient is not eating. Dehydration and renal failure are common at the end of life and caution is necessary with certain opioids in this setting, such as morphine, codeine, and tramadol. Pethidine (meperidine), because of its short half-life requiring frequent dosing and the presence of active metabolites, should never be used for chronic pain. Methadone, fentanyl, and hydrocodone, because they do not have active metabolites, do not produce cumulative toxicity in renal failure. Oxycodone should be used with caution in renal failure. Opioid toxicities in terminal cancer patients may yield to opioid rotation, as shown by one study in which pain scores improved at less than equianalgesic doses after rotation.[96]

SUMMARY

Pain is a common and feared symptom in the dying person. It is important to recognize that in the dying person pain may arise not only from physiologic causes but also from emotional, psychological, and spiritual causes, and thus the total treatment of pain requires a comprehensive assessment of the sources of pain and treatment directed at all etiologies. Often in the dying person such treatment requires the involvement of a team of clinicians with expertise in addressing the myriad issues and sources of pain and suffering experienced by the dying person in addition to physical pain. Palliative care teams can be especially helpful to the dying person, their family, and their clinicians. The care of the dying poses certain challenges in addition to multiple sources of pain. Very often the dying person is not able to communicate, making pain assessment difficult. Furthermore, patients who are dying may no longer wish to pursue investigations of the physiologic sources of pain and simply want pain control. Finally, the presence of many other symptoms such as dyspnea, fatigue, nausea, and others can contribute to pain and suffering and require treatment. Fortunately, there are many effective medications to relieve pain in the dying person and there is always more one can do to treat pain and other symptoms at the end of life, relieve suffering, and promote comfort and dignity. The skillful clinician may derive enormous personal satisfaction from helping patients and their families at this important time of life.

ACKNOWLEDGMENTS

We are grateful for the assistance of Emily Philipps who helped with editing and evidence scoring and Salina Ng who worked on the figures.

REFERENCES

1. Froggatt K, Payne S. A survey of end-of-life care in care homes: issues of definition and practice. *Health and Social Care in the Community*. 2006; **14**: 341–8.
2. Rogg L, Graugaard PK, Loge JH. Physicians' interpretation of the prognostic term "terminal": a survey among Norwegian physicians. *Palliative and Supportive Care*. 2006; **4**: 273–8.
3. Christakis NA, Lamont EB. Extent and determinants of error in doctors' prognoses in terminally ill patients: prospective cohort study. *British Medical Journal*. 2000; **320**: 469–72.
4. Oster MW, Vizel M, Turgeon LR. Pain of terminal cancer patients. *Archives of Internal Medicine*. 1978; **138**: 1801–02.
* 5. Grond S, Zech D, Schug SA *et al.* Validation of World Health Organization guidelines for cancer pain relief during the last days and hours of life. *Journal of Pain and Symptom Management*. 1991; **6**: 411–22.
6. Rolnick SJ, Jackson J, Nelson WW *et al.* Pain management in the last six months of life among women who died of ovarian cancer. *Journal of Pain and Symptom Management*. 2007; **33**: 24–31.
7. Weiss SC, Emanuel LL, Fairclough DL, Emanuel EJ. Understanding the experience of pain in terminally ill patients. *Lancet*. 2001; **357**: 1311–15.
8. Greer DS, Mor V, Morris JN *et al.* An alternative in terminal care: results of the National Hospice Study. *Journal of Chronic Diseases*. 1986; **39**: 9–26.
9. Lamont EB, Christakis NA. Complexities in prognostication in advanced cancer: "to help them live their lives the way they want to". *Journal of the American Medical Association*. 2003; **290**: 98–104.
10. Lichter I, Hunt E. The last 48 hours of life. *Journal of Palliative Care*. 1990; **6**: 7–15.
11. Fainsinger R, Miller MJ, Bruera E *et al.* Symptom control during the last week of life on a palliative care unit. *Journal of Palliative Care*. 1991; **7**: 5–11.
12. Hinton JM. The physical and mental distress of the dying. *Quarterly Journal of Medicine*. 1963; **32**: 1–21.
13. Saunders C. *The management of terminal disease*. London: Edward Arnold, 1978.
14. Strang P, Strang S, Hultborn R, Arner S. Existential pain – an entity, a provocation, or a challenge? *Journal of Pain and Symptom Management*. 2004; **27**: 241–50.
15. Abraham A, Kutner JS, Beaty B. Suffering at the end of life in the setting of low physical symptom distress. *Journal of Palliative Medicine*. 2006; **9**: 658–65.
* 16. Hearn J, Higginson IJ. Do specialist palliative care teams improve outcomes for cancer patients? A systematic literature review. *Palliative Medicine*. 1998; **12**: 317–32.
17. Schrader SL, Horner A, Eidsness L *et al.* A team approach in palliative care: enhancing outcomes. *South Dakota Journal of Medicine*. 2002; **55**: 269–78.
18. Higginson IJ, Finlay IG, Goodwin DM *et al.* Is there evidence that palliative care teams alter end-of-life

experiences of patients and their caregivers? *Journal of Pain and Symptom Management.* 2003; **25**: 150–68.

19. Morrison RS. Health care system factors affecting end-of-life care. *Journal of Palliative Medicine.* 2005; **8**: S79–87.

20. Takesaka J, Crowley R, Casarett D. What is the risk of distress in palliative care survey research? *Journal of Pain and Symptom Management.* 2004; **28**: 593–8.

∗ 21. Lynn J, Teno JM, Phillips RS *et al.* Perceptions by family members of the dying experience of older and seriously ill patients. SUPPORT Investigators. Study to understand prognoses and preferences for outcomes and risks of treatments. *Annals of Internal Medicine.* 1997; **126**: 97–106.

22. Tolle SW, Tilden VP, Hickman SE, Rosenfeld AG. Family reports of pain in dying hospitalized patients: a structured telephone survey. *Western Journal of Medicine.* 2000; **172**: 374–7.

23. Trask PC, Teno JM, Nash J. Transitions of care and changes in distressing pain. *Journal of Pain and Symptom Management.* 2006; **32**: 104–09.

24. Steinhauser KE, Christakis NA, Clipp EC *et al.* Factors considered important at the end of life by patients, family, physicians, and other care providers. *Journal of the American Medical Association.* 2000; **284**: 2476–82.

25. Hauser JM, Chang CH, Alpert H *et al.* Who's caring for whom? Differing perspectives between seriously ill patients and their family caregivers. *American Journal of Hospice and Palliative Care.* 2006; **23**: 105–12.

26. Hinton J. How reliable are relatives' retrospective reports of terminal illness? Patients and relatives' accounts compared. *Social Science and Medicine.* 1996; **43**: 1229–36.

27. McPherson CJ, Addington-Hall JM. Evaluating palliative care: bereaved family members' evaluations of patients' pain, anxiety and depression. *Journal of Pain and Symptom Management.* 2004; **28**: 104–14.

28. Ellershaw J, Smith C, Overill S *et al.* Care of the dying: setting standards for symptom control in the last 48 hours of life. *Journal of Pain and Symptom Management.* 2001; **21**: 12–7.

29. Ventafridda V, Ripamonti C, De Conno F *et al.* Symptom prevalence and control during cancer patients' last days of life. *Journal of Palliative Care.* 1990; **6**: 7–11.

30. SUPPORT. A controlled trial to improve care for seriously ill hospitalized patients. The study to understand prognoses and preferences for outcomes and risks of treatments. The SUPPORT Principal Investigators. *Journal of the American Medical Association.* 1995; **274**: 1591–8.

31. Cain JM, Hammes BJ. Ethics and pain management: respecting patient wishes. *Journal of Pain and Symptom Management.* 1994; **9**: 160–5.

32. Yurk R, Morgan D, Franey S *et al.* Understanding the continuum of palliative care for patients and their caregivers. *Journal of Pain and Symptom Management.* 2002; **24**: 459–70.

∗ 33. Curtis JR, Wenrich MD, Carline JD *et al.* Patients' perspectives on physician skill in end-of-life care:

differences between patients with COPD, cancer, and AIDS. *Chest.* 2002; **122**: 356–62.

34. Back AL, Arnold RM, Tulsky JA *et al.* On saying goodbye: acknowledging the end of the patient–physician relationship with patients who are near death. *Annals of Internal Medicine.* 2005; **142**: 682–5.

35. O'Mahony S, Blank AE, Zallman L, Selwyn PA. The benefits of a hospital-based inpatient palliative care consultation service: preliminary outcome data. *Journal of Palliative Medicine.* 2005; **8**: 1033–9.

∗ 36. Ray A, Block SD, Friedlander RJ *et al.* Peaceful awareness in patients with advanced cancer. *Journal of Palliative Medicine.* 2006; **9**: 1359–68.

37. Seale C, Addington-Hall J. Euthanasia: why people want to die earlier. *Social Science and Medicine.* 1994; **39**: 647–54.

38. Georges JJ, Onwuteaka-Philipsen BD, van der Wal G *et al.* Differences between terminally ill cancer patients who died after euthanasia had been performed and terminally ill cancer patients who did not request euthanasia. *Palliative Medicine.* 2005; **19**: 578–86.

∗ 39. Bascom PB, Tolle SW. Responding to requests for physician-assisted suicide: "These are uncharted waters for both of us...". *Journal of the American Medical Association.* 2002; **288**: 91–8.

40. Georges JJ, Onwuteaka-Philipsen BD, van der Heide A *et al.* Requests to forgo potentially life-prolonging treatment and to hasten death in terminally ill cancer patients: a prospective study. *Journal of Pain and Symptom Management.* 2006; **31**: 100–10.

41. Hudson PL, Kristjanson LJ, Ashby M *et al.* Desire for hastened death in patients with advanced disease and the evidence base of clinical guidelines: a systematic review. *Palliative Medicine.* 2006; **20**: 693–701.

42. Ganzini L, Nelson HD, Schmidt TA *et al.* Physicians' experiences with the Oregon Death with Dignity Act. *New England Journal of Medicine.* 2000; **342**: 557–63.

43. Lawlor PG. Delirium and dehydration: some fluid for thought? *Supportive Care in Cancer.* 2002; **10**: 445–54.

44. Quill TE. Principle of double effect and end-of-life pain management: additional myths and a limited role. *Journal of Palliative Medicine.* 1998; **1**: 333–6.

∗ 45. Fainsinger RL, Waller A, Bercovici M *et al.* A multicentre international study of sedation for uncontrolled symptoms in terminally ill patients. *Palliative Medicine.* 2000; **14**: 257–65.

∗ 46. Cherny NI. Sedation for the care of patients with advanced cancer. *Nature Clinic Practice. Oncology.* 2006; **3**: 492–500.

47. Gevers JK. Terminal sedation: between pain relief, withholding treatment and euthanasia. *Medicine and Law.* 2006; **25**: 747–51.

∗ 48. Lo B, Rubenfeld G. Palliative sedation in dying patients: "we turn to it when everything else hasn't worked". *Journal of the American Medical Association.* 2005; **294**: 1810–16.

* 49. Quill TE. Perspectives on care at the close of life. Initiating end-of-life discussions with seriously ill patients: addressing the "elephant in the room". *Journal of the American Medical Association*. 2000; **284**: 2502–07.

50. Duggleby W. The language of pain at the end of life. *Pain Management Nursing*. 2002; **3**: 154–60.

* 51. Herr K. Pain assessment in cognitively impaired older adults. *American Journal of Nursing*. 2002; **102**: 65–7.

52. Chibnall JT, Tait RC. Pain assessment in cognitively impaired and unimpaired older adults: a comparison of four scales. *Pain*. 2001; **92**: 173–86.

* 53. Tonelli MR. Waking the dying: must we always attempt to involve critically ill patients in end-of-life decisions? *Chest*. 2005; **127**: 637–42.

54. Feldt KS. The checklist of nonverbal pain indicators (CNPI). *Pain Management Nursing*. 2000; **1**: 13–21.

55. Block SD. Perspectives on care at the close of life. Psychological considerations, growth, and transcendence at the end of life: the art of the possible. *Journal of the American Medical Association*. 2001; **285**: 2898–905.

56. Gonzales GR, Elliott KJ, Portenoy RK, Foley KM. The impact of a comprehensive evaluation in the management of cancer pain. *Pain*. 1991; **47**: 141–4.

57. Levy MH. Pharmacologic treatment of cancer pain. *New England Journal of Medicine*. 1996; **335**: 1124–32.

58. Zech DF, Grond S, Lynch J *et al.* Validation of World Health Organization guidelines for cancer pain relief: a 10-year prospective study. *Pain*. 1995; **63**: 65–76.

* 59. Ventafridda V, Tamburini M, Caraceni A *et al.* A validation study of the WHO method for cancer pain relief. *Cancer*. 1987; **59**: 850–6.

60. Jacox A, Carr DB, Payne R. New clinical-practice guidelines for the management of pain in patients with cancer. *New England Journal of Medicine*. 1994; **330**: 651–5.

61. Fineberg IC, Wenger NS, Brown-Saltzman K. Unrestricted opiate administration for pain and suffering at the end of life: knowledge and attitudes as barriers to care. *Journal of Palliative Medicine*. 2006; **9**: 873–83.

62. Forbes K. Opioids: beliefs and myths. *Journal of Pain and Palliative Care Pharmacotherapy*. 2006; **20**: 33–5.

63. Portenoy RK, Sibirceva U, Smout R *et al.* Opioid use and survival at the end of life: a survey of a hospice population. *Journal of Pain and Symptom Management*. 2006; **32**: 532–40.

64. Bercovitch M, Waller A, Adunsky A. High dose morphine use in the hospice setting. A database survey of patient characteristics and effect on life expectancy. *Cancer*. 1999; **86**: 871–7.

65. Bercovitch M, Adunsky A. High dose controlled-release oxycodone in hospice care. *Journal of Pain and Palliative Care Pharmacotherapy*. 2006; **20**: 33–9.

66. Weschules DJ, Bain KT, Reifsnyder J *et al.* Toward evidence-based prescribing at end of life: a comparative analysis of sustained-release morphine, oxycodone, and transdermal fentanyl, with pain, constipation, and caregiver interaction outcomes in hospice patients. *Pain Medicine*. 2006; **7**: 320–9.

67. Jakobsson M, Strang P. Fentanyl patches for the treatment of pain in dying cancer patients. *Anticancer Research*. 1999; **19**: 4441–2.

68. Wong JO, Chiu GL, Tsao CJ, Chang CL. Comparison of oral controlled-release morphine with transdermal fentanyl in terminal cancer pain. *Acta Anaesthesiologica Sinica*. 1997; **35**: 25–32.

* 69. Nicholson AB. Methadone for cancer pain. *Cochrane Database of Systematic Reviews*. 2004; **CD003971**.

70. Daeninck PJ, Bruera E. Reduction in constipation and laxative requirements following opioid rotation to methadone: a report of four cases. *Journal of Pain and Symptom Management*. 1999; **18**: 303–09.

71. Moulin DE, Palma D, Watling C, Schulz V. Methadone in the management of intractable neuropathic noncancer pain. *Canadian Journal of Neurological Sciences*. 2005; **32**: 340–3.

* 72. Davis MP, Walsh D. Methadone for relief of cancer pain: a review of pharmacokinetics, pharmacodynamics, drug interactions and protocols of administration. *Supportive Care in Cancer*. 2001; **9**: 73–83.

73. Mathew P, Storey P. Subcutaneous methadone in terminally ill patients: manageable local toxicity. *Journal of Pain and Symptom Management*. 1999; **18**: 49–52.

74. Moryl N, Kogan M, Comfort C, Obbens E. Methadone in the treatment of pain and terminal delirium in advanced cancer patients. *Palliative and Supportive Care*. 2005; **3**: 311–17.

75. Payne R. Recognition and diagnosis of breakthrough pain. *Pain Medicine*. 2007; **8**: S3–7.

* 76. Anderson SL, Shreve ST. Continuous subcutaneous infusion of opiates at end-of-life. *Annals of Pharmacotherapy*. 2004; **38**: 1015–23.

77. Cools HJ, Berkhout AM, De Bock GH. Subcutaneous morphine infusion by syringe driver for terminally ill patients. *Age and Ageing*. 1996; **25**: 206–08.

78. Davis MP, Walsh D, LeGrand SB, Naughton M. Symptom control in cancer patients: the clinical pharmacology and therapeutic role of suppositories and rectal suspensions. *Supportive Care in Cancer*. 2002; **10**: 117–38.

79. Fine PG. Low-dose ketamine in the management of opioid nonresponsive terminal cancer pain. *Journal of Pain and Symptom Management*. 1999; **17**: 296–300.

80. Ferrini R. Parenteral lidocaine for severe intractable pain in six hospice patients continued at home. *Journal of Palliative Medicine*. 2000; **3**: 193–200.

81. Goodman LS, Gilman A, Hardman JG *et al. Goodman & Gilman's the pharmacological basis of therapeutics*, 9th edn. New York: McGraw-Hill, Health Professions Division, 1996; xxi: 1905.

82. Twycross R. The risks and benefits of corticosteroids in advanced cancer. *Drug Safety*. 1994; **11**: 163–78.

83. Strasser F, Bruera ED. Update on anorexia and cachexia. *Hematology/Oncology Clinics of North America*. 2002; **16**: 589–617.

* 84. Feuer DJ, Broadley KE. Corticosteroids for the resolution of malignant bowel obstruction in advanced gynaecological

and gastrointestinal cancer. *Cochrane Database of Systematic Reviews.* 2000; **CD001219**.

85. Reisfield GM, Wilson GR. Intrathecal drug therapy for pain #98. *Journal of Palliative Medicine.* 2004; **7**: 76.

86. Exner HJ, Peters J, Eikermann M. Epidural analgesia at end of life: facing empirical contraindications. *Anesthesia and Analgesia.* 2003; **97**: 1740–2.

87. Fine PG. Palliative radiation therapy in end-of-life care: evidence-based utilization. *American Journal of Hospice and Palliative Care.* 2002; **19**: 166–70.

88. Cohen ST, Block S. Issues in psychotherapy with terminally ill patients. *Palliative and Supportive Care.* 2004; **2**: 181–9.

89. Correa-Velez I, Clavarino A, Barnett AG, Eastwood H. Use of complementary and alternative medicine and quality of life: changes at the end of life. *Palliative Medicine.* 2003; **17**: 695–703.

* 90. Pan CX, Morrison RS, Ness J *et al.* Complementary and alternative medicine in the management of pain, dyspnea, and nausea and vomiting near the end of life. A systematic review. *Journal of Pain and Symptom Management.* 2000; **20**: 374–87.

91. Shlay JC, Chaloner K, Max MB *et al.* Acupuncture and amitriptyline for pain due to HIV-related peripheral neuropathy: a randomized controlled trial. Terry Beirn Community Programs for Clinical Research on AIDS. *Journal of the American Medical Association.* 1998; **280**: 1590–5.

92. McCaffery M, Wolff M. Pain relief using cutaneous modalities, positioning, and movement. *Hospice Journal.* 1992; **8**: 121–53.

93. Ouslander JG. Drug prescribing for the elderly. *Western Journal of Medicine.* 1981; **135**: 455–62.

94. Page J, Henry D. Consumption of NSAIDs and the development of congestive heart failure in elderly patients: an underrecognized public health problem. *Archives of Internal Medicine.* 2000; **160**: 777–84.

95. Mavity L. Constipation near the end of life. *Journal of Palliative Medicine.* 2006; **9**: 1502–03.

96. de Stoutz ND, Bruera E, Suarez-Almazor M. Opioid rotation for toxicity reduction in terminal cancer patients. *Journal of Pain and Symptom Management.* 1995; **10**: 378–84.

29

Pain in cancer survivors

W PAUL FARQUHAR-SMITH

Introduction	399	Radiotherapy-induced pain	405
Chemotherapy-induced neuropathic pain	399	Conclusion	406
Pain after cancer surgery	402	References	406

KEY LEARNING POINTS

- Surgery, chemotherapy, and radiotherapy can cause chronic pain in cancer survivors that has detrimental effects on function and quality of life.
- Pain in cancer survivors is underrecognized and undertreated.
- The adverse symptoms of chemotherapy-induced peripheral neuropathy (CIPN) can be dose limiting or even stop treatment.
- Most CIPN presents as a length-dependent, symmetrical sensory neuropathy in a "stocking-glove" distribution after cumulative chemotherapy.
- Management of CIPN is compromised by a lack of standardization of assessment and a paucity of research into preventative and treatment strategies.

- Postbreast cancer surgery pain (PBCSP) exemplifies the problem of chronic pain following cancer surgery.
- Incidence of PBCSP could be reduced by recognition and reduction of remediable risk factors.
- Although less common due to refinement of radiotherapy, radiation-induced neuropathy remains a debilitating and problematic pain to treat.
- More research is required into the specific neuropathic pain of these examples of pain in cancer survivors, since current management is extrapolated from existing neuropathic pain treatments.

INTRODUCTION

Patients with cancer can experience pain from a number of sources:

- the cancer itself by direct tumor involvement with bone, soft tissues, viscera, and nerves;
- incidental noncancer pain that may be problematic and impact significantly on quality of life;
- pain associated with cancer treatment.

Surgery, radiotherapy, and chemotherapy form the basis of treatment of most cancers and are associated with persistent pain that may be difficult to treat long after the cancer is in remission or cured. This problem is likely to grow due to increasing cancer survival rates.[1] Pain has

added significance since persistence or return of pain after apparent treatment often provokes the patient to assume cancer recurrence.[2] This chapter will focus on pain associated with surgery, radiotherapy, and chemotherapy.

CHEMOTHERAPY-INDUCED NEUROPATHIC PAIN

Presentation and mechanisms of chemotherapy-induced peripheral neuropathy

Many antineoplastic chemotherapies are neurotoxic (**Box 29.1**). Peripheral neuropathy can lead to significant

Box 29.1 Selection of chemotherapuetic agents associated with sensory peripheral neuropathy

- Platinum analogs*
  - cisplatin
  - carboplatin
  - oxaliplatin
- Vinca alkaloids*
  - vincristine
  - vinblastine
- Taxanes*
  - paclitaxel
  - docetaxel
- Thalidomide*
- Bortezomib*
- Doxorubicin
- Etoposide
- Gemcitabine
- Ifosfamide
- Interferon-α

*Higher risk agents

Box 29.2 Diagnostic features of CIPN

- Length dependency
  - Distal parts of limb long nerves affected ("stocking-glove distribution")
- Symmetrical symptoms
  - Onset temporally related to administration of neurotoxic chemotherapy
  - Onset can be rapid, delayed or after cessation of treatment ("coasting")
- Signs and symptoms of neurosensory dysfunction
  - Including paresthesias and pain
- Sparing of motor function compared to sensory symptoms

N.B. Presentation of oxaliplatin CIPN may be different. Reproduced with permission from Hausheer et al.[7]

functional impairment. Neurotoxicity may be dose limiting or even warrant the cessation of treatment, potentially jeopardizing optimal treatment.[3] Although chemotoxicity can affect the central nervous system, peripheral neuropathy is most prevalent affecting from 10 up to 100 percent of patients depending on patient factors, chemotherapeutic agent, and dose.[4, 5] Longer duration of therapy and higher cumulative dose increases the risk of neuropathy. Preexisting neuropathy from previous chemotherapy or of other etiologies, such as diabetes, increases risk of further peripheral neurotoxicity and pain. Chemotherapy-induced peripheral neuropathy (CIPN) also impacts negatively on quality of life measures and activities of daily living in a population that may have thought these aspects would improve after successful cancer treatment. As with other chronic pain in cancer survivors, symptoms of CIPN and pain are underreported.[6] This is compounded by the heterogenicity of scoring and diagnostic criteria and limited effective treatment and preventative strategies.

Chemotherapeutic agents act by different mechanisms, yet there is a remarkable similarity in the patterns of CIPN (**Box 29.2**). Most CIPNs are predominantly sensory, although motor systems may be affected at a subclinical level. The distribution of pain and sensory dysfunction is symmetrical, principally in the "stocking–glove" distribution indicative of "length dependence." The final common mechanism of chemotherapy-induced neuropathy is interference with microtubule-mediated axonal transport.[7, 8] Distal parts of long nerves in the

limbs are susceptible due to lack of nutrient transport and are therefore preferentially affected. However, animal models of CIPN propose biochemical alterations in nerve function are central to pain and hyperalgesia rather than gross anatomical damage. Clinical observation of rapidly induced CIPN could be explained by chemotherapy-induced degeneration of receptor terminals in skin and increases in perineural proinflammatory cytokines.[4] Alterations in neuronal excitability may also be involved in pain generation.[9] Other pathologies, such as mitochondrial abnormality, may be involved.[10] Nevertheless, combination neurotoxic chemotherapies increase the risk of neuropathy, as would be expected by a functional or anatomical common final pathway. Other mechanisms of damage include axonal Wallerian degeneration,[11] direct injury to dorsal root ganglion (DRGs) cells,[12] and, infrequently, demyelination.[13]

AXONOPATHY AND NEURONOPATHY

Axonal and DRG damage are termed axonopathy and neuronopathy, respectively.[7] A neuronopathy is less common, usually occurs after higher doses of taxanes and platins,[8, 14] and involves a more rapid (hours to days) development of symmetrical length-dependent sensory peripheral neuropathy. The symptoms are constant, persistent, and more often involve loss of deep tendon reflexes.[7] Axonopathies present more insidiously, gradually increasing in severity after multiple chemotherapy treatments. Lower limbs are affected before the upper limbs but in the same length-dependent "stocking–glove" distribution. Although clinical presentation may fluctuate, continuing neurotoxic chemotherapy increases damage whilst stopping treatment may allow recovery.

Occasionally, "coasting" occurs whereby symptoms continue to deteriorate after cessation of treatment.[15]

Assessment of CIPN

THE ROLE OF QUANTITATIVE SENSORY TESTING

Although clinical presentation may be similar with different chemotherapies, quantitative sensory testing (QST) exposes variations in sensory abnormalities.[4, 16] For example, cisplatin- and vincristine-induced CIPN reveal elevated cold pain threshold, whilst paclitaxel patients report burning sensation with cold stimulus.[4] However, QST findings do not consistently reflect clinical symptoms, nor correlate with cumulative dose of chemotherapy, nor is there evidence to suggest that QST identifies CIPN earlier than clinical history and examination.[17, 18] However, the addition of assessment of vibration sense may facilitate CIPN diagnosis and surveillance, such as is encompassed in the total neuropathy score.[19, 20]

CIPN ASSESSMENT

The numerous and disparate grading scales for CIPN hinder obfuscate clear diagnostic and comparable data. Several scales including the World Health Organization (WHO),[21] Eastern Cooperative Oncology Group (ECOG),[22] and National Cancer Institute common toxicity criteria (NCIC-CTC)[23] range from 0 to 4 and include subjective and objective measures (**Table 29.1**). These are predominantly clinician based and are not relevant to all CIPN. Comparison of these scales exposes large discrepancies in interobserver assessment, especially where

interpretation of subjective parameters is required.[24] Realization that patient-centered terms such as "intolerable" and "disabling" would be better quantified by patients and that function and quality of life issues are paramount, has led to the development of more patient-based evaluation.[7, 25] Investigators of other neuropathic pains have attempted to standardize assessment,[26] yet currently there is no accepted valid and reliable scale that encompasses the combination of clinician and patient appraisal, subjective and objective assessment, and function and quality of life issues. The deficiency of a unifying scale also impairs the ability to assess recovery and natural history of CIPN.

CIPN for selected specific agents

PLATINUM-BASED CHEMOTHERAPY

Cisplatin, carboplatin, and oxaliplatin are chemotherapeutic agents that act by damaging DNA. They differ in the incidence of CIPN, probably due to pharmacokinetic factors.[20] Cisplatin causes axonopathy after cumulative dosing, predominantly affects large fibers and exhibits "coasting" after cessation of treatment.[27, 28] "Coasting" may be related to persistence of cisplatin in DRGs.[3] Resolution of symptoms (in approximately 80 percent) may take months or years, though permanent objective signs can remain. The clinical presentation and incidence of CIPN are similar after carboplatin.[29] Oxaliplatin is more likely to cause acute self-limiting neurotoxicity, but affects hands, feet, and perioral regions and is aggravated by cold.[30] However, it may also induce a longer duration, cumulative CIPN.[30, 31]

Table 29.1 Grading of CIPN.

Scale	Grade 0	Grade 1	Grade 2	Grade 3	Grade 4
WHO[21]	None	Paresthesias and/or decreased tendon reflexes	Severe paresthesias and/or mild weakness	Intolerable paresthesias and/or motor loss	Paralysis
ECOG[22]	None	Decreased tendon reflexes, mild paresthesias, mild constipation	Absent deep tendon reflexes, severe constipation, mild weakness	Disabling sensory loss, severe peripheral neuropathic pain, severe weakness, bladder disfunction	Respiratory dysfunction, secondary to weakness, paralysis confining patient to bed/wheelchair
NCIC-CTC[23]	None	Loss or deep tendon reflexes or paresthesias (including tingling) but not interfering with function	Mild/moderate objective sensory loss or paresthesia (including tingling) interfering with function, but not interfering with activities of daily living	Sensory loss or paresthesia interfering with activities of daily living	Permanent sensory loss that interferes with function

After Quasthoff and Hartung.[3]

TAXANES

Paclitaxel and docetaxel act by increasing aggregation of microtubules, although the mechanism of neurotoxicty may also involve changes in membrane excitability. Paclitaxel CIPN is cumulative, dose-dependent and often dose-limiting, especially in conjunction with other CIPN-inducing agents.[19] Paclitaxel induces symptoms typical of a length-dependent, symmetrical sensory axonopathy that start within days of treatment, increasing in incidence with subsequent cycles and may exhibit "coasting."[11] Weekly compared to three-weekly dosing schedules and more rapid infusion are associated with a higher incidence of CIPN, possibly due to less interdose recovery time and higher peak dose.[7, 32] The supposition that the vehicle Cremaphor EL (polyoxyethylated castor oil) generates CIPN rather than paclitaxel is unfounded.[7] Docetaxel induces clinically identical CIPN, but is less neurotoxic than paclitaxel as demonstrated in combination with carboplatin for ovarian cancer after six three-weekly cycles.[33]

BORTEZOMIB

Bortezomib is a proteasome inhibitor used for the treatment of several malignancies and is licensed for relapsed multiple myeloma. Bortezomib causes axonopathy.[34] In a randomized trial (APEX), 36 percent of patients developed bortezomib-induced CIPN and 8 percent discontinued treatment because of CIPN.[35] Evidence of preexisting peripheral neuropathy was present in 69 percent at baseline and was a risk factor for severe neuropathy.[34, 35, 36] Fifty-one percent with grade 2 CIPN or above improved with a median time of 107 days.[35] Another controlled trial identified cumulative, dose-related sensory neuropathy as the most important adverse event.[37] Here, 12 percent required dose reduction and cessation of treatment in 4 percent, although the majority experienced some improvement of CIPN symptoms.[37] The timeline of clinical progression or resolution is still unclear, but 71 percent of the patients that developed CIPN improved after 1 to 529 days.[36]

THALIDOMIDE

Thalidomide is also used for refractory multiple myeloma and may act by tumor necrosis factor modulation. It causes distal axonal degeneration presenting with the familiar constellation of symptoms of symmetrical, length-dependent sensory neuropathy.[38] In contrast to other CIPN there is no clear cumulative dose–response and symptoms may occur after brief or extended therapy or present well after cessation of treatment.[39] Over a two-year period, 50 percent of patients receiving thalidomide exhibited evidence of CIPN which was proportional to daily dose rather than duration of treatment.[40] Thalidomide-induced CIPN is common, often dose limiting, and is less likely to recover.[41]

Prevention and treatment of CIPN

PREVENTION

Amifostine has proven efficacy as a cytoprotective agent against many chemotherapies in animal models. However, amifostine only achieved nonsignificant reduction of cisplatin-induced neuropathy, and had no effect on paclitaxel-induced neuropathy but caused frequent side effects.[8, 14] Accordingly, the American Society of Clinical Oncology does not support its use.[42] The nonessential amino acid glutamine has been shown to reduce painful high dose paclitaxel-induced neuropathy, albeit in a trial without blinding, randomization, or placebo.[43] Inexpensive and with possible sensitization of tumor to chemotherapy qualities, glutamine warrants further investigation.[44] Glutathione protects against oxidative damage and in several underpowered trials prevented CIPN activity, especially after oxaliplatin.[14] Acetyl-L-carnitine is another agent that has shown neuroprotective promise.[45] More data are required to identify a preventative treatment for CIPN without affecting anticancer efficacy and without appreciable adverse effects.

TREATMENT

Patient education and nonpharmacological interventions are important elements of CIPN treatment. Few studies have specifically examined pharmacological treatments for CIPN and most of the available data are gleaned from neuropathic pain studies where postherpetic neuralgia and diabetic neuropathy are overrepresented.[46] Extrapolation would suggest treating painful CIPN as other neuropathic pain using evidence-based guidelines.[46, 47] However, CIPN and neuropathies of disparate etiologies may be mechanistically distinct and the extrapolation should be made cautiously. Indeed, in a recent randomized, crossover, controlled trial, gabapentin had no significant effect on painful or sensory symptoms of CIPN[48] nor did it reduce oxaliplatin-induced CIPN in patients treated for colorectal cancer.[49] Experimental revelation of mechanistic details of CIPN may allow development of novel treatments.

PAIN AFTER CANCER SURGERY

Chronic pain following surgery is a major cause of pain morbidity. Surgery was recognized as a causative factor in 20 percent of patients attending chronic pain clinics.[50] Chronic pain is more common after breast surgery for cancer than breast surgery for benign conditions.[51] Incidence of chronic pain after breast cancer surgery varies from 4–6 percent[52] to 25 percent,[53] and up to 52 percent.[54] The variation in prevalence may reflect changing patterns of surgical procedure and the disparity of classification of pain syndromes. For example, to label chronic pain after breast conserving surgery, "postmastectomy pain" is misleading. The use of the term "postbreast cancer surgery pain" (PBCSP) encompasses and consolidates the myriad of existing terms.

Not all local pain following breast surgery will necessarily be related to the surgery *per se*.[55] For example, the fear of pain can result in immobility leading to secondary shoulder pain.[52] Similar to other pains in cancer survivors, PBCSP is underreported and underestimated by clinicians.[56] Patients may be unwilling to report pain that they believe indicates recurrence, or reluctant to complain about a symptom perceived to be less important than life-threatening disease.[57]

Etiology and classification

Pain can be experienced in the scar, chest wall, arm, or in the breast itself after mastectomy or breast conserving surgery. The pain is often associated with sensory disturbance,[53] and the predominant etiology of PBCSP is injury to peripheral nerve fibers.[58] This is consistent with observations of spontaneous pain, allodynia, and sensory loss and it is likely the mechanisms of peripheral and central sensitization following nerve injury are involved.[59] A number of breast surgery-related pain syndromes have been coined based on pain character, location, and timing postsurgery. Pain can occur after mastectomy, lumpectomy with or without axillary dissection and with or without radiotherapy or chemotherapy.[60]

A classification of neuropathic pain following breast surgery has been proposed delineated by mechanism, epidemiology, and treatment: phantom breast pain, intercostobrachial neuralgia, neuroma pain, and "other."[61] Although these terms identify specific subsets, diagnosis of neuropathic pain by putative mechanism is problematic in the clinical setting. Furthermore, at present the evidence for treatment of neuropathic pain does not support the use of specific agents for any of the four mechanistically different groups.

Risk factors

Various authors have stressed the need to recognize risk factors in order to prevent chronic pain following breast cancer surgery. Several factors have been identified but not all studies have demonstrated their association with chronic pain. Younger patients are more likely to complain of PBCSP.[57, 62, 63, 64, 65, 66] A retrospective survey identified 65 percent of patients aged 30–49 who reported "postmastectomy pain syndrome" compared to 26 percent in those over 70 years.[57] However, other retrospective surveys of breast cancer survivors have not recognized age as a risk factor.[52, 60] Anxiety and depression have been suggested as risk factors for PBCSP and are more

prevalent in younger patients.[63, 66, 67] Younger age is associated with more aggressive disease and treatment, including radiotherapy and chemotherapy, which may contribute to the development of chronic pain.[63] These interventions cause nerve damage, increase vulnerability to surgical insult, and therefore neuropathic pain. Indeed, several studies have demonstrated an association of chemotherapy and radiotherapy with the development of PBCSP[53, 66, 68, 69] and with the severity of that pain.[64] However, not only have some workers failed to confirm this association,[60, 65] but the interdependence of treatment modality with age makes it difficult to ascribe chemotherapy and radiotherapy as independent risk factors.[57]

Surgical factors

INTERCOSTOBRACHIAL NEURALGIA AND AXILLARY DISSECTION

Damage and dysfunction in the intercostobrachial nerve (ICBN) has been proposed as a contributing or principal etiology of PBCSP.[55, 70] However, although the anatomy of the ICBN is varied, PBCSP after surgery remote from the axilla is unlikely to be ICBN dysfunction. Nevertheless, three months after preservation of ICBN during axillary dissection, 61 percent of patients had no pain symptoms, compared to 29 percent where the nerve had been sacrificed.[71][III] Although sensory disturbances were increased after ICBN severance, less pain in the nerve preservation group was only evident at time of discharge and not at three months.[72][III] However, here the ICBN was only spared in 65 percent of the preservation group, occasionally cut to achieve adequate surgical access.[72][III] Pain was reported by 59 percent of patients with ICBN transection 30 months or more after axillary surgery compared to 31 percent when the nerve was spared,[73][III] yet a similar trial showed no advantage of ICBN preservation three years after axillary surgery.[74][II] Other studies have failed to identify axillary dissection as a conclusive risk factor for pain.[75] The observation of 30 percent developing pain with ICBN preservation, and 30 percent not developing pain after ICBN section requires additional explanatory mechanisms. Nevertheless, axillary surgery may contribute to PBCSP[65] and ICBN preservation is a pragmatic surgical technique that could help reduce short- and long-term pain. Sentinel node biopsy is less likely to threaten the ICPN and is associated with less pain than axillary dissection.[76]

CONSERVING AND RADICAL SURGERY – THE INFLUENCE OF ACUTE PAIN

Does conserving compared to more radical surgery, such as mastectomy, or reconstructive surgery influence the development of chronic pain? Surgical factors are interrelated with intensity of acute pain previously identified as a risk factor in other postsurgical chronic pains.[50, 58] Indeed, in a retrospective survey of 509 patients 10–58 months after breast cancer surgery, acute postoperative pain and type of surgery were identified as pivotal to chronic pain development.[68] More invasive surgery results in greater acute pain and pain at 30 days postbreast cancer surgery.[63] Chronic pain at one year was less in patients treated in a unit more experienced in breast cancer surgery and who were more likely to have breast conserving surgery.[77][III] Recall of more severe acute postoperative pain correlated with chronic pain,[77][III] although patients with chronic pain may overestimate the memory of acute pain.[78] However, a prospective study not reliant upon recall linked acute postoperative pain intensity with intensity of chronic pain.[64] Nevertheless, others have found chronic pain unrelated to invasiveness of breast surgery[2] and some even identified increased chronic pain after conservative compared to radical breast surgery.[65, 67] Indeed, conservative breast surgery is associated with a 40 percent incidence of chronic PBCSP.[79] Increased likelihood of adjuvant radiotherapy after conservative surgery may negate any potential benefits of conservative surgery. Severity of acute pain may be the delineating factor and not type of surgery *per se*.

The influence of acute postoperative pain in the genesis of chronic pain is compatible with mechanisms of peripheral afferent input driving central sensitization. The association of surgical complications with chronic pain may be pain related.[53] Sensory testing on patients with PBCSP revealed results consistent with central sensitization and ongoing peripheral input to the spinal cord.[80] Therefore, control of acute pain should be an effective prevention strategy. Local anesthetic paravertebral blockade not only reduced postoperative pain after breast cancer surgery,[81][II] but reduced pain one year later.[82] [III] Patients who had received patient-controlled analgesia (PCA) following mastectomy had significantly lower acute pain scores and reported less persistent pain four years later.[75]

RECONSTRUCTION

Implant reconstruction has been implicated as a risk factor for postsurgical chronic pain in cancer patients as well as use of implants in nonmalignant surgery.[51] There are few data concerning chronic pain after reconstructions using latissimus dorsi flaps, transverse rectus abdominis muscle (TRAM), or deep inferior epigastic perforator (DIEP) free flaps which are frequently used for breast reconstruction. DIEP flap reconstructions may provoke less postoperative pain than latissimus dorsi flaps and perhaps be associated with less chronic pain.[83] Although the evidence is not conclusive, identification of risk factors could facilitate the prevention and treatment of PBCSP and at least increase awareness of a chronic pain

that is highly prevalent and underdiagnosed. Some factors such as age are intransigent, and therefore efforts should be concentrated on remedial factors such as ensuring good postoperative pain control and allaying preoperative anxiety.

Phantom breast pain

Phantom breast sensations and pain occur frequently postmastectomy although less commonly than phantom limb phenomena.[84, 85] A lesser cortical representation of the breast has been postulated to account for these observations.[86] Reported prevalence ranges from more than 60 to 15 percent for sensation and from 0 to 44 percent for phantom pain.[85] In contrast to phantom limb pain, phantom breast pain may have a delayed onset and tends to remain constant in intensity rather than decrease over time.[86, 87] Phantom mastectomy pain may be mechanistically related to phantom limb pain whereby somatosensory cortical reorganization is driven by preoperative pain[88] and perioperative pain may also be a risk factor for phantom breast pain.[86, 87] Other studies have not supported this notion.[84] Potential risk factors such as radiotherapy, chemotherapy, and reconstruction also do not seem to influence the development of phantom breast pain.[84]

Treatment of PBCSP

Not only is PBCSP underreported, but there is evidence to suggest it is also poorly treated.[52] PBCSP has a negative impact on quality of life. Pain was reported as being more detrimental to quality of life measures than perceived disfigurement.[89] Even when disfigurement is reduced by conservative surgery, pain adversely affects quality of life more than the benefit of improved body image.[79] Nonpharmacological and psychological therapies may be of value, including pain management programs.[90] However, relatively few patients with PBCSP use analgesic medicines.[51, 52, 65] Only 29 percent of patients with PBCSP received prescribed therapy, and only 44 percent obtained relief.[52] Qualitative surveys imply this may be due to a reluctance to take ineffective medication that causes side effects, and development of pain coping strategies.[2, 62] Practitioner unfamiliarity and lack of knowledge of PBCSP as a neuropathic pain state could explain the absence of antineuropathic agents in patients treatments.[52]

There is a paucity of controlled trials of treatments for PBCSP. Although the burning sensation of capsaicin may have compromised blinding, a small randomized trial using 0.075 percent capsaicin cream showed 62 percent achieved at least 50 percent pain relief.[91][II] Amitriptyline reduced pain intensity in 8 out of 15 patients with neuropathic pain after breast cancer surgery in a randomized, double-blind crossover study.[92][II] However, analysis was not on an intention to treat basis since four patients who withdrew due to adverse effects were not included.[92][II] Similar criticism could be levied at a methodologically comparable study using venlafaxine to treat PBCSP.[93][II] There was no effect on average daily pain intensity and although the secondary outcomes of average pain relief and maximum pain intensity were reduced by venlafaxine, 2 of the 15 patients withdrew (one because of side effects), and 2 of the remaining 13 could not tolerate the higher 75 mg dose.[93][II] In a separate study, venlafaxine given a day before and two weeks after breast cancer surgery reduced pain scores on movement and specifically pain in the axilla, chest wall, and arm, six months later.[94][II] A multimodal approach including gabapentin reduced pain in the postoperative period and at three and six months.[95][II] Perioperative application of topical local anesthetic (EMLA) did not alter acute pain scores yet reduced PBCSP at three months.[96][II]

Analogous to the paucity of CIPN treatment data, PBCSP is not well represented in the neuropathic pain evidence-base. A similar extrapolation has to be made that disregards the disparity of etiologically distinct neuropathic pain states. Further controlled trials are required. However, it is important to avoid the perpetuation of the continuing reluctance to consider opioid medication in the treatment of neuropathic pain when the evidence of efficacy is well established.[97][I]

RADIOTHERAPY-INDUCED PAIN

Physical nature of radiotherapy

Radiotherapy is frequently used for many cancer treatments, both as primary treatment and as an adjunct, with chemotherapy and surgery. Ionizing radiation is thought to create free radicals that interfere with nuclear function and induce cell death. Radiotherapy is focused onto tumor to reduce the potential for damage to normal tissues. Ionizing radiation can lead to many potential complications depending on the site of application and susceptible normal tissues which are exposed, such as skin and mucous membranes. Some radiation damage results in well-described pain syndromes such as radiotherapy for bowel cancer, which is associated with later development of abdominal pain and intestinal obstruction.[98] Pelvic radiotherapy for carcinoma of the endometrium and cervix is also implicated in long-term chronic pain.[99] The deleterious effects of these pains are reflected in the global reduction in of quality of life measures.[99]

Brachial plexus neuropathy

Radiotherapy adversely affects nerve function acutely and in the long term. Brachial plexus neuropathy (BPN) is well characterized.[100] This may develop decades after the radiotherapy and is secondary to slowly developing fibrosis following endarteritis obliterans after slow depletion of proliferating cells.[101, 102] In the 1960s, the developing use of breast conserving strategies and higher energy radiation directed below the skin reduced dose-limiting skin damage but led to higher total doses and greater risk of plexopathy.[103] Dose rationalization, sophistication of administration, and fractionation of radiotherapy treatments have reduced BPN since repeated smaller doses of radiation are less damaging than larger fractions for a given total dose.[104] Increased incidence of BPN from patients treated in the 1960s was clearly associated with larger fractions.[105] A recent review of hypo-fractionated adjuvant radiotherapy for breast cancer identified BPN prevalence of 1.7 to 73 percent after fractions of 2.2 to 4.58 Gy and total doses between 43.5 and 60 Gy.[106] Fractions of 2.2 to 2.5 Gy and total doses between 34 and 40 Gy were associated with less than 1 percent prevalence of BPN.[106] Some studies have suggested an increased incidence with chemotherapy, and that BPN occurs in younger patients.[107]

Rarely, BPN occurs concomitantly or soon after radiotherapy,[108] yet most radiation-induced plexopathy occurs more than six months after treatment. Higher doses have a reduced latency for BPN.[106] Progressive forelimb weakness characterizes this plexopathy with variable deficits of sensation and pain. Pain is much more common in tumor-related plexopathy,[102, 109] although pain has been described as anything from a rare symptom[110] to almost a universal one in radiation-induced BPN.[111]

Other features that may identify radiation-induced neuropathy compared to tumor-related neuropathy are:

- initial involvement of upper plexus divisions;
- slow progression;
- long duration.[102]

Examination of 100 patients with BPN identified 78 as being caused by tumor and 22 secondary to radiotherapy.[109] The lower trunk (C7–8, T1) was involved in 72 percent of the tumor-induced BPN whilst 78 percent of radiotherapy-induced BPN involved the upper trunk (C5–6).[109] In collusion with clinical symptoms and signs, investigations such as magnetic resonance imaging (MRI) can aid in correct diagnosis of the plexopathy.[112][II]

The risk of radiation BPN increases with time. Following a total of 60 Gy supraclavicular lymph node irradiation, the frequency severe plexopathy was present in 2 percent after 5 years, 5.5 percent after 10 years, 11.8 percent after 15 years, and 19.1 percent after 19 years.[113] Moreover, the increasing incidence was due to patients presenting initially with lower grade plexopathy progressing in severity.[113] Indeed, patients apparently problem free at five years still have an appreciable risk of late plexopathy complications.[105]

Treatment of radiation-induced BPN

Modulation of radiotherapy regimes forms the mainstay of preventative strategies. Hyperbaric oxygen treatment failed to prevent or slow the progression of BPN.[114]

There is a paucity of data concerning the treatment of painful BPN. As for other neuropathic pain, extrapolation of evidence from postherpetic neuralgia and diabetic neuropathy trials guides pharmacological treatment. The use of "antineuropathic" medications and opioids have been suggested.[115] At a median follow-up time of 9.5 years, 17 out of 33 patients with radiation-induced BPN were receiving long-term morphine for pain.[111] Surgical techniques have also been used, such as covering the plexus with myocutaneous flaps[116] and percutaneous cervical cordotomy.[117] Although cordotomy has an evidence-base in treatment of tumor-related pain (e.g. mesothelioma[118] and breast cancer[119]), its role in radiation-induced BPN is unclear. When present, pain not only infers the anxiety of tumor recurrence but is often refractory to treatment. A multidisciplinary, multimodal approach is often required. Pain can also contribute to the resentment felt by some to the damaging effects of their radiotherapy. Pressure groups such as Radiotherapy Action Group Exposure (RAGE) serve as a reminder of the need for regular appraisal and refinement of potentially damaging treatments.[110, 120]

CONCLUSION

Surgery, chemotherapy, and radiotherapy all cause chronic pain problems that have a major negative impact on quality of life and are often thought to herald returning disease. These chronic pains are underreported by patients and practitioners and consequently undertreated. Identification and reduction of risk factors and continuing modulation and refinement of anticancer therapies can be effective preventative measures. Pain in cancer survivors such as PBCSP, painful CIPN, and radiation-induced neuropathy, are exemplars of neuropathic pain poorly represented in the literature. Research into effective treatments is necessary to address this growing chronic pain problem.

REFERENCES

1. Peto R, Boreham J, Clarke M et al. UK and USA breast cancer deaths down 25% in year 2000 at ages 20–69 years. Lancet. 2000; 355: 1822.
2. Carpenter JS, Andrykowski MA, Sloan P et al. Postmastectomy/postlumpectomy pain in breast cancer survivors. Journal of Clinical Epidemiology. 1998; 51: 1285–92.
 * 3. Quasthoff S, Hartung HP. Chemotherapy-induced peripheral neuropathy. Journal of Neurology. 2002; 249: 9–17.
 * 4. Cata JP, Weng HR, Lee BN et al. Clinical and experimental findings in humans and animals with chemotherapy-induced peripheral neuropathy. Minerva Anestesiologica. 2006; 72: 151–69.
5. Chaudhry V, Rowinsky EK, Sartorius SE et al. Peripheral neuropathy from taxol and cisplatin combination chemotherapy: clinical and electrophysiological studies. Annals of Neurology. 1994; 35: 304–11.
6. Stephens RJ, Hopwood P, Girling DJ, Machin D. Randomized trials with quality of life endpoints: are doctors' ratings of patients' physical symptoms interchangeable with patients' self-ratings? Quality of Life Research. 1997; 6: 225–36.
 * 7. Hausheer FH, Schilsky RL, Bain S et al. Diagnosis, management, and evaluation of chemotherapy-induced peripheral neuropathy. Seminars in Oncology. 2006; 33: 15–49.
8. Openshaw H, Beamon K, Synold TW et al. Neurophysiological study of peripheral neuropathy after high-dose Paclitaxel: lack of neuroprotective effect of amifostine. Clinical Cancer Research. 2004; 10: 461–7.
9. Siau C, Xiao W, Bennett GJ. Paclitaxel- and vincristine-evoked painful peripheral neuropathies: Loss of epidermal innervation and activation of Langerhans cells. Experimental Neurology. 2006; 201: 507–14.
10. Flatters SJ, Bennett GJ. Studies of peripheral sensory nerves in paclitaxel-induced painful peripheral neuropathy: evidence for mitochondrial dysfunction. Pain. 2006; 122: 245–57.
11. Lipton RB, Apfel SC, Dutcher JP et al. Taxol produces a predominantly sensory neuropathy. Neurology. 1989; 39: 368–73.
12. Screnci D, McKeage MJ, Galettis P et al. Relationships between hydrophobicity, reactivity, accumulation and peripheral nerve toxicity of a series of platinum drugs. British Journal of Cancer. 2000; 82: 966–72.
13. Sahenk Z, Barohn R, New P, Mendell JR. Taxol neuropathy. Electrodiagnostic and sural nerve biopsy findings. Archives of Neurology. 1994; 51: 726–9.
 * 14. Ocean AJ, Vahdat LT. Chemotherapy-induced peripheral neuropathy: pathogenesis and emerging therapies. Supportive Care in Cancer. 2004; 12: 619–25.
15. Grunberg SM, Sonka S, Stevenson LL, Muggia FM. Progressive paresthesias after cessation of therapy with very high-dose cisplatin. Cancer Chemotherapy and Pharmacology. 1989; 25: 62–4.
16. Dougherty PM, Cata JP, Cordella JV et al. Taxol-induced sensory disturbance is characterized by preferential impairment of myelinated fiber function in cancer patients. Pain. 2004; 109: 132–42.
17. Forsyth PA, Balmaceda C, Peterson K et al. Prospective study of paclitaxel-induced peripheral neuropathy with quantitative sensory testing. Journal of Neuro-oncology. 1997; 35: 47–53.
18. Berger T, Malayeri R, Doppelbauer A et al. Neurological monitoring of neurotoxicity induced by paclitaxel/cisplatin

chemotherapy. *European Journal of Cancer*. 1997; **33**: 1393–9.

19. du BA, Schlaich M, Luck HJ *et al*. Evaluation of neurotoxicity induced by paclitaxel second-line chemotherapy. *Supportive Care in Cancer*. 1999; **7**: 354–61.

✳ 20. Cavaletti G, Marmiroli P. Chemotherapy-induced peripheral neurotoxicity. *Expert Opinion on Drug Safety*. 2004; **3**: 535–46.

21. Miller AB, Hoogstraten B, Staquet M, Winkler A. Reporting results of cancer treatment. *Cancer*. 1981; **47**: 207–14.

22. Oken MM, Creech RH, Tormey DC *et al*. Toxicity and response criteria of the Eastern Cooperative Oncology Group. *American Journal of Clinical Oncology*. 1982; **5**: 649–55.

23. Postma TJ, Heimans JJ. Grading of chemotherapy-induced peripheral neuropathy. *Annals of Oncology*. 2000; **11**: 509–13.

24. Postma TJ, Heimans JJ, Muller MJ *et al*. Pitfalls in grading severity of chemotherapy-induced peripheral neuropathy. *Annals of Oncology*. 1998; **9**: 739–44.

25. Postma TJ, Aaronson NK, Heimans JJ *et al*. The development of an EORTC quality of life questionnaire to assess chemotherapy-induced peripheral neuropathy: the QLQ-CIPN20. *European Journal of Cancer*. 2005; **41**: 1135–9.

26. Cruccu G, Anand P, Attal N *et al*. EFNS guidelines on neuropathic pain assessment. *European Journal of Neurology*. 2004; **11**: 153–62.

27. Mollman JE. Cisplatin neurotoxicity. *New England Journal of Medicine*. 1990; **322**: 126–7.

28. Siegal T, Haim N. Cisplatin-induced peripheral neuropathy. Frequent off-therapy deterioration, demyelinating syndromes, and muscle cramps. *Cancer*. 1990; **66**: 1117–23.

29. Rosell R, Gatzemeier U, Betticher DC *et al*. Phase III randomised trial comparing paclitaxel/carboplatin with paclitaxel/cisplatin in patients with advanced non-small-cell lung cancer: a cooperative multinational trial. *Annals of Oncology*. 2002; **13**: 1539–49.

30. Extra JM, Marty M, Brienza S, Misset JL. Pharmacokinetics and safety profile of oxaliplatin. *Seminars in Oncology*. 1998; **25**: 13–22.

31. Cersosimo RJ. Oxaliplatin-associated neuropathy: a review. *Annals of Pharmacotherapy*. 2005; **39**: 128–35.

32. Williams C, Collingwood M, Simera I, Grafton C. Short versus long duration infusions of paclitaxel for any adenocarcinoma. *Cochrane Database of Systematic Reviews*. 2003; **CD003911**.

33. Vasey PA, Jayson GC, Gordon A *et al*. Phase III randomized trial of docetaxel-carboplatin versus paclitaxel-carboplatin as first-line chemotherapy for ovarian carcinoma. *Journal of the National Cancer Institute*. 2004; **96**: 1682–91.

34. Stubblefield MD, Slovin S, Gregor-Cortelli B *et al*. An electrodiagnostic evaluation of the effect of pre-existing peripheral nervous system disorders in patients treated with the novel proteasome inhibitor bortezomib. *Clinical Oncology (Royal College of Radiologists)*. 2006; **18**: 410–18.

35. Richardson PG, Sonneveld P, Schuster MW *et al*. Bortezomib or high-dose dexamethasone for relapsed multiple myeloma. *New England Journal of Medicine*. 2005; **352**: 2487–98.

36. Richardson PG, Briemberg H, Jagannath S *et al*. Frequency, characteristics, and reversibility of peripheral neuropathy during treatment of advanced multiple myeloma with bortezomib. *Journal of Clinical Oncology*. 2006; **24**: 3113–20.

37. Richardson PG, Barlogie B, Berenson J *et al*. A phase 2 study of bortezomib in relapsed, refractory myeloma. *New England Journal of Medicine*. 2003; **348**: 2609–17.

38. Tseng S, Pak G, Washenik K *et al*. Rediscovering thalidomide: a review of its mechanism of action, side effects, and potential uses. *Journal of the American Academy of Dermatology*. 1996; **35**: 969–79.

39. Tosi P, Zamagni E, Cellini C *et al*. Neurological toxicity of long-term (>1 yr) thalidomide therapy in patients with multiple myeloma. *European Journal of Haematology*. 2005; **74**: 212–16.

40. Bastuji-Garin S, Ochonisky S, Bouche P *et al*. Incidence and risk factors for thalidomide neuropathy: a prospective study of 135 dermatologic patients. *Journal of Investigative Dermatology*. 2002; **119**: 1020–6.

41. Eriksson T, Bjorkman S, Hoglund P. Clinical pharmacology of thalidomide. *European Journal of Clinical Pharmacology*. 2001; **57**: 365–76.

42. Schuchter LM, Hensley ML, Meropol NJ, Winer EP. 2002 update of recommendations for the use of chemotherapy and radiotherapy protectants: clinical practice guidelines of the American Society of Clinical Oncology. *Journal of Clinical Oncology*. 2002; **20**: 2895–903.

43. Vahdat L, Papadopoulos K, Lange D *et al*. Reduction of paclitaxel-induced peripheral neuropathy with glutamine. *Clinical Cancer Research*. 2001; **7**: 1192–7.

44. Savarese DM, Savy G, Vahdat L *et al*. Prevention of chemotherapy and radiation toxicity with glutamine. *Cancer Treatment Reviews*. 2003; **29**: 501–13.

45. Pisano C, Pratesi G, Laccabue D *et al*. Paclitaxel and cisplatin-induced neurotoxicity: a protective role of acetyl-L-carnitine. *Clinical Cancer Research*. 2003; **9**: 5756–67.

✳ 46. Finnerup NB, Otto M, McQuay HJ *et al*. Algorithm for neuropathic pain treatment: an evidence based proposal. *Pain*. 2005; **118**: 289–305.

✳ 47. Attal N, Cruccu G, Haanpaa M *et al*. EFNS guidelines on pharmacological treatment of neuropathic pain. *European Journal of Neurology*. 2006; **13**: 1153–69.

48. Wong GY, Michalak JC, Sloan JA, Lorprinzi CL. A phase III, double blinded, placebo controlled randomised trial of gabapentin in patients with chemotherapy-induced peripheral neuropathy. A North Central Cancer Group Study. *Journal of Clinical Oncology*. 2005; **23** (Suppl. 729), Abstract 8001.

49. Mitchell P, Goldstein D, Michael M et al. Addition of gabapentin to a modified FOLFOX regimen does not reduce neurotoxicity in patients with advanced colorectal cancer. *Journal of Clinical Oncology.* 2006; **23** (Suppl. 266), Abstract 3581.

50. Macrae WA. Chronic pain after surgery. *British Journal of Anaesthesia.* 2001; **87**: 88–98.

51. Wallace MS, Wallace AM, Lee J, Dobke MK. Pain after breast surgery: a survey of 282 women. *Pain.* 1996; **66**: 195–205.

52. Stevens PE, Dibble SL, Miaskowski C. Prevalence, characteristics, and impact of postmastectomy pain syndrome: an investigation of women's experiences. *Pain.* 1995; **61**: 61–8.

53. Tasmuth T, von SK, Hietanen P et al. Pain and other symptoms after different treatment modalities of breast cancer. *Annals of Oncology.* 1995; **6**: 453–9.

54. Fassoulaki A, Sarantopoulos C, Melemeni A, Hogan Q. Regional block and mexiletine: the effect on pain after cancer breast surgery. *Regional Anesthesia and Pain Medicine.* 2001; **26**: 223–8.

55. Vecht CJ, Van de Brand HJ, Wajer OJ. Post-axillary dissection pain in breast cancer due to a lesion of the intercostobrachial nerve. *Pain.* 1989; **38**: 171–6.

56. Foley KM. Pain syndromes in patients with cancer. *Medical Clinics of North America.* 1987; **71**: 169–84.

57. Smith WC, Bourne D, Squair J et al. A retrospective cohort study of post mastectomy pain syndrome. *Pain.* 1999; **83**: 91–5.

＊ 58. Kehlet H, Jensen TS, Woolf CJ. Persistent postsurgical pain: risk factors and prevention. *Lancet.* 2006; **367**: 1618–25.

59. Coderre TJ, Katz J, Vaccarino AL, Melzack R. Contribution of central neuroplasticity to pathological pain: review of clinical and experimental evidence. *Pain.* 1993; **52**: 259–85.

60. Carpenter JS, Sloan P, Andrykowski MA et al. Risk factors for pain after mastectomy/lumpectomy. *Cancer Practice.* 1999; **7**: 66–70.

＊ 61. Jung BF, Ahrendt GM, Oaklander AL, Dworkin RH. Neuropathic pain following breast cancer surgery: proposed classification and research update. *Pain.* 2003; **104**: 1–13.

62. Macdonald L, Bruce J, Scott NW et al. Long-term follow-up of breast cancer survivors with post-mastectomy pain syndrome. *British Journal of Cancer.* 2005; **92**: 225–30.

63. Katz J, Poleshuck EL, Andrus CH et al. Risk factors for acute pain and its persistence following breast cancer surgery. *Pain.* 2005; **119**: 16–25.

64. Poleshuck EL, Katz J, Andrus CH et al. Risk factors for chronic pain following breast cancer surgery: a prospective study. *Journal of Pain.* 2006; **7**: 626–34.

65. Caffo O, Amichetti M, Ferro A et al. Pain and quality of life after surgery for breast cancer. *Breast Cancer Research and Treatment.* 2003; **80**: 39–48.

66. Gulluoglu BM, Cingi A, Cakir T et al. Factors related to post-treatment chronic pain in breast cancer survivors: the interference of pain with life functions. *International Journal of Fertility and Women's Medicine.* 2006; **51**: 75–82.

67. Tasmuth T, von SK, Kalso E. Pain and other symptoms during the first year after radical and conservative surgery for breast cancer. *British Journal of Cancer.* 1996; **74**: 2024–31.

68. Tasmuth T, Kataja M, Blomqvist C et al. Treatment-related factors predisposing to chronic pain in patients with breast cancer – a multivariate approach. *Acta Oncologica.* 1997; **36**: 625–30.

69. Ishiyama H, Niino K, Hosoya T, Hayakawa K. Results of a questionnaire survey for symptom of late complications caused by radiotherapy in breast conserving therapy. *Breast Cancer.* 2006; **13**: 197–201.

70. Wood KM. Intercostobrachial nerve entrapment syndrome. *Southern Medical Journal.* 1978; **71**: 662–3.

71. Torresan RZ, Cabello C, Conde DM, Brenelli HB. Impact of the preservation of the intercostobrachial nerve in axillary lymphadenectomy due to breast cancer. *Breast Journal.* 2003; **9**: 389–92.

72. Abdullah TI, Iddon J, Barr L et al. Prospective randomized controlled trial of preservation of the intercostobrachial nerve during axillary node clearance for breast cancer. *British Journal of Surgery.* 1998; **85**: 1443–5.

73. Taylor KO. Morbidity associated with axillary surgery for breast cancer. *ANZ Journal of Surgery.* 2004; **74**: 314–17.

74. Freeman SR, Washington SJ, Pritchard T et al. Long term results of a randomised prospective study of preservation of the intercostobrachial nerve. *European Journal of Surgical Oncology.* 2003; **29**: 213–15.

75. Legeby M, Segerdahl M, Sandelin K et al. Immediate reconstruction in breast cancer surgery requires intensive post-operative pain treatment but the effects of axillary dissection may be more predictive of chronic pain. *Breast.* 2002; **11**: 156–62.

76. Barranger E, Dubernard G, Fleurence J et al. Subjective morbidity and quality of life after sentinel node biopsy and axillary lymph node dissection for breast cancer. *Journal of Surgical Oncology.* 2005; **92**: 17–22.

77. Tasmuth T, Blomqvist C, Kalso E. Chronic post-treatment symptoms in patients with breast cancer operated in different surgical units. *European Journal of Surgical Oncology.* 1999; **25**: 38–43.

78. Tasmuth T, Estlanderb AM, Kalso E. Effect of present pain and mood on the memory of past postoperative pain in women treated surgically for breast cancer. *Pain.* 1996; **68**: 343–7.

79. Amichetti M, Caffo O. Pain after quadrantectomy and radiotherapy for early-stage breast cancer: incidence, characteristics and influence on quality of life. Results from a retrospective study. *Oncology.* 2003; **65**: 23–8.

80. Gottrup H, Andersen J, Rendt-Nielsen L, Jensen TS. Psychophysical examination in patients with post-mastectomy pain. *Pain.* 2000; **87**: 275–84.

81. Kairaluoma PM, Bachmann MS, Korpinen AK et al. Single-injection paravertebral block before general anesthesia enhances analgesia after breast cancer surgery with and

without associated lymph node biopsy. *Anesthesia and Analgesia.* 2004; **99** 1837–43, table.

82. Kairaluoma PM, Bachmann MS, Rosenberg PH, Pere PJ. Preincisional paravertebral block reduces the prevalence of chronic pain after breast surgery. *Anesthesia and Analgesia.* 2006; **103**: 703–08.

83. Misra A, Chester D, Park A. A comparison of postoperative pain between DIEP and extended latissimus dorsi flaps in breast reconstruction. *Plastic and Reconstructive Surgery.* 2006; **117**: 1108–12.

84. Rothemund Y, Grusser SM, Liebeskind U *et al.* Phantom phenomena in mastectomized patients and their relation to chronic and acute pre-mastectomy pain. *Pain.* 2004; **107**: 140–6.

85. Nikolajsen L, Jensen TS. Phantom limb pain. *British Journal of Anaesthesia.* 2001; **87**: 107–16.

86. Kroner K, Krebs B, Skov J, Jorgensen HS. Immediate and long-term phantom breast syndrome after mastectomy: incidence, clinical characteristics and relationship to pre-mastectomy breast pain. *Pain.* 1989; **36**: 327–34.

87. Kroner K, Knudsen UB, Lundby L, Hvid H. Long-term phantom breast syndrome after mastectomy. *Clinical Journal of Pain.* 1992; **8**: 346–50.

88. Flor H, Elbert T, Knecht S *et al.* Phantom-limb pain as a perceptual correlate of cortical reorganization following arm amputation. *Nature.* 1995; **375**: 482–4.

89. Stanton AL, Krishnan L, Collins CA. Form or function? Part 1. Subjective cosmetic and functional correlates of quality of life in women treated with breast-conserving surgical procedures and radiotherapy. *Cancer.* 2001; **91**: 2273–81.

90. Robb KA, Williams JE, Duvivier V, Newham DJ. A pain management program for chronic cancer-treatment-related pain: a preliminary study. *Journal of Pain.* 2006; **7**: 82–90.

91. Watson CP, Evans RJ. The postmastectomy pain syndrome and topical capsaicin: a randomized trial. *Pain.* 1992; **51**: 375–9.

92. Kalso E, Tasmuth T, Neuvonen PJ. Amitriptyline effectively relieves neuropathic pain following treatment of breast cancer. *Pain.* 1996; **64**: 293–302.

93. Tasmuth T, Hartel B, Kalso E. Venlafaxine in neuropathic pain following treatment of breast cancer. *European Journal of Pain.* 2002; **6**: 17–24.

94. Reuben SS, Makari-Judson G, Lurie SD. Evaluation of efficacy of the perioperative administration of venlafaxine XR in the prevention of postmastectomy pain syndrome. *Journal of Pain and Symptom Management.* 2004; **27**: 133–9.

95. Fassoulaki A, Triga A, Melemeni A, Sarantopoulos C. Multimodal analgesia with gabapentin and local anesthetics prevents acute and chronic pain after breast surgery for cancer. *Anesthesia and Analgesia.* 2005; **101**: 1427–32.

96. Fassoulaki A, Sarantopoulos C, Melemeni A, Hogan Q. EMLA reduces acute and chronic pain after breast surgery for cancer. *Regional Anesthesia and Pain Medicine.* 2000; **25**: 350–5.

97. Eisenberg E, McNicol E, Carr DB. Opioids for neuropathic pain. *Cochrane Database of Systematic Reviews.* 2006; **CD006146**.

98. Birgisson H, Pahlman L, Gunnarsson U, Glimelius B. Adverse effects of preoperative radiation therapy for rectal cancer: long-term follow-up of the Swedish Rectal Cancer Trial. *Journal of Clinical Oncology.* 2005; **23**: 8697–705.

99. Bye A, Trope C, Loge JH *et al.* Health-related quality of life and occurrence of intestinal side effects after pelvic radiotherapy – evaluation of long-term effects of diagnosis and treatment. *Acta Oncologica.* 2000; **39**: 173–80.

*100. Schierle C, Winograd JM. Radiation-induced brachial plexopathy: review. Complication without a cure. *Journal of Reconstructive Microsurgery.* 2004; **20**: 149–52.

101. Johansson S, Svensson H, Denekamp J. Timescale of evolution of late radiation injury after postoperative radiotherapy of breast cancer patients. *International Journal of Radiation Oncology, Biology, Physics.* 2000; **48**: 745–50.

*102. Johansson S. Radiation induced brachial plexopathies. *Acta Oncologica.* 2006; **45**: 253–7.

103. Powell S, Cooke J, Parsons C. Radiation-induced brachial plexus injury: follow-up of two different fractionation schedules. *Radiotherapy and Oncology.* 1990; **18**: 213–20.

104. Jung BF, Herrmann D, Griggs J *et al.* Neuropathic pain associated with non-surgical treatment of breast cancer. *Pain.* 2005; **118**: 10–14.

105. Johansson S, Svensson H, Denekamp J. Dose response and latency for radiation-induced fibrosis, edema, and neuropathy in breast cancer patients. *International Journal of Radiation Oncology, Biology, Physics.* 2002; **52**: 1207–19.

106. Galecki J, Hicer-Grzenkowicz J, Grudzien-Kowalska M *et al.* Radiation-induced brachial plexopathy and hypofractionated regimens in adjuvant irradiation of patients with breast cancer – a review. *Acta Oncologica.* 2006; **45**: 280–4.

107. Olsen NK, Pfeiffer P, Johannsen L *et al.* Radiation-induced brachial plexopathy: neurological follow-up in 161 recurrence-free breast cancer patients. *International Journal of Radiation Oncology, Biology, Physics.* 1993; **26**: 43–9.

108. Olsen NK, Pfeiffer P, Mondrup K, Rose C. Radiation-induced brachial plexus neuropathy in breast cancer patients. *Acta Oncologica.* 1990; **29**: 885–90.

*109. Kori SH, Foley KM, Posner JB. Brachial plexus lesions in patients with cancer: 100 cases. *Neurology.* 1981; **31**: 45–50.

110. Cross NE, Glantz MJ. Neurologic complications of radiation therapy. *Neurologic Clinics.* 2003; **21**: 249–77.

111. Fathers E, Thrush D, Huson SM, Norman A. Radiation-induced brachial plexopathy in women treated for carcinoma of the breast. *Clinical Rehabilitation.* 2002; **16**: 160–5.

112. Qayyum A, MacVicar AD, Padhani AR *et al.* Symptomatic brachial plexopathy following treatment for breast cancer:

utility of MR imaging with surface-coil techniques. *Radiology.* 2000; **214**: 837–42.

113. Bajrovic A, Rades D, Fehlauer F *et al.* Is there a life-long risk of brachial plexopathy after radiotherapy of supraclavicular lymph nodes in breast cancer patients? *Radiotherapy and Oncology.* 2004; **71**: 297–301.

114. Pritchard J, Anand P, Broome J *et al.* Double-blind randomized phase II study of hyperbaric oxygen in patients with radiation-induced brachial plexopathy. *Radiotherapy and Oncology.* 2001; **58**: 279–86.

115. Stubblefield MD, Custodio CM. Upper-extremity pain disorders in breast cancer. *Archives of Physical Medicine and Rehabilitation.* 2006; **87**: S96–9.

116. Lu L, Gong X, Liu Z *et al.* Diagnosis and operative treatment of radiation-induced brachial plexopathy. *Chinese Journal of Traumatology.* 2002; **5**: 329–32.

117. Kori SH. Diagnosis and management of brachial plexus lesions in cancer patients. *Oncology (Williston Park).* 1995; **9**: 756–60.

118. Jackson MB, Pounder D, Price C *et al.* Percutaneous cervical cordotomy for the control of pain in patients with pleural mesothelioma. *Thorax.* 1999; **54**: 238–41.

119. Sanders M, Zuurmond W. Safety of unilateral and bilateral percutaneous cervical cordotomy in 80 terminally ill cancer patients. *Journal of Clinical Oncology.* 1995; **13**: 1509–12.

120. Sikora K. Enraged about radiotherapy. *British Medical Journal.* 1994; **308**: 188–9.

30

Cancer pain management in the community setting

MARGARET GIBBS, VICKY ROBINSON, NIGEL SYKES, AND CHRISTINE MIASKOWSKI

Setting the scene	411	Out-of-hours palliative care medication provision	416
Palliative care – the specialty	412	Case history	417
Medication provision at home	414	Conclusions	419
The use of drugs outside their license	415	References	420
Specialist versus generalist prescribing in the community	416		

KEY LEARNING POINTS

- Cancer pain management at home is an important issue because that is the setting in which most people with cancer spend most of their illness and in which most wish to die.
- Successful pain control in the home requires flexible interworking and excellent communication between members of the primary healthcare team and the multiprofessional resources of the treating oncologist and/or specialist palliative care service. A crucial aspect of this cooperation is the effective provision of out-of-hours care and drugs for symptom control.

- In the UK, the Department of Health is pursuing a number of relevant policy initiatives, including implementation of the Gold Standards Framework and improved end of life care education for care home staff.
- In the United States, a number of states (e.g. California, Oregon) have passed legislation that requires that physicians have continuing education in pain management and palliative care.
- The recommendations of the fourth report of the Shipman Inquiry have resulted in new regulations for the UK governing the supply, handling, and disposal of controlled drugs in the community.

SETTING THE SCENE

The control of cancer pain at home depends on five fundamental principles.

1. The availability of specialist advice and support to primary care practitioners.
2. A skilled and educated workforce.
3. Team work that includes the patient and family (see Chapter 7, Teamworking in cancer pain management).
4. The availability of medicines for optimum pain and symptom control.
5. A system that ensures that the *right* medication reaches the *right* patient at the *right* time.

Since the publication in the UK of the National Cancer Plan[1] and, more recently, the Supportive and Palliative Care Guidance for Adults with Cancer from the UK National Institute for Health and Clinical Excellence (NICE)[2][I], there have been major advances in all of these areas. Part one of this chapter (Palliative care – the specialty) begins with a brief history and definition of palliative care and how it is provided at home in the UK. Next, it moves on to how medicines are provided at home (Medication provision at home), with particular emphasis on the development of guidance since publication of the Fourth Shipman Report in 2004.[3] Some of the challenges of local formularies and out of hours care are discussed (Out-of-hours palliative care medication provision). Part two takes the form of a case history illustrating the use of the above four principles in the care of a patient at home with cancer pain. Differences in perspectives and approaches from the United States are provided within each of the sections of this chapter.

PALLIATIVE CARE – THE SPECIALTY

Dame Cicely Saunders, the founder of the modern hospice movement, brought together the importance of sound research and good education as essential components of skilled and compassionate care of the dying. Her early work was in the efficacy of oral morphine in cancer pain, for which she developed the approach of regular preemptive administration that has proved revolutionary in cancer pain control. She also pioneered the insight that pain is a psychosocial and spiritual phenomenon as well as a physical one, and hence required a multi-professional team approach in order to be tackled adequately. Latterly, it has been recognized that these principles can be applied throughout the course of the cancer journey, in so-called "supportive care."[4][I] The World Health Organization first issued a definition of palliative care in 1990 and its most recent (2003) definition[5] is shown in **Box 30.1**.

In the United States, several initiatives have been undertaken to improve the management of cancer pain. In 1992, the Agency for Health Care Policy and Research published a clinical practice guideline on the management of cancer pain.[6] Recently, this guideline was updated by an interdisciplinary committee of the American Pain Society.[7] The intended users of these clinical practice guidelines are oncology patients, primary care providers, as well as specialists in oncology and palliative care. The importance of patient and family caregiver education is emphasized in these national guidelines. In addition, the Joint Commission for the Accreditation of Health Care Organizations (i.e. an organization that voluntarily accredits healthcare organizations in the United States) has published pain standards that have raised clinicians awareness of the need to assess and manage acute and chronic pain in all types of patients.[8] An important consideration with these initiatives is to evaluate the actual impact of guidelines and standards on patient care.

How can palliative care help cancer pain earlier in the disease process?

Figure 30.1 shows how the interface between acute and palliative care has evolved in the last 40 years. After the initial use of a sequential model **Figure 30.1a** in which palliative care took over completely from acute care, but only in the last stages of life, there has been a growing

---

> ### Box 30.1 Extracts from the 2003 World Health Organization definition of palliative care
>
> Palliative care… is an approach that improves the quality of life of patients and their families facing the problems associated with life-threatening illness, through the **prevention and the relief of suffering** by means of early identification and impeccable assessment and treatment of pain and other problems, physical, psychosocial, and spiritual.[5] It:
>
> - affirms life and regards dying as a normal process;
> - provides relief from pain and other symptoms;
> - intends neither to hasten nor postpone death;
> - integrates psychological and spiritual aspects of care;
> - offers a support system to help patients to live as actively possible until death;
> - offers a support system to help the family cope during the patient's illness and in their own bereavement;
> - uses a team approach to address the needs of patients and families, including bereavement counselling if indicated;
> - enhances the quality of life, and may also positively influence the course of illness;
> - is applicable early in the course of illness, in conjunction with other therapies that are intended to prolong life, such as chemotherapy or radiation therapy, and includes those investigations needed to better understand and manage distressing clinical complications.
>
> Reprinted with permission from the World Health Organization.

---

acceptance that acute and palliative modes of care should work together. In the case of steadily progressive disease there may be a corresponding gradual transfer of emphasis from the acute to the palliative **Figure 30.1b**. However, the increasing chronicity of cancer and the application of palliative care to nonmalignant conditions have meant that it is often appropriate for the involvement of palliative care to be a fluctuating one, responding flexibly to new needs and withdrawing again to some degree as these are met **Figure 30.1c**.

Palliative home care teams – UK experience

Most people with cancer want to stay at home for as long as possible.[9][III] Hospice and palliative home care teams

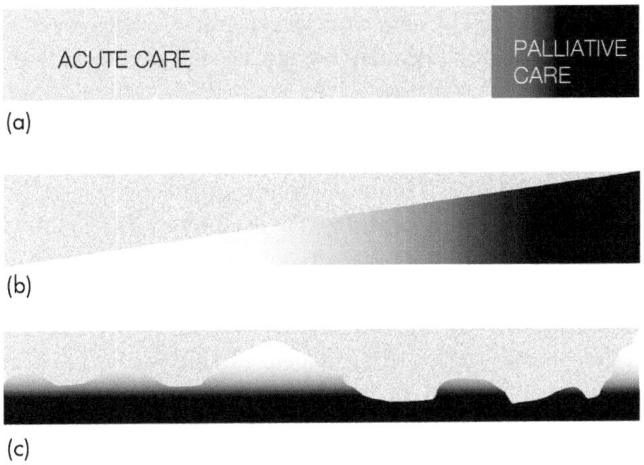

ACUTE CARE PALLIATIVE CARE

(a)

(b)

(c)

Figure 30.1 The landscape of palliation. (a) Acute care finally gives up and hands over to palliative care. (b) Acute care and palliative care work together, the balance between them changing as the disease progresses. (c) Palliative care works alongside acute care in a flexible way responsive to the varying balance of need. Redrawn with permission from Cooper J (ed.). *Stepping into palliative care.* Oxford: Radcliffe Publishing Ltd, 2000: Fig 2.1, page 20.

help people to achieve this by working alongside the patient's general practitioner (GP or family physician) and district nurse. In the UK in 2006, there were 327 home care teams, who cared for over 100,000 new patients.

These teams, consisting mainly of specialist nurses each with a case load, provide advice and support to patients and families, district nurses, and GPs. Each specialist nurse will have access to other palliative care specialists – doctors, social workers, counsellors, occupational therapy, physiotherapy, spiritual care. Resourcing these teams has for many years been a highly political issue, dependent on the priorities set locally. Despite some financial contribution from the Department of Health in England and recommendations from NICE, provision across the UK remains inequitable.

Hospice and palliative home care teams are also responsible for providing education and training to staff who work in the independent care home sector where more and more people in the UK are being cared for and will die. For this reason, the care home sector is an increasing focus of government attention in relation to end of life provision.[10][V]

Palliative home care teams – US experience

Unfortunately, no national initiative to provide palliative care services to cancer patients at home exists in the United States. However, recent efforts to build capacity in palliative care are proving fruitful. For example, between 2000 and 2005, the number of hospitals with palliative care services grew by 96 percent, from 632 to 1240 based on data from the 2007 American Hospital Association Annual

Survey of Hospitals. In addition, in 2006, the Accreditation Council for Graduate Medical Education (ACGME) in the United States decided to begin accrediting hospice and palliative medicine fellowship programs. Starting in 2008, physicians will for the first time be able to become board certified in hospice and palliative care and the first fellowship programs will be able to seek ACGME accreditation.[11] In addition, in terms of nursing education, End-of-Life Nursing Education Consortium (ELNEC-Oncology) in partnership with the Oncology Nursing Society has educated over 50,000 nurses around the United States in the principles and practices of palliative care.[12]

These types of initiatives, grounded in clinician education, should help the 85 percent of US residents who report that they would prefer to die at home to be able to do so. Currently, only about 50 percent do die at home. However, recent reports suggest that between 1990 and 2000, the number of deaths in US hospitals decreased by 17 percent.[11]

Perhaps, like the UK, the US will one day have a national initiative to provide palliative care services at home. In many instances, home care agencies within the US do provide palliative care services. However, the level of training afforded to clinicians who provide these services is not consistent across home care agencies.

So who does what?

When it comes to the assessment and management of cancer pain at home teamworking is vital (see Chapter 7, Teamworking in cancer pain management). In the UK the overall clinical responsibility for patients at home sits with the GP, unless a "shared care" protocol has been drawn up. Later in the chapter are examples of a flexible approach to teamworking in assessment, prescribing, and management. However, without a fundamental commitment to communication between professionals and the patient and families, care can become confused and professionals suspicious of one another's motives. Thus, the relationship between the specialist (palliative care service) and the generalist (the GP and community nurse) requires investment of time at referral to formulate a management plan together. An example of this forms part of the case history related in part two of this chapter (see under Case history below). Here, thirty minutes spent by the clinical nurse specialist face to face with the patient's GP in his surgery represented the foundation of good communication.

In the US, the primary responsibility for pain management in the home can rest with any number of clinicians (e.g. primary care provider, oncologist, palliative care physician if home hospice care is being provided to the patient). The need for team work in this setting is critical. In many instances, the home care nurse and/or the patient's family caregiver is involved in the coordination of pain management services.

MEDICATION PROVISION AT HOME

To enable people with cancer to remain at home, the relationship with their GP, district nurse, and community pharmacist is key. Another factor, for most patients, is the judicious use of medication. Two recurring issues have made the provision of appropriate medication for people dying at home a problem: first, the medication required at the end of life often needs to be in injectable form, which is not routinely stocked in local pharmacies, and second, although it is often possible to plan ahead, unpredictable and unexpected deterioration does occur and if not managed well can spoil many months of excellent palliative care, leaving relatives and professionals feeling despondent.

These issues have long been recognized and many local schemes and procedures have been introduced to improve access to the necessary drugs. The medication list for cancer pain patients inevitably includes controlled drugs (CDs), but the legislation governing their management, the Misuse of Drugs Act 1971 and the Medicines Act 1968, was written when practice was different. It became outdated and so in order to be workable some schemes fell into legal gray areas.

Over the last few years, a number of initiatives in the UK have sought to clarify and unify the provision of care, including medication, to palliative care patients, and now we have the necessary guidance and frameworks to start to make real improvements. This section will look at some of this guidance, some of the specific drug-related problems, and the strategies for managing out-of-hours care for our patients.

The development of guidance

The legal status of CDs is the main complicating issue in end of life analgesia management, and hence additional guidance has been welcomed. The ability of Dr Harold Shipman to obtain and use CDs inappropriately over a number of years led to a thorough inquiry, headed by Dame Janet Smith, the fourth of whose six reports addressed the issue of CD regulation in the community.[3] The inquiry exposed gaps in the governance arrangements for CDs and the government responded with a command paper "Safer Management of CDs," which generally accepted the inquiry's recommendations. While procedures and record-keeping were tightened up, it was reassuring for palliative care to see that the "need for patients to have timely access to CDs" was one of the aims of the resultant work program. The main focus of the strengthened safety measures was in primary care but further work has been carried out to ensure that these are extended into secondary care (January 2007) and the regulation of health professionals (February 2007). Standard operating procedures are being put in place in all environments where CDs are held. Overseeing the

procedures will be a network of accountable officers (AO), one in each establishment using CDs and overseen by the AO at the local primary care trust (PCT). These officers have two responsibilities: first to ensure that CDs are managed correctly in their workplace and second to form a local task force, if required, to investigate and act on any areas of concern regarding CDs in the locality.

Amongst the changes set out by the Department of Health (January 2007) for practice in the community, CD prescriptions on specific forms (called FP10) may be electronically generated. Private prescriptions for CDs can no longer be written on notepaper but must be on a specific FP10 (PCD), which means these prescriptions will also be processed at the Prescription Pricing Division who send back data to PCT prescribing teams. In this way, prescribing patterns and anomalies should be easier to detect. Prescribing of CDs has been restricted to no more than 30 days supply and each FP10 is only valid for 28 days from issue. A prescriber identifier number will now appear on each FP10, again enabling individual prescribing trends to be recognized quickly (**Table 30.1**).

The record-keeping and monitoring process will enable an audit trail to be kept for the process of prescribing and dispensing. It has been suggested that patients are issued with a patient record card for continuing audit and safety purposes. Each time injectable CDs are dispensed, the total would be entered on to the card and healthcare professionals would use it as a record of administration and running balance in the home. The feasibility of this system has yet to be confirmed.

With or without this card, one loophole that still exists is the safe collection and destruction of unwanted CDs after a patient's death at home. It is extremely difficult to envisage a foolproof method of containing this end of the audit trail. The "controlled" status of the drugs changes once they have been supplied to a patient, as they become the patient's property and no longer the responsibility of any external authority. Meanwhile, healthcare professionals (mainly nurses) find themselves removing drugs and returning them to pharmacies when they are able, but without any supporting paperwork. It is perfectly legal for a healthcare professional to be in possession of CDs in these circumstances, but some sort of returns system needs to be devised to safeguard everyone involved.

The changes described above have been brought in over a very short space of time as a response to a series of tragic events. It is hoped that while increasing safety they will not deter any practitioner from prescribing opioids when necessary and that patients will not be subject to any unnecessary delays in receiving their medication.

Medication provision at home – the US experience

Unlike the UK, the US does not have a national health insurance plan. Therefore, while the broad issues

Table 30.1 New governance arrangements for controlled drugs in the community in the UK (2007).

Area	New arrangements
Prescription writing	Handwriting requirements removed – will all be electronic eventually
	Written on FP10 or FP10 (PCD) if private
	GPs may not prescribe for themselves, close family, or friends
Prescription validity	28 days from issue
	Not more than 30 days supply
Patient responsibility	Patient or representative collecting CDs must sign the back of the prescription
Record keeping	Community pharmacy records should be electronic eventually
	Running balances to be recorded
	Prescriber and identifier number to be recorded
	Patient returns to be recorded
Monitoring	Accountable officers responsible for each organization using CDs
	Standard operating procedures to be written and used in all areas using CDs
Inspection	The Healthcare Commission to lead national CD group and manage and monitor self-assessment of CDs in trusts and independent health care
	Pharmaceutical Society inspectors to include CD monitoring in their inspection of community pharmacies
Additional changes	Pharmacists will be able to amend small technical errors on CD prescriptions as long as the prescriber's intentions were clear
	PCTs to look at safe systems for disposal of patient returns
	More people will be authorized to witness destruction of returned and out of date CDs

surrounding the provision of analgesic medications, particularly CDs, may be similar, the specifics regarding these issues are somewhat different. For example, rather than dealing with a national formulary of CDs, each insurance plan (whether public or private) in the US has its own formulary of approved medications. Clinicians who care for patients who require palliative care need to have a working knowledge of their various medications that are approved by the health insurance plans that cover their patients.

In addition to the availability of specific analgesics on a health plan's formulary, the issue of payment or co-payment for these medications is an important consideration for many patients and clinicians. Depending on the patient's level of co-pay for generic and brand name medications, as well as the total amount of medication expenses that are covered per year, may determine which medication the physician prescribes. In addition, it may determine whether the patient fills the prescription for their analgesic medication, their anticancer medication (if any is prescribed), or buys groceries that week and pays the rent. These types of decisions are becoming more common among the poor and the middle class in the US given the rising cost of health care.

The lack of availability of CDs in some pharmacies in the US has been the subject of study.[13, 14, 15] In these studies, pharmacies in neighborhoods where patients were more likely to be from a minority group were less likely to stock the opioid analgesics required for palliative care patients. For example, in one study[14] Michigan pharmacies in minority zip codes were 52 times less likely

to carry sufficient amounts of opioid analgesics than pharmacies in white zip codes regardless of the residents' income.

While federal regulations in the US govern the prescription of CDs, each state has additional requirements that affect how clinicians prescribe CDs to palliative care patients and how prescriptions for CDs are monitored. In general, clinicians in the US are advised to monitor all patients on CDs using the four "As." Patients need to be assessed in terms of the following: **Analgesia** (i.e. degree of pain relief), **Adverse effects** (i.e. the occurrence and severity of side effects), **Activities of daily living** (i.e. is the patient's functional abilities maintained or optimal given the context of care), and **Abuse concerns**.[16] Assessment of these four areas and documentation of these four areas are considered the best approaches to safeguard clinicians if they were to come under investigation or regulatory scrutiny.

THE USE OF DRUGS OUTSIDE THEIR LICENSE

Palliative care is an area of prescribing where long-term safety considerations may be less crucial when making a prescribing decision. The most important consideration in this patient group is making sure the patient is as free from pain or other unwanted symptoms as possible. Therefore, individual patient factors dominate the decision-making process.

Additionally, in this speciality many drugs are used outside the terms of their product license. The use of drugs in palliative care has historically been regarded as adventurous, leading many healthcare professionals to feel that they are being asked to take an unknown amount of risk in prescribing, dispensing, or administering drugs. However, the vast majority of treatment decisions made in palliative care involve the use of familiar, established medications. Statements on the use of drugs outside their license in palliative care have been published by the Association for Palliative Medicine and the matter is also covered in the introductory pages of the *Palliative care formulary*.[17, 18][V]

Licensing is basically a commercial issue and a prescriber is always ultimately responsible for any prescription decision. In essence, and really the only difference in prescribing a licensed drug for an indication outside its license, is that if something were to go wrong the company would not accept any liability for the consequences. Using familiar drugs, such as amitriptyline or sodium valproate for neuropathic pain or antipsychotic drugs such as haloperidol for nausea and vomiting, is likely to present the same adverse effect profile whatever the indication. Additionally, market forces mean that as many of the drugs used in palliative care are also well used for their licensed indication or are available only as generics, there is virtually no chance of any manufacturer considering the costly process of funding research in order to apply for a license for the small palliative care usage of their drug.

There has been encouragement from the Healthcare Commission to discuss the use of drugs outside their license with patients before commencing treatment. Whilst informing patients about their treatment is without doubt a worthy aim, such discussions are difficult and, if not worded carefully, may lead to confusion. The use of terminology such as "outside the terms of a drug's license" may sound more worrying that it need be. Patients should be made aware of the potential confusion that may arise when they read the patient information leaflet supplied with their medication, as this may not be appropriate to the indication it is being used for. Providing an additional information leaflet explaining the use of the most commonly used palliative care drugs outside license can be very reassuring. Examples of these are available at www.palliativedrugs.com, the website associated with the *Palliative care formulary*.[18][V]

The same issues enumerated above would apply in the US.

SPECIALIST VERSUS GENERALIST PRESCRIBING IN THE COMMUNITY

Another barrier to seamless care for palliative care patients can occur in some Strategic Health Authorities and PCTs where a list of "specialist only" drugs is in use. These lists can vary from area to area but generally include some of the more costly drugs that are likely to be

recommended for pain and other aspects of symptom control. GPs are discouraged from taking clinical responsibility for prescribing and monitoring the listed drugs for their patients at home and the specialist who has recommended the treatment is asked to continue to arrange provision and care. This can present practical complications for patients and families as they cannot obtain the drug(s) they need locally, but it also has financial implications for the independent (i.e. non-NHS but not for profit) specialist palliative care units which constitute the majority of UK specialist palliative care provision. The drugs budget provided to such units is intended only for the care of in-patients so individual negotiation is necessary to facilitate reimbursement from the patient's PCT as an "exceptional circumstance."

In a small number of cases, the only means of providing effective analgesia is by using a continuous epidural infusion, and if such a patient is to be cared for at home the highest level of communication and training for the professionals involved is needed and, again, a discussion with the PCT on how their needs are to be managed. It is possible to obtain prefilled cassettes from pharmaceutical specialist providers on FP10, but the clinical responsibilities and funding must be quite clear before embarking on such a discharge. It is quite unacceptable to send such a patient home without being confident that all the necessary parties are competent and confident in managing their care.

While "specialist only drugs" do not exist in the United States, except for some rare exceptions, most primary care clinicians, and oncologists for that matter, do not have experience with specialized techniques (e.g. chronic administration of spinal opioids) for severe pain. Therefore, as in the UK, the coordination of healthcare services for these patients is critical. In many cases, specialists in pain management or palliative care recommend and initiate these complex pain management regimens. In many cases, these specialty services reside in academic medical centers. When patients return home, the management of their pain is carried out by primary care clinicians and home care nurses. To ensure a successful transition of care, education of clinicians, patients, and family caregivers is a critical component of the pain management plan.

OUT-OF-HOURS PALLIATIVE CARE MEDICATION PROVISION

It is not always appreciated that around 75 percent of any week is actually "out of hours" and the importance of this has only recently been addressed nationally. With changes to the contract for GPs in the UK, The Department of Health (DH) recognized in 2000 that out-of-hours provision of care was in need of a complete review.[19] Palliative care, along with pediatrics and psychiatry, was recognized as one of the three specific therapeutic areas for special consideration when drawing up guidance. In her comprehensive report on out of hours palliative care in the community, Thomas discussed the main problems and offered some solutions and examples of good practice.[20][V] PCTs have been charged with accrediting out-of-hours medical services and one of the provisos for obtaining accreditation is having access to the national out-of-hours formulary drugs. These include a useful range of the injectable drugs most likely to be needed for palliative care patients and elsewhere in the formulary are other standard, oral preparations. One of the new principles in the Department of Health out-of-hours plans is that patients should not need to carry the burden for obtaining drugs as they should be available at the same time and place as the out of hours consultation.

For ambulant patients, this standard can be met by ensuring that the drugs are stocked at the out-of-hours center but for dying patients, it is essential that the prescriber or administrator of medicines should have them to hand as quickly as possible after the need for them has been identified. Enabling this is not simple as the law is very specific on who is legally permitted to possess, store, prescribe, record, and supply drugs – particularly CDs. It is not possible to write a "one fits all" procedure for these processes, as standard operating procedures and personnel must be specific to each different locality. Examples of working practices are being collected on the DH out-of-hours website and practical guidance has been produced by the National Prescribing Centre[21][V] and the National Pharmacy Association.[22][V] A limited amount of service and procedure sharing is possible between neighboring organizations. Ideally, the out-of-hours doctor should be in a position to administer a first dose of a drug and if possible supply further doses to hold the situation until the next working day.

Complementary to this immediate response, many areas have a rotational on-call service from local pharmacies who agree to stock a range of palliative care drugs. However, two practical issues need to be addressed in order for this to be helpful. First, the prescription still needs to be written and available for the pharmacist at some stage before the drugs are supplied and someone needs to make the journey to enable that to happen. Second, the need for urgent palliative care drugs is far from an everyday occurrence, so these services need to be well publicised, supported, and financed in order to be useful to all concerned.

It is possible to minimize the need for emergency supply even further if patients are supplied with a "crisis pack" containing the basic drugs likely to be required in their last days or hours. The principle of a "just-in-case" pack is also recommended in the Gold Standards Framework[23] and supported by many community pharmacists.[24][V] Identifying palliative care patients on GPs' lists acts as a prompt for their GP to prescribe a small quantity of injectable drugs to be kept in the home for use if needed to manage potential pain, nausea, agitation, and retained secretions. If injections are supplied, the accompanying paperwork to enable another healthcare professional to administer the drugs is required. The timing of this process is probably the most difficult issue, as the appropriate dose range needs to be prescribed in order to be useful and this can be difficult to predict. Also, it could be argued that it is poor practice to prescribe any medication for a patient who is not in need of it imminently. For this reason, regular reviews of the existing prescription and drugs are necessary. Prescribing the drugs for the individual patient takes away all the complex legal and procedural issues that are involved when drugs are kept as "stock" by the out of hours service or pharmacy. A pilot "just in case" scheme in Hertfordshire in 2005 prevented 16 hospital admissions at a total drug cost of just £10 per patient.[24][V]

The establishment of Cancer and Supportive Care Networks and now the End of Life Strategy in the UK[25] has been another good opportunity to coordinate some of these initiatives and find local, workable solutions with the minimum of duplication. The networks have also been important in providing suitable education and paperwork to facilitate generalists to prescribe and administer the necessary medication safely.

The provision of medication to dying patients at home has long been in need of review and rationalization. The coincidental timing of the outcome of Shipman's actions and the national focus on providing good out-of-hours service has hastened the task of clarifying and simplifying some of these processes.

Considerations to the policies and procedures described in this section have not been explored on a national level in the United States. They would be a welcome approach to improving the pain management of palliative care patients in the US.

CASE HISTORY

I understand that patients will need some strong pain killers for their cancer pain, it's just that we are working in the shadow of Harold Shipman. For instance, I no longer feel able to leave a supply of morphine in a patient's house.

George's GP, December 2006

This was said during a conversation about George, a patient newly referred to the hospice home care team for pain and symptom control. Thirty minutes was spent with his GP, explaining the role of the specialist palliative care service as supporters and partners in care, listening to his concerns, and formulating a management plan for this patient's pain. It was 30 minutes well spent.

George was a 76-year-old man diagnosed with Duke's C rectal carcinoma in March 2003. He underwent an abdominoperineal resection and chemotherapy, recovered well and was stable until two years later when he developed hip pain. A computed tomography (CT) scan identified presacral recurrence, which responded well to radiotherapy. Eighteen months later, he again developed hip pain. Biopsy and CT scan identified a mass eroding the right sacrum. The oncology team at the hospital decided that further chemotherapy or radiotherapy was not an option. This meant that future treatment would be totally palliative.

George was devastated by the news that there was no further "curative" treatment available and agreed to a referral to the hospice home care team (HCT) for pain and symptom control. The Clinical Nurse Specialist (CNS) visited him at home.

George's overriding symptom was pain. He described a constant ache in his right buttock with episodes of sharp shooting pain radiating down the back of his right leg to his heel, worse on movement. He also had pins and needles from the right heel to the toes with loss of function, altered sensation, and limited mobility in his right leg. George verbally rated his pain intensity as about seven out of a maximum of ten. He was also very constipated, with no colostomy action for several days.

George lived alone in a first floor one bedroom flat. Because of his poor mobility, he was no longer able to manage the stairs. This caused him a great deal of distress – he had always been physically fit (he worked as a delivery man for a large brewery). He was not particularly religious but still had many questions as to "why has the cancer returned?"

Managing George's pain

At referral to the HCT, George was taking oral morphine 5–10 mg prn, and amitriptyline 10 mg at night. These had been commenced at his hospital appointment. He was gaining only modest relief of his pain from this regime: the neuropathic stabbing element of the pain had improved but the deep ache was little changed. However, despite the low dose of amitriptyline, George reported that his mouth was dry and that he was experiencing some urinary hesitancy. After a telephone discussion with the hospice doctor and George's GP, it was decided to stop the amitriptyline and replace it with gabapentin, at a starting dose of 100 mg tds, rising to 300 mg tds over the next two weeks.

To make it easier for George, it was agreed with the local pharmacist that his medication would be dispensed in a compliance aid.[26][V] It was also decided to establish and titrate a regular morphine dose in order to explore its effectiveness for the two elements of George's pain. In addition, he was prescribed some laxatives and, since he was feeling rather nauseated, metoclopramide as an antiemetic. The CNS explained this to George and checked his understanding of this plan. She offered to visit again the next day. Contact numbers were given and George was invited to contact the HCT at any time.

On her way back to the office the CNS called in to see George's GP at his surgery to see if he would be available to visit George with her the following day. He agreed to do this. When she returned to the office she contacted the community nursing service, explained her findings and asked them to begin visiting George at home. Her assessment of his condition told her that he would need regular contact from the community nurses as he deteriorated further.

George's nonphysical pain

George was anxious and concerned about his increasing disability. His wife had died ten years previously and he had lived alone since then. He had always been very active and was emotionally very upset at the prospect of not being able to get down the stairs again without help. He cried during this first visit. George accepted a referral to the hospice social worker for emotional support and the occupational therapist for assistance with mobility.

Joint visits – what value?

His GP and the CNS saw George at home together the next afternoon. George's medication had just been delivered by the local community pharmacy. He had received a call from the district nurse that morning and was expecting her the following day. There had been some improvement in the aching component of his pain. He was still in discomfort from lancinating pain in the leg, but understood that the new medicine would take a few days to start working. He was willing to wait that long. Together with George they drew up a management plan. He wanted to be at home for as long as possible, and was adamant that he wanted no further hospital admissions. Nor was he willing to consider a hospice admission for pain control – "I'd rather put up with some pain." George was happy with the suggestion that he would need weekly visits – alternating between the CNS and the GP (Note: if a doctor has not seen a patient within two weeks of death, he is unable to issue a death certificate. If no other doctor can issue a certificate, a referral to the coroner is necessary to establish cause of death.)

The CNS wrote down for him the names of the people due to visit him during the next few days (the district nurse, the social worker, and the occupational therapist). The following week when the CNS visited, his pain was under control on an average of 120 mg morphine every 24 hours. However, George was complaining of unpleasant dreams that had worsened as the morphine had been titrated upwards. This problem was discussed with the palliative care team doctor and it was decided to switch his opioid to oxycodone at an equivalent dose. The GP agreed to prescribe a supply of oxycodone.

At the GP's next visit George's pain control had been maintained and his nightmares had much improved. For patient convenience, he therefore converted the four-hourly oxycodone regime into 30 mg bd of a long-acting preparation (Oxycontin), with 10 mg immediate-release oxycodone for breakthrough pain.

After the visit, George's GP asked the CNS for information on the Gold Standards Framework.[23] She provided him with the contact details of the local facilitator. Over the following weeks, George's pain continued to fluctuate (two to five out of ten) and his final Oxycontin dose was 50 mg bd, with 400 mg tds of gabapentin.

Dying

Six weeks later the on-call CNS was called late one evening by George's daughter Sue. His pain had been fairly well controlled, but he had now become profoundly weak, and had taken to his bed. He had not been interested in food for over a week and was only drinking small sips of tea. George's regular CNS was due to visit the next day. Sue lived some distance away, but had come up earlier that day to stay for a week with her father. She did not think a home visit was necessary that night, but would appreciate a home visit as soon as possible the next day.

At the HCT's multidisciplinary meeting the next morning the team agreed that is sounded as if George was beginning to die. Medicines were prescribed and a small supply dispensed from the hospice to be given via a syringe driver, given at equivalent doses to those he had been taking orally. The CNS telephoned the GP's surgery and the district nurse to tell them what had happened. The GP would not be able to visit until the afternoon but the district nurse was able to meet the CNS at the house.

When she arrived at George's home, the district nurse had been there a few minutes. It was clear to them both that George was dying. He was very drowsy but rousable and able to respond to simple questions. Together they made their assessment. He was in some pain, as he had not managed to take his analgesia that morning. He did not want to be moved anywhere. He understood that he was now in the last few days of his life. Sue was in the room during the conversation and although desperately upset was glad that there was a plan to keep him at home to die.

The CNS gave George a subcutaneous injection of oxycodone 10 mg together with haloperidol 0.5 mg for his nausea, and then set up a subcutaneous infusion from a syringe driver, set to deliver oxycodone 60 mg, haloperidol 1 mg, and clonazepam 1 mg per 24 hours, the last being added because of George's neuropathic pain component.

Out-of-hours care

Once again on her way back to the office the CNS decided to call in on the GP surgery. She wanted to make sure that her actions and the management plan were communicated to both her GP and the out-of-hours service. The district nurse agreed to complete an out-of-hours handover form which would be faxed through to the out-of-hours GP service and the night nursing service. This would ensure that George would receive the care prescribed should he need a visit out of hours. This information would prevent an unnecessary admission to hospital out of hours.

George died at home peacefully a couple of days later. His family were with him.

CONCLUSIONS

Achieving good control of pain and other symptoms at home is vital to the hopes of the majority of people with cancer and to the memories (and hence future assumptions about health care) of those close to them. This task needs the back up of inpatient facilities, but failures of symptom management in the community lead to unnecessary admissions with consequent emotional and financial costs. Pain control at home does not, by and large, entail much technology but it does need apparently simple things to be done well – and that, in practice, is difficult.

In the UK, everyone has a right to access a GP and the associated community nursing and social services, but people with cancer pain make up only a small proportion of these professionals' workload. Time is short and so, sometimes, is expertise. The devolution of responsibility for out-of-hours services to PCTs has removed continuity of care. A specialist community palliative care service that is flexible in its responses, proactive in communication with the primary healthcare team, and available 24 hours a day can bridge these gaps and improve both pain control and the entire patient experience.[27][I] The case history in this chapter has provided a practical example of this work in action.

The UK government is continuing to pursue a number of central initiatives aimed at enhancing community palliative care. The Gold Standards Framework[23] applies a method of identification of all palliative care patients within and across palliative care, as well as helping GPs with the essentials of generic palliation. The Preferred Place of Care Assessment[28][III] is yet to be fully implemented but aims to facilitate communication between professionals and patients about end of life issues, including the place where the patient would like to receive their care – a preference which of course tends to change with time and circumstances.[9][III] Third, the Liverpool Integrated Care Pathway[29][III] provides a tool to assist the continuation of effective symptom control during the final stages of life, and is increasingly being used in the community and in care homes, as well as in hospital and hospice settings.

The full effects of revisions to the governance of the supply, handling, and disposal of controlled drugs in the community have yet to emerge, but there is an explicit official recognition of the importance of opioids to pain control of people living at home with cancer and a commitment to continuing efforts to make these medications available in an appropriate and timely fashion.

Britain has led the world in palliative care, yet in practice there is still a long way to go before every person with cancer pain who wishes to remain at home can be sure of receiving the help they need when they need it. However, the issue has caught the attention of both government and the health professions as never before, raising the hope that a future edition of this book will be able to report significant progress in this vital, but so often overlooked, area of care.

In reflections on the case described above, a question that came to mind was how many patients and family members in the UK and US would be able to describe that type of experience if they chose to die at home. At the present time, it is almost impossible to know the answer to that question – because the answer is dependent on so many factors. Not just governmental policies that govern who does and does not have health care within a nation, but interpersonal factors that govern the interactions between clinicians, patients, and family caregivers. The large number of issues that were raised in this chapter and the case study provide "food for thought" for clinicians who are interested in improving the care that palliative care patients receive. Perhaps a worthy activity in both the UK and the US, and other places in the world, would be to use this chapter as a springboard for discussions and planning to achieve the best possible care for palliative care patients within a local community. In each community, depending on specific circumstances, different approaches will need to be designed to achieve optimal levels of care for palliative care patients.

REFERENCES

1. Department of Health. *The NHS cancer plan*. London: Department of Health, 2000.
* 2. National Institute for Clinical Excellence. *Improving supportive and palliative care for adults with cancer*. London: National Institute for Clinical Excellence, 2004.
3. Smith J. The Shipman Inquiry Fourth Report: The regulation of controlled drugs in the community, July 2004. Accessed June 24, 2007. Available from: www.the-shipman-inquiry.org.uk/fourthreport.asp
4. National Institute for Clinical Excellence. *Improving supportive and palliative care for adults with cancer*. London: National Institute for Clinical Excellence, 2004: 18–20.
5. World Health Organization. www.who.int/cancer/palliative/definition/en/, cited June 24, 2007.

6. Miaskowski C, Jacox A, Hester NO, Ferrell B. Interdisciplinary guidelines for the management of acute pain: implications for quality improvement. *Journal of Nursing Care Quality*. 1992; **7**: 1–6.
7. Miaskowski C, Cleary J, Burney R *et al*. *Guideline for the management of cancer pain in adults and children*, Vol. 3. Glenview, IL: American Pain Society, 2005.
8. Berry PH, Dahl JL. The new JCAHO pain standards: implications for pain management nurses. *Pain Management Nursing*. 2000; **1**: 3–12.
9. Hinton J. Which patients with terminal cancer are admitted from home care? *Palliative Medicine*. 1994; **8**: 197–210.
10. Henry C, Young E. National Council for Palliative Care/The NHS End of Life Care Programme. Introductory guide to end of life care in care homes. Last updated April 2006; cited January 25, 2008. Available from: http://eolc.cbcl.co.uk/eolc/eolcpublications/Guide%20To%20EoLC%20care%20homes%20lo.pdf
* 11. Kuehn BM. Hospitals embrace palliative care. *Journal of the American Medical Association*. 2007; **298**: 1263–5.
* 12. Coyne P, Paice JA, Ferrell BR *et al*. Oncology End-of-Life Nursing Education Consortium training program: improving palliative care in cancer. *Oncology Nursing Forum*. 2007; **34**: 801–07.
13. Green CR, Ndao-Brumblay SK, West B, Washington T. Differences in prescription opioid analgesic availability: comparing minority and white pharmacies across Michigan. *Journal of Pain*. 2005; **6**: 689–99.
14. Lin S, Crawford SY, Warren Salmon J. Potential access and revealed access to pain management medications. *Social Science and Medicine*. 2005; **60**: 1881–91.
15. Morrison RS, Wallenstein S, Natale DK *et al*. "We don't carry that" – failure of pharmacies in predominantly nonwhite neighborhoods to stock opioid analgesics. *New England Journal of Medicine*. 2000; **342**: 1023–6.
16. Passik SD, Kirsh KL, Whitcomb L *et al*. A new tool to assess and document pain outcomes in chronic pain patients receiving opioid therapy. *Clinical Therapeutics*. 2004; **2**: 552–61.
17. Interface Pharmacist Network Specialist Medicines. Palliative Care Shared Care Guidelines 2005. Last updated March 2005; cited January 25, 2008. Available from: www.ipnsm.n-i.nhs.uk/library/Palliative%20SCGs.html
18. Twycross RG, Wilcock A, Thorp S. *Palliative care formulary 2*. Abingdon: Radcliffe, 2003.
19. Department of Health. *Raising standards for patients. New partnerships in out of hours care*. London: Department of Health, 2000.
* 20. Thomas K. *Out of hours palliative care in the community*. London: Macmillan Cancer Relief, 2001.
* 21. National Prescribing Centre. A guide to good practice in the management of controlled drugs in primary care (England) – 2nd edition. Liverpool: National Prescribing Centre. Last updated February 2007; cited January 25,

2008) Available from: www.npc.co.uk/controlled_drugs/cdpublications.htm (National Prescribing Centre).

22. NPA (National Pharmaceutical Association) PSNC (Pharmaceutical Serices Negotiating Committee), RPSGB (Royal Pharmaceutical Society of Great Britain) and CCA (Company Chemists' Association). *Achieving safe practice – A guide for PCTs and organised providers.* 2005.

23. Thomas K. The Gold Standards Framework (GSF) England. Department of Health. Last updated 2005; cited January 25, 2008. Available from: www.goldstandardsframework.nhs.uk/

24. Amass C, Allen M. How a 'just in case' approach can improve out of hours palliative care. *Pharmaceutical Journal.* 2005; **275**: 22–3.

25. Department of Health. www.dh.gov.uk/en/Policyandguidance/Organisationpolicy/Endoflifecare/index.htm, cited June 24, 2007.

26. Raynor DK, Nunney JM. Medicine compliance aids are partial solution not panacea. *British Medical Journal.* 2002; **324**: 1338.

27. Gysels M, Higginson I, Rajasekaran M *et al. Improving supportive and palliative care for adults – research evidence.* London: NICE, 2004: 213–66.

∗ 28. Pemberton C, Storey L, Howard A. The preferred place of care document: an opportunity for communication. *International Journal of Palliative Nursing.* 2003; **9**: 439–41.

∗ 29. Ellershaw J, Wilkinson S. *Care of the dying: a pathway to excellence.* Oxford: Oxford University Press, 2003.

Index

This index covers the chapters in this volume only. A combined index covering all four volumes in the *Clinical Pain Management* series is available as a pdf on the accompanying website: www.clinicalpainmanagement.co.uk

An *F* following a page reference indicates that the reference is to a figure; a *T* indicates that the reference is to a table.

Notes
To save space in the index, the following abbreviations have been used:
CBT – cognitive-behavioral therapy
ICU – intensive care unit
NSAIDs – nonsteroidal anti-inflammatory drugs
PCA – patient-controlled analgesia
TENS – transcutaneous electrical nerve stimulation

abdominal pain, pancreatic cancer 35
absorption, drug 107
accountable officers (AO) 414
Accreditation Council for Graduate
    Medical Education (ACGME),
    palliative care accreditation 413
acetaminophen *see* paracetamol
    (acetaminophen)
acetyl-L-carnitine 402
acetylsalicylic acid *see* aspirin
    (acetylsalicylic acid)
*Achieving a balance in national opioids
    control policy: guidelines for
    assessment* 84
acid phosphatase test 257
acquired tolerance 105
acupressure (Shiatsu) 272,
    277–8
acupuncture 271–4
  acute pain 272
  breast cancer 273
  chemotherapy-induced nausea 274
  clinical trial evidence 272–3
  complications 274
  contraindications 274
  dyspnea 274
  historical aspects 271–2
  mechanism of action 273
  meridian theories 273
  metastatic disease 273
  neurophysiology 273
  non-pain symptoms 273–4

postoperative 272
procedure-related pain 216
traditional Chinese approach
    271
treatment course 272
western medical approach 271
acute interstitial nephritis,
    NSAID-induced 136
acute pain, TENS 236 *T*
acute renal failure (ARF),
    NSAID-induced 135–6
  mechanisms 135–6, 136 *F*
  reduced circulation volumes 136
acute tolerance (tachyphylaxis) 105
adaptation 49–50
addiction
  children 354–5
  definition 106, 157
  induction fears 106
  opioids *see* opioid addiction
adrenocorticotrophic (ACTH)
    hormone, acupuncture 273
advance statements 96–7
affective changes, opioid-induced
    154
affinity, drug 105
Africa, palliative care services 86, 88–9,
    90 *F*
  historical aspects 88–9
  initiatives 88
  opioid usage 89, 90 *F*
  organizational provision 89, 89 *T*

agitation
  end of life care 335
  pain misinterpretation 43
agonist 105
agonist–antagonist 105
airway obstruction, tumors 312
alcohol abuse
  history taking 39
  as prognostic factor 42–3
  screening 42–3
alcohol neurolysis 227, 228 *T*
  concentration effects 227, 227 *T*
  nerve regeneration 227
  neurolytic celiac plexus blockade 228
  phenol neurolysis *vs.* 228
alcohol toxicity, intrathecal
    neurolysis 231 *T*
alfentanil
  dyspnea 313
  procedure-related pain 217
alkaline phosphatase tests 257
AL-TENS 237–8, 239 *T*, 240 *F*
alvimopan 324
Alzheimer's disease, nonverbal pain
    assessment 370–1
AM404 125
amethocaine 217
amifostine 402
amitriptyline
  elderly 369
  neuropathic pain 205
  postbreast cancer surgery pain 404–5

ammonium compounds, neurolysis 228
amphetamines
    contraindications 184–5
    depression 332
    fatigue 329
    opioid-induced sedation 184
analgesia/analgesics
    adjuvant
        breakthrough pain 290
        children 351–4
    administration routes 110–1
        children 349–50
    "as required" 111
    in elderly see elderly
    opioid-induced 154
        tolerance 156
    oral administration 109–11
        children 349
    pediatric cancer pain 347–9
    postbreast cancer surgery pain 404
    reduced effect, increased nociceptive
        inputs 106
    refusal 94
        by relatives 96
    stimulation-induced see stimulation-
        induced analgesia
    sublingual administration,
        breakthrough pain 291
    substance abuse patients 384–5
    see also individual drugs
anastrazole 265
anemia 311
anesthesia/anesthetic, elderly 368
anger
    assessment 56
    management strategies 56
angular cheilitis 316
animal models/studies
    bone pain 4–5
    chemotherapy-induced peripheral
        neuropathy 8, 400
    neuropathic pain 7–8
    somatic pain 4
    visceral pain 9
anorexia and cachexia see anorexia
    cachexia syndrome (ACS)
anorexia cachexia syndrome
    (ACS) 326–8
    causes 326
    clinical findings 327
    investigations 327
    management 327
        nonpharmacological 327
        pharmacological 327–8
        potential therapies 328
    neurohormonal mechanisms 327, 327 F
    noncancer illness 326

pathophysiology 326–7
    starvation vs. 327
antagonist 105
antiarrhythmics 208
anticholinergics 335
anticonvulsants
    children 354
    elderly 369
    side effects 369
    see also antiepileptics; individual drugs
antidepressants
    anxiety 333
    children 351–3
    clinical pharmacology 205
    depression 332
    elderly 369
    mechanism of action 205
    neuropathic pain 205–6
    see also individual drugs/drug classes
antidiarrheals 326 T
antiemetics, opioid therapy and 113,
    191
antiepileptics
    adverse effects 206
    clinical pharmacology 206
    mechanism of action 206
    neuropathic pain 206–7
        new drugs 207
        older drugs 206
antihistamines
    cough 315
    opioid-induced pruritus 192
"antineuropathic" medication, brachial
    plexus neuropathy 406
antipsychotics
    agitation 335
    delirium 334
        opioid-induced 187
antitussives 315
anxiety 332–3
    etiology 332–3
    family's future 49
    management 333
    predisposing factors 57
    prevalence 332
    quality of life 49
    risk assessment 57–8
    symptoms 57
anxiety scores, family caregiver
    65
anxiolytics
    dyspnea 313–4
    elderly 368
    opioid therapy and 113–4
appraisal support, professional
    teams 75
aprepitant 320 T

aromatherapy 277–8
    elderly 370
β artificial saliva, xerostomia 316
Asia Pacific region, palliative care
    services 86
aspirin (acetylsalicylic acid)
    children 348
    elderly 365
    gastrointestinal injury risk 129, 131–3
assessment/measurement (of
    pain) 38–47
    dementia patients 43
    Down syndrome 371
    dying person 392, 392 F
    elderly 361–2
    intensity evaluation 41–2, 43 T
        graphic display 42
        instruments 41
    investigations 40
    measurement 38–47
    multidimensional 42, 42–3
    nonverbal behavior 370–1, 392
    by nurses 364, 371
    pain, other symptom integration 44
    see also specific scales
Association for Palliative Medicine,
    outside license drug use 415–6
ASTRONAUT study 366
attentional distraction 300
auriculoacupuncture 272
    elderly 370
    neuropathic pain 272

back pain
    children 346
    meningeal carcinomatosis 32
    pancreatic cancer 35
baclofen 209
bacterial infections, oral 317
βarrestin2 gene, opioid response 174
barriers, to pain relief see pain relief
    barriers
Barriers questionnaire, family
    caregivers 64–5
base of skull metastases, pain
    syndromes 29–30
    clinical features 29, 31 T
    radiographic investigations 30,
        31 F
behavioral pain scales, dementia/
    delirium patients 43
benzodiazepines
    agitation 335
    anxiety 333
    delirium 334
        opioid-induced 187
    elderly 365

bereavement support 334
bethanecol 316
bile duct dilation, opioid-induced 192
biliary spasm, opioid-induced 192
biliary tract, opioid effects 155
bioavailability (F) 107
    subcutaneous 110
biopsychosocial model for pain 297
bisphosphonates
    bone metastases 265–6
    breakthrough pain 290
    elderly 369
    hypercalcemia 321
    metastatic bone pain 290, 369
bladder, opioid effects 192
bladder pain, phantom 36
bladder spasm 36
body fluid screening, substance
    abuse 381
body temperature regulation 331
bone metabolism affecting drugs,
    elderly 369
bone metastases
    diagnostic criteria 257–8
    hypercalcemia 319
    incidence 257 T
    osteoblasts 256–7
    osteoclast activation 256–7
    pathophysiology 256–7
    sacral 29 T
    vertebral see vertebral metastases
bone pain
    animal models 4–5
    blood-borne metastasis 256
    causes 257 T
    clinical presentation 257
    diagnostic criteria 257–8
    dorsal horn alteration 5
    etiology 256–7
    hormone treatment 265–6
    management 256–69, 267 F
        evidence-based evaluation 258–64
        incidence pain 258
        pharmacological 258
        surgery 266–7
    metastatic see metastatic bone pain
    neuropathic 5
    pathological features 5, 6 F
    pathophysiology 4–5, 256–7
    peripheral activation 5
    prognosis 266 F, 267
    radiotherapy see radiotherapy
    response to drugs 5
    syndromes 28–9
    tumor infiltration 256
bone scans, patient assessment 40
borborygmi 323

bortezomib 402
bowel obstruction, advanced
    cancer 321–3
    clinical features 322
    incidence 321
    management 322–3
        "dip and suck" indispensable
            322
        nonsurgical 322–3
        surgical intervention 322
    pathophysiology 321
    vomiting management 322, 323 F
bowel toxicity, radiotherapy-
    induced 259
brachial plexopathy 32
    causes 32
brachial plexus neuropathy (BPM),
    radiotherapy-induced 405
    incidence 405
    time–incidence relationship 405
    treatment 406
    tumor-induced neuropathy vs. 405
brain tumors, primary
    pediatric cancer pain 346
    radiotherapy 252–3
branched chain amino acids
    (BCAA) 328
breakthrough pain
    as prognostic indicator 288
    baseline therapy
        optimization 289–90, 290 F
    bone 28
    characteristics 287–8
    children 346
    definition 43, 287
    management 286–95
        antineoplastic treatment 289
        comorbid condition
            treatment 289
        dying person 393
        elderly 368
        nonpharmacologic therapies 292,
            292 T
        parenteral formulations 292
        precipitating factor treatment 289
        primary interventions 288
        strategies 288 T
        symptomatic
            interventions 289–91
        transmucosal formulations
            291–2
    model 287 F
    opioid titration 43
    prevalence 287
    rescue dosing 114, 290, 290 F
        oral 291, 291 F
    subtypes 287

breast, phantom pain 404
breast cancer
    acupuncture 273
    elderly 360
    metastatic
        hypnosis 276, 301
        pain prevalence 18
        radiotherapy 254
    metastatic bone pain
        chemotherapy 264
        hormone treatment 265
    postoperative chronic pain see
        postbreast cancer surgery pain
        (PBCSP)
    supportive psychotherapy 298–9
    TENS 241–242 T
breast reconstruction, postoperative
    pain 404
breathing, noisy, end of life 335
breathlessness see dyspnea
Brief Pain Inventory (BPI) 42
bronchial carcinoma
    radiotherapy 252
    unilateral facial pain 32
bronchoalveolar carcinoma 315
bronchodilators, dyspnea 314
bronchorrhea, bronchoalveolar
    carcinoma 315
bulking agents 324
buprenorphine 159–60, 169 T
    bioavailability 159
    breakthrough pain 291
    cancer pain use 159–60
    elderly 367
    neuropathic pain 204, 206
        clinical studies 204
    pharmacodynamics 159
    pharmacokinetics 159
    pharmacology 204
    routes of administration/
        formulations 159
    side effects 159
    tolerance 159–60
    transdermal patches 159–60
        elderly 368
buspirone
    anxiety 333
    dyspnea 314
butorphanol 162

cachexia see anorexia cachexia
    syndrome (ACS)
caffeine, opioid-induced sedation 185
CAGE, alcoholism diagnosis 42–3
calcitonin
    elderly 369
    hypercalcemia 321

camphor 330
cancer
    global burden 81
        non-pain symptoms control 310–42
            gastrointestinal problems 316–7
            psychiatric problems 331–4
            psychological problems 331–4
            respiratory symptoms 311
            see also individual symptoms
Cancer and Supportive Care
    Networks 417
cancer-directed therapy, pain
    induction 7
cancer-induced bone pain (CIBP) see
    bone pain
cancer pain syndromes 27–37
cancer-related suicide 57
    management 332
    psychiatrist referral 57
    risk evaluation 57
    risk factors 21–3, 332
Cancer Relief India 87
cancer survivors, pain 399–410
candidiasis, oral 316–7
    risk factors 316
    treatment 316–7
cannabinoids 275
    anorexia cachexia syndrome 328
CanSupport 87
capsaicin
    neuropathic pain 209
    pain relief 275
    postbreast cancer surgery pain
        404–5
    pruritus 330
carbamazepine
    elderly 369
    side effects 369
carbocisteine 315
carboplatin 401
cardiovascular system
    NSAID-induced adverse effects
        136–8
    opioid effects 155
caregiving, definition 63–4
carers see family caregiver
catechol-O-methyltransferase (COMT),
    opioid response variability 174
categorical-rated scale (CRS),
    elderly 361
cathartic drugs 190
cauda equina compression see spinal
    cord compression
causality 98
cavernous sinus syndrome 31 T
ceiling effect 105
    nonopioid drugs 111

celecoxib
    cardiovascular risk 137
    elderly 366
Cental Europe, palliative care
    services 86
central hypogastric pain 35
central nervous system (CNS), opioid
    effects 154–5
central neuropathic pain 200
cerebral metastasis, headache
    management 253
characterization (of pain) 41,
    41 T
    multiple sites 41
Checklist of Nonverbal Pain
    Indicators 392
chemical neurolysis 225–34
    agents 226 T, 227–8
        see also individual agents
    clinical applications 228–31
    historical aspects 225–6, 226 T
    pathophysiology 226–7, 227 T
    surgical sectioning vs. 226, 226 T
chemotherapy
    metastatic bone pain 264–5,
        264 T
        indications 264
    nausea and vomiting see nausea and
        vomiting
    neuropathic pain induction see
        chemotherapy-induced
        peripheral neuropathy (CIPN)
    neurotoxic agents 400
    neurotoxicity 399–400
chemotherapy-induced peripheral
    neuropathy (CIPN) 399–402
    animal models 8, 400
    assessment 401
        standardization 401
    axonopathy 8, 400–1
    "coasting" 400–1
    diagnostic features 400
    grading scales 401, 401 T
    mechanisms 399–401
    neuroimmune responses 8
    neuronopathy 400–1
    neurotoxic agents 400, 401–2
    pain distribution 400
    pathophysiology 7
    presentation 399–401
    prevention 402
    treatment 8–9, 402
    as unique pain syndrome 4
chest pain, radiotherapy 252
chest radiography, dyspnea 311
Child Depression Inventory,
    breakthrough pain 346

children
    cancer pain see pediatric cancer pain
    desire to protect 54
    helping parents talk to 54–5
    with ill relative, behavioral changes
        54
    opioid adverse effects 351,
        353 T
    opioid tolerance 354–5
    PCA 350
    psychological evaluation 54–5
    psychosocial needs 54
Chinese herbs 275
cholecystokinin (CCK)
    acupuncture 273
    opioid effectiveness 202–3
cholestasis 330
cholestyramine 330
choline magnesium trisalicylate
    (Trilisate), children 348
chronic pain
    adult survivors, childhood
        cancers 346
    TENS 236 T
chronic renal failure, NSAID-induced
    135
CINODs (COX inhibitors and NO
    donors; NO-NSAIDs) 138
Cipla Cancer Palliative Care Centre 87
cirrhosis, effects on
    pharmacokinetics 108
cisplatin, neuropathy induction 7,
    401
clearance (Cl), drugs
    definition 107
    elderly 365
    hepatic function and 108
Clinical Nurse Specialist (CNS) 418
clivus syndrome 31 T
clodronate 265–6
clonazepam
    elderly 369
    opioid-induced myoclonus 188
coanalgesic drugs 113
    adverse effects 181
    opioid adverse effect
        management 181–2
codeine 157
    cancer pain use 157
    children 348, 352 T
    cough 315
    elderly 367
    pharmacodynamics 157
    pharmacokinetics 157
    routes of administration/
        formulations 157
    side effects 157

cognitive-behavioral therapy
(CBT) 299–303
acute *vs.* chronic pain 303
anxiety 333
assumptions 299
children 306, 347
general anesthesia *vs.* 306
components 300
coping skills/techniques 299,
305–6
depression 332
efficacy, evidence for 301–2
individual studies 301
systemic reviews/meta-analyses
301–2
goals 299
maladaptive thoughts 299
models 303
procedure-related pain 216
children 216, 305–6
efficacy 305–6
strategies 300
symptom limitations 304
tailoring 302–3
cognitive failure
history taking 39
opioid-induced 185
cognitive impairment
pain assessment 371
dying person 392, 392 *F*
strong opioids 113
cognitive restructuring 300
colon, visceral pain 9
colorectal cancer, radiotherapy
254
colored analog scale (CAS) 371
Commission of Specialist in Pain
Therapy and Palliative Care,
Romania 84–5
Commission on Narcotic Drugs,
Economic and Social Council 83
communication, unhelpful 52
community setting pain
management 411–21
case history 417–9
at home medication provision
414–5
United Kingdom 414
United States 414–5
out-of-hours medication
provision 416–7
case history 419
"crisis pack" 417
drug access problems 417
"just-in-case" pack 417
on-call pharmacy services 417
work practices 417

outside license drug use 415–6
"specialist only" drugs 416
specialist *vs.* generalist prescribing 416
United Kingdom 416
United States 416
see also palliative care
competitive antagonist 105
complementary therapies 270–85
children 270–1
definition 270
dying person 394
elderly 369–70
medical profession's attitude to 271
reasons for use 271
usage 270–1
see also individual therapies
complex regional pain
syndromes 229–30
computed tomography (CT)
base of skull metastases 30, 31 *F*
malignant bone tumors 257
malignant psoas syndrome 34 *F*
patient assessment 40
pulmonary emboli 311–2
confidentiality, psychological
evaluation 51
confusion
causes, terminally ill patients 333–4
opioid-induced, children 353 *T*
Confusion Assessment Method
(CAM) 186
conscious sedation 218–9
complications 219
contraindications 219
definition 218–9
precautions/guidelines 219
consent 94–5
drug testing 385
informed *see* informed consent
constipation 323–4
clinical findings 323
definition 189
dying person 394–5
investigations 323
management 324
opioid-induced 155, 189–90, 323
children 351, 353 *T*
clinical presentation/findings 189
diagnostic criteria 189–90
elderly 367
epidemiology 181 *T*, 189
etiology 189
investigations 189–90
management 190
pathophysiology 189
prevention 190
pathophysiology 323

continuous subcutaneous
administration, analgesia 110
controlled drugs (CDs)
United Kingdom
audit trail 414
guidance development 414,
415 *T*
legislation 414
prescriptions 414
record-keeping/monitoring 414
unwanted, collection/
destruction 414
United States
insurance plans 414–5
lack of availability 415
payment/co-payment issues
415
prescription regulations 415
controlled release (CR)
oxymorphone 161
coping 49–50
definition 50
mechanisms assessment 55–6
coproxamol 367
cordotomy 406
Cornell scale for depression in
dementia (CSDD) 371
corticosteroid(s)
airway obstruction 312
anorexia cachexia syndrome 327–8
bowel obstruction 322–3
breakthrough pain 290
children 354
dying person 394
nausea and vomiting 320 *T*
cough 314–5
antineoplastic treatment 314–5
clinical findings 314
history/examination 314
management 314
palliative treatment 315
cough suppression, opioids 155,
315
counterirritants, pruritus 330
cranial nerve pain syndromes 29–30
cross-tolerance
definition 105
opioids 106
incomplete 156
cryoanalgesia 231
advantages/disadvantages 232 *T*
cyclizine 320 *T*
cyclooxygenase(s)
single nucleotide polymorphisms 127
splice variants 127
cyclooxygenase 1 (COX-1) 126–7
in inflammation 126

cyclooxygenase 2 (COX-2) 126–7
cyclooxygenase 2 (COX-2) inhibitors
  cardiovascular risks 136–7
  children 348
  definition 127
  gastrointestinal adverse effect risk 133
  thrombotic risk 136
cyclooxygenase 3 (COX-3) 127
  paracetamol effect 124
cyclooxygenase-inhibitors and
    NO-donors (CINODs;
    NO-NSAIDs) 138
CYP2D6 enzyme, opioid
    metabolism 173
cytochrome P450 3A4 (CYP3A4),
    opioid metabolism 173
cytokines, cancer-induced bone pain 5

danthron 325 *T*
decision-making
  by healthcare professional 96
  patient's involvement 95
  patients who have capacity, western
    society 95
  patients who lack capacity 96–7
  by relatives
    patients who have capacity 95–6
    patients who lack capacity 96
    process 67 *T*
deep brain stimulation (DBS) 246
deep inferior epigastric perforator
    (DIEP) free flaps 404
deep sedation 219
dehydration, dying person 394–5
delirium 333
  agitated 186
  causes, terminally ill patients 333–4
  clinical features 333
  definition 185–6
  elderly 361
  environmental manipulation 333
  hypoactive 186
  management 333
    pharmacological 333–4
  mixed 186
  opioid-induced 185–7
    clinical presentation 186
    diagnostic criteria 186
    epidemiology 186
    etiology 186
    examination 186
    management, evidence-based
      evaluation 186–7
    pathophysiology 186
    prognosis 187
  pain assessment 43
  pain overestimation 186

Delirium Rating Scale (DRS) 40
delta-opioid agonists, intraspinal
    administration 154
delta receptors 152
dementia patients, pain assessment 43
denial assessment 55–6
depression 331–2
  depressed mood *vs.* 56
  diagnosis 331–2
  elderly 369
  history taking 39
  management 332
  predisposing factors 56
  prevalence 21, 331–2
  risk assessment 56–7
    diagnostic instruments 56–7
  somatic features 331–2
depression scores, family caregiver 65
dexamethasone
  airway obstruction, tumors 312
  anorexia cachexia syndrome
    327–8
  children 354
  dying person 394
  superior vena caval obstruction
    312
dexamphetamine
  children 353–4
  opioid-induced sedation 184
dextroamphetamine *see*
    dexamphetamine
dextromethorphan 315
dextropropoxyphene 367
Diagnostic and Statistical Manual
    (DSM) IV
  delirium definition 185
  substance abuse definition 380
dialysis, pharmacokinetic effects 108
diamorphine
  cough 315
  neuropathic pain 204
diarrhea 324–6
  clinical findings 324
  history taking 324
  investigations 324
  management 324–6, 326 *T*
  pathophysiology 324
diazepam
  agitation 335
  dyspnea 314
diclofenac
  opioid-sparing effect 181–2
  thrombogenicity 136, 137–8
dietary fiber, constipation 324
dipyrone 125
  agranulocytosis associations 125
  in cancer pain 125

dissociation 300–1
distraction 277, 300
  attentional 300
  children 277, 347
  efficacy 301
  elderly 370
docetaxel 402
doctors
  attitudes to pain in elderly 362
  pain estimation 364
doctrine of double effect 97–8
  conditions 98
  end of life issues 391
  euthanasia 98
  foreseen harms 98
  intention 98
  pain relief-life shortening issues
    97
domperidone 320 *T*
donepezil 185
dorsal horn alterations, cancer-induced
    bone pain 5
dose–response curves 105, 105 *F*
Down syndrome, pain assessment 371
doxepin 330
driving
  opioid-induced cognitive failure 185
  spinal cord stimulation
    patients 245–6
drug(s)
  absorption 107
  addiction *see* addiction
  affinity 105
  clearance *see* clearance (Cl), drugs
  efficacy (intrinsic activity) 105
  lipid solubility, age-related
    changes 365
  potency 105
  side effects, patient information 94
drug abuse, history taking 39
drug seeking behavior 107
drug transporters, opioid response
    variability 107
dry mouth *see* xerostomia
dual channel TENS 243
dying person 389–98
  case history 419
  dying trajectory 390, 390 *F*
  family caregiver 390–1
  interdisciplinary team 390
  nonpain symptom management 394
  opioids 392–3
  pain
    adverse effects 394–5
    etiology 390
    prevalence 390
    sensory aspects 391

pain assessment 392, 392 *F*
  nonverbal patients 392
pain management
  adjuvant drugs 393–4
  challenges in 391–2
  clinical interventions,
        efficacy 390–1
  communication in 391
  drug routes of administration 393–4
  nonpharmacological 394
  treatment choices 393–5
  polypharmacy 393–4
  quality of life 391, 392
  "total pain" 390, 392
  unique care 389–91
dying state 389–90
dynorphin receptors, cancer-induced
        bone pain 5
dynorphins 153
dysesthesia
  brachial plexopathy 32
  intrathecal neurolysis-induced
        231 *T*
  malignant paraplegia 30–1
  spinal cord compression 30–1
dyspepsia, NSAID-induced 128–9
dysphagia 317–8
  clinical findings 317
  etiology 317
  investigations 317
  management 317–8
  neurogenic 317
  neurological problems and 317
dysphoria, opioid-induced 154
  children 353 *T*
dyspnea 311
  acupuncture 274
  causes 311–3
  clinical findings 311
    emotional component 311
  definition 311
  drug treatment 313–4
    nebulized drugs 314
  history/examination 311
  investigations 311–2
  management 312–3
    supportive care 312
  palliation 313–4
  pathophysiology 311

ear acupuncture *see*
        auriculoacupuncture
Eastern Europe, palliative care
        services 86
ecomaps, psychological evaluation 51
Edmonton Classification System for
        Cancer Pain (ECS-CP) 44, 45 *T*

Edmonton Symptom Assessment
        System (ESAS)
  anxiety diagnosis 39
  depression diagnosis 39
  pain intensity 42
education
  family 52–3
  family caregiver 67–8, 363
  healthcare professionals
    analgesic drug use 82
    pain control issues 94
  patients *see* patient education
efficacy (intrinsic activity), drugs
        105
eicosapentaenoic acid (EPA) 328
elderly 359–78
  ageist attitudes 360
  analgesia
    additional 368–70
    misconceptions 363
    simple 365–6
  assessment 361–2
  carers
    knowledge/experience 363–4
    pain overestimation 363
  etiology 360
  hospital admissions 360
  nighttime pain 361
  nonpharmacological
        management 369–70
  nonverbal patients 370–1
  nursing home patients 371–2
    pain prevalence 371
    undertreatment risk 371
  opioids *see* opioid(s)
  pain characteristics 360–1
  pain control 362–3
    doctors' attitudes 362
    healthcare professionals'
          attitudes 362–3
    nurses' attitudes 362–3
    patients' attitudes 362
  pain definitions 360
  pain incidence 360
  pain measurement instruments
        361
  pain relief measurement 361
  palliative care interventions 360
  patient knowledge/experience 364
  pharmacodynamics 365
  pharmacokinetics 365
  quality of life 360, 361, 363
  reluctance to report 362
  residential home patients 371–2
    resignation to pain 372
  terminal dependency period 360
  tolerance to pain 360

electroacupuncture 272
elimination half-life ($t_{1/2}$) 107
emetic (vomiting) pattern
        generator 318, 318 *F*
EMLA
  postbreast cancer surgery pain
        404–5
  procedure-related pain 216
    children 349–50
emotional distress, pain and 303
empowerment, patient 297
end of dose failure 287
  epidemiology 288
end of life care 334–5
  agitation management 335
  home care 334
  multiprofessional care team
        334
  pain relief 334
  prognosis estimations 334
  secretion management 335
  symptoms control 334
End-of-Life Nursing Education
        Consortium (ELNEC-Oncology)
        413
End of Life Strategy 417
endometrial carcinoma
  hormone treatment 265
  metastatic bone pain
        management 265
endomorphin-1 153
endorphins 153
endoscopic retrograde
        cholangiopancreatography
        (ERCP) 218
endothelins (ET), cancer-induced bone
        pain 5
enkephalins 153
enteropathy, NSAID-induced 134
Entonox, procedure-related pain *see*
        nitrous oxide mixture, procedure-
        related pain
epidemiology 13–26
  assessment tools 14
  future challenges 23
  pain measurement 14
  pain, other factors relationship 18–21
epidural infusions, children 354
epidural neurolytic blockade 230–1
  phenol 230
epidural spinal cord compression 29 *T*
epileptiform neuralgia 206
episodic pain *see* breakthrough pain
erythromycin 320 *T*
erythropoietin
  fatigue 329
  uremic itch 331

esophageal candidiasis 316
esophageal stents 215 *F*
Essaic 274
ethamsylate 315
ethical issues 93–100
  consent *see* consent
  healthcare professional, moral
    obligations 97
  intrusive questioning 95
  pain management 93–100
    blame 99
    dying person 391
  prolongation of life 97–9
    common-sense approach 97
    "double effect" 97
    foreseen harms 98
    intention 98
    media's role 97
    moral failures 98–9
    public acceptance 98
  psychological evaluation 51
  substance abuse and pain
    management 384, 386
  total pain 95
  see also decision-making
ethosuxamide 8–9
etiology (of pain) 28 *T*, 151
etoricoxib 137
European Association for Palliative
  Care (EAPC)
  opioid adverse effect management
    guidelines 181
  opioid switching
    recommendations 169
European Organization for Research
  and Treatment of Cancer
  (EORTC), elderly pain
  assessment 361
euthanasia 98, 391
exercise programs, fatigue 329
external beam radiotherapy, bone
  pain 258–9

faces pain scale (FPS), cognitive
  impairment 371
facet join pain, radiofrequency
  lesioning 232
facial affective scale (FAS), cognitive
  impairment 371
facial pain, bronchial cancer 32
failed back surgery syndrome (FBSS)
  deep brain stimulation 246
  spinal cord stimulation 244
falls, elderly 361
family
  as "attorney" 96
  carers *see* family caregiver

as co-clients 53
conflict of needs 54
education needs 52–3
emotional risk, predisposing
  factors 53
importance of 52–3
needs 53
palliative care concerns 52–3
psychological evaluation 53–4
psychological state 53
psychosocial assessment 52
family caregiver
  anxiety scores 65
  burden of caring 52
  definition 63–4
  demographics 364
  depression scores 65
  dying person 390–1
  financial burden 65
  health status scores 65
  pain education program 67–8,
    363
  pain experience
    communication problems 64
    impact of cancer 65
    perceptions 64
  pain management 63–70
    barriers to 64–5
    clinical practice implications 68
    implementation difficulties 66,
      66 *T*
    processes 66–7, 67 *T*
    research implications 68
    skills 66–8, 67 *T*
  pain overestimation 64, 363
  pain underestimation 64
  palliative care patient, impact of
    caring for 65
  psychosocial assessment 52
  quality of life 65
  strain on 65
famotidine 133
fatigue 328–9
  management 329
  treatable causes 328
fear(s)
  addiction 106
  opioid-related *see* opioid(s)
  tolerance 106
fentanyl 160, 169 *T*
  breakthrough pain 291
  children 349, 352 *T*
  dyspnea 313
  elderly 368
  interindividual response
    variability 174
  metabolism 203

Middle East usage 88
neuropathic pain 202, 203–4
  clinical studies 203–4
pharmacodynamics 160
pharmacokinetics 160
pharmacology 203
procedure-related pain 217
routes of administration/
  formulations 110, 160
side effects 160
  elderly 368
  sedation 184
sublingual formulations 291
transdermal 203
  children 349
  elderly 367
  nausea induction 191
uses 160
fentanyl buccal tablet (FBT) 160
  breakthrough pain 292
fever, dying person 394
first pass clearance 107
  elderly 365
flecainide 208–9
fluconazole 316–7
fluid intake, constipation 324
fluid retention, NSAID-induced 135
fluoxetine 205
FP10 414
funicular pain, spinal cord
  compression 30
furosemide 314

gabapentin
  cancer-induced bone pain 5
  chemotherapy-induced peripheral
    neuropathy 8–9, 402
  neuropathic pain 206, 207
  postbreast cancer surgery pain 404–5
  pruritus 330
gallium nitrate 321
ganglion impar block 230
gas exchange, dyspnea 311
gastric emptying times, prolonged 108
gastric erosions, NSAID-induced 128–9
  Helicobacter pylori 128
gastric outlet obstruction 318
gastrointestinal bleeding
  aspirin-induced 129
  NSAID-induced 129
  paracetamol-induced 125
gastrointestinal system
  nonpain-related symptom
    control 316–7
  NSAIDs adverse effects *see* NSAID-
    induced gastrointestinal effects
  opioid effects 155, 189

general anesthesia, children, CBT *vs.* 306
genomaps, psychological evaluation 51
ghrelin 328
gliomas 252–3
glove anesthesia technique 300–1
glutamine 402
glutathione 402
glycerol neurolysis 228, 228 *T*
P-glycoprotein, opioid response variability 170–3
glycopyrronium bromide 335
government policy, pain management 82
granisetron 320 *T*
group psychotherapy, distress 303
growth factors, cancer-induced bone pain 5
guided imagery 277, 299–300
gut transit time 323

H1 antihistamines 330
H2 blockers 133
haloperidol
    delirium 187, 334
    nausea and vomiting 191, 320 *T*
hands-on care provision, family caregiver 67 *T*
headache
    base of skull metastases 29–30, 31 *T*
    meningeal carcinomatosis 32
    radiotherapy 252–3
healing (therapeutic touch) 278
healthcare professionals
    decision-making 96
    education *see* education
    elderly pain control, attitudes to 362–3
    ethical issues 97
    opioid use fears 115
Helicobacter pylori, NSAID-induced gastric erosions 128
helium/oxygen mixtures, dyspnea 314
hematological malignancy, children 346
hemibody radiotherapy, bone pain *see* wide field irradiation, bone pain
hemoptysis 315
hepatic function, drug clearance and 108
hepatic pain 35
hepatomegaly
    lower rib cage discomfort 35
    pain 35
herbal medicine 274–5
    antitumor potential 274
    preparation quality 275
    side effects 275
    see also individual medicines

herpetic infections, oral 317
highly selective COX-2 inhibitors *see* cyclooxygenase 2 (COX-2) inhibitors
history taking 39–40, 39 *T*
    alcohol/drug abuse 39
    cognitive failure 39
    concurrent medical conditions 40
    mood disorders 39
    previous treatments 39
    sexual 55
holistic assessment framework 51 *F*
homecare service, palliative care
    India 87
    Middle East 87
home care team (HCT) 418
home environment, pain management difficulties 66, 66 *T*
homeopathy 275
hormone treatment, bone pain 265–6
Horner's syndrome, vertebral metastases 28–9
hospice movement development 85, 412
    Africa 88–9
    poorer countries 85
Hospital Anxiety and Depression Scale (HADS) 39, 56–7
hot flashes *see* hot flushes
hot flushes
    acupuncture 274
    clinical findings 331
    management 331
hydration, opioid-induced delirium 187
hydromorphone 161, 169 *T*
    breakthrough pain 291
    cancer pain use 161
    children 349, 352 *T*
    elderly 368
    pharmacodynamics 161
    pharmacokinetics 161
    routes of administration/ formulations 161
    side effects 161
hyoscine butylbromide 335
hyoscine hydrobromate (scopolamine) 191, 320 *T*
hyoscine hydrobromide 335
hyperalgesia, opioid-induced 188–9
    clinical presentation 189
    diagnostic criteria 189
    epidemiology 189
    etiology 188
    management, evidence-based evaluation 189
    pathophysiology 188

hypercalcemia 319–21
    management 319–21
    symptoms 319
hypertension, NSAID-induced 135
hyperthermia, therapeutic 231–2
hypertonic solution neurolysis 228
hyperventilation 311
hypnosis 275–7, 299–300
    children 304–5, 347
        direct suggestions 304
        indirect suggestions 305
        procedure-related pain 276, 305
        techniques 304–5
    components 300
    definition 275, 299
    efficacy 300, 301–2
        children 305
        individual studies 301, 305
        systemic reviews/meta-analyses 301–2, 305
    elderly 369–70
    mechanisms of action 276–7
    nomenclature confusion 276
    non-pain symptoms 276
    pain relief aims 275
    procedure-related pain 216
    side effects 276, 302
    techniques 300–1
hypnotic responsiveness 300
hypnotic suggestibility 300
hypnotizability 300
hypogastric pain, central 35
hypoglossal nerve pain syndrome 30
hypogonadotrophic hypogonadism, opioid-induced 192
hypothalamus, temperature regulation 331
hypothermia, therapeutic 231
hypotonic solution neurolysis 228

ibandronate 321
ibuprofen
    thrombogenicity 137–8
    upper GI injury risk 131–3
iliac fossae pain 35
illicit drug users, opioids 106–7
imagery 299–300
    children 304–5
    efficacy 301
    elderly 369–70
    guided 277, 299–300
immediate release tablets 110–1
immune system
    cancer-induced bone pain 5
    opioid effects 156, 192
immunosuppression, opioid-induced 156

incident pain
  bone 258
  definition 287
  epidemiology 288
  rescue analgesics 114
  see also breakthrough pain
India
  cancer incidence 86
  opioid use regulations 84
  palliative care services 86–7
    government-funded centers 87
    historical aspects 86
    homecare service 87
    sources of provision 86
Indian Association of Palliative Care
    (IAPC) 87
"individual" 50, 51 F
induction heating 231–2
indwelling needles, acupuncture 272
  clinical trial evidence 273
infection(s)
  pain induction 36
  treatment, breakthrough pain 289
inferior mesenteric plexus, neurolytic
    block 230
informal carers 52–3
informational support, professional
    teams 75
informed consent 94
  patient's risk/harm assessment 95
  side effects 94
instrumental support, professional
    teams 75
intense TENS 238, 239 T, 240 F
intention, ethical issues 98
intercostal nerve cryoneurolysis 231
intercostobrachial neuralgia, postbreast
    cancer surgery pain 403
interdisciplinary care 74
interleukins, cancer-induced bone
    pain 5
intermittent bolus, loading dose
    calculation 108
International Narcotics Control Board
    (INCB) 82–3
International Observatory on End of
    Life Care (IOELC), access to
    cancer pain relief findings
    85–6
International Symposium on Cancer
    Pain, first 82
intestinal linitis plastica 321
intimacy 55
intramuscular drug administration
    110
  children 350
intrapelvic pain 35–6

intrathecal neurolysis 230
  complications 230, 231 T
  patient positioning 230
  technique 230
intravenous drug administration
    110
  children 350
  dying person 393–4
  loading dose calculation 108
intrinsic activity (efficacy), drugs 105
iodine, metastatic bone pain 263–4
[131I]iodine-metaiodobenylguanidine
    ([131I]MIGB) 354
ion trapping, NSAID adverse
    effects 130
ipratropium bromide 314
Iscador 274
ISCD-10, delirium definition 185
Island Hospice 88–9
isotope bone scan, malignant bone
    tumors 257
Israel, palliative care services 87
Italy, opioid use regulations 83–4
itch see pruritus
itraconazole 316–7

jugular foramen syndrome 31 T

kappa opioid receptors 152
Katz Activities of Daily Living,
    elderly 361
ketamine
  bioavailability 208
  cancer pain use 208
    intravenous "burst" 208
  elderly 368
  multiple receptor activity 207
  opioid sensitivity and 202–3
  pharmacodynamics 207
  pharmacokinetics 207–8
  procedure-related pain 218
    advantage/disadvantages 218
  side effects 207
  terminal sedation, children 354
ketoconazole 316–7
ketorolac 181–2
kidneys, NSAID adverse effects 128 T,
    135–6, 135 F

lanreotide 320 T
large intestine
  obstruction see bowel obstruction
  opioid effects 155
  toxicity, NSAID-induced 135
lasers
  acupuncture 272
  neurolysis 232

Latin America, palliative care
    services 86
laxatives
  constipation 190, 324, 325 T
  dying person 394–5
  opioid therapy and 113–4, 190
  rectal 324
learned responses, nausea and
    vomiting 318
learned tolerance 105
levomepromazine
  agitation 335
  nausea and vomiting 320 T
levorphanol 162
licofelone 138
lidocaine
  adverse effects 208
  cough 315
  dyspnea 314
  neuropathic pain 208
  patches 209
limbic system, acupuncture 273
linear analog scale (LAS), elderly 361
lipid solubility, age-related changes 365
lipoxygenase (LOX) 125 F, 138
liver disease, chronic
  opioid bioavailability 108
  pharmacokinetic effects 108
liver pain, radiotherapy 253
living wills 96–7
loading dose 108
local anesthetic(s)
  neuropathic pain 208–9
    systemic agents 208–9
  procedure-related pain 217
    practical aspects 217
    toxicity 217
  pruritus 330
loin pain, radiotherapy 253
loperamide 326
lorazepam
  dyspnea 314
  nausea and vomiting 320 T
  opioid-induced delirium 187
LOX-COX inhibitors 138
lumbar discogenic pain 232
lumbar metastatic pain 28–9, 29 T
lumbosacral nerve roots, phenol
    "saddle" blocks 230
lumbosacral plexopathy 33–5
  presacral recurrence 35
  upper 33
lumbosacral plexus, radiotherapy
    infiltration 254
lumiracoxib
  thrombogenicity 137
  withdrawal 127

lung cancer, elderly 360
lymphangitis carcinomatosa 312
lymphedema 329

magnetic resonance imaging (MRI)
   malignant bone tumors 257
   meningeal carcinomatosis 33 F
   patient assessment 40
   spinal cord compression 31, 32 F
   vertebral metastases 28, 30 F
maintenance dose calculation 108
major depressive episode 56
malignant bone pain see bone pain
malignant pericardial effusions 312–3
malignant pleural effusions 312–3
malignant psoas syndrome 34–5
   features 34, 34 F
   pain distribution 34
malnutrition, elderly 361
massage 277–8
   definition 277
   dormant cancer cell mobilization
      risk 278
   dying person 394
   elderly 370
   physical effects 278
mast cells, pruritus 329
mastectomy, nerve trauma/damage 7
maximal androgen blockade, prostate
   cancer 265
McGill Pain Questionnaire (MPQ) 42
   elderly 361–2
mean transit time (MMT-S),
   opioid-induced
   constipation 189–90
measurement of pain see assessment/
   measurement (of pain)
mechanisms (of pain) 27–8
media, end of life issues reporting 97
medical gases, dyspnea 314
medical oncologists, elderly pain
   control 362
medroxyprogesterone 328
megestrol acetate
   anorexia cachexia syndrome 328
   hot flushes 331
melatonin 328
meloxicam 136
Memorial Delirium Assessment Scale
   (MDAS) 40, 186
Memorial Pain Assessment Card 42
Memorial Symptom Assessment Scale
   10-18 (MASAS 10-18),
   children 346
meningeal carcinomatosis 31–2
   causes 31
   diagnosis 32

pain syndromes 29 T, 31–2
radiological investigation 32,
   33 F
spinal symptoms/signs 32 T
Mental Capacity Act 2005, England
   96
menthol 330
merpethidine see pethidine
mesothelioma 252
metastatic bone pain
   breakthrough 290
   NSAIDs 128
   radiotherapy 259, 260 F
metastatic disease, children 346
methadone 160–1, 169 T
   accumulation 160
   breakthrough pain 291
   cancer pain use 160–1
   children 349, 352 T
      "as needed" dosing 349
   cough 315
   dose conversion 393
   dying person 393
   morphine vs. 393
   neuropathic pain 204
   pharmacodynamics 160
   pharmacokinetics 160
   pharmacology 204
   routes of administration/
      formulations 160
   side effects 160
      sedation 184
   substance abuse patients 385
   unacceptability 393
methotrimeprazine 354
methylnaltrexone
   cholestasis 330
   constipation 324
methylphenidate
   children 353–4
   fatigue 329
   opioid-induced sedation 184
metimazole see dipyrone
metoclopramide 320 T
midazolam
   agitation 335
   delirium 334
      opioid-induced 187
   procedure-related pain 218
Middle East
   opioid availability 88
   palliative care services 86, 87–8
      education/training 88
      home care services 87
      hospice inpatient care units 88
      service development barriers
      88

Middle East Cancer Consortium
   (MECC) 87
   opioid availability 88
   physician prescribing powers 88
Mini-Mental State Examination
   (MMSE) 39–40, 186
miosis, opioid-induced 155
mirtazepine
   depression 332
   pruritus 330
misoprostol 133
mistletoe 274
mood disorders, history taking 39
morphine 158–9, 169 T
   affective response changes 158
   analgesic action onset 158
   brachial plexus neuropathy,
      radiotherapy-induced 406
   breakthrough pain 291
   cancer-induced bone pain 5
   cancer pain use 159
   children 348
      clearance 348
      dosages 348, 352 T
   conjugation 158
   continuous subcutaneous
      administration 110
   cough 315
   dying person 393
   dyspnea 313
      starting dose 313
   effects, in absence of pain 158
   elderly 367
      adverse effects 367
      prescription 362
   limitations 113
   metabolism 158
      children 348
   methadone vs. 393
   neuropathic pain 202, 203
      clinical studies 203
   pharmacodynamics 158
   pharmacokinetics 158
   pharmacology 203
      children 348
   rectal administration 110
   respiratory depression induction
      191
      delayed 191
   routes of administration/
      formulations 159
   side effects 158
      delayed 158
      sedation 184
   switching 169
   transdermal, nausea induction 191
   WHO analgesic ladder 113

morphine-3-glucuronide (M3G) 158,
    203
  elderly 367
morphine-6-glucuronide (M6G) 158,
    203
motility disorders 321
motor cortex stimulation 246
motor paresis, neurolysis-induced 231 T
mucolysis 315
mucositis 317
  dysphagia 317
multidrug resistance gene 1 (MDR-1),
    opioid response variability 170–3
Multinational Etoricoxib and
    Diclofenac Arthritis Long-term
    (MEDAL) program 366
multiple myeloma 264
mu (μ) opioid-receptors
  A118G nucleotide substitution
    173–4
  knockout mice 173
  response variability 173–4
  stimulation 152
  structure 152
  subtypes 152
muscle tone, opioid effects 155
music therapy 278–9
myoclonus
  definition 187
  opioid-induced 187–8
    children 353 T
    clinical presentation/findings 188
    diagnostic criteria 188, 188 T
    epidemiology 187–8
    etiology 187
    management, evidence-based
      evaluation 188
    pathophysiology 187
  patterns 187
myofascial trigger points 273

nabilone 320 T
nabumetone 133
  gastrointestinal adverse effects 133
nalbuphine 162
nalfurafine 331
nalmefene 163
naloxone 162
naltrexone 163
naproxen
  cardiovascular risks 136–7
  elderly 366
  metastatic bone pain 258
  thrombogenicity 137–8
narcotic drugs
  export regulations 83
  import regulations 83

international regulations 82–3
  manufacture regulations 83
  see also individual drugs
Narcotic Drugs and Psychotropic
    Substances Act 1985, India 84
nasogastric tubes, drug
    administration 110–1
National Cancer Control Programme,
    India 86
National Council for Palliative Care,
    psychosocial care definition 50–1
national opium agency 83
nausea and vomiting 318–9
  bowel obstruction 322, 323 F
  causes 318, 319 T
  chemotherapy-induced
    acupuncture 274
    hypnosis 276
    management plan 322 F
    TENS 243
  clinical findings 318
  management 319
    nonpharmacological 319
    pharmacological 320 T
    plans 321 F, 322 F
  opioid-induced 155, 190–1
    children 353 T
    epidemiology 190
    etiology 190
    management, evidence-based
      evaluation 190–1
    pathophysiology 190
  pathophysiology 318, 318 F
  postoperative, acupuncture 273–4
  prevalence 318
nefopam 126
Neighbourhood Network in Palliative
    Care (NNPC), India 87
nephrotic syndrome, NSAID-induced
    135
nerve blocks
  chemical neurolytic agents see
    chemical neurolysis
  physical neurolytic agents see physical
    neurolysis
nerve of Arnold, bronchial cancer
    pain 32
nerve pain, radiotherapy treatment 254
  indications 252, 252 T
nerve trauma, surgery-induced 7
neuroleptics
  children 354
  elderly 368
neurolysis
  chemical see chemical neurolysis
  pathophysiology 226–7
  selective 226–7

neurolytic celiac plexus block
    (NCPB) 228–9
  alcohol use 228
  complications 229
  controversies 229, 230 T
  efficacy 229, 229 T
  indications 229
  procedure 229
neurolytic sympathetic blocks 229–30
neuropathic itch 329
neuropathic pain
  assessment 43
  bone metastasis 260
    radiotherapy 260, 261 F
  central 200
  chemotherapy-induced see
    chemotherapy-induced
    peripheral neuropathy (CIPN)
  definitions 41, 200
  drug sequencing 209
  drug synergy 209
  drug treatment 200–12
    dosing schedules 201 T
    topical 209
  etiology 201
  models 7–9
    limitations 7
    pain behaviors 7–8
    reproducible tumor confinement 7
  nerve compression 7
    models 7–8
  paroxysmal 290
  pathological 200
  pathophysiology 5–7, 201
  peripheral 200
  physiological 200
  prevalence 5–6, 200
  secondary 7
  symptoms 7
  therapy-related 7
  WHO management guidelines 209
nitric acid, NSAID-induced peptic
    ulceration 134
nitrogen/oxygen mixtures, dyspnea
    314
nitrous oxide mixture, procedure-
    related pain 218
  advantages/disadvantages 218
nitrovasodilators 134
NMDA receptor 207
NMDA receptor antagonists,
    neuropathic pain 207–8
nociceptive inputs 3
nociceptive pain 41
nociceptors, tumor-related pain
    345–6
noncompetitive antagonist 105

Non-Government Organization (NGO),
    palliative care services
    Israel 87
    Palestinian Authority 87
nonopioids 123–50
    end of life care 334–5
    WHO analgesic ladder 111–2
    see also individual drugs
nonprofessional caregivers see family
    caregiver
NO-NSAIDs (CINODs) 138
nonsmall cell lung cancer (NSCLC) 264
nonsteroidal anti-inflammatory drugs
    (NSAIDs) 126–38
    adverse effects 128, 128 T
        cardiovascular risks 136–8
        elderly 366
        gastrointestinal risks see NSAID-
            induced gastrointestinal effects
        renal problems 128 T, 135–6, 135 F
        thrombotic risks 136–8
    anorexia cachexia syndrome 328
    bone pain 258
    breakthrough pain 289–90
        rescue dosing 290
    children 348
    classification 127–8, 127 T
    clinical use 128
    as coanalgesics
        opioid toxicity 181
        positive effects 181–2
    elderly 365–6
    future developments 138
    mechanism of action 125 F,
        126–7
        single nucleotide
            polymorphisms 127
        splice variants 127
    metastatic bone pain 128
    paracetamol vs. 124
    procedure-related pain 218
    response to, interindividual
        variability 127
    sweating 331
    worldwide usage 126
    see also individual drugs
nonverbal behavior, pain
    assessment 370–1
    dying person 392
norketamine 208
normeperidine 349
North America, palliative care
    services 86
NSAID-induced gastrointestinal
    effects 128–9, 128 T
    damage mechanisms 129–30
    elderly 366

ion trapping 130
peptic ulcers see peptic ulceration,
    NSAID-induced
    risk factors 130–3
        age 131 T
        concomitant conditions 132 T
        concomitant medicine use 132 T
        gender 131 T
        identification 130, 131 T, 132 T
        peptic ulcers 131 T
    risk management 130
    risk reduction strategies 130–4
        COX-2 inhibitors 130, 133
        drug choice 130, 132 T
        lowest effective dose 132 T
    safe drugs 131–3, 132 T
    topical theory 130
numerical rating scores 14
nurses
    attitudes to pain in elderly 362–3
    pain estimation 364
        nonverbal assessment 371
nystatin 316

occipital condyle syndrome 31 T
Oceania, palliative care services 86
octreotide
    diarrhea 326
    nausea and vomiting 320 T
odontoid process fracture 29 T
olanzapine
    nausea and vomiting 320 T
    opioid-induced delirium 187
older people see elderly
omeprazole 366
ondansetron
    cholestasis 330
    nausea and vomiting 320 T
        opioid-induced 191
opiate 202
opioid(s)
    addiction see opioid addiction
    adjuvant drugs 113–4
        adverse effect management 181–2
    adverse effects 179–99, 156–7
        administration route changes
            183
        children 351, 353 T
        classification 180
        combination drugs 183
        dose response 180
        epidemiology 180, 181 T
        etiology 180
        fear of 151–2
        genetic variability 180
        management strategies 180–3
        nonopioid receptors in 180

pathophysiology 180
symptomatic management 182
see also individual effects
as antidiarrheals 326
blood–brain barrier 154
bone pain 258
breakthrough pain 289, 290 F
children
    adverse effects 351, 353 T
    dose escalation 350, 351
    dosing schedules 350, 352 T
classification 153–4
    agonist–antagonists 154
    partial agonist 153–4
    pure agonists 153
    pure antagonists 154
controlled-release preparations 384–5
cough suppression 315
cross-tolerance 106
definition 153
dose conversion tables 183 T,
    184 T
dual pharmacology 115
dying person 392–3
dyspnea 313
elderly 366–8
    at home delivery systems
        368
    continuous infusion 368
    drug combinations 367
    end of life care 334–5
endogenous 153
    binding characteristics 153 T
    precursor molecules 153
fear of
    dying person 393
    elderly 366
    by healthcare professionals 115
    by patients 115
illicit use 106–7
in individuals without pain 154
inhaled, breakthrough pain 286
long-acting, dying person 393
nasal administration, breakthrough
    pain 292
neuropathic pain 202–4
    controversies in 202–3
    dosing schedules 201 T
    genetic variations 202–3
pharmacological effects 154–6
    age-related changes 367
    cardiovascular system 155
    central nervous system 154–5
    gastrointestinal system 155
    immune system 156, 192
    increased muscular tone 155
    neuroendocrine 155

opioid(s) (*continued*)
    renal system 155–6
    respiratory system 154–5
    skin 156
    pharmacology 151–67
    physical dependence 156–7,
        191
    regulations/legislation
        Indian 84
        Italian 83–4
    rescue dosing *see* rescue analgesia/
        dosing
    response, interindividual variability
        candidate genes 170–4
        causes 170
        drug metabolism 173
        drug transporters 170–3
        genetics 170–4
        pain pathway interactions 174
        receptors 173–4
        receptor signaling 174
        scientific rationale 170
    rotation *see* opioid rotation
    routes of administration, dying
        person 393
    strong
        adverse effects 113
        elderly 367
        immediate use 116
        procedure-related pain 217
        respiratory depression 113
        sedation 113
        starting dose 114
        WHO analgesic ladder 113
    substance abuse patients 384–5
    switching *see* opioid switching
    therapeutic uses 157–63
        mild to moderate pain 157–8
        mixed agonist–antagonists 162
        moderate to severe pain 158–62
    tolerance *see* opioid tolerance
    topical, procedure-related pain 217
    underprescription 115
    volume of distribution 107
    weak
        elderly 366–7
        legislation 112
    withdrawal symptoms 156–7
    see also individual drugs
opioid addiction 157, 191
    cancer patients 157
    children 355
    parental fears 355
opioid antagonists 162–3
    cholestasis 330
    constipation 324
    newer compounds 163

opioid irrelevant pain 116
opioid receptor(s) 152–3
    action on pain pathway
        152–3
    acupuncture 273
    distribution 152, 202
    opioid activities 202 *T*
    receptor-specific actions 152
    signaling response variability
        174
    signal transduction 153
    structure 152
    subtypes 152
    TENS 238
    see also specific receptors
opioid rotation 182–3
    children 351
    cross-tolerance 106
    definition 182
    delirium 187
    dose conversions 183 *T*, 184 *T*
    effectiveness 182
    guidelines 183
    opioid-induced myoclonus 188
    opioid switching *vs.* 169
    WHO analgesic ladder in 182
opioid switching 168–78
    adverse effect profiles 169–70
    children 350–1
        equianalgesic dose 350–1
    clinical rationale 169–70
    dose calculations 169
    dose-ration ranges 169
    evidence base 170
        studies 171–172 *T*
    opioid rotation *vs.* 169
    refractory nausea 191
opioid tolerance 156, 191
    children 354–5
    clinical features 106
    management 156
    mechanisms 156
opiophobia 115
oral drug administration
    children 349
    dying person 393–4
    loading dose calculation 108
    WHO guidelines, efficacy 109–11,
        116
oral problems 316–7
oral transmucosal fentanyl citrate
    (OTFC)
    breakthrough pain 291–2
    cancer pain 160, 203
    children 349
    procedure-related pain 217
orexin 328

organic hallucinosis
    definition 185
    opioid-induced 185
        children 353 *T*
        clinical findings 185
        clinical presentation 185
        management 185
oropharyngeal pain 317
orphanin NQ/nociceptin 153
osmotic laxatives 325 *T*
osteoblasts, bone metastases 256–7
osteoclast-activating factors
    (OAFs) 256–7
osteoclasts, bone metastases 256–7
osteoporosis, vertebral metastases *vs.* 28
osteoprotogerin (OPG) 256–7
ovarian cancer, radiotherapy 254
oxaliplatin 401
oxycodone 161, 169 *T*
    breakthrough pain 291
    cancer-induced/related neuropathic
        pain 204
    cancer pain use 161
    children 348, 352 *T*
    constipation induction 190
    elderly 368
    nausea induction 191
    pharmacodynamics 161
    pharmacokinetics 161
    pharmacology 204
    routes of administration/
        formulations 161
    side effects 161
oxygen, dyspnea 314
    withholding treatment 314
oxymorphone 161
oxytocin, acupuncture 273

paclitaxel, neuropathy induction 7, 402
    animal models 8
pain
    components 50 *F*
    definition 13
    psychology 297
Pain and Palliative Care Clinic,
    Kerala 87
Pain and Policy Study Group
    (PPSG) 84
    opioid policy assessment
        guidelines 84
        workshop approach 84
    research areas 84
    Romanian work 84–5
pain appraisal, cognitive processes
    in 297
pain assessment *see* assessment/
    measurement (of pain)

pain assessment in advanced dementia (PAINAD) 371
pain clinics, India 87
pain evaluation 41–4
pain flare *see* breakthrough pain
pain history *see* history taking
pain management
    barriers to *see* pain relief barriers
    clinical guidelines 116–7, 117 *T*
        criticism 116–7
        online 117 *T*
        WHO *see* World Health Organization (WHO)
    ethics *see* ethical issues
    historical aspects 82
    psychological interventions *see* psychological interventions, pain management
    teamworking *see* teamworking
pain management inventory (PMI), elderly 362
pain related behaviors 392
pain relief barriers
    drug availability 82–4
        economic factors 82
        Indian regulations 84
        Italian regulations 83–4
        narcotic drug regulations 82–3
    family caregivers 64–5
    international perspective 81–92
    principle of balance 84–5
    service development patterns 85–9
pain scales, cognitive impaired 392 *F*
Palestinian Authority, palliative care services 87
palliative care 412–3
    acute care–palliative care interface 412, 413 *F*
    emotional pain alleviation, ethics 95
    global development 85
    model 389–90, 390 *F*
    services, worldwide distribution 86
    social pain alleviation, ethics 95
    United States 412
    WHO definition 412
Palliative Care Formulary, non-licensed drug use 415–6
palliative home care teams
    team members roles 413
    United Kingdom 412–3
    United States 413
palonsetron 320 *T*
pamidronate 265–6
Pancoast tumor 254
pancreatic cancer 35

pancreatic pain, cancer-induced 35
para-aortic lymphadenopathy 253–4
paracentesis 215 *F*
paracetamol (acetaminophen) 124–5
    adverse effects 125
        gastrointestinal bleeds 125
        renal failure 125
    breakthrough pain 289–90
    children 347–8
        contraindications 347–8
        dosing 347–8
        safety 348
    development 124
    elderly 365, 367
    mechanism of action 124–5, 125 *F*
        COX-3 124
        COX inhibition 124
    NSAIDs *vs.* 124
    overdosage 125
    popularity 124
    sweating 331
parathyroidectomy, uremic itch 330
parathyroid hormone-related peptide (PTHrP), hypercalcemia 319
parenteral drug administration 110
Parkinson's disease, communication in 370–1
paroxetine
    cancer-induced/related neuropathic pain 205
    pruritus 330
partial agonist
    ceiling effect 105
    definition 105
pathological fractures 266–7
pathological neuropathic pain 200
pathophysiology (of pain) 3–12
patient(s)
    analgesics, reluctance to take 94
    assessment 38–47
        historical aspects 38
    drug use misunderstandings 94
    evaluation 39–40
patient-controlled analgesia (PCA)
    children 350
    postbreast cancer surgery pain 404
patient education 297–8
    children 304
    components 297
    efficacy, evidence for 298
    family members 298
    medication compliance 298
    nonpharmacological interventions 297

opioid fear reductions 298
pain assessment 297
pain control issues 94
patient empowerment 297
pharmacological 297
patient record card, controlled drugs 414
pediatric cancer pain 345–58
    analgesics 347–9
        adjuvant 351–4
        postoperative pain models 347
        routes of administration 349–50
        studies 347
    anesthetic management approaches 354
    breakthrough pain 346
    complementary therapy use 270–1
    epidemiology 346
    etiology 345–6
    nonpharmacological control 346–7
        environmental 347
    pharmacological management 347–54
    psychological interventions 304–5
    terminal sedation 354
pelvic pain, radiotherapy 254
pentazocine
    cancer pain 162
    mechanism of action 105
peptic ulceration, NSAID-induced 129
    absolute risk 129
    prophylaxis 130, 133–4
        drug choice 134
        prostaglandin replacement 133–4
        stomach acid reduction 133
    relative risk 129
    trends 129
percutaneous balloon pericardiotomy 313
pericardial effusions, malignant 312–3
peripheral neuropathic pain 200
peripheral neuropathy 34–5
    chemotherapy-induced *see* chemotherapy-induced peripheral neuropathy (CIPN)
    paraneoplastic manifestation 34–5
    tumor invasion 35
peristaltic actions, gut 323
periventricular and periaqueductal gray matter, deep brain stimulation 246
pethidine 162
    cancer pain use 162
    children 349, 352 *T*
    dying person 394–5
    pharmacodynamics 162
    pharmacokinetics 162
    procedure-related pain 217

pethidine (*continued*)
routes of administration/
formulations 162
side effects 162
toxicity 162
petrissage 277–8
P-glycoprotein, opioid response
variability 170–3
phantom pain
bladder 36
breast 404
post-rectal excision 36
pharmacodynamics 105–7
definition 364–5
elderly 365
long-term exposure effects 105–7
receptor effects 105
pharmacodynamic synergy 209
pharmacodynamic tolerance 105
pharmacokinetics 107–8
definition 364–5
dosing regimen calculation 108
elderly 365
distribution 365
factors influencing 108
terminology 107
pharmacokinetic synergy 209
pharmacokinetic tolerance 105
phenobarbital 335
phenol
neurolysis 227–8, 228 *T*
alcohol neurolysis *vs.* 228
epidural blockade 230
patient positioning 227
pruritus 330
phenothiazines 314
phenytoin
cancer-induced/related neuropathic
pain 206
elderly 369
side effects 369
pholcodine 315
phosphate, hypercalcemia 321
phospholipase-A$_2$ inhibitors (PLA$_2$)
138
phosphorus, metastatic bone pain 264
physical dependence
agents 226 *T*
children 354–5
definition 106, 156–7
opioids 156–7, 191
physical examination 40
physical neurolysis 225–34
agents 231–3
pathophysiology 226–7, 226 *T*
surgical sectioning *vs.* 226, 226 *T*
see also individual agents/techniques

physiological neuropathic pain
200
phytotherapy *see* herbal medicine
pilocarpine 316
pituitary ablation 254
plain x-ray
malignant bone tumors 257
malignant psoas syndrome 34 *F*
patient assessment 40
spinal cord compression 31
platinum-based chemotherapy,
peripheral neuropathy
induction 401
pleural disease, radiotherapy 252
pleural effusions, malignant
312–3
pleurodesis 312–3
polypharmacy
delirium 186
dying person 393–4
positive mental images 299–300
efficacy 301
positron emission tomography (PET)
hypnosis 277
malignant bone tumors 257
postbreast cancer surgery pain
(PBCSP) 402–5
acute pain influences 403–4
axillary dissection 403
breast reconstruction 404
classification 403
etiology 403
intercostobrachial neuralgia 403
PCA 404
risk factors 403
surgical factors 403–4
treatment 404–5
"posthypnotic suggestion" 275
postmastectomy pain syndrome
(PMPS) 205–6
postoperative nausea,
acupuncture 273–4
post-surgical pain 402–5
potency, drug 105
"potentization," homeopathy
275
prednisolone 327–8
preferential COX-2 inhibitors
127
pregabalin 206
premedication, procedure-related
pain 214
prevalence (of pain) 14–8
advanced cancer 14–8, 19–21 *T*, 28 *T*
assessment 13–4
bereaved carer studies 14–8, 19–21 *T*
recall bias 14–8

early disease 14, 15–18 *T*
metastatic disease effects 18
primary tumor site 18, 22 *T*, 28 *T*
terminal cancer 28 *T*
time of diagnosis 14
primary care physicians, pain control in
elderly 362
principle of balance, opioid
analgesics 84–5
procedure-related pain
analgesia provision 213–4
approaches to 214–5
assessment 216 *T*
children
causes 346
incidence 213
psychological interventions 304
control 213–21
future directions 219–20
incidence 213
local techniques 216–7
mild to moderate 214 *T*
moderate to severe 213, 214 *T*.
nonpharmacological
interventions 215–6
patient factors 214, 216 *T*
physician factors 214–5
procedural preparations 216
procedures causing 214 *T*
sedating drugs 218–9
system factors 215
topical techniques 216–7
profile-tailored cognitive-behavioral
therapy 302–3
progestogens
anorexia cachexia syndrome 328
side effects 328
Programme for Cancer Pain Relief,
WHO 82
promethazine 314
propofol
agitation 335
procedure-related pain 218
prostate cancer
hormone treatment 265
strontium 263
prostate specific antigen (PSA), bone
metastasis 257
protein binding, age-related
changes 365
proton pump inhibitors (PPIs)
elderly 366
NSAID-induced peptic ulcer
prophylaxis 133
pruritus 329–31
causes 329
clinical findings 329–30

management 330
  general measures 330
  systemic treatments 330–1
  topical treatments 330
  opioid-induced 156, 192
    children 353 *T*
  pathology 329
pseudoaddiction 107
  substance abuse 381
pseudomembranous stomatitis 316
psychiatric problems, non-pain
    related 331–4
psycho-education *see* patient education
psychological dependence *see* addiction
psychological distress 303
  pain interactions 48–9
  prevalence 21
psychological evaluation
  confidentiality 51
  coping mechanisms 55–6
  effective communication skills 52
  ethical issues 51
  family 48–62
    practical steps 53–4
  moral issues 51
  objectives 50–1
  patient 48–62
psychological interventions, pain
    management 296–309
  adult populations 297–303
  children 304–5
  see also individual interventions
psychological problems, non-pain
    related 331–4
psychomotor performance, opioid-
    induced cognitive failure 185
psycho-oncology 380
psychosocial assessment 50–2
  carers 52
  family 52
  friends 52
  individual 51
  physical resources 52
  social resources 52
psychosocial care 50–1
psychosocial support groups, substance
    abuse 383
psychostimulants
  adverse effects 184–5
  children 353–4
  opioid-induced sedation 184
psychotherapy
  depression 332
  group, distressed patients 303
  supportive *see* supportive
    psychotherapy
public attitudes (to pain) 49

pulmonary edema, opioid-induced 192
pulmonary emboli 311–2

quantitative sensory testing (QST),
    CIPN 401

radiation damage, late 259
radiation-induced fibrosis 7
radiation tolerance dose 259
radicular pain, spinal cord
    compression 30
radiofrequency lesioning (RF) 232
  advantages/disadvantages 232, 232 *T*
  clinical applications 232–3
  complications 233
  definition 232
  sympathetic chain 233
radioisotope therapy
  bone pain 262–4, 262 *T*
  elderly 370
  see also individual radioisotopes
radionuclides, children 354
radiotherapy 251–5
  airway obstruction, tumors 312
  analgesic action mechanisms 251
  bone pain 258–64
    dose 259–61, 260 *F*
    efficacy 267
    elderly 370
    immobilization 258
    localization 258–9
    localized pain 258–9
    metastatic 258
    multiple sites 261
    neuropathic 260, 261 *F*
    pain relief onset 259, 260 *F*
    planning 259
    postoperative 266–7
    retreatment rates 260–1, 261 *F*
    side effects/complications 259
    spine 259
    superficial bones 259
    treatment delivery 259
    wide field irradiation *see* wide field
      irradiation, bone pain
  brachial plexus neuropathy induction
    see brachial plexus neuropathy
    (BPM), radiotherapy-induced
  breakthrough pain 289
  elderly 370
  hemoptysis 315
  indications 251–2
  nerve pain 254
  pain induction 405–6
  physical nature 405
  soft tissue pain 252–4
  superior vena caval obstruction 312

Radiotherapy Action Group Exposure
    (RAGE) 406
raised intracranial pressure, nausea and
    vomiting 318, 321 *F*
ranitidine 366
receptors, drug effects 105
rectal administration, analgesia 110
  breakthrough pain 291
  children 350
  dying person 393–4
rectal cancer
  case history 417–8
  postoperative pain recurrence 36
rectal fullness sensation 36
rectal laxatives 324
rectal pain 36
refractory nausea, opioid switching
    191
Reiki healing 278
relatives, as "attorney" 96
relaxation 277, 299–300
  efficacy 301, 302
  elderly 369–70
renal cancer
  radiotherapy 253
  recurrence, lumbosacral
    plexopathy 33
renal disease, pharmacokinetic
    effects 108
renal failure
  dying person 394–5
  pain management 40
  paracetamol-induced 125
renal impairment
  opioid use, elderly 367
  pharmacokinetic effects 108
renal system, opioid effects 155–6
rescue analgesia/dosing 111, 114
  breakthrough pain 290, 291
    children 350
    oral 291
  definition 290
  elderly 368
  ideal medication 290, 290 *F*
  time–action relationship 291, 291 *F*
resource access, family caregiver 67 *T*
respiratory depression, opioid-
    induced 154–5, 191
  children 353 *T*
  tolerance 156
respiratory system
  non-pain symptoms control 311
  opioid effects 154–5
*Responding to patients who are
    silent* 371
retroperitoneal sarcoma,
    radiotherapy 253

revised Edmonton Staging System (rESS) 44, 45 *T*
rhenium 264
rib fractures, pathological 29
rib metastases 29
rifampicin 330
risperidone 187
rofecoxib
  cardiovascular risk 137
  elderly 366
  gastrointestinal adverse effects 133
  withdrawal 127
Romania, opioid availability 84–5
root pain, spinal cord compression 30
rule of double effect *see* doctrine of double effect
ryodoraku 272

sacral metastases 29 *T*
Safe management of CDs 414
salbutamol 314
salivary flow, acupuncture 274
salt retention, NSAID-induced 135
samarium
  bone pain 263
  gamma camera imaging 263, 263 *F*
Saunders, Cicely 85, 412
  "total pain" concept 85
scopolamine (hyoscine hydrobromate) 191, 320 *T*
sedation
  conscious *see* conscious sedation
  deep 219
  opioid-induced 154, 184–5
    children 353 *T*
    clinical presentation 184
    epidemiology 184
    etiology 184
    management 184–5
    pathophysiology 184
    psychostimulants 184
    strong opioids 113
    tolerance 184
  procedure-related pain 218–9
seizures, opioid-induced 187–8
selective neurolysis 226–7
selective serotonin reuptake inhibitors (SSRI)
  cancer-induced/related neuropathic pain 205
  depression 332
self-hypnosis 276
  children 305
  efficacy 301
senile pruritus 329
senna 325 *T*

serotonin and noradrenergic reuptake inhibitors (SNRI) 205–6
serotonin release, acupuncture 273
sexual counseling programs 55
sexual history taking 55
sexuality 55
sexual problems 55
Shanti Avedna Ashram 87
Shiatsu (acupressure) 272, 277–8
Shipman, Dr Harold 414
Single Convention on Narcotic Drugs 115
  remit 82–3
Single Convention on Narcotic Drugs 1961 (amended 1972) 82
single nucleotide polymorphisms (SNPs), NSAIDs and 127
skeletal muscle relaxants 209
skin
  opioid effects 156
  radiotherapy side effects 259
skin care, lymphedema 329
skin patches, analgesia delivery 110
sleep, opioid effects 154
small cell lung cancer (SCLC) 264
small intestine
  NSAID-induced toxicity 134–5
    management 135
    pathophysiology 134–5
  obstruction *see* bowel obstruction
  opioid effects 155
social support
  patient 49
  professional team 75
sodium cromoglycate 330
sodium valproate 206
soft tissue pain, radiotherapy 252–4
  indications 252, 252 *T*
somatic pain
  cancer-induced
    animal models 4
    pathophysiology 4–5
  definition 41
somatization, as prognostic factor 43
South African hospice development 88–9
Special Prescription Form, Italy 83–4
sphenoid sinus syndrome 31 *T*
sphincters
  intrathecal neurolysis effects 231 *T*
  opioid effects 192
spinal cord
  opioid effects 152–3
  radiotherapy side effects 259
spinal cord compression
  causes 30
  children 346

imaging 31, 32 *F*
  pain syndromes 30–1
spinal cord stimulation (SCS) 243–5
  clinical effectiveness 244
  clinical technique 244–6
  contraindications 245–6
  cost-effectiveness 244
  electrode placement 244–5
  indications 245 *T*
  mechanism of action 243–4
  MRI compatibility 245–6
  rationale 243–4
spinal cord tumors, children 346
spironolactone, elderly 365
splenic pain management, radiotherapy 253
spontaneous pain, epidemiology 288
squashed stomach syndrome 318
  management 321 *F*
staging (of pain) 43–4
starvation, anorexia cachexia syndrome *vs.* 327
St Christopher's Hospice 85
stellate ganglion neurolytic block 229–30
steroids *see* corticosteroid(s)
stimulation-induced analgesia 235–50
  definition 235
  historical aspects 235
  recent techniques/developments 246
  see also individual techniques
stimulation-produced analgesia *see* stimulation-induced analgesia
"stocking-glove" distribution, chemotherapy-induced peripheral neuropathy 400
stomach, opioid effects 155
stool analysis of transit time (SST), opioid-induced constipation 189–90
stroke, communication in 370–1
strontium, metastatic bone pain 263
subarachnoid infusion, children 354
subcutaneous drug administration
  children 350
  dying person 393–4
substance abuse, pain management 379–88
  analgesic therapy 384–5
  case example 385–6
  clinician–patient trust 381
  definitions 380
  drug testing/screening 381, 382, 385
    body fluids tested 385, 386 *T*
    consent 385
    result interpretation 385, 386 *T*

health care resources utilized 379
impact on 380–1
incidence 383, 383 T
institutional policy 381–2
management guidelines 381–5
medicolegal issues 384, 386
multidisciplinary care team 381
multidisciplinary program 381–2, 382 T
nonpharmacologic approaches 382, 385
patient assessment 381, 382 T
patient identification 381
psychosocial support groups 383
structure 384
research directions 386
treatment outcomes 383
undertreatment 380
written care agreements 383–4
dismissal from treatment 384
example 384
initiation criteria 383–4
noncompliance consequences 384
outcomes 383 T
substance dependence see addiction
sufentanil 217
suicide
cancer-related see cancer-related suicide
risk, elderly 363
superior hypogastric plexus block 230
superior vena caval obstruction (SVCO) 312
supportive care 412
supportive psychotherapy 298–9
breast cancer 298–9
components 298
definition 298
efficacy 298–9
SUPPORT study 391
suprascapular nerve entrapment 32–3
risk factors 32–3
surgery
breakthrough pain 289
breast cancer, postoperative pain see postbreast cancer surgery pain (PBCSP)
nerve trauma risk 7
sweating 331
investigations 331
management 331
opioid-induced 156
pathology 331
Swedish massage see massage
sympathetic blocks, neurolytic 229–30

symptom clusters, psychological interventions 303–4
symptom substitution 300

tachyphylaxis (acute tolerance) 105
tamoxifen 265
tapotement 277–8
taste alterations 317
taxanes 402
teamworking 71–80
absent planning 76
bad teamwork scenario 71–2, 77–9
Charing Cross experience 76
colleague relationship problems 76
communication breakdown 76
with patients 76
conflicts 76
management strategies 79 F
downside/failure 76
effectiveness 74
experienced team scenario 72–3, 79–80
inexperienced team scenario 71–2, 77–9
maintenance problems 76
member variety 74–5
need for 73–4
clinician issues 73–4
patient issues 73
professional companionship 73
organizational development (OD) 77, 78 T
definition 77
teambuilding 77
peer supervision 75
planning 77
local needs survey 77
power/status problems 76
roles in 75, 75 T
social support 75
successfulness 74–5, 74 T
clarity 74
development time 75–6
support 75–6
team definition 74
team development 77, 77 T
stages 78 T
tension 76
theory 74–7
views on 71
temperature regulation 331
terminal sedation 391
children 354
delta 9-tetrahydrocannabinol (THC) 328
thalamic ablation 254

thalidomide
anorexia cachexia syndrome 328
chemotherapy-induced peripheral neuropathy 402
pruritus 330
sweating 331
therapeutic dependence 107
therapeutic touch (healing) 278
thioridazine 331
third-party assessment, dementia/ delirium patients 43
thoracocentesis 312–3
thrombosis
COX-2 mediated 136, 137 F
NSAID-induced 136–8
COX-2 inhibitors 136
epidemiology 136–7, 137 T
mechanism 136
non-selective NSAIDs 136
tizanidine 209
tolerance
acquired 105
acute (tachyphylaxis) 105
children 354–5
definition 105, 156, 191
fear of 106
learned 105
opioids see opioid tolerance
pharmacodynamic 105
pharmacokinetic 105
topical anesthesia
children 349–50
practical aspects 217
procedure-related pain 216
total body clearance, drugs 107
total pain
dying person 390, 392
ethical issues 95
tramadol 157–8
cancer-induced/related neuropathic pain 204
clinical studies 204
cancer pain use 158
children 348
constipation induction 190
elderly 367
pharmacodynamics 157
pharmacokinetics 157
pharmacology 204
routes of administration/ formulations 158
side effects 157–8
WHO analgesic ladder 112–3
tranexamic acid 315
transcranial magnetic stimulation (TMS) 246

transcutaneous electrical nerve
    stimulation (TENS) 236–43
    administration 236
    chemotherapy-induced nausea 243
    clinical effectiveness 238–43,
        241–242 T
    clinical technique 243
    concerns 237
    contraindications/precautions 243,
        245 T, 370
    controls 238 F
    conventional 237, 240 F
    devices 236, 237 F, 237 T
    elderly 370
    electrode positioning 243, 244 F
    historical aspects 235
    non-pain related effects 239 T
    optimal settings 236, 237 T
    procedure-related pain 216
    pruritus 330
    rationale 237–8
    short-term effects 243
    techniques 237, 239 T
    treatable conditions 239 T
    tumor growth and 237
transcutaneous spinal electroanalgesia
    (TSE) 238
transdermal delivery systems
    analgesia 110
    opioids, dying person 393
transient pain see breakthrough pain
transitory pain see breakthrough pain
transmucosal drug administration 111
treatment-related side effects,
    behavioral interventions 302
tricyclic antidepressants
    cancer-induced/related neuropathic
        pain 205
    children 351–3
        pre-treatment investigations 353
    depression 332
    elderly 369
trigeminal neuralgia, radiofrequency
    lesioning 233
Trilisate (choline magnesium
    trisalicylate), children 348
Trivandurum Regional Cancer
    Centre 87
tropisetron 191, 320 T
tumor-induced pain
    children 346
    etiology 345–6
    TENS 241–242 T

Uganda, morphine use 89
UGT2B7 expression, opioid response
    variability 173

ultraviolet light, pruritus 330
undertreatment 115
upper limb pain management,
    radiotherapy 254
uremic itch 330–1
uridine-diphosphoglucuronosyl-
    trasferase (UGT) system 173
urinary incontinence, strontium
    contraindication 263
urinary retention
    dying person 394
    opioid-induced 155–6
        children 353 T
uterine cancer, radiotherapy
    254

valdecoxib
    cardiovascular risk 137
    withdrawal 127, 137
venlafaxine
    cancer-induced/related neuropathic
        pain 205–6
    chemotherapy-induced neuropathy
        treatment 8–9
    postbreast cancer surgery pain
        404–5
    postmastectomy pain
        syndrome 205–6
venting gastrostomy
    bowel obstruction 322
    nausea and vomiting 319
verbal rating scale (VRS), elderly
    361
vertebral collapse 266
vertebral metastases
    C7-T1 28–9, 29 T
    MRI 28, 30 F
    pain syndromes 28–9, 29 T
        differential diagnosis 28
        osteoporosis vs. 28
VIGOR trial 133
vincristine-induced neuropathy
    animal models 8
    pathophysiology 7
    treatment 8–9
visceral pain
    cancer-induced 9
    definition 41
visual analog scale (VAS)
    depression 39
    dying person 392
    elderly 361
visualization 277
volume of distribution (V_d)
    definition 107
    initial-steady state differences 107,
        108

loading dose calculations 108
    opioids 107
vomiting see nausea and vomiting
vomiting (emetic) pattern generator
    (VPG) 318, 318 F

wallerian degeneration 226
warfarin, elderly 365
Western Asia, palliative care services
    86
Western Europe, palliative care
    services 86
WHO analgesic ladder 111–4, 112 F
    adjuvant drugs 111, 113–4
    breakthrough pain 289
    children 347
    coanalgesic drugs 111, 113
    interventional therapies 111
    limitations 82
    in opioid rotation 182
    principles 109
    step one: use of nonopioids
        111–2
    step two: use of weak opioids
        112–3
        validity 112
    step three: use of strong opioids
        113
wide dynamic neurons (WDR), cancer-
    induced bone pain 5
wide field irradiation, bone pain 261–2,
    262 F
    doses 261–2
    efficacy 262
    toxicity 262 T
"wind up" phenomenon, opioid
    effectiveness 202–3, 207
wire stents
    airway obstruction 312
    superior vena caval obstruction
        312
withdrawal symptoms 106
    children 355
    opioids 156–7
    prevention 106
World Health Organization (WHO)
    cancer pain relief guidelines 104
        aims 109, 114
        apparent failure 116
        attention to detail 109, 114–5
        availability 110 T
        children 345
        by the clock 109, 111
        efficacy 115–6
        evaluation 115–6
        history/examination 109
        implementation difficulties 115

for the individual 109, 114
by the ladder *see* WHO analgesic
    ladder
by the mouth 109–11, 116
prescription modifications
    114–5
principles 108–15
reassessment 114–5
written instructions 114

"foundation measures" 82
palliative care definition 412
Programme for Cancer Pain Relief
    82

xerostomia 316
    causes 316 *T*
    definition 192
    opioid-induced 192

epidemiology 192
etiology 192
management, evidence-based
    evaluation 192
pathophysiology 192
treatment 316
x-rays *see* plain x-ray

zolendronate 321

T - #0960 - 101024 - C0 - 276/219/20 - PB - 9781138372436 - Gloss Lamination